Manual of Small Animal Soft Tissue Surgery

Manual of Small Animal Soft Tissue Surgery

Second Edition

Karen Tobias, DVM, MS, Diplomate ACVS

Professor of Small Animal Surgery
Department of Small Animal Clinical Sciences
College of Veterinary Medicine
University of Tennessee Institute of Agriculture
Knoxville TN, USA

WILEY Blackwell

This edition first published 2017

© 2017 John Wiley and Sons, Inc. (except illustrations © Karen Tobias, unless where stated otherwise)

Edition History
Wiley-Blackwell (1e, 2009)

All rights reserved. No part of this publication may be reproduced, stored in a retrieval system, or transmitted, in any form or by any means, electronic, mechanical, photocopying, recording or otherwise, except as permitted by law. Advice on how to obtain permission to reuse material from this title is available at http://www.wiley.com/go/permissions.

The right of Karen Tobias to be identified as the author of this work has been asserted in accordance with law.

Registered Office(s)

John Wiley & Sons, Inc., 111 River Street, Hoboken, NJ 07030, USA

Editorial Office

111 River Street, Hoboken, NJ 07030, USA

For details of our global editorial offices, customer services, and more information about Wiley products visit us at www.wiley.com.

Wiley also publishes its books in a variety of electronic formats and by print-on-demand. Some content that appears in standard print versions of this book may not be available in other formats.

Limit of Liability/Disclaimer of Warranty

The contents of this work are intended to further general scientific research, understanding, and discussion only and are not intended and should not be relied upon as recommending or promoting scientific method, diagnosis, or treatment by veterinarians for any particular patient. In view of ongoing research, equipment modifications, changes in governmental regulations, and the constant flow of information relating to the use of medicines, equipment, and devices, the reader is urged to review and evaluate the information provided in the package insert or instructions for each medicine, equipment, or device for, among other things, any changes in the instructions or indication of usage and for added warnings and precautions. While the publisher and authors have used their best efforts in preparing this work, they make no representations or warranties with respect to the accuracy or completeness of the contents of this work and specifically disclaim all warranties, including without limitation any implied warranties of merchantability or fitness for a particular purpose. No warranty may be created or extended by sales representatives, written sales materials or promotional statements for this work. The fact that an organization, website, or product is referred to in this work as a citation and/or potential source of further information does not mean that the publisher and authors endorse the information or services the organization, website, or product may provide or recommendations it may make. This work is sold with the understanding that the publisher is not engaged in rendering professional services. The advice and strategies contained herein may not be suitable for your situation. You should consult with a specialist where appropriate. Further, readers should be aware that websites listed in this work may have changed or disappeared between when this work was written and when it is read. Neither the publisher nor authors shall be liable for any loss of profit or any other commercial damages, including but not limited to special, incidental, consequential, or other damages.

Library of Congress Cataloging-in-Publication Data

Names: Tobias, Karen M., author.
Title: Manual of small animal soft tissue surgery / Karen Tobias.
Description: Second edition. | Hoboken, NJ : John Wiley & Sons Inc., 2017. |
Includes bibliographical references and index.
Identifiers: LCCN 2017009000 | ISBN 9781119117247 (cloth)
Subjects: LCSH: Veterinary surgery. | Soft tissue injuries–Surgery. | MESH:
Surgery, Veterinary–methods | Animals, Domestic–surgery
Classification: LCC SF911 .T63 2017 | NLM SF 911 | DDC 636.089/7–dc23 LC record
available at https://lccn.loc.gov/2017009000

Cover Design: Wiley

Cover Images: (Background) © Max Krasnov/Shutterstock; (Image insets) Courtesy of Karen Tobias

Set in 10.5/13 pt SabonLTStd-Roman by Thomson Digital, Noida, India
Printed and bound by CPI Group (UK) Ltd, Croydon, CR0 4YY

C9781119117247_190224

To Jacob Calder Tobias and Jessica Lee Tobias, who have grown into fine adults. You are intelligent, thoughtful, fascinating people. I'm so glad to have you in my life!

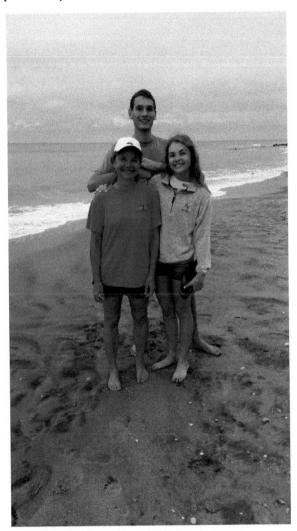

To Jacob Calder Tobias and Jessica Lee Tobias, who have grown into fine adults. You are intelligent, thoughtful, fascinating people. I'm so glad to have you in my life!

Contents

Contributors

Karen Tobias, DVM, MS, Diplomate ACVS
Professor of Small Animal Surgery
Department of Small Animal Clinical Sciences
College of Veterinary Medicine
University of Tennessee Institute of Agriculture
Knoxville TN

Thomas Chen, DVM, Diplomate ACVO
Clinical Assistant Professor of Ophthalmology
Department of Small Animal Clinical Sciences
College of Veterinary Medicine
University of Tennessee Institute of Agriculture
Knoxville TN

Acknowledgements

The following veterinarians, as third-year students, contributed chapters to the first edition of the *Manual of Small Animal Soft Tissue Surgery*. These folks are now well established in practices across the country, and several have even become surgical specialists. Their contributions have been invaluable!

Catherine Ashe, DVM
Scrotal Urethrostomy

Paige Brock, DVM
Rectal Prolapse

Jessica Carbonell, DVM
Ovariohysterectomy

Erika Gallisdorfer, DVM
Cystotomy

Kandace Henry, DVM
Cystostomy Tubes

Rebecca Tolbert Hodshon, DVM
Feline Perineal Urethrostomy

Cam Hornsby, DVM
Urethral Prolapse

Katherine Kottkamp, DVM
Perineal Hernia

Sarah Lane, DVM
Prepubertal Gonadectomy

Marina Manashirova, DVM
Prescrotal Urethrostomy

Ashley McKamey, DVM
Episioplasty

Martha Patterson, DVM
Prostatic Omentalization

Tara Read, DVM
Renal Biopsy Techniques

Robert Simpson, DVM
Abdominal Incision

Sharon Stone, DVM
Pyometra

Rachel Tapp, DVM
Anal Sacculectomy

Amy Joy (Wood) Hodshon
Cryptorchidectomy

Preface

When the *Manual of Small Animal Soft Tissue Surgery* was first published in 2010, its purpose was to provide practical information on common surgical conditions, clear instructions on surgical procedures, and intraoperative photographs to illustrate techniques and make them easier to understand.

The success of the text wildly exceeded my expectations: at the time of this writing, the book has been published in eight languages and has served as a reference for countless practitioners. Some of those veterinarians contacted me with tips and tricks of their own, such as how to improve suture placement for perineal or scrotal urethrostomy, or introduced me to alternative techniques, such as subcostal muscular gastropexy. I've incorporated many of their suggestions into this new edition.

Other improvements include the addition of eight new chapters on limb and toe amputations and ophthalmic surgery, better explanations and photos for some techniques (e.g., vertical ear canal resection and tensioning sutures), and expanded information about wound management and dressing selection. Additionally, literature searches were performed on each topic, so that the text and bibliographies are pertinent and up to date.

As with the first edition, I look forward to hearing your comments and suggestions and learning more from you!

Section 1 Surgery of the Skin

Chapter 1
Primary Wound Closure

Wound healing starts almost immediately after skin incision. Initially, blood clots form to seal the wound and provide a scaffold for cell migration. The inflammatory phase of healing starts about 6 hours after injury. White blood cells migrate into the wound to begin debridement. They also release cytokines, growth factors, and other chemicals that stimulate vessel ingrowth and tissue repair. Three to five days after injury, granulation tissue begins to replace the fibrin plug that fills the wound. Up to this point, wound strength is relatively poor. As collagen content increases, the wound gradually becomes stronger. The greatest rate of collagen accumulation occurs between 7 and 14 days after injury. After 2 to 3 weeks, the wound begins to mature as collagen content and fiber orientation change.

In clean, incised, sutured wounds, epithelium migrates across the gap within 48 hours. Epithelium will also grow downward into the incision and around sutures, making tracts that can give the appearance of infection. By 10 to 15 days after wounding, these epithelial ingrowths regress.

Wound healing can be affected by a variety of factors, including motion, tension, poor blood supply, anemia, malnutrition, corticosteroids, radiation, and antineoplastic drugs. Systemic diseases such as diabetes mellitus, hepatic or renal dysfunction, feline leukemia, or hyperadrenocorticism may delay healing. Healing is also prolonged when wounds are edematous or infected or contain foreign material or necrotic debris. The use of lasers to incise the skin will increase inflammation and risk of necrosis and decrease wound tensile strength and cosmesis compared with scalpel blade incisions. Rate of wound healing varies with species; for instance, incised wounds in cats gain strength more slowly than in dogs.

In general, primary wound closure is more likely to be successful when Halsted's principles of surgery are followed. These include gentle tissue handling, accurate hemostasis, preservation of adequate blood supply, strict asepsis, avoidance of tension, careful tissue approximation, and obliteration of dead space. In dogs and cats, skin wounds are often closed in two layers. The subcutaneous tissue is closed to reduce bleeding, dead space, and tension, and the dermis is apposed to promote rapid epithelialization.

Manual of Small Animal Soft Tissue Surgery, Second Edition. Karen Tobias.
© 2017 John Wiley & Sons, Inc. Published 2017 by John Wiley & Sons, Inc.

Preoperative management

Diagnostics and supportive care depend on the individual patient's status. Prophylactic antibiotics (one dose administered intravenously at induction and a second dose 1.5 to 6 hours later) should be considered for prolonged surgical procedures, since infection rates double when surgery time increases from 60 to 90 minutes. Wounds should be widely clipped and prepped, especially when drain placement or skin advancement is required.

Surgery

Subcutaneous and skin closure can be performed with interrupted or continuous suture patterns. Interrupted patterns are preferred when wounds are under tension or tissue integrity is questionable. Continuous patterns are faster to perform and, when used in the subcutis, leave less foreign material within the wound. Skin sutured in a continuous pattern is more likely to dehisce if the site is traumatized after surgery or the sutures cut through the tissues. A cruciate suture pattern provides the benefits of an interrupted closure while decreasing surgical time. Cruciate sutures can be tied with a gap between the first and second throw to permit postoperative relaxation if tissues swell.

Skin apposition with a buried intradermal pattern may provide a more cosmetic appearance compared with a simple interrupted pattern. Intradermal patterns are difficult to perform on thin skin or long or irregular incisions. Short incisions, such as ovariohysterectomy and castration sites, can be rapidly closed with a running subcutaneous-to-intradermal pattern. With this technique, the subcutaneous closure is continued directly into an intradermal pattern, which is tied off to the original subcutaneous suture end.

In most animals, subcutaneous tissues are closed with 3-0 absorbable monofilament suture material on a taper needle. Intradermal patterns are performed with 3-0 or 4-0 absorbable suture material on a cutting or taper needle. In large dogs, the intradermal layer can also be closed with 2-0 monofilament absorbable suture on a taper needle. Suture materials that absorb in ≤120 days are preferred. Skin is usually closed with 3-0 nylon or another nonabsorbable material. The size of the suture bites and the distance between sutures depend on the thickness of the skin.

During knot tying, sutures may inadvertently form half hitches when uneven tension is placed on the suture ends. Frequently, a right-handed person pulls too hard on the right end of the suture (usually the short or looped end) because of a tendency to overuse the dominant hand. Also, many surgeons throw the needle holder into the suture when tying a knot. This lifts up on the suture, hitching a previously square throw. A half-hitched throw is easy to identify: one end of the suture will stand straight up while the other end lies flat. With a square throw, both suture ends will lie flat. Surgeon's knots, in which the first throw is doubled, are harder to hitch than knots made of single throws, since the double throw provides more friction and resists tension. Surgeon's knots provide the same security as simple square knots. Hitching can be prevented by placing the needle holder directly over the incision line, wrapping the suture around the needle holder with the nondominant hand, and pulling the suture ends evenly while watching the throw settle directly over the incision line. The throw should remain in a horizontal orientation as it is being tightened. With some monofilament sutures, it may be necessary to pull harder with the nondominant hand to square a throw.

Surgical technique: subcutaneous-to-intradermal closure

1. Start the subcutaneous suture at the far end of the incision, opposite from where you would normally start your intradermal pattern. For example, closure of the subcutis of an abdominal incision would start at the left end of the incision for a right-handed surgeon standing on the dog's right.
2. In the subcutaneous tissues, take a bite perpendicular to the incision line at one end of the surgical wound.
3. Tie two knots, leaving the free end at least 2.5 cm long. Place a hemostat on the free end of the suture to keep it out of the way (fig. 1-1).
4. Perform a simple continuous subcutaneous closure.
    a. For incisions with minimal subcutaneous tissue, take full-thickness bites that include the cut edge of the subcutaneous tissue on each side.
    b. For incisions with wide areas of exposed subcutaneous fat, use a pattern similar to a Lembert. On one side of the incision, insert the needle in and out of the subcutaneous fat near, and perpendicular to, the skin edge. Take a similar bite on the opposite side of the incision. This will invert the cut edge of the subcutis, leaving a smooth closure.
5. Continue the subcutaneous closure to the end of the incision.
6. Once the near end of the incision is reached, begin the intradermal pattern from that end (fig. 1-1), taking long, overlapping bites oriented parallel to the skin margin (fig. 1-2).
    a. No knot is needed. The first bite starts at the crotch of the incision.
7. At the end of the incision line, take a final dermal bite from superficial to deep (fig. 1-3). The bite should enter the dermis and exit out the subcutaneous tissue next to the free end of the original knot.
8. Using four single throws, tie two knots, pulling parallel to the incision line (fig. 1-4). Cut the free end of the suture short.
9. If the knots do not bury, pass the needle end of the suture through the gap in the incision near the knot (fig. 1-5), under the subcutis, and out the skin lateral to the incision line (fig. 1-6) before cutting the needle end.

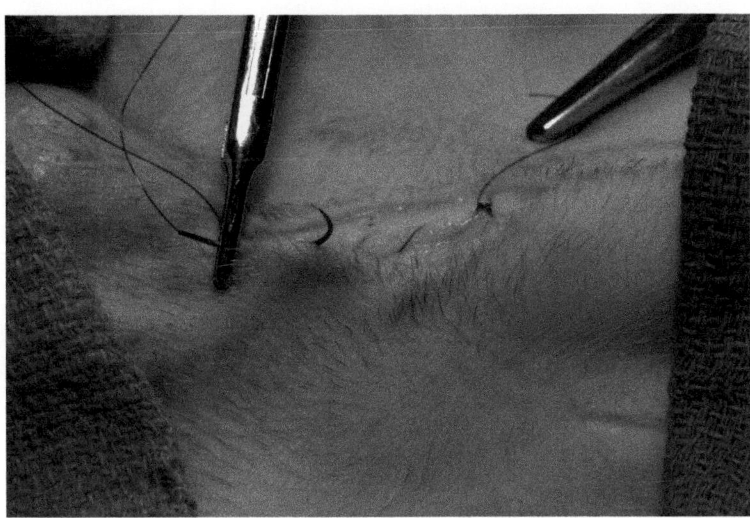

Figure 1-1 Subcutaneous-to-intradermal pattern. Start the subcutaneous pattern at the far end, leaving the knot end long (hemostat attached in photo). Once you reach the near end of the incision, start immediately into an intradermal pattern.

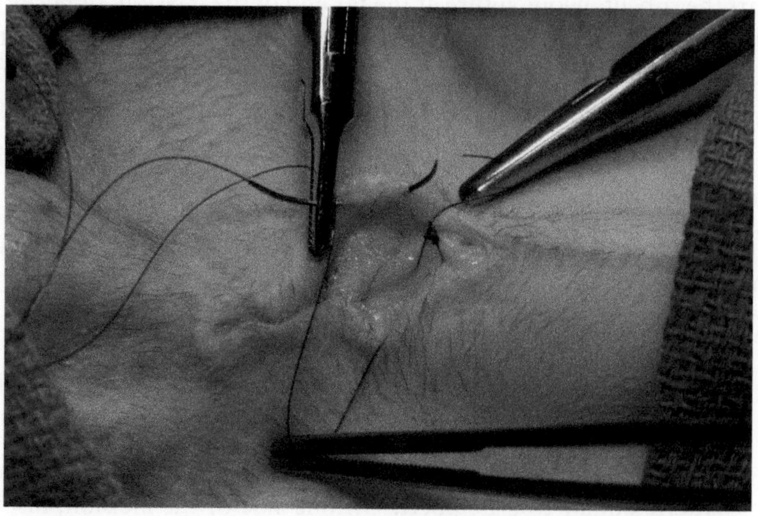

Figure 1-2 Take long bites in the intradermal layer, slightly overlapping with the bites on the contralateral side.

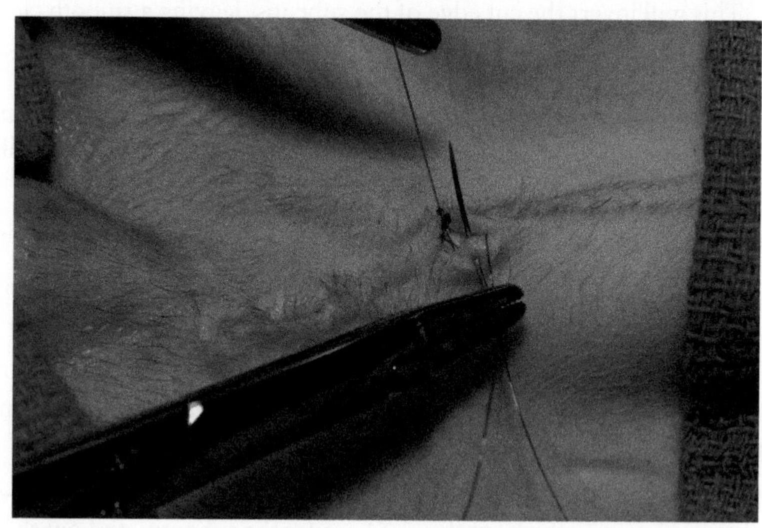

Figure 1-3 Take a final bite at the far end of the incision line from superficial to deep, entering at the intradermal layer and exiting below the subcutis. Make sure that the needle end and knot end of the sutures are adjacent to each other.

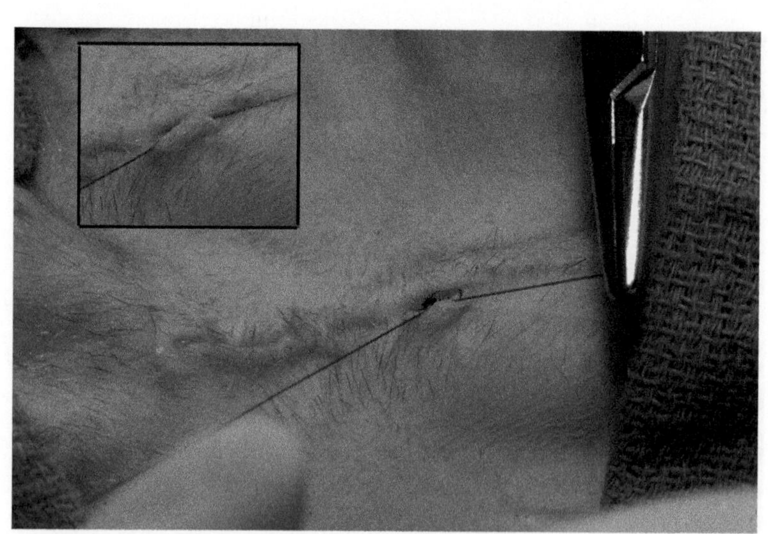

Figure 1-4 Tie four simple throws, pulling lengthwise along the incision line to appose skin edges (inset) and bury the knots.

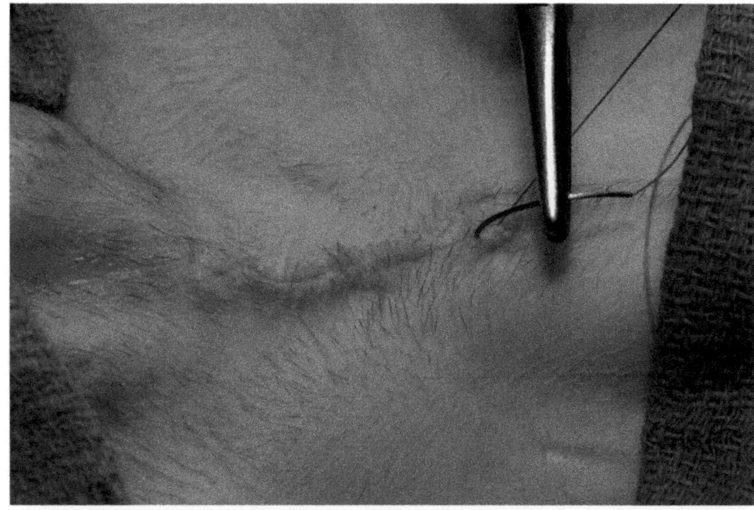

Figure 1-5 To further bury the knot, pass the needle through the gap in the incision near the knot and under the subcutis.

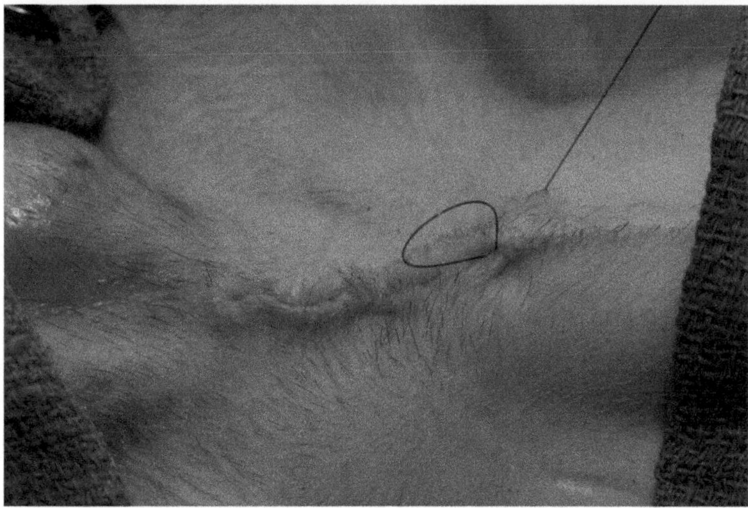

Figure 1-6 Exit the needle from the skin laterally and place tension on the suture to pull the knot down and under the subcutis.

Surgical technique: intradermal pattern

1. For an incision that is parallel to the long axis of the dog (e.g., an ovariohysterectomy incision), begin the closure at the end of the incision closest to the hand driving the needle holder. In other words, if you are a right-handed surgeon, start at the right end of the incision.
2. In the incision edge closest to you, take a bite from deep to superficial, passing the needle from below the subcutis and up and out of the dermis (fig. 1-7). Position the needle perpendicular to the skin edge during the bite.
3. Cross over to the opposite side and take a bite from superficial to deep, starting at the dermis and passing through and under the subcutis (fig. 1-7).
4. Verify that the two suture ends are adjacent to each other and exiting in front of the portion of the suture that crosses the incision line (on the side of the crossover suture that is away from the end of the incision). The knot will not bury if the crossover suture is between the two suture ends.

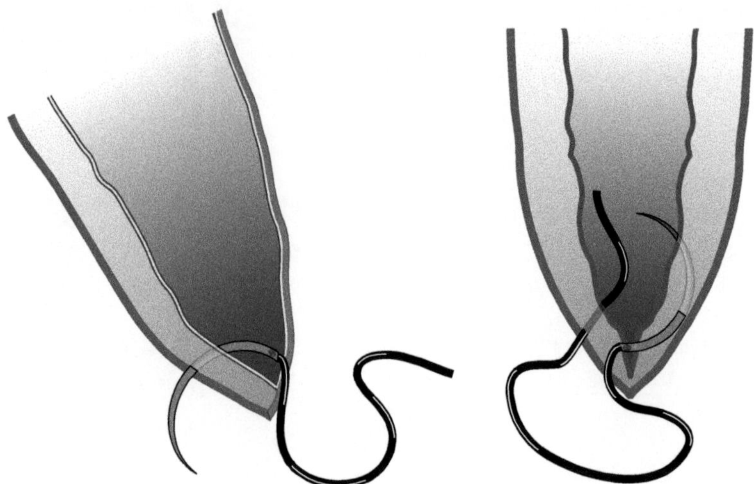

Figure 1-7 To start the intradermal pattern, take a bite from superficial to deep (left), starting at the dermis and exiting below the subcutis. Take a second bite from deep to superficial (right), starting below the subcutis and exiting at the dermis.

5. Tie four single square throws, pulling horizontally and parallel to (along) the incision line to bury the knots under the subcutis (see fig. 1-4).
6. Take intradermal bites along the incision.
   a. Gently evert the skin to expose the dermis and facilitate proper suture placement (see fig. 1-2). If possible, grasp the subcutis with thumb forceps instead of the skin when everting.
   b. Take a bite at least 5 mm long and keep the needle within the dermal layer for the entire bite (fig. 1-2).
   c. Take a bite on the opposite side of the incision. Start the bite at a level just behind the exit point of the previous bite on the opposite side (fig. 1-8). This will cause the sutures to angle backwards slightly as they cross the incision line, improving apposition.
7. End the last dermal bite 0.5 cm from the end of the incision in animals with thin skin and 1cm from the end of the incision in animals with thick skin.
8. Take a bite on one skin margin from superficial to deep, passing the needle through the dermis and exiting under the subcutis (fig. 1-9). Position the needle perpendicular to the skin edge during the bite.
9. Leave a 2- to 4-cm loop of suture and take a bite on the opposite skin margin from deep to superficial, starting below the subcutis and exiting

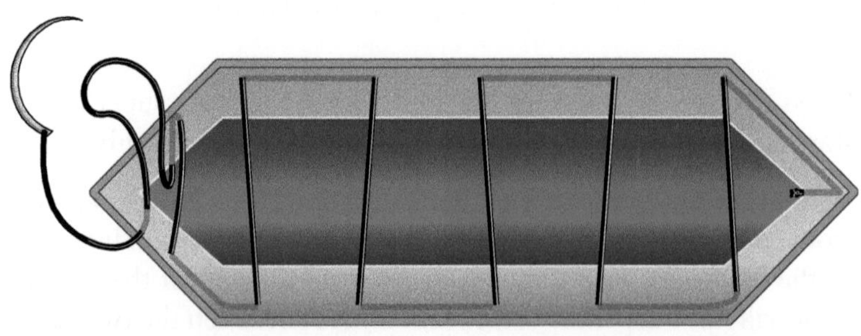

Figure 1-8 Take bites parallel to the skin margins, slightly overlapping with bites on the contralateral side. To begin tying the final knot, take a bite from superficial to deep and then deep to superficial, leaving a loop between the bites.

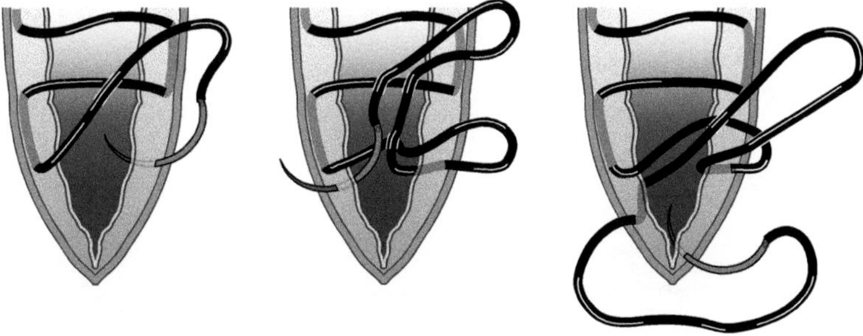

Figure 1-9 To bury the final knot, take a bite from superficial to deep (left); leave a loop and take a second bite from deep to superficial (center). Take another bite from superficial to deep (right), and tie this end to the loop.

out the dermis (figs. 1-8 and 1-9). Both ends of the loop will now be deep to the subcutis.

10. Cross over to the other side, and take another bite from superficial to deep. Make sure that the needle exits below the subcutis next to the suture loop and the crossover stitch does not come between the loop and needle end (fig. 1-9).
11. Using four single throws, tie two knots, pulling parallel to (along) the incision line (fig. 1-4).
12. If the knots are not buried, tuck the knot under the subcutis before cutting the needle end.
    a. Cut off the free end of the knot.
    b. Reload the needle.
    c. Palm the needle holder and insert the needle, pointed straight down, adjacent to the knot so that the needle passes into the incisional gap (fig. 1-5).
    d. Pass the needle under the subcutaneous tissues.
    e. Bring the needle up and out of the skin to one side of the incision (fig. 1-6).

Lift firmly up on the suture to pull the knot down through the incisional gap. Cut off the remaining suture end.

Surgical technique: cruciate pattern

1. Take a bite through the far skin margin 0.5 to 1 cm from the edge. Exit out the near skin margin the same distance from the edge, and pull most of the suture through the skin.
2. Take a second, similar bite, 0.5 to 1 cm parallel to the first (figs. 1-10 and 1-11).
3. Tie a surgeon's throw, tightening the suture so that it is in contact with the skin without compressing it (fig. 1-12).
4. Tie a second throw, leaving a small loop between it and the surgeon's throw as you tighten.
5. Tie the third and fourth throws to the second throw to form a secure knot above the loop (figs. 1-12 and 1-13).

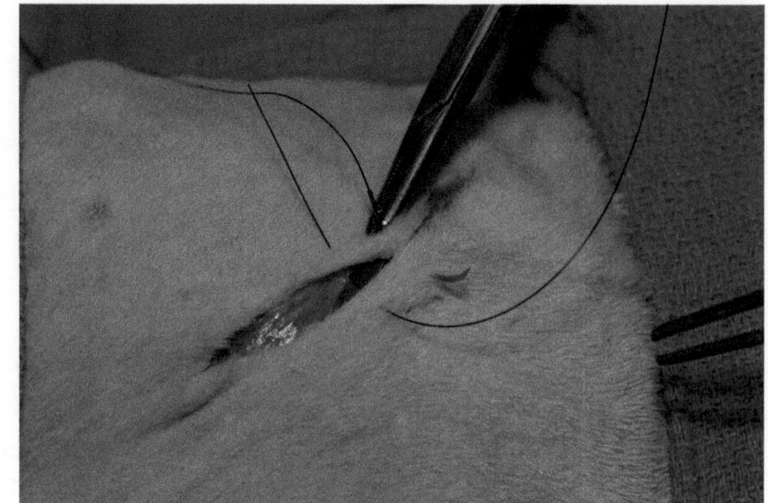

Figure 1-10 Cruciate suture. Take bites perpendicular to the skin edges.

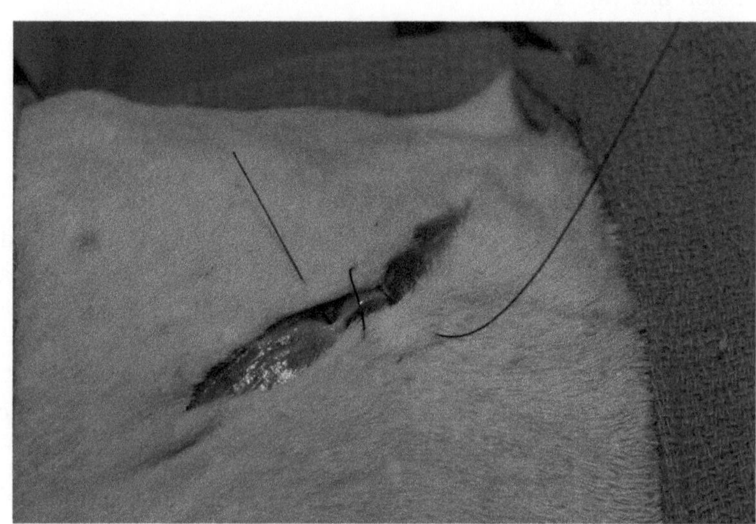

Figure 1-11 The second bite is parallel to the first.

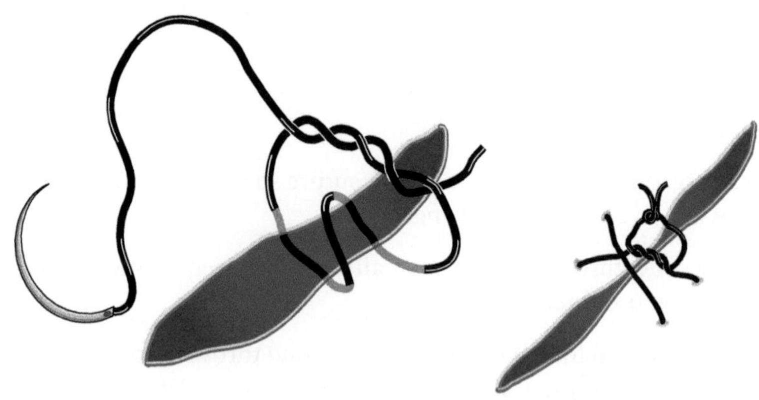

Figure 1-12 If there is tension on the skin line, tie a surgeon's throw to appose skin margins and leave a small loop between the surgeon's throws and the remaining throws.

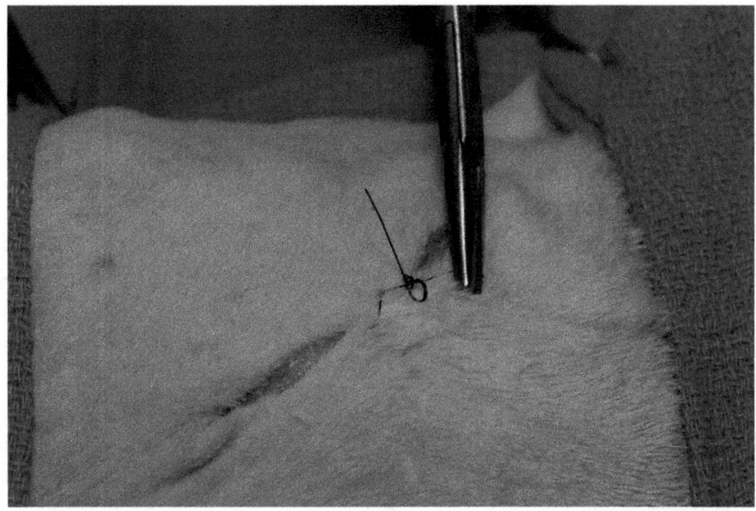

Figure 1-13 Final appearance. The skin should lie flat.

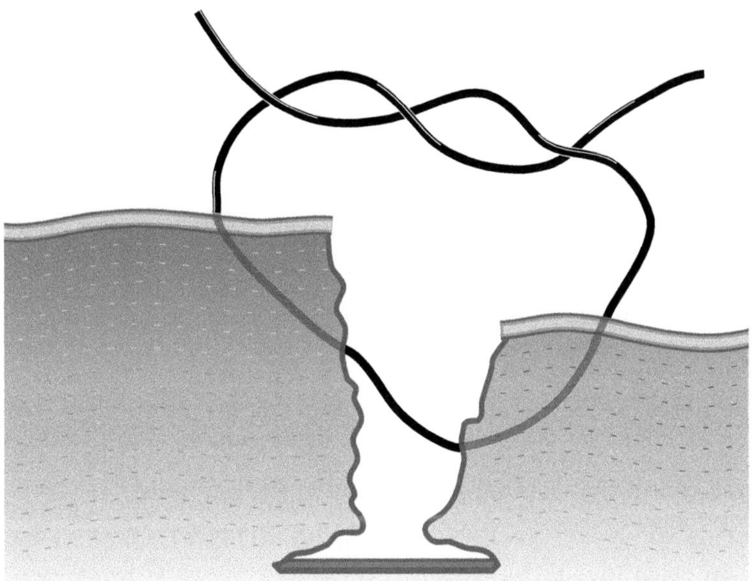

Figure 1-14 To level out uneven skin edges, take a deeper bite of the depressed side and shallower bite of the elevated side.

6. To close skin with uneven edges because of variable skin thickness or uneven subcutaneous closure, take a shallower bite of the elevated side and a deeper bite of the depressed side (fig. 1-14). This will actually provide bites of the same thickness that will level the skin when the first throw is tightened.

Surgical technique: Ford interlocking pattern for a right-handed surgeon

1. Starting at one end of the incision, take a bite across the incision line. For a right handed surgeon, the needle should pass from right to left and perpendicular to the incision line. Tie 2 knots.
2. Lay the suture on the left side of the incision so that it is lateral to the incision line and to where the needle will exit with each suture bite (fig. 1-15).

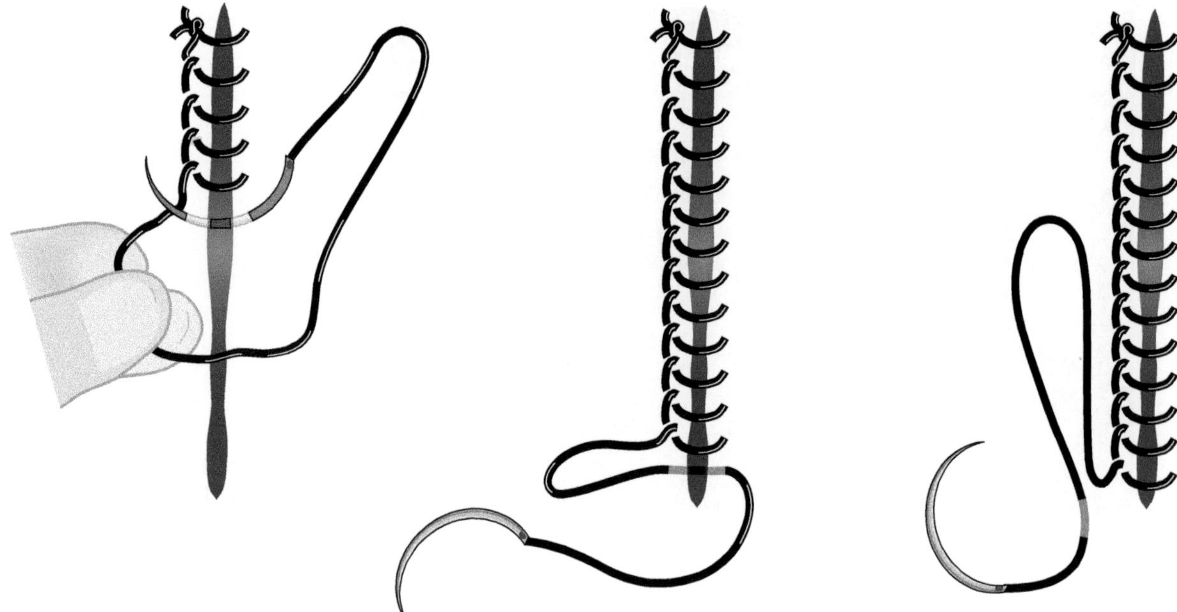

Figure 1-15 Retract the suture laterally as you take skin bites, so the needle comes up within the loop of the suture. Take the last suture bite from the opposite direction (middle figure) or a skin bite lateral to the final suture (right figure) to make a narrow loop for tying off the pattern.

3. Take a suture bite from right to left across the incision line so that the needle exits the tissue within the loop of suture.
4. Tighten the suture so that it lies against the skin without compressing it (fig. 1-16).
5. Continue the pattern to the end of the incision line. Take bites 0.5 to 1 cm from the edge and 0.5 to 1 cm apart, depending on skin thickness.
6. At the end of the incision, tie the suture end to a loop.
    a. Pass the needle from left to right on the last bite to make a narrow loop for tying (fig. 1-15).

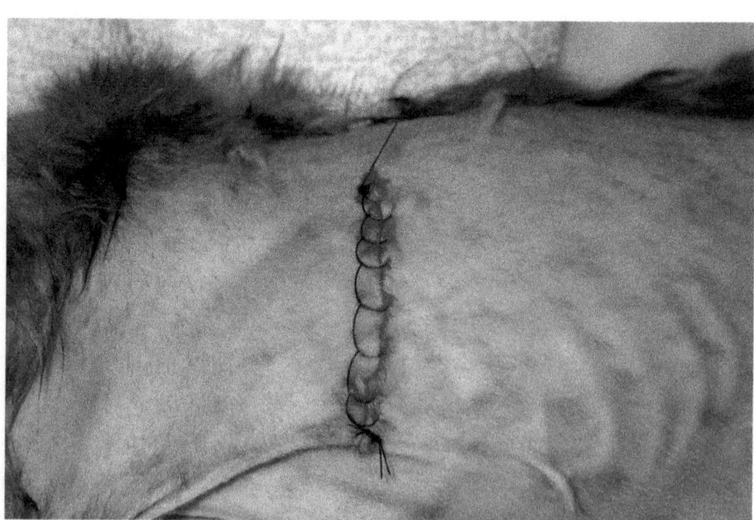

Figure 1-16 A Ford interlocking pattern should lie gently against the skin.

b. Alternatively, take a bite of the skin lateral to the incision, starting near the suture exit site and ending 0.5 to 1 cm away to make a narrower loop for tying (fig. 1-15).

Postoperative considerations

Nonabsorbable skin sutures are usually removed 10 to 14 days after placement. Sutures may be left in longer in patients that have conditions that could delay wound healing (e.g., mast cell tumor excision). An Elizabethan collar or protective bandage should be placed as needed to protect the site until it is healed.

Complications of incisional closure are often related to technique. During closure, subcutaneous tissues may appear ruffled or buckled if sutured with large appositional bites instead of a Lembert type of pattern. Skin sutures that are too tight (fig. 1-17) or too loose can result in ischemia or wound contamination, respectively. Skin edges may fail to appose with intradermal patterns for several reasons. If bites on opposite sides of the incision do not overlap slightly, gaps may occur. In this case, sutures crossing the incision line can be seen advancing at a forward angle, instead of perpendicular or slightly backward, before the suture is tightened. Gaps may also be present if the suture enters or exits through subcutis instead of remaining in the dermis for its entire path. Buckling of the skin during intradermal closure may be caused by too much overlapping of contralateral bites. Buckling can also occur if bites are not parallel to the skin surface (e.g., bites that enter and exit the dermis but, midway, pass through the subcutis). Skin can purse string if the intradermal suture is pulled too tightly when the ending knot is tied.

Failure to bury intradermal knots can occur for several reasons. Knots that are too close to the end of the incision can be trapped above a web of subcutis, since the subcutaneous incision is often shorter than the skin incision. To prevent knot prolapse out of the incision, the subcutaneous incision should be extended to the end of the dermal incision or the knot should be started farther from the incision end. Knots can accidentally be pulled out of the incision line if the suture is tightened perpendicular to the incision line or is lifted up when the knot is being tied. Crossover sutures can accidentally be included in or under

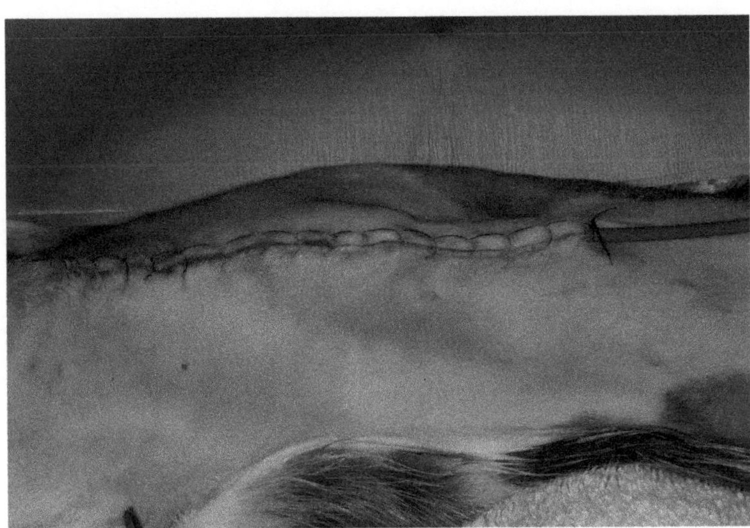

Figure 1-17 This cat underwent diaphragmatic hernia repair; the red rubber chest tube was exited out through the diaphragmatic and abdominal closures. In this cat the Ford interlocking pattern is pulled too tightly, resulting in ridges in the skin.

the knot when the final sutures are being placed or the tucking maneuver is performed. During the tucking maneuver, passage of the needle through the superficial subcutis instead of through the incisional gap will prevent the knot from burying.

Corticosteroids, cytotoxic agents, and radiation will delay wound healing. The greatest effect is seen during the early stages of wound repair; however, later stages may also be affected. Specific recommendations cannot be made regarding postoperative use of these agents. Cytotoxic or radiation therapy is usually delayed for 7 to 14 days until the wound strength has increased and the incision appears to be healed.

Bibliography

Amalsadvala T and Swaim SF: Management of hard-to-heal wounds. Vet Clin Small Anim Pract 2006;36:693–711.

Mison M.B. et al: Comparison of the effects of the CO_2 surgical laser and conventional surgical techniques on healing and wound tensile strength of skin flaps in the dog. Vet Surg 2003;32:153–160.

Pavletic MM: Basic principles of wound healing. In Atlas of Small Animal Wound Management & Reconstructive Surgery. Ames Ia., Wiley-Blackwell, 2010: pp. 18–29.

Rajbabu K. et al: To knot or not to knot? Sutureless haemostasis compared to the surgeon's knot. Am R Coll Surg Engl 2007;89:359–362.

Rosine and Robinson GM: Knot security of suture materials. Vet Surg 1989; 18:269–273.

Smeak DD: Buried continuous intradermal suture closure. Compend Contin Educ Pract Vet 1992;14:907–918.

Sylvester A. et al: A comparison of 2 different suture patterns for skin closure of canine ovariohysterectomy. Can Vet J 2002;43:699–702.

Chapter 2
Lumpectomy and Primary Closure

Removal of small benign skin masses is relatively simple. When masses are large or malignant, however, extensive resection may be necessary. Direct closure of large wounds may require tension-relieving techniques such as walking or stent sutures or skin stretchers. When direct closure is not an option, flaps, grafts, or other tension-relieving techniques may be necessary (see Chapters 3–6).

Preoperative management

Staging for metastases should be performed in animals with malignant masses. In most animals, this would include three-view thoracic radiographs; in animals with mast cell tumors, abdominal ultrasound is more critical. If preoperative cytology confirms a mast cell tumor, the animal should receive intravenous diphenhydramine before surgical clipping and prepping to reduce mast cell degranulation, and the site should be prepped gently to prevent swelling.

Before resection, masses should be measured and local skin tension evaluated to develop a plan for wound closure. If possible, incisions should be made parallel to the lines of tension to facilitate closure. Incision size depends on the type of mass present. Recommended margins for mast cell tumor removal are 2 cm laterally and at least one fascial plane deep. Surgical margins for high grade soft tissue sarcomas and vaccine-induced fibrosarcomas should be at least 3 cm laterally from the palpable tumor and two fascial planes deep. Synthetic monofilament suture with absorption time ≤120 days is often used for subcutaneous closure, since fibrous tissue around long-lasting suture material may be palpable for months, making postoperative assessment of recurrence more challenging.

Size of resection and method of closure should be considered when clipping and positioning the animal. In some animals, a "hanging skin prep" (suspension of skin by towel clamps) provides more laxity during closure. If the surgical procedure is expected to last longer than an hour, prophylactic antibiotics are recommended. For patients undergoing placement of continuous suction drains or infusion catheters at surgery, the site for drain or catheter

Manual of Small Animal Soft Tissue Surgery, Second Edition. Karen Tobias.
© 2017 John Wiley & Sons, Inc. Published 2017 by John Wiley & Sons, Inc.

exit should be planned in advance so that it can be bandaged easily after surgery. If radiation therapy is to be considered at a later date, the drain exit site should be near enough the surgical incision to be included in the radiation field, and hemoclips should be placed in the subcutaneous boundaries of the excision site to help guide radiation planning. Once the mass is removed, its subcutaneous surface and cut edges should be marked with blue or green ink and allowed to dry before being placed in formalin. This will allow the pathologist to evaluate margins during histologic examination.

Surgery

In animals with tumors, either the tumor or proposed incision site can be outlined with a sterile pen (fig. 2-1). Skin and subcutaneous tissues are usually incised or transected with a blade and scissors to prevent damage to tissue margins. When skin is incised by radio wave radiosurgery, CO_2 laser, or monopolar electrosurgery, char will penetrate the skin biopsies 0.16 to 0.22 mm, and char will extend into the surrounding skin up to 0.26 mm. During dissection, an interrupted suture can be placed through all tissue layers

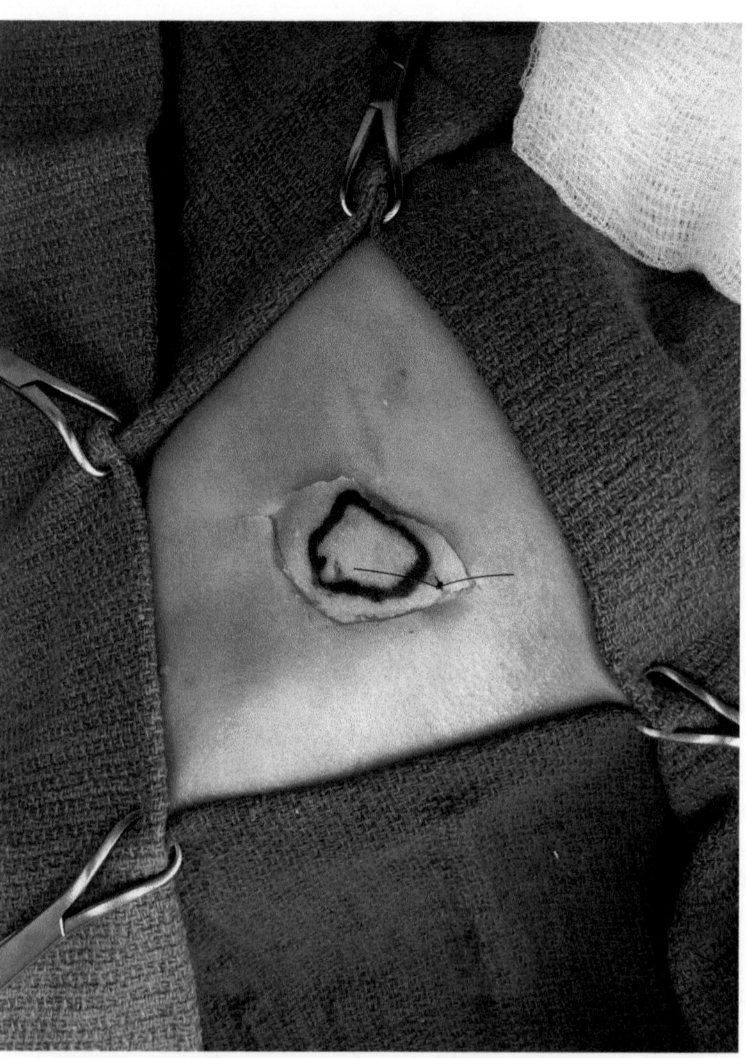

Figure 2-1 Benign mass outlined with a sterile marker. At one end of the incision, a simple interrupted suture has been placed through the skin and underlying tissues to hold the layers together during dissection and excision.

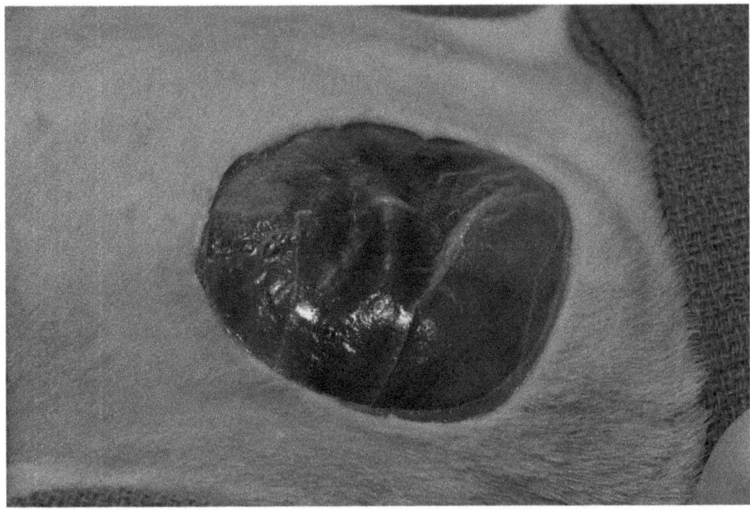

Figure 2-2 Circular wound.

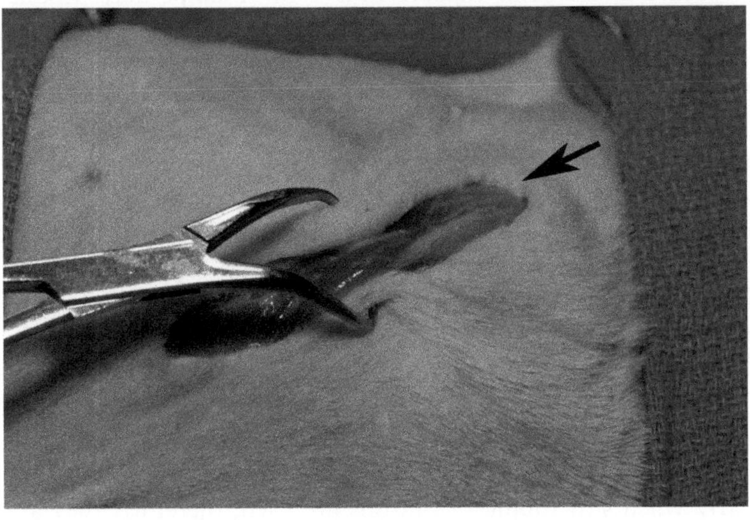

Figure 2-3 If skin laxity is sufficient, circular wounds can be closed in a linear manner. This may result in excess skin (*arrow*) or a "dog ear" at one or both ends of the incision.

at one end of the incision (fig. 2-1). This will hold the layers together and also serve as a directional marker for the pathologist.

Elliptical or elongated wounds can be apposed in a linear fashion. The subcutaneous tissues are elevated along the wound margins to facilitate closure. When the resection site is large or irregular, the first skin suture is placed across the center of the wound to evaluate skin position, and then additional skin sutures are placed across the middle of each remaining half of the incision. Alternatively, towel clamps can be used to temporarily appose skin margins of wide wounds. Subcutaneous sutures are then placed between the skin sutures or towel clamps to reduce tension before the remaining skin sutures are placed.

Circular wounds (fig. 2-2) can be turned into an ellipse and then closed in a linear fashion (fig. 2-3) or closed in a T, Y, or X shape (fig. 2-4). As mentioned earlier, the central sutures are placed first to evaluate final skin position. Tension is greatest in the center of the wound where the tips of the Y or X come together. A buried horizontal mattress suture can be run circumferentially through the subdermal layer to reduce the stress on the skin suture line (fig. 2-4), or the three skin edges can be pulled together with a half buried

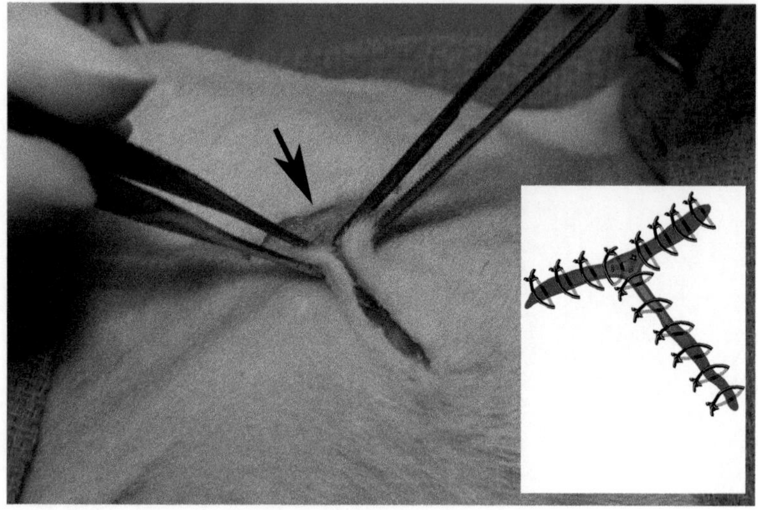

Figure 2-4 To make a Y-shaped closure, pull the skin edges along one half of the defect together from side to side (thumb forceps) and pull the remaining arc of the skin edge (arrow) centrally. Pull together the subcutaneous tissues at the tips of the Y with a buried purse-string suture before adding the remaining sutures (inset).

mattress suture in the skin. Closure in a Y or X shape may produce skin puckers or folds ("dog ears"); if these are small, they can be left in place.

Subcutaneous elevation and apposition will reduce tension on skin sutures. To stretch and advance skin before closure, walking sutures can be applied from the wound bed to the subcutaneous tissues under the skin. Besides relieving tension, walking sutures also close dead space and advance the skin margins to allow primary apposition. Dimples in the skin produced by these sutures will usually resolve in 2 to 3 weeks. Walking sutures are not recommended in flaps because they damage blood supply and cause local necrosis. They are also contraindicated in infected wounds, thin skin, or areas of motion.

Stent sutures reduce tension by spreading pressure out over a large area. The primary skin incision is apposed, and tension is reduced by placement of vertical mattress sutures that cross over soft tubing or rolled gauze (fig. 2-5). If left in place for long periods, stent sutures can cause necrosis at pressure points, particularly when stiff tubing or buttons are used; therefore, they are often removed within 2 to 3 days of placement.

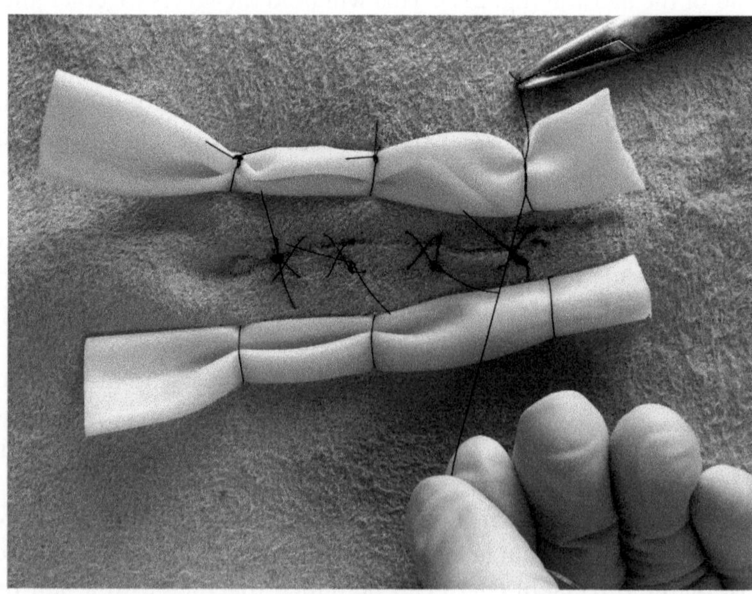

Figure 2-5 Stent sutures made with Penrose drains and vertical mattress pattern.

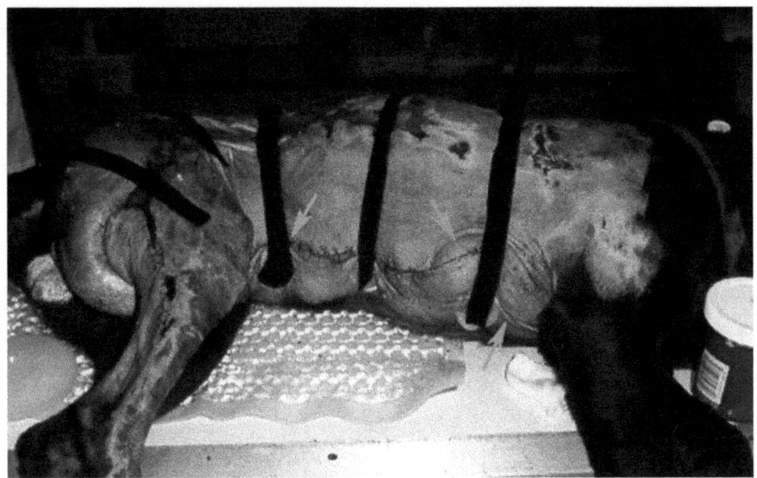

Figure 2-6 Skin-stretching device. The elastic bands have been temporarily tightened to demonstrate the stretching effects (arrows) on the skin. Once the skin has been cleaned, bandage dressings will be placed over the wound bed before securing the elastic bands to the Velcro dorsally. This dog underwent a caudal superficial epigastric flap (180° rotation) to cover a burn wound on the hip.

Skin can be stretched before or after lumpectomy with tie-over bandages or elastic skin stretchers (fig. 2-6). Skin stretching devices are made with Velcro® self-adherent pads, 1-inch-wide sewing elastic, and cyanoacrylate ("superglue"). The hair is clipped and the skin is cleaned with soap and alcohol and allowed to dry completely. Several pads are glued at least 5 to 10 cm from the margins on either side of the wound, using the "hook" portion of the pad. Application of a thin layer of superglue to the contact surface of the pad improves adhesion to the skin. The pile surface of the elastic bands will secure the elastic to the hooks on the pads. A dressing is placed under the bands if a wound or incision is present. Initially the elastic bands should be under moderate tension; tension is increased every 6 to 8 hours to stretch the skin. In most patients, skin is stretched significantly in 4 days, with the greatest gains in the first 48 to 72 hours. When no longer needed, pads can be removed by peeling them off the skin or using a glue solvent.

Surgical technique: lumpectomy

1. With a sterile ruler and marking pen, measure and draw appropriate margins around the mass.
2. Make an incision through the skin and subcutaneous tissues along the marked line (fig. 2-7).
3. If a mast cell tumor is present, continue dissection at least one fascial plane below the tumor. For high-grade soft tissue sarcomas in dogs and injection site sarcomas in cats, remove wider margins (fig. 2-8).
4. Place a suture full thickness through the fascia, subcutis, and skin to hold the layers together and to mark one edge of the resection (see fig. 2-1).
5. Place two full-thickness sutures along a second edge of the resected tissues, 90 degrees from the first suture, so that orientation of the mass will be marked (note these suture placements on the histology submission form) and the tissue layer orientation will be maintained (a tissue "sandwich").
6. Using sharp and blunt dissection, remove the mass. Cauterize or ligate associated blood vessels.

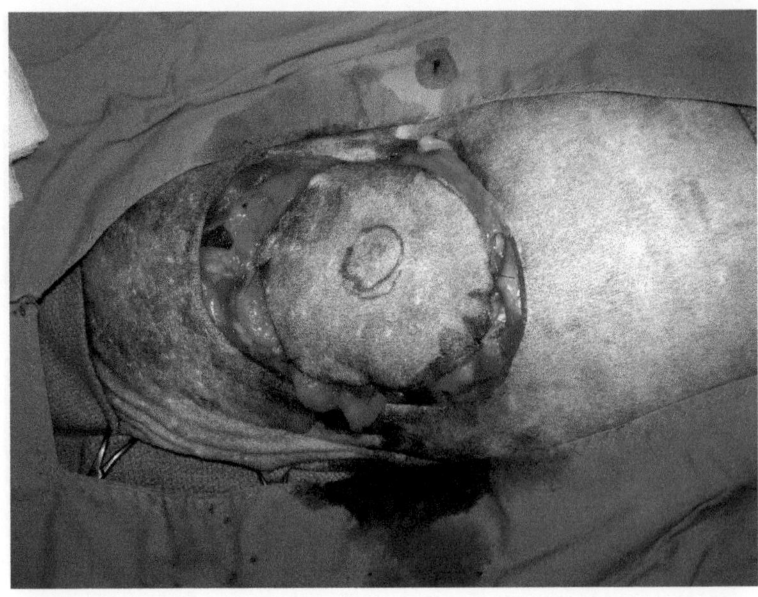

Figure 2-7 Incise the skin at least 2 cm around the margin of a mast cell tumor and at least 3 cm around the margin of a high-grade or vaccine-associated sarcoma. In this dog, the skin was incised 5 cm lateral to the mass (inner purple circle), which was previously diagnosed as a fibrosarcoma.

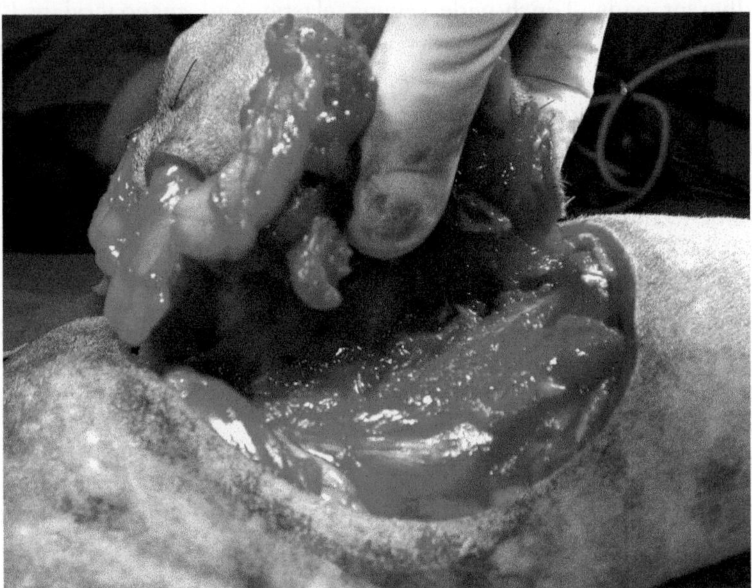

Figure 2-8 Dissect at least one fascial plane below mast cell tumors, if possible, and at least 2 fascial planes below high-grade sarcomas. In this dog the dorsal spinous processes were removed along with the adjacent muscle.

7. If possible, appose any incised fascial or muscle edges with interrupted or continuous sutures of 2-0 or 3-0 rapidly absorbable material (fig. 2-9).
8. Carefully undermine the skin margins with blunt and sharp dissection at the level of the loose areolar fascia or deep to the panniculus muscle. Leave any direct cutaneous vessels intact. Large wounds may require undermining for 8 to 14 cm laterally along the skin margin.
9. Place a continuous suction drain as needed, exiting the drain through healthy skin at a site that will be easily covered with a bandage (e.g., away from the prepuce or anus).
10. To stretch the skin toward the midline of the defect and secure it in place, insert subcutaneous walking sutures with 3-0 or 4-0 rapidly absorbable suture (fig. 2-10).

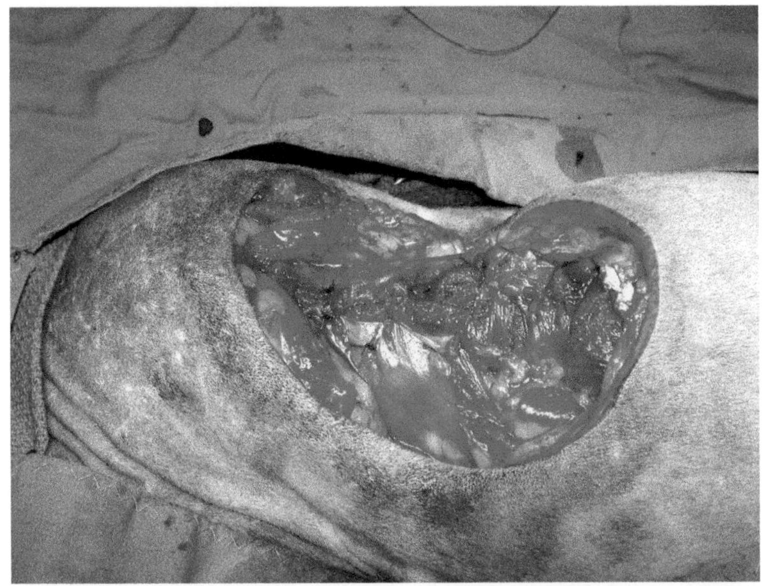

Figure 2-9 Close fascia with interrupted sutures if under tension.

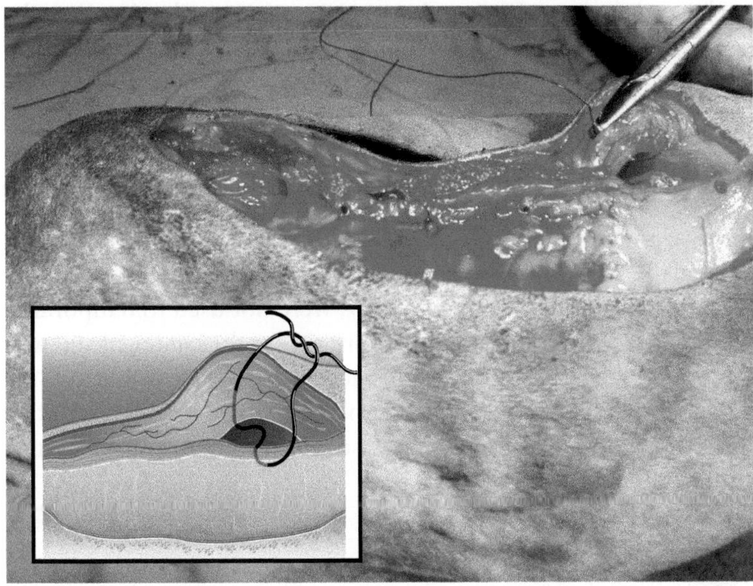

Figure 2-10 To place walking sutures, take a bite of the subcutaneous tissues close to the base of the elevated skin, then take a bite of the wound bed fascia closer to midline (inset). The resultant suture will pull the skin closer to midline.

a. Near the junction of the elevated skin base and subcutis, take a bite of subdermal fascia or deep dermal tissue in the skin parallel to the direction of advancement.

b. Take a bite in the wound bed a few centimeters closer to the wound center than the skin bite, and tie the suture. In some animals, the first row of walking sutures may need to be preplaced before tying.

c. Continue to place several walking sutures in a row, spacing them at least 3 cm apart, and placing as few sutures as possible.

d. Repeat the process on the opposite side of the incision.

e. Place additional staggered rows of walking sutures successively closer to the skin margin, with the wound bed bites closer to midline than the skin bites so that the skin is stretched toward midline as it is tacked in place.

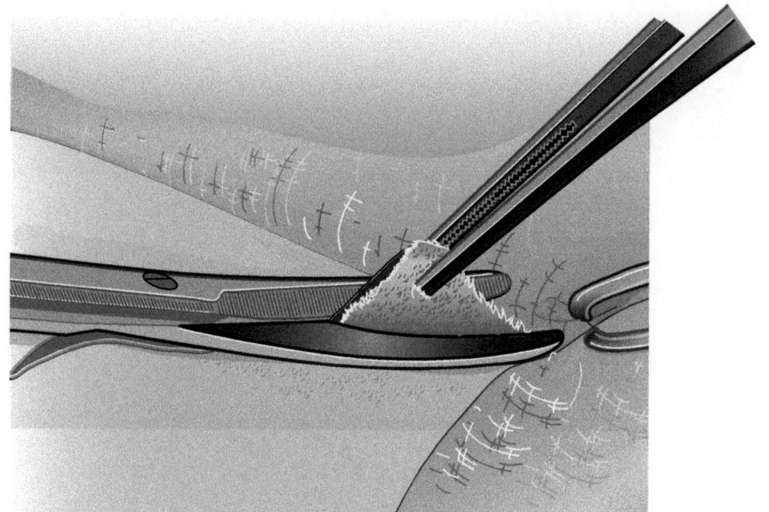

Figure 2-11 Excise large dog ears by transecting them at their base with scissors or a blade.

11. For large defects or those under tension, temporarily place towel clamps across the wound to appose the skin edges (fig. 2-3).
12. Appose the subcutaneous fat with simple interrupted or simple continuous sutures of 3-0 rapidly absorbable material.
13. Excise large dog ears by cutting across the elevated tissue several mm above its base with sharp scissors or a blade (fig. 2-11).
14. Appose the skin with staples or simple interrupted or cruciate sutures of 3-0 nylon (fig. 2-12). If towel clamps were not used to temporarily close the wound, place the first skin suture across the center of the wound to appose the skin. If skin position is acceptable, place a skin suture across the widest part of each half of the wound, then fill in the gaps. Interrupted buried intradermal sutures can also be placed before skin sutures to further reduce tension.

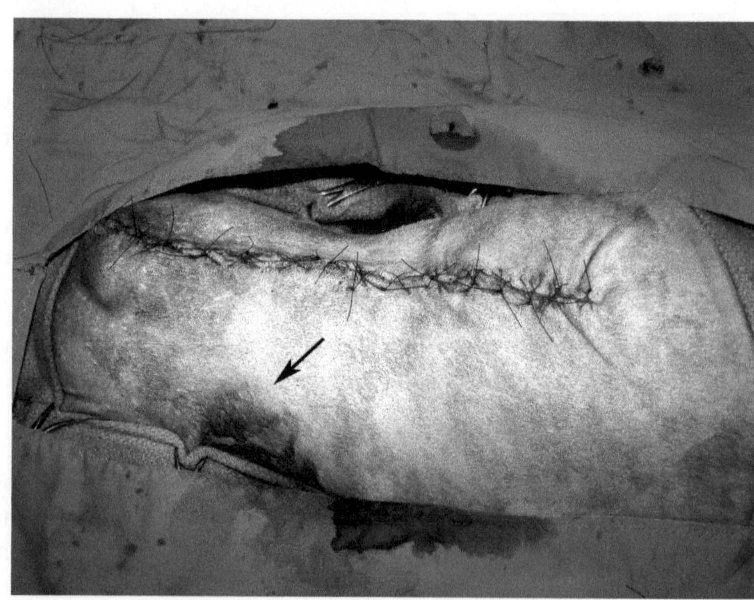

Figure 2-12 Final appearance. Note how recruitment of skin from the flank fold resulted in exposure of unclipped areas (arrow). These areas were kept covered with additional drapes until skin closure was complete; however, a wider prep is preferable.

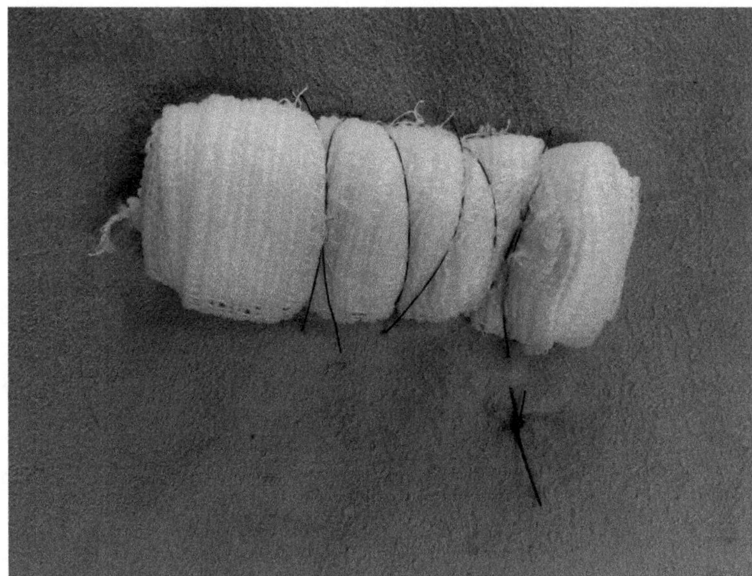

Figure 2-13 Bolster for relieving tension. Vertical mattress sutures (interrupted or continuous pattern) are placed in the skin to either side of the bolster (roll gauze) and tied to keep the bolster in place.

15. For added relief of tension along the skin closure, place temporary stent sutures, a tie-over bandage, a bolster (fig. 2-13), or other tension relieving mechanism. To place a bolster,
    a. Place a tightly rolled gauze or pad over the incision line.
    b. Place vertical mattress sutures (interrupted or continuous pattern) over the bolster and through the skin to either side of the bolster.
    c. Tie the suture over the material firmly enough to release tension on the skin closure without crushing the skin under the material or within the suture bites.
    d. Leave in place for 1-3 days.
16. If tension is excessive, consider flaps, grafts, or tensioning closures instead (see chapters 3–6)

Postoperative considerations

Elizabethan collars and exercise restriction are recommended, particularly in wounds with tension. Bandages may be required to protect drain exit sites or reduce mobility. Postoperative analgesics are critical, especially in patients with walking sutures or wounds under tension. In animals undergoing mast cell tumor resection, skin sutures are left in place for up to 3 weeks, since healing is prolonged. Administration of antineoplastic agents or high dose corticosteroids should be delayed until the wound is healed enough for suture removal.

Common complications after mass removal include seroma or hematoma formation, dehiscence, infection, or tumor recurrence from incomplete resection. Seroma formation and dehiscence are common in dogs after mast cell tumor resection because of local tissue reaction and delayed healing. Walking sutures may disrupt blood supply to advanced skin, and stent sutures may cause ischemia under the devices. When Velcro skin stretchers are used, improperly applied adhesive pads may loosen prematurely.

Bibliography

Amalsadvala T and Swaim S: Management of hard-to-heal wounds. Vet Clin Small Anim Pract 2006;36:693–711.

Bray JP, Polton GA, McSporran KD, et al: Canine soft tissue sarcoma managed in first opinion practice: outcome in 350 cases. Vet Surg 2014;43:774–782.

Fulcher RP et al: Evaluation of a two-centimeter lateral surgical margin for excision of grade I and grade II cutaneous mast cell tumors in dogs. J Am Vet Med Assoc 2006;228:210–215.

Hedlund CS: Large trunk wounds. Vet Clin N Am Small Anim Pract 2006;36: 847–872.

Pavletic MM: Use of external skin-stretching device for wound closure in dogs and cats. J Am Vet Med Assoc 2000;217:350–354.

Silverman EB et al: Histologic comparison of canine skin biopsies collected using monopolar electrosurgery, CO_2 laser, radiowave radiosurgery, skin biopsy punch, and scalpel. Vet Surg 2007;36:50–56.

Chapter 3
Basic Flaps

Development of local flaps may be necessary when primary skin closure results in excessive tension. Local skin flaps ("random pedicle flaps") rely on the blood supply within the subdermal plexus, the extent of which varies with body location. Flaps can either be advanced so that the direction of the skin is relatively unchanged, or they can be pivoted up to 90 degrees to cover an adjacent defect (fig. 3-1).

Advancement or "sliding" flaps are easiest to perform because they do not produce a second wound. Flaps can be advanced unilaterally to produce a U-shaped closure or bilaterally to produce an H- or I-shaped closure. Alternatively, a relaxing incision can be made parallel to the long axis of the wound to produce a bipedicle advancement flap that is slid across the wound. The resultant wound at the donor site is either closed primarily or left to granulate in.

Because closure of wounds with advancement flaps depends on stretching the skin, local structures such as eyelids and lips can be distorted with wound closure. A rotational flap, which pivots local skin into the region, will reduce this distortion. Triangular-shaped wound beds can be closed with unilateral or bilateral semicircular rotational flaps. Although semicircular rotational flaps do not produce a secondary defect, they require movement of a greater proportion of skin and therefore are used less commonly than transposition and advancement flaps. With a transposition flap, the advancing skin is rotated over and beyond intervening normal skin into a nearby wound bed. Rectangular flaps of skin can be rotated up to 90 degrees to close an adjacent defect.

Preoperative management

Wound beds that are contaminated with debris, contain devitalized tissue, or are infected should either be debrided extensively or managed as open wounds before flaps are performed. Wide clipping and prepping should be performed for any large mass removal or wound closure. The area around the recipient site should be evaluated for skin laxity, which will determine whether the donor site can be closed once the flap has been elevated and moved. The skin adjacent to the defect is picked up with thumb and forefingers; if a ridge of skin can be created, the donor site can most likely be closed. A template of the flap can be cut from flexible material, manually held in place at the proposed flap base, and its free end rotated to the recipient site to estimate the amount of

Manual of Small Animal Soft Tissue Surgery, Second Edition. Karen Tobias.
© 2017 John Wiley & Sons, Inc. Published 2017 by John Wiley & Sons, Inc.

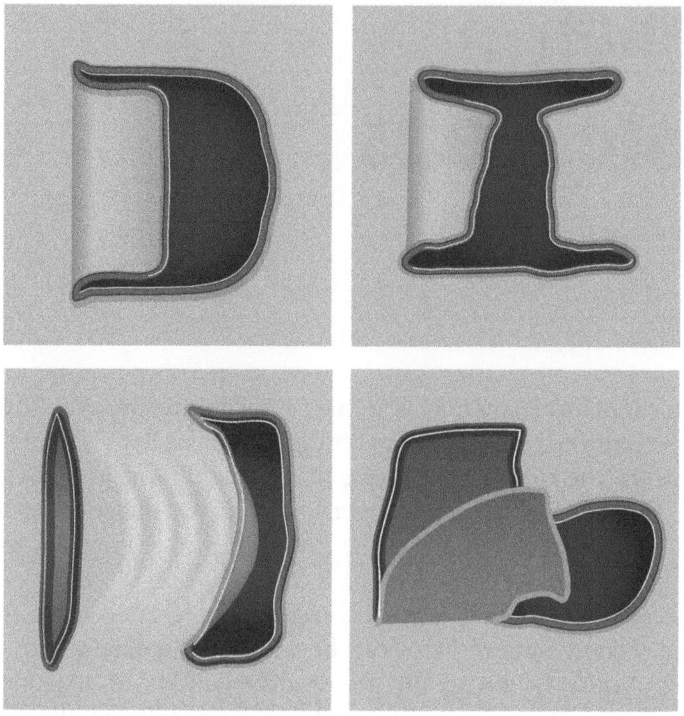

Figure 3-1 Common random pedicle flaps (top left to bottom right) include unilateral single pedicle advancement, bilateral single pedicle advancement, bipedicle advancement, and transposition flaps.

coverage available. Animals should be positioned so that extra skin is pulled up near the surgery site (see fig. 7-1).

Surgery

Because blood supply varies, a specific ratio of flap length to width cannot be determined. In general, flaps should be as short as possible to cover the wound without tension and have a base that is slightly wider than the remaining flap width. Flaps that are too wide, however, lose mobility, so clinical judgment is important for determining flap size. Occasionally a flap with a length at least twice the width will survive if the blood supply is adequate. Flaps must be handled gently to prevent damage to the subdermal plexus.

Surgical technique: unilateral or bilateral single pedicle advancement flap

1. With an index finger, push the skin along the wound margin toward the wound to determine the direction of flap advancement (fig. 3-2). The flap should come from the area that has the loosest skin and should be developed perpendicular to the lines of tension along the wound. If the wound is very large or tension is high, use bilateral flaps.
2. If desired, use a sterile marking pen to outline the proposed flap.
3. Make two skin incisions, perpendicular to the long axis of the wound, starting at each end of the recipient bed (fig. 3-3). Skin incisions should diverge slightly so that the flap base will be wider than the tip. For a U-shaped advancement flap, the skin incisions will extend from one side of the wound bed. For an H- or I-shaped (bilateral) advancement flap, the skin incisions will extend from both sides of the wound bed (see fig. 3-1).

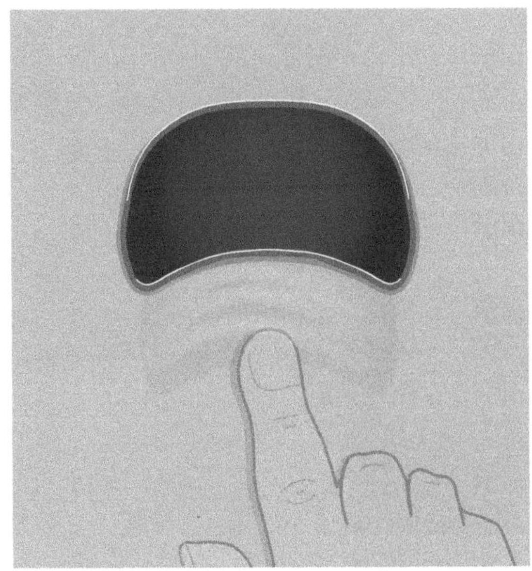

Figure 3-2 Push the skin along the wound margin to find the skin with the greatest mobility.

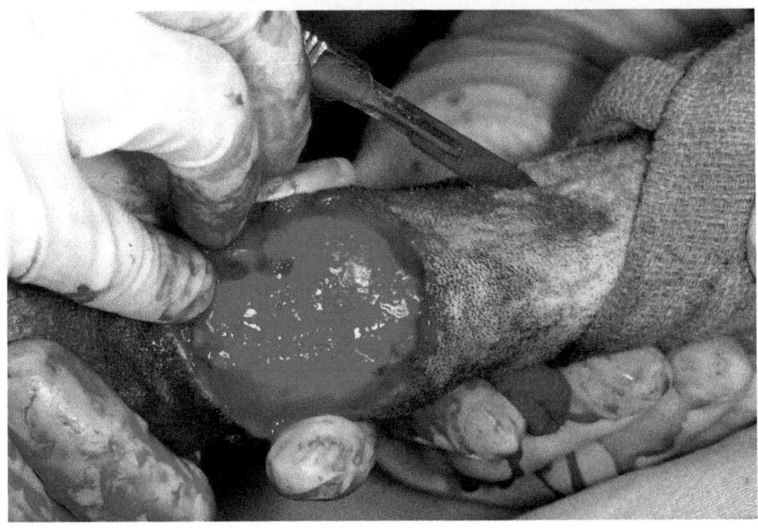

Figure 3-3 Incise the skin along the sides of the proposed flap.

4. Incise through the subcutaneous fat below the skin incisions.
5. Ligate or carefully cauterize any bleeding vessels along the cut edges of the flap or in the wound bed.
6. Starting at the wound margin, undermine the flap carefully toward its base (fig. 3-4), staying below any panniculus muscle. Leave any direct cutaneous vessels to the flap intact. Handle the flap gently; place stay sutures at the corners if needed to provide retraction.
7. Undermine the skin margins around the recipient bed, staying below the subcutaneous fat and any superficial muscle (e.g., cutaneous trunci, platysma).
8. With stay sutures or skin hooks, pull the corners of the flap to the opposite wound edge to check flap position. If tension on the flap is too great, undermine more of the skin around the wound. If necessary, make the flap longer or make a second flap.

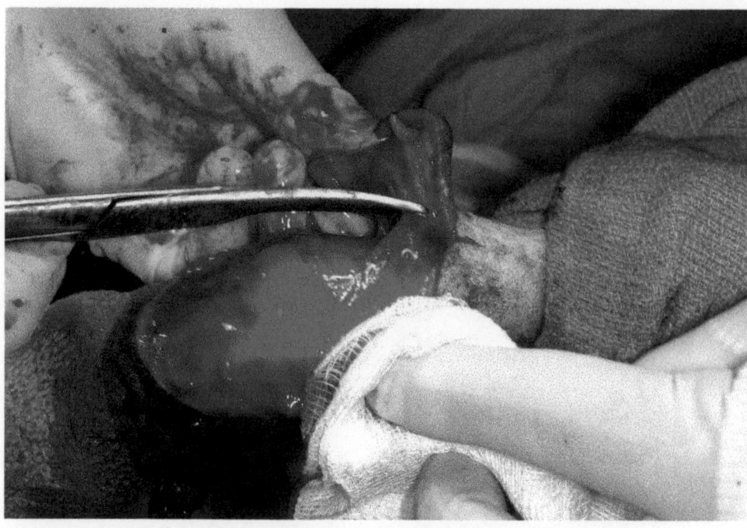

Figure 3-4 Elevate the subcutaneous tissues of the flap below the level of any panniculus muscle and preserving any direct cutaneous vessels.

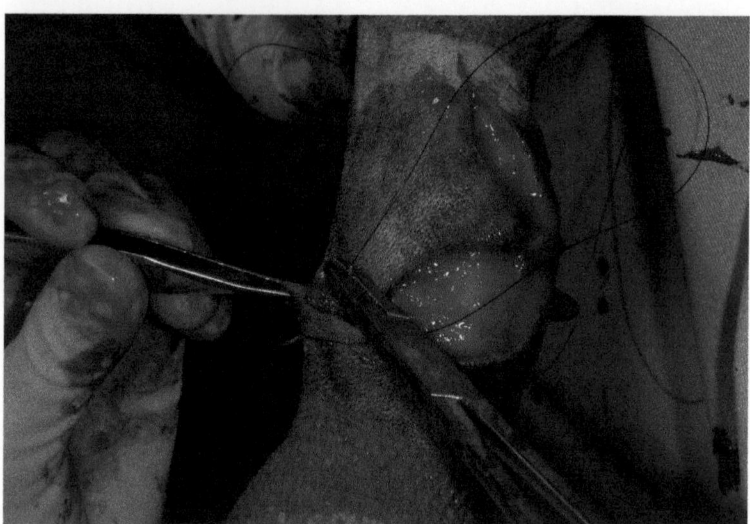

Figure 3-5 Suture the corners in place.

9. If extensive dead space is present, place a continuous suction drain under the flap, exiting out of the skin away from the flap.
10. Place two or three interrupted skin sutures to hold the flap in its final position (fig. 3-5).
11. Appose the subcutaneous tissue with simple interrupted, inverted (buried), or simple continuous sutures of rapidly absorbable monofilament.
12. Close the skin with simple interrupted or cruciate sutures of nylon or with staples (fig. 3-6). Leave small dog ears near the base of the flap in place. If dog ears are large, they can be removed parallel or at an angle to the flap.

Surgical technique: releasing incision with bipedicle flap

1. Make a slightly curved releasing incision parallel to the near skin edge of the wound, leaving the resultant flap attached at both ends ("bipedicle") and slightly narrower at the center than the bases. The length of the flap should be no more than 4 times its width.

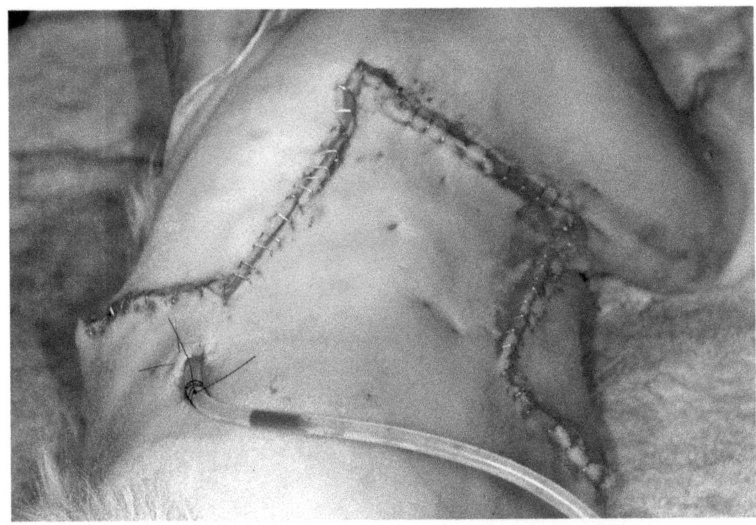

Figure 3-6 Single pedicle advancement flap. Dog ears that formed at each side of the base were removed at right angles to the flap. A continuous suction drain was placed under the flap to decrease seroma formation.

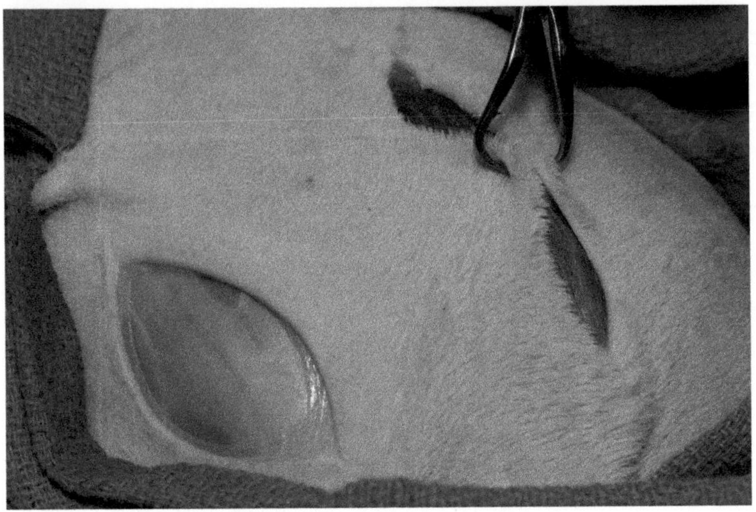

Figure 3-7 Releasing incision with bipedicle flap. Hold the skin over the wound together with a towel clamp to facilitate suture placement at that site.

2. Undermine the skin flap and the skin around the recipient site, staying below any panniculus muscle.
3. Slide the flap over the recipient bed (fig. 3-7) and hold it in place with a suture or towel clamp.
4. If tension forms at the corners near the base of the flap, make the flap longer or make a second flap along the opposite side of the wound.
5. Appose the flap to the surrounding skin as described for a single pedicle advancement flap.
6. Close the donor site primarily in a linear fashion or T-shape, or allow it to heal by second intention. If primary closure is performed, elevate the skin around the donor site to improve skin mobility.

Surgical technique: transposition flap

1. With a sterile marker, draw the flap.
    a. Lift and release the skin to determine skin laxity. The flap is usually developed on the side of the wound with the least skin tension.

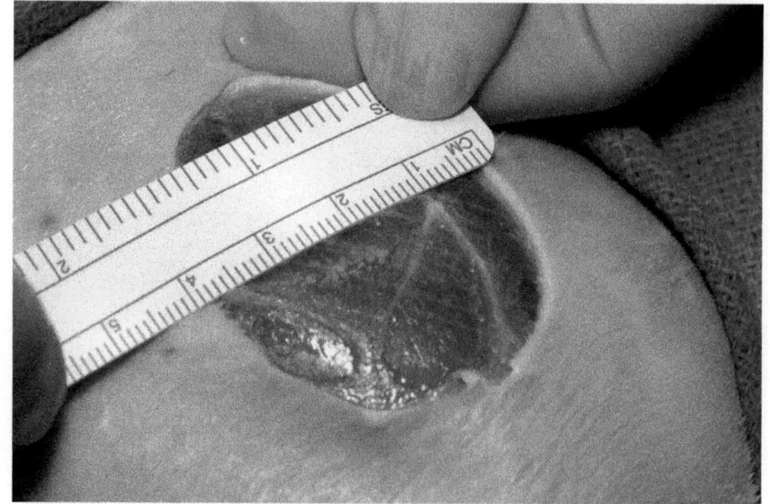

Figure 3-8 Before developing a transposition flap, measure wound width to determine flap width.

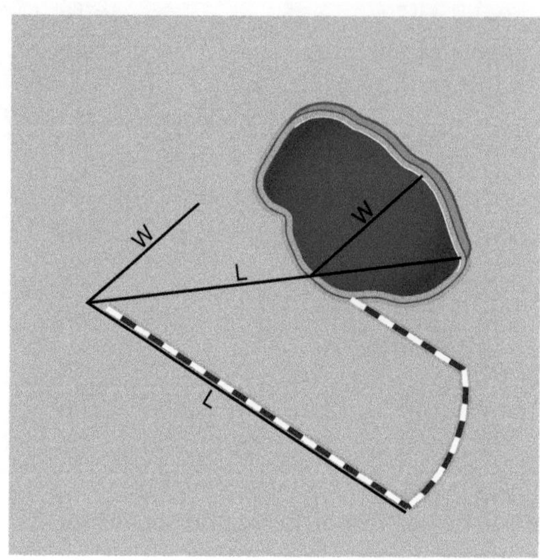

Figure 3-9 Measure the distance from the pivot point to the farthest point on the wound to determine flap length (L). Incise the flap so that the width of the narrowest part of the flap equals the width of the wound (W).

b. Measure the width of the wound, which is equivalent to flap width (fig. 3-8).

c. Mark the flap width along the proposed baseline, on the side of the wound that has the loosest skin. This will determine the pivot point on which the flap rotates.

d. Measure from the pivot point to the farthest point on the wound (fig. 3-9). This will be the flap length.

e. Draw two parallel lines, perpendicular to the proposed flap base, to outline the flap width and length. One line will start along the wound margin (fig. 3-9). Connect them with a third line.

2. Incise through the skin and subcutaneous tissues at the marked line.
3. Gently elevate the skin and subcutaneous tissues of the flap with Metzenbaum scissors, staying below any panniculus muscle.
4. Rotate the flap (up to 90 degrees) along its pivot point to cover the wound (fig. 3-10).

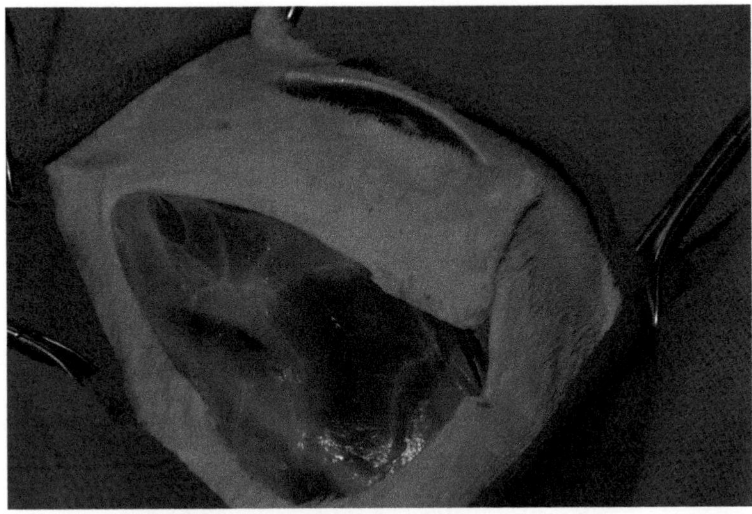

Figure 3-10 Rotate the flap to cover the wound.

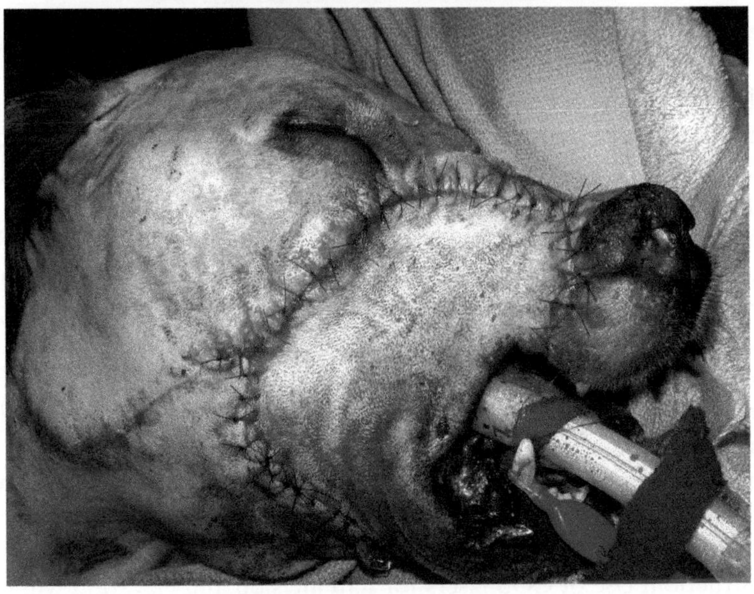

Figure 3-11 Transposition flap. This dog underwent partial maxillectomy and lip resection to remove a fibrosarcoma. A full thickness flap, based rostrally, was developed from the cheek and lower lip and rotated to fill in a defect in the upper lip.

5. Undermine the skin around the recipient bed.
6. Place interrupted sutures between the corners of the distal flap end and the wound margin to check skin position.
7. Fill in the gaps with interrupted subcutaneous sutures, inverting (burying) the sutures if the skin is thin, before completing the skin closure (fig. 3-11).
8. Place a continuous suction drain if dead space is present.
9. Elevate skin and subcutaneous tissues around the donor site and close the wound. Closure of the donor site is often in an L- or T-shape, although use of a single pedicle advancement flap occasionally is required.

Postoperative considerations

Elizabethan collars are recommended for 7 to 10 days after surgery. Non-compressive bandages are particularly important to protect flaps over bony prominences or in areas of high motion. If a bandage is placed, it should be

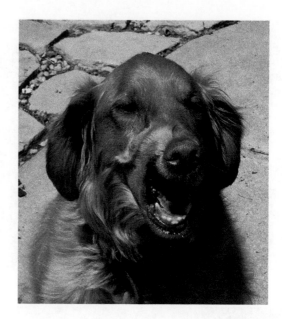

Figure 3-12 Appearance 1 year after transposition. The dog had an unusual hair pattern and lip conformation on the operated side.

thickly padded to prevent compression and subsequent ischemia of the flap. Splints may be necessary in areas of excessive mobility. Bandages should be changed at least 1, 3, and 6 days after surgery to check the health of the flap. Flap necrosis may not be evident for up to 6 days after surgery.

In general, mean skin flap survival rate for random pedicle flaps is 83% to 89%. Flap necrosis is more likely when flaps are excessively long or narrow, experience tension or excessive motion, or are traumatized during tissue elevation, surgical manipulation, or after surgery. Necrotic portions of the flap should be resected and the remaining wound allowed to heal by second intention or managed by delayed primary closure with additional flaps or grafts.

Other complications include dehiscence, infection, hematoma formation, and distortion of local tissues. Complication rates are higher in patients that receive radiation therapy, particularly when it is administered prior to wound reconstruction. Use of CO2 lasers for flap incision and elevation will prolong healing and reduce wound tensile strength. Final appearance of the patient may be altered because of differences in hair growth (fig. 3-12).

Bibliography

DeCarvalho Vasconcellos CH et al: Clinical evaluation of random skin flaps based on the subdermal plexus secured with sutures or sutures and cyanoacrylate adhesive for reconstructive surgery in dogs. Vet Surg 2005;34:59–63.

Degner DA: Facial reconstructive surgery. Clin Tech Small Anim Pract 2007;22:82–88.

Hedlund CS: Large trunk wounds. Vet Clin N Am Small Anim Pract 2006;36: 847–872.

Hunt GB et al: Skin-fold advancement flaps for closing large proximal limb and trunk defects in dogs and cats. Vet Surg 2001;30:440–448.

Mison MB et al: Comparison of the effects of the CO2 surgical laser and conventional surgical techniques on healing and wound tensile strength of skin flaps in the dog. Vet Surg 2003;32:153–160.

Pope ER: Head and facial wounds in dogs and cats. Vet Clin N Am Small Anim Pract 2006;36:793–817.

Schmidt K. et al: Reconstruction of the lower eyelid by third eyelid lateral advancement and local transposition cutaneous flap after "en bloc" resection of squamous cell carcinoma in 5 cats. Vet Surg 2005;34:78–82.
Seguin B. et al: Tolerance of cutaneous or mucosal flaps placed into a radiation therapy field in dogs. Vet Surg 2005;34:214–222.

Chapter 4
Tension-Relieving Techniques

Skin necrosis and dehiscence may occur when wounds are apposed primarily under excessive tension. Tension can be relieved by relaxing and lengthening the skin surrounding these sites with a variety of means, including Z-plasty, meshing, tensioning sutures, and devices such as tie-over bandages (discussed in Chapter 8).

A Z-plasty transposes two interdigitating flaps of skin to increase skin length along lines of tension while shortening it perpendicularly. Z-plasty is especially useful for small to medium-sized skin wounds on the lower legs and large wounds on the trunk. It can also be used for lengthening and relaxing scars, contractures, and circular stenosis or strictures (e.g., anal strictures). The amount of skin lengthening depends on the size of the Z incision, the angles of the limbs on the Z, and the amount of local skin elasticity. When the limbs of the incised Z are the same length and at 60-degree angles, the skin will lengthen 40% to 60% along the lines of tension. Wider angles will produce more tension. Angles less than 45 degrees produce narrow flaps with an insufficient blood supply. Longer limbs will produce greater skin relaxation; however, blood supply to the flaps could be affected.

For lower-extremity wounds, skin tension can also be relieved with single or multiple relaxing or releasing incisions. Relaxing incisions will gape open, allowing the skin to shift and stretch so that the original wound can be closed primarily. Skin defects produced by relaxing incisions can be closed primarily or allowed to heal by contraction and re-epithelialization. A single relaxing incision, which produces a bipedicle flap, provides significant tension relief (see p. 28). Compared to multiple relaxing incisions, it is less likely to damage direct cutaneous vessels and is therefore preferred for large wounds.

Use of multiple relaxing incisions, or mesh expansion, is similar to a free mesh graft except that some of the local blood supply is maintained along the skin attachment. Skin should be meshed only in sites where the underlying tissue is healthy and has sufficient blood supply to provide nutrition and vascular ingrowth to the overlying skin. After healing, multiple relaxing incision sites have an acceptable cosmetic appearance as long as the original defect was no more than one-fourth of the limb circumference.

Tensioning sutures rely on mechanical creep and stress relaxation of local skin to gradually stretch and mobilize the skin surrounding wound edges.

Manual of Small Animal Soft Tissue Surgery, Second Edition. Karen Tobias.
© 2017 John Wiley & Sons, Inc. Published 2017 by John Wiley & Sons, Inc.

Tensioning sutures are often performed in concert with open wound management (see Chapter 8) and are usually placed at least 2 to 3 days before wound closure. Once in place, the sutures are gently tightened 1 to 3 times a day and in many cases produce enough relaxation for primary wound closure. Once the wound edges can be apposed without tension, the tensioning sutures are removed and the wound closed routinely in 2 or 3 layers.

Preoperative management

Animals should be clipped and prepped widely for any large mass excision or when incisional tension is expected. The surgery site should first be evaluated to determine whether other tension-relieving techniques, such as advancement or rotational flaps, can be used. If a Z-plasty or relaxing incision technique is performed, the skin adjacent to the original incision should be healthy and have adequate blood supply.

Surgery

To determine whether a Z-plasty is feasible, the skin surrounding the tight incision should be grabbed parallel to the closure (perpendicular to the lines of tension) to see if there is any give in that direction. If the skin cannot be stretched or relaxed parallel to the incision, a Z-plasty will not work because tension release relies on "borrowing" laxity perpendicular to the lines of tension. Meshing, grafting, short-term open wound management with tie-on bandages, or other techniques should then be considered.

When performing a Z-plasty, the original wound can be closed before or after the Z is made. If relaxing incisions are used, skin tension is tested as the relaxing incisions are made. The skin along each segment of the original wound is closed as the tension is relieved. The initial prep for tensioning sutures should be wide enough to prevent wound contamination and permit effective bandage placement. The skin and subcutis (and panniculus muscle, when present) must be freely moveable from underlying tissues for relaxing incisions and tensioning sutures to be effective.

Surgical technique: Z-plasty

1. Verify that there is sufficient skin laxity perpendicular to the lines of tension to allow flap rotation before starting a Z-plasty (see note above).
2. With a sterile marking pen and ruler, draw the central limb of the Z parallel to the lines of tension (perpendicular to the wound closure), starting 1 to 3 cm away from the wound, depending on location and size of the Z.
3. Draw the top and bottom limbs of the Z at 60 degrees from the central limb. The corners of the Z can be slightly curved to round the flap tips and improve blood supply.
4. Make full-thickness skin incisions at the drawn lines (fig. 4-1).
5. Undermine the triangular flaps of the Z and the surrounding skin. Handle the tips of the flaps carefully with stay sutures or skin hooks

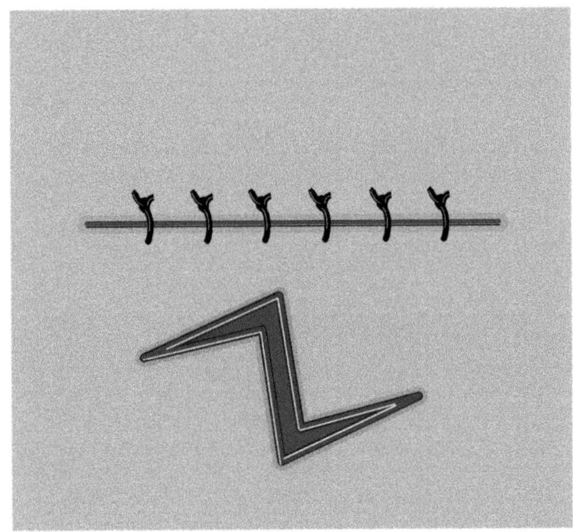

Figure 4-1 Z-plasty. Incise the central limb perpendicular to the wound and parallel to the lines of tension, and make the two arms at 60° from the central limb.

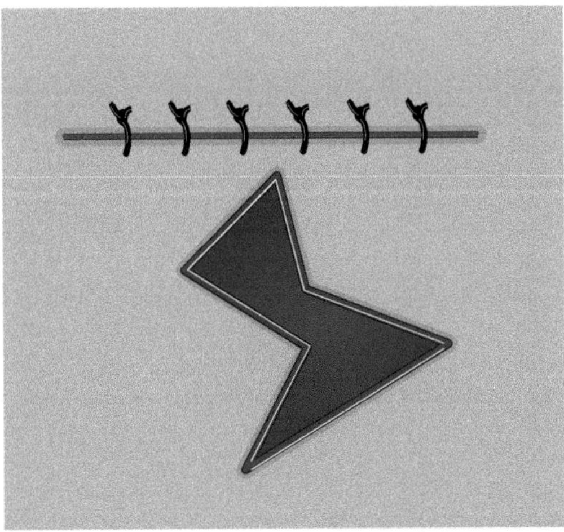

Figure 4-2 Undermine the flaps and transpose them.

to prevent damage. The Z incision will lengthen, the incisional gap widen, and the triangular flaps start to transpose automatically as the flaps are elevated.

6. Transpose the triangular flaps of the Z (fig. 4-2). This will change the direction of the central limb 90 degrees so that it is now parallel to the original wound.
7. Appose the tip of each transposed flap to its new location with an interrupted mattress or purse-string suture in the subcutaneous tissues. If there is insufficient subcutis, secure the flap tips in their new locations with simple interrupted skin sutures. If the tips are under excessive tension, undermine more of the local tissues or lengthen the limbs of the Z.
8. If dead space is expected, place a subcutaneous continuous suction drain before Z-closure (fig. 4-4) and exit it through healthy skin away from the surgery site.
9. Close the subcutaneous tissues, if present, with buried interrupted sutures of 3-0 or 4-0 rapidly absorbable monofilament suture material.
10. Close the skin in an interrupted pattern (figs. 4-3 and 4-4).
11. Multiple Z-plasties can be performed for reconstruction of strictures or contractures (figs. 4-5 and 4-6).

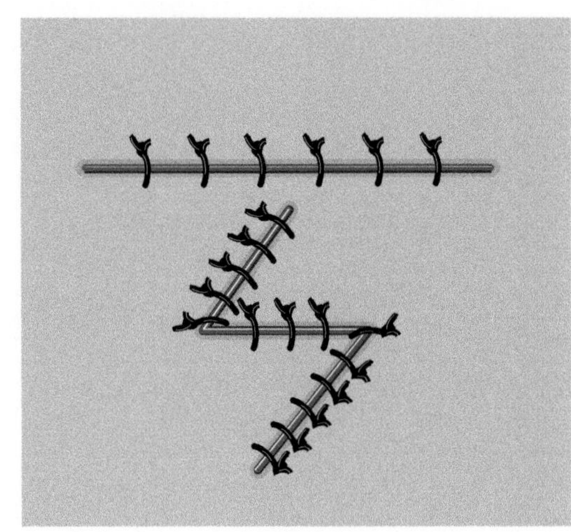

Figure 4-3 Suture the flaps into their new positions. The central limb of the new Z will be parallel to the wound margin and perpendicular to the lines of tension.

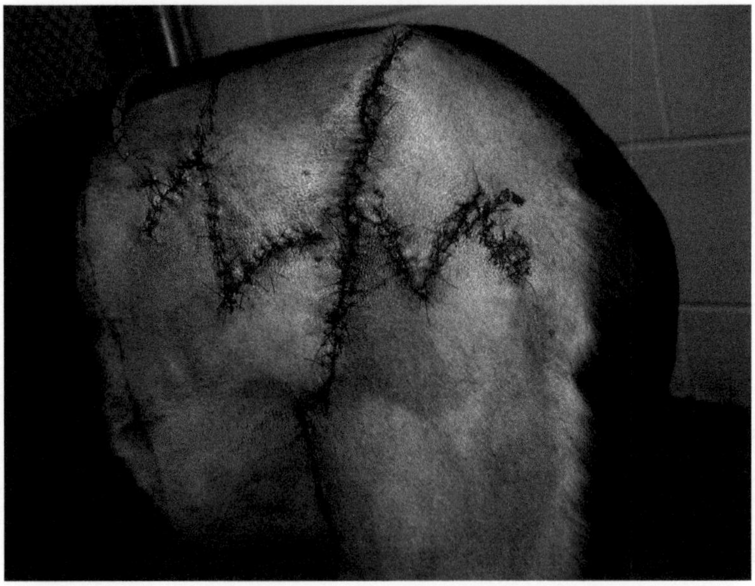

Figure 4-4 Final appearance 1 day after resection of a large soft tissue sarcoma of the lateral flank and bilateral Z plasties to reduce tension. A continuous suction drain was placed during surgery to reduce seroma formation and tension on the closure.

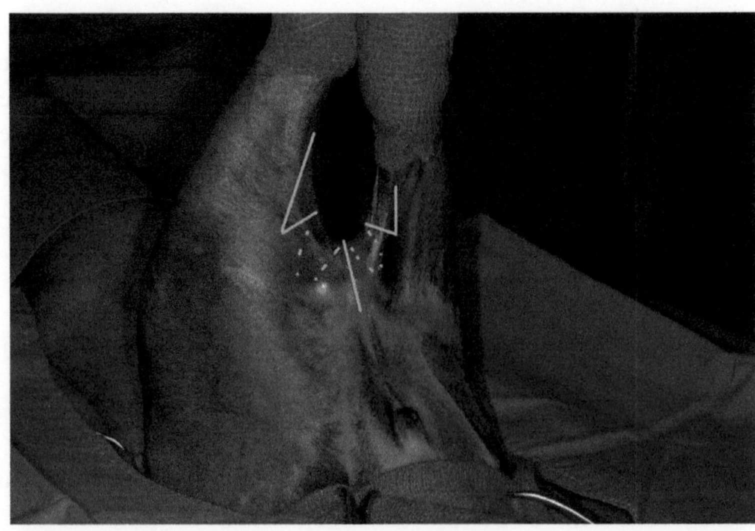

Figure 4-5 Inguinal skin contracture after massive wound closure in a cat. The central limbs of the proposed Z-plasties (green lines) will be perpendicular to the lines of tension and thus will transect the scars along the medial surface of the pelvic limbs.

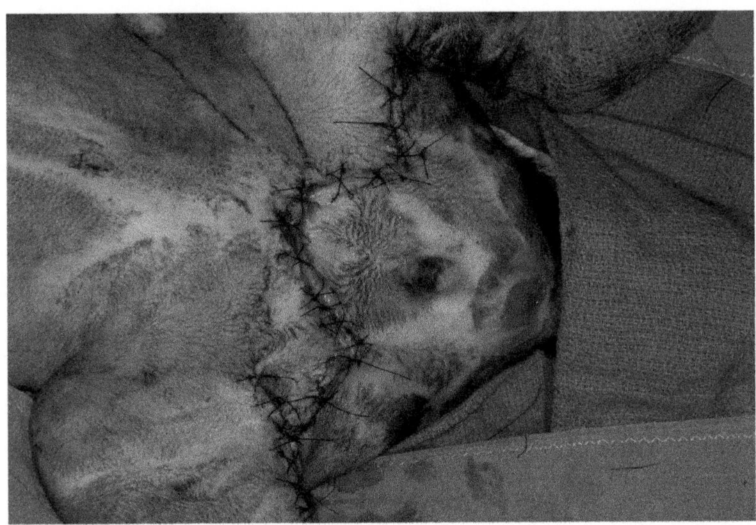

Figure 4-6 Final appearance of cat in fig. 4-5.

Surgical technique: multiple relaxing incisions

1. Undermine the skin around the primary wound.
2. If direct appositional closure is not possible or produces too much tension, make several 1- to 2-cm-long incisions parallel to and approximately 1 to 2 cm away from the edges of the original wound (depending on wound location). Ends of incisions should be at least 1 cm apart.
3. With skin hooks, towel clamp, or a preplaced intradermal tension suture (an adjustable suture left untied at one or both ends), appose the edges of the original wound (fig. 4-7). If the wound edges will not appose or are under tension, make a second, staggered row of relief incisions 2 cm abaxial (lateral) to the first row wherever the skin is under tension (fig. 4-8).
4. If an intradermal suture was used for apposition, tie each end off but leave the knot and suture ends visible for later suture removal. If no intradermal pattern was used, appose the skin edges of the primary wound with a simple interrupted cutaneous pattern.

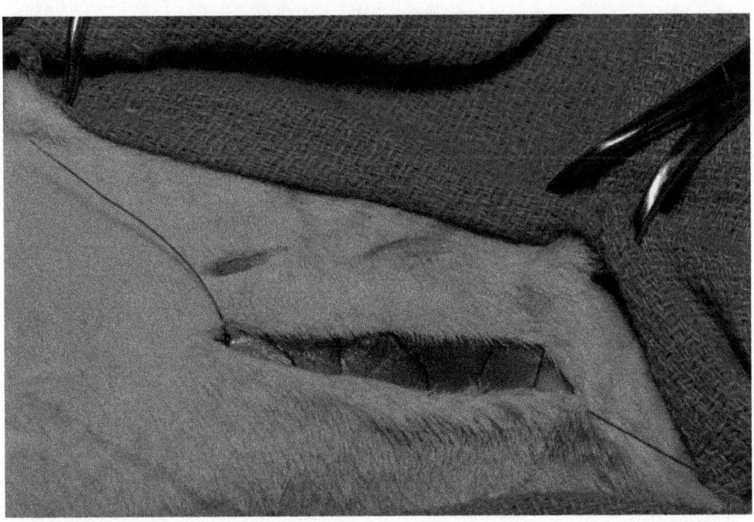

Figure 4-7 Undermine the skin surrounding the wound and make several 1- to 2-cm-long incisions parallel to and 1 to 2 cm away from the wound margin. Preplace an intradermal suture and tighten; add more relaxing incisions if needed to appose skin margins.

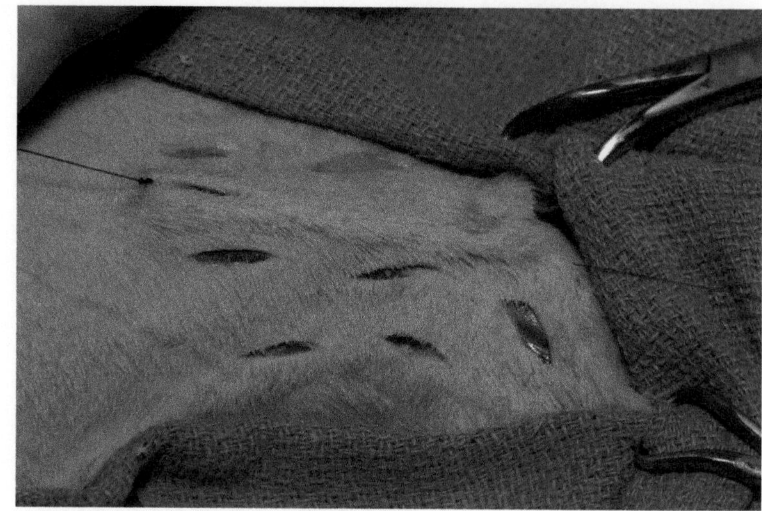

Figure 4-8 Tighten the intradermal suture completely. The relaxing incisions should gape open to relieve tension along the primary wound margin.

Surgical technique: tensioning suture

1. Elevate the skin (including subcutis and, when present, panniculus muscle) from any attachments to the wound bed and undermine it abaxial to the wound bed.
2. With 0 polypropylene or nylon on a cutting needle, take a full thickness bite of skin across (perpendicular to) the end of the wound and tie two knots.
3. Taking wide (≥1 cm), full thickness bites, place a loose simple continuous pattern in the skin (fig. 4-9). Place bites ≥1 cm apart.
4. If the wound is too large to span with a continuous pattern from a single suture, end the first pattern near the center of the wound's length and secure it with a hemostat (see fig. 4-9). Start a second simple continuous pattern from the opposite end of the wound and work toward the center [note: you start the bites of the second pattern from the side of the wound

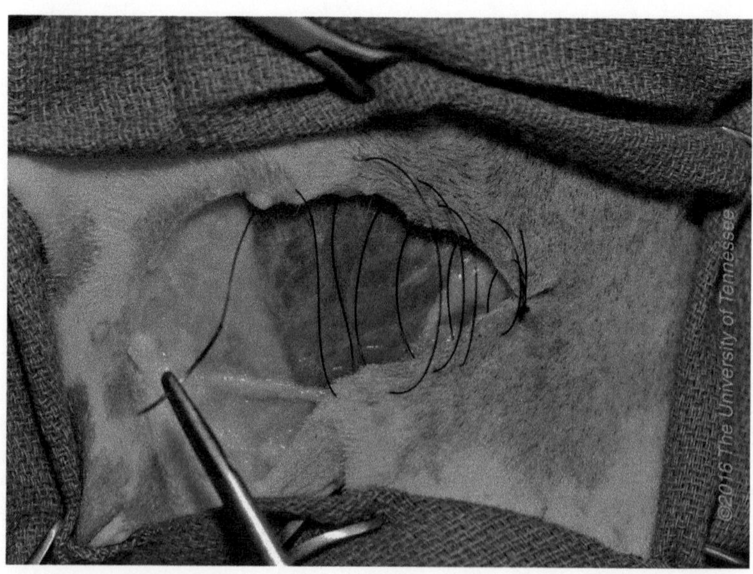

Figure 4-9 Start a simple continuous pattern of monofilament nonabsorbable suture from one end of the wound. Take bites at least 1 cm wide and 1 cm apart, and leave the pattern loose.

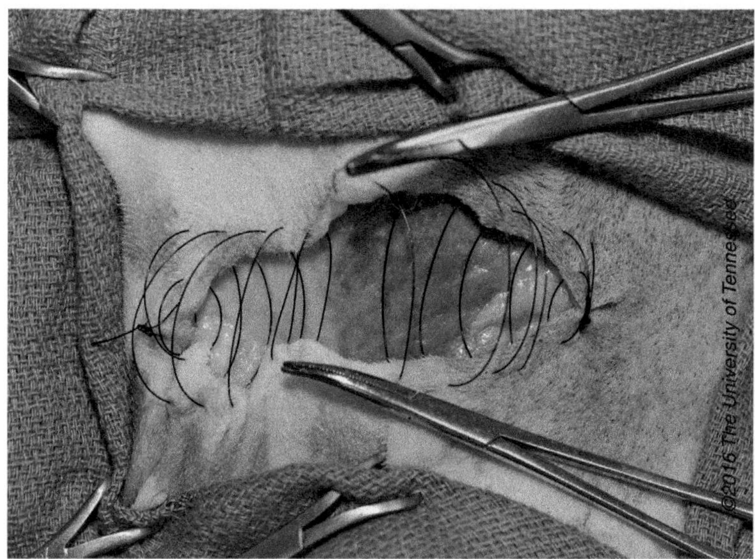

Figure 4-10 For large wounds, start a second continuous pattern from the opposite end of the wound, ending in the center of the wound. Secure the suture ends with hemostats or by knotting them together. © 2016 The University of Tennessee.

opposite to that of the first pattern]. Secure the two free ends with hemostats (fig. 4-10) or by knotting them together.

5. If the wound is small enough to span with a continuous pattern from a single suture, tie the pattern off at the far end (fig. 4-11).
6. Insert the appropriate dressing in the wound bed, making sure it is tucked under all the sutures crossing the bed (fig 4-12). This prevents the sutures from cutting into the wound bed. To facilitate dressing placement, slide a scalpel handle under all crossing sutures, then insert the dressing below the scalpel handle.
7. Gently "load" the tensioning pattern by lifting up on the central suture(s) and gradually tightening from each end to take up slack, and secure the central suture loop or ends with a split-shot fishing sinker or other device (fig. 4-13). Final tension should be mild so that sutures are not cutting into

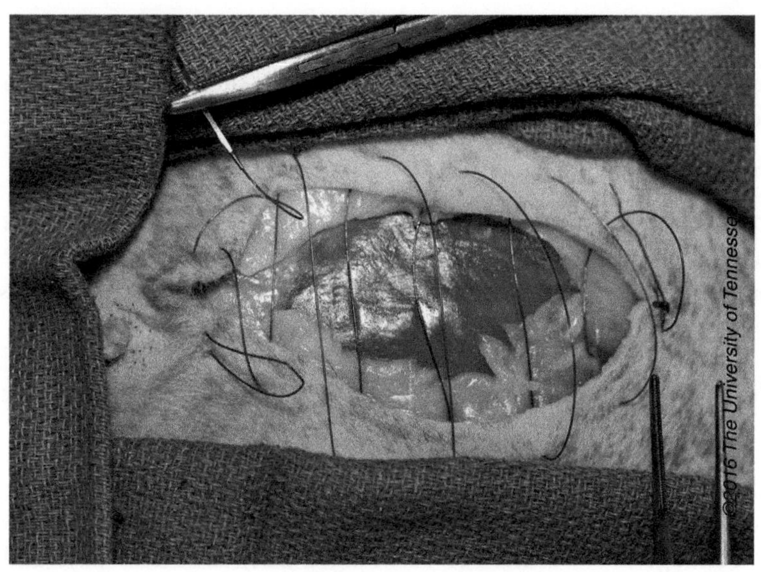

Figure 4-11 For small wounds, continue the initial pattern to the opposite end of the wound and tie it off, leaving the pattern loose centrally. In this figure, a backhand bite was taken at the end of the wound to make a narrower loop for knot tying. © 2016 The University of Tennessee.

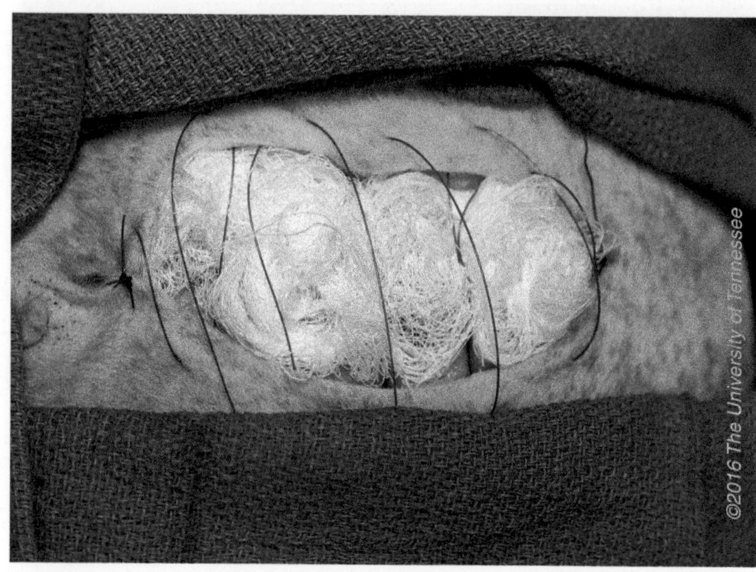

Figure 4-12 Tuck the dressing under all the crossing sutures so that it is held in the wound pocket against the wound bed. © 2016 The University of Tennessee.

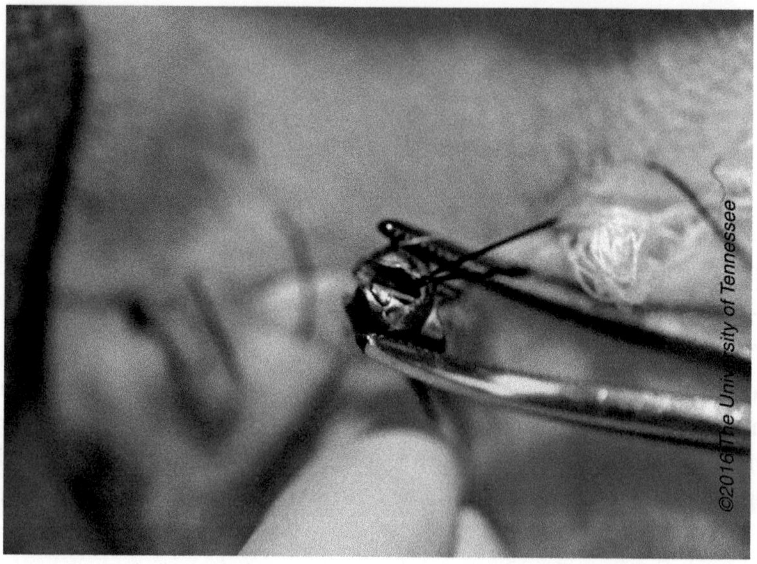

Figure 4-13 Gently tighten the pattern from the ends toward the center to provide mild tension, and secure the central sutures together with a split-shot fishing sinker. © 2016 The University of Tennessee.

the skin (fig. 4-14). If possible, place the split shot so it is resting on the dressing rather than the skin.

8. Cover the site with a bandage.
9. Change the dressing and tension at least once a day: remove the split-shot sinker and relax the sutures. Remove and replace the dressing as described above, then gradually tighten the tensioning suture to further appose the skin, and place a bandage.

Postoperative considerations

Elizabethan collars are recommended to prevent self-trauma. Care and healing for multiple relaxing incisions are similar to that for mesh grafting (see p. 50). Meshed areas should be covered with a nonadherent dressing and absorptive padded bandage that will need to be changed daily for 5 to 7 days and then

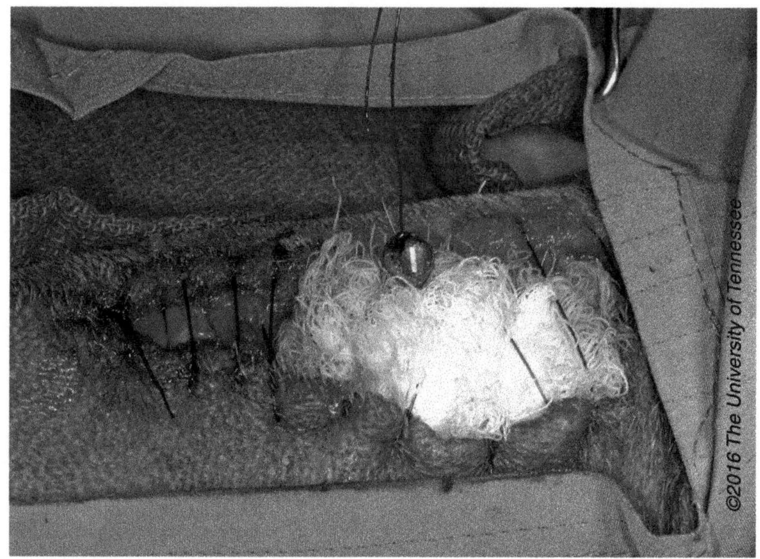

Figure 4-14 In this patient, the sinker is resting on the gauze to prevent pressure necrosis of the skin; however, the right half of the pattern has been pulled too tightly, resulting in excessive skin compression. The sinker should be removed and the pattern loosened to prevent tissue damage. © 2016 The University of Tennessee.

every 2 to 3 days until the site is healed. Noncompressive bandages are placed at Z-plasty sites to cover any drain exit wounds or reduce mobility. A variety of dressings can be used within wound beds under a tensioning suture (see p. 74); usually the site is covered with an absorptive secondary layer and a protective tertiary layer.

Complications of tension-relieving techniques are skin necrosis, dehiscence, and infection. Dehiscence of Z-plasty most commonly occurs when surrounding skin has limited laxity or the Z limb lengths or angle sizes are too large. Necrosis may occur if Z angles are too narrow. Meshed skin may necrose if meshing is extensive and underlying tissues lack sufficient vascularity to provide nutrition and vessel ingrowth. Tensioning sutures will damage the skin if pulled too tightly, either by cutting into it or by compressing vessels and lymphatics and thus interfering with blood and lymphatic flow. The amount the tensioning sutures can be "loaded" depends on many variables, including species of the patient, wound location, and skin health; to prevent damage to local skin, it is best to be conservative when applying tension and to consider applying smaller loads more frequently.

Bibliography

Bosworth C and Tobias KM: Skin reconstruction techniques: Z-plasty as an aid to tension-free wound closure. Vet Med 2004;99:892–897.

Fowler D: Distal limb and paw injuries. Vet Clin Small Anim 2006;36:819–845.

Song AH and Tobias KM: Tensioning sutures for open wounds. Clinician's Brief 2017;15:33–38.

Vig MM: Management of experimental wounds of the extremities in dogs with Z-plasty. J Am Anim Hosp Assoc 1992;28:553–559.

Vig MM: Management of integumentary wounds of extremities in dogs: an experimental study. J Am Anim Hosp Assoc 1985;21:187–192.

Chapter 5
Full-Thickness Mesh Grafts

Skin grafting may be necessary when wounds cannot be closed with direct apposition or covered with local or regional flaps. Solid sheets of free skin can be placed over wounds; however, fluid collection under the graft inhibits "graft take" (revascularization). A mesh graft is a full- or partial-thickness sheet of skin that has been fenestrated to allow drainage and expansion. Mesh grafts are useful in many locations on the body because of their ability to conform to uneven surfaces. Full-thickness mesh grafts are preferred to partial-thickness grafts because, once healed, the grafted skin is relatively resistant to trauma and provides a reasonably cosmetic appearance.

Survival and "take" of a mesh graft depends on early vascularization from the underlying tissues. Mesh grafts should therefore be placed on vascular, noninfected beds. If wounds are infected, contaminated, or have a poor blood supply, mesh grafting is delayed for 5 to 10 days until a healthy granulation bed is present. Mesh grafts can also be placed on fresh surgical wounds (e.g., a tumor resection site) over healthy muscle or an omental flap that has been extended from the abdominal cavity into a wound.

For at least 48 hours, mesh grafts will appear cyanotic while the transplanted tissue relies on "plasmatic imbibition" (fluid absorption from the wound bed) for nourishment. Blood circulation and lymphatic drainage are usually present by the fifth day after surgery as long as the graft has appropriately adhered to an underlying vascular bed. The open wounds left in the mesh graft heal by contraction and re-epithelialization in 1 to 2 weeks.

Preoperative management

In animals with chronic or infected wounds, grafting should be delayed until infection is resolved and blood supply is improved. In these animals, punch biopsies of the wound bed should be submitted for culture and sensitivity. If new epithelium is already advancing along the edges of the wound, then the bed is probably ready to be grafted. If the wound bed is pale and thick, tissue samples can also be submitted for histologic evaluation. Wound beds that consist primarily of fibrous tissue and minimal vasculature may need to be excised. An incision is made around the fibrous wound bed adjacent to the skin

Manual of Small Animal Soft Tissue Surgery, Second Edition. Karen Tobias.
© 2017 John Wiley & Sons, Inc. Published 2017 by John Wiley & Sons, Inc.

margins, and its subcutaneous attachments are transected with Metzenbaum scissors. The fresh wound is managed with dressings and bandages until healthy granulation tissue appears.

Animals with chronic wounds or infection may be hypokalemic, hypoproteinemic, anemic, or dehydrated. Fluid and electrolyte imbalances and severe anemia should be corrected before surgery. Hetastarch will provide oncotic support in hypoalbuminemic animals. Cachectic animals may require feeding tubes and nutritional support. Some clinicians will apply an antimicrobial dressing (e.g., gentamicin ointment) over the wound bed for 24–48 hours before grafting to reduce the bacterial load within the granulation tissue.

Before surgery, the wound should be filled with a sterile water-soluble lubricant and the surrounding skin clipped and vacuumed. The lubricant is then flushed out with water to remove any loose hairs from clipping. The wound bed can be scrubbed gently with antiseptic soap and gauze sponges to remove topical contaminants and debride the surface. The donor site is also clipped and prepped.

Surgery

If possible, the donor and recipient sites should be on the same side of the animal so that both areas can be reached simultaneously during surgery. Donor skin is usually obtained from the lateral thoracic and abdominal walls. At these locations, the skin is relatively abundant and of reasonable thickness. Hair color, texture, and length can also be matched to the recipient site to improve cosmesis. Meshing will allow expansion of the graft along its width but will concurrently make the graft shorter. Therefore, skin harvested for an expanded mesh graft does not need to be as wide as the wound bed, but it does need to be longer.

The graft can be secured to healthy skin edges with interrupted sutures, a continuous pattern, or a combination of both or by staples. Placement of a petroleum-impregnated mesh, secured to healthy skin with staples, around the graft, will help prevent movement of the graft during subsequent bandage changes. The graft can be evaluated through the mesh and antimicrobial ointment applied to the mesh over open wounds before the bandage is replaced.

Surgical technique: full-thickness mesh graft

1. Measure the wound bed for estimated graft dimensions or make a template of the wound using a sterile glove wrapper or other material (fig. 5-1).
2. With a sterile marker, mark the direction of hair growth at the donor and recipient sites (fig. 5-2).
3. Using the template or measurements, outline the skin graft so that it is about one-third longer than the defect and at least half its width. Make sure to orient the template or dimensions so that the hair growth at the donor and recipient sites will match.
4. With a sterile marker, outline the graft on the donor site. Grasp the site with your fingers and temporarily elevate the surrounding skin to verify that the donor site can be closed easily.

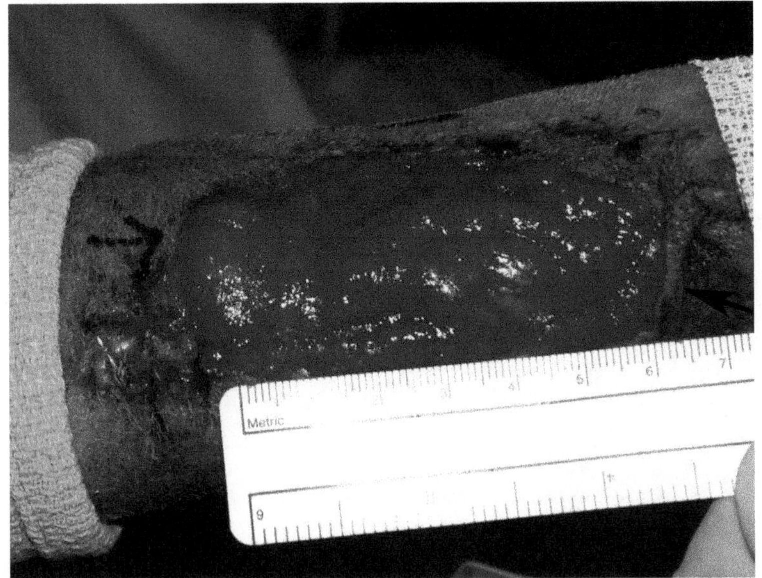

Figure 5-1 Mark the direction of hair growth around the wound and measure the wound bed.

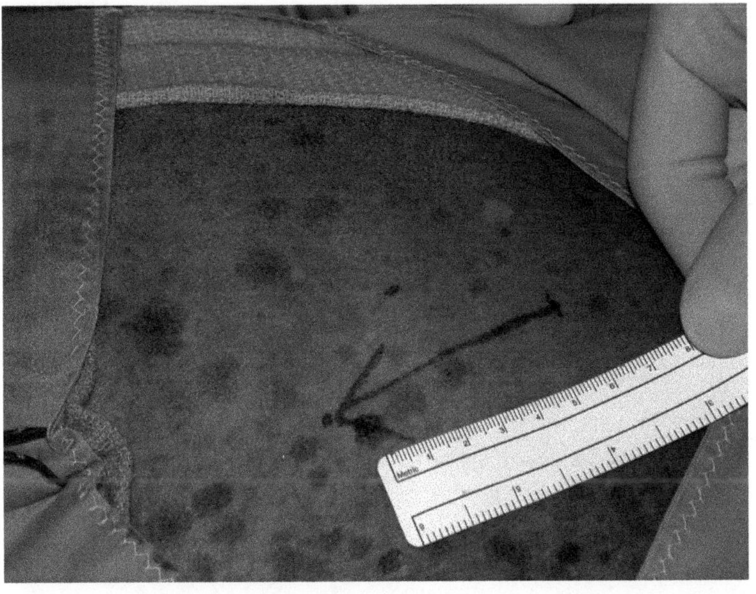

Figure 5-2 Mark the direction of hair growth at the donor site and outline a graft. Grafts that will be expanded should be longer than the recipient bed.

5. Resect any islands of epithelium on the recipient bed that will be covered by the graft.
6. Cover the prepared graft bed with moistened gauze.
7. Harvest the donor skin, and remove the attached subcutaneous tissue during (fig. 5-3) or after donor skin removal (fig. 5-4).
   a. To remove subcutaneous tissues as the graft is being developed:
      i. Incise the full-thickness graft along three edges.
      ii. With Metzenbaum scissors, use blunt and sharp dissection to elevate the skin.
      iii. Drape the skin, subcutaneous side up, over your finger, a folded laparotomy pad, or a gauze sponge.

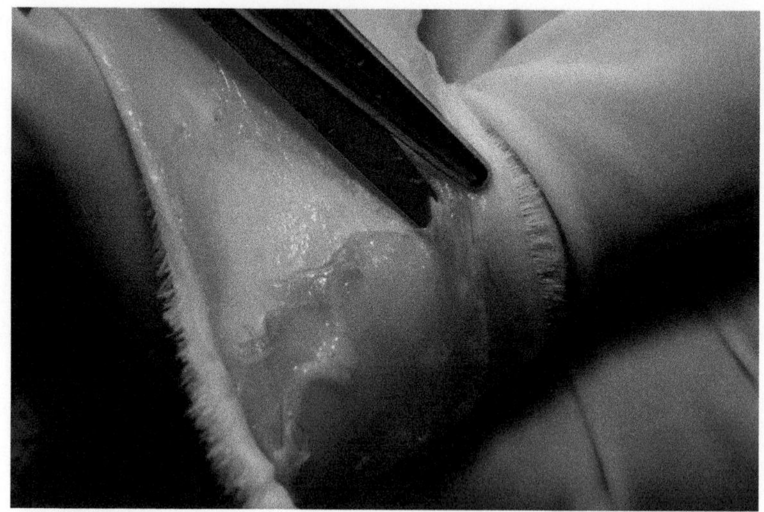

Figure 5-3 Incise the donor skin along three margins, then roll it over your finger or a gauze sponge to expose the subcutis. Remove the subcutaneous fat from the graft with fine-tipped scissors.

iv. While holding the skin under tension, resect the subcutaneous fat and panniculus muscle from the graft (fig. 5-3) using Metzenbaum or tenotomy scissors.

v. Transect the remaining skin attachments.

vi. Rinse the graft and examine it for remaining fragments of fat. The dermal surface of the graft should have a cobblestone appearance.

b. To remove subcutaneous tissues after graft development:

i. Incise the graft along all of the marked borders.

ii. With Metzenbaum scissors, transect any subcutaneous attachments and remove the graft from the donor site.

iii. With the dermal surface facing up, stretch the skin and secure it to a sterile roll of coadhesive wrap with skin staples (fig. 5-4) or to a piece of sterile cardboard with hypodermic needles or suture.

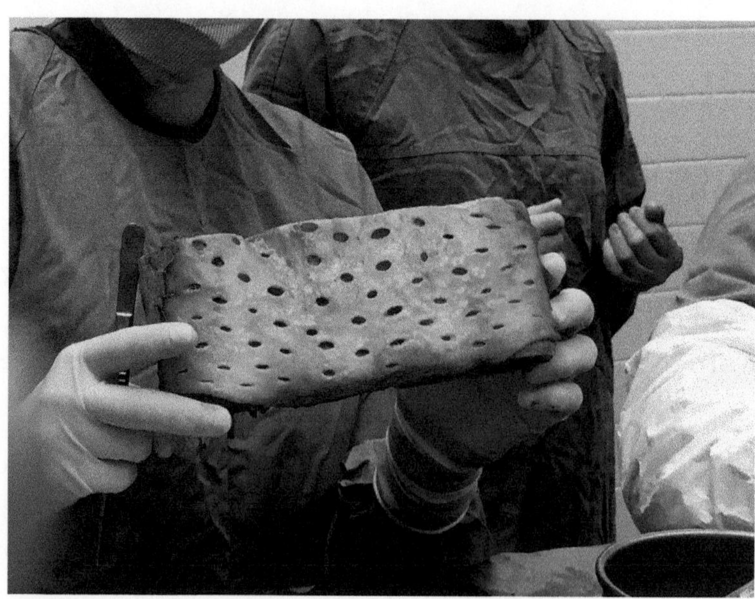

Figure 5-4 This large graft was secured, subcutaneous side up, with skin staples to several rolls of cohesive wrap. The subcutaneous fat was removed with tenotomy scissors, and the skin was meshed while still on the rolls. If further expansion is needed, the mesh openings can be enlarged.

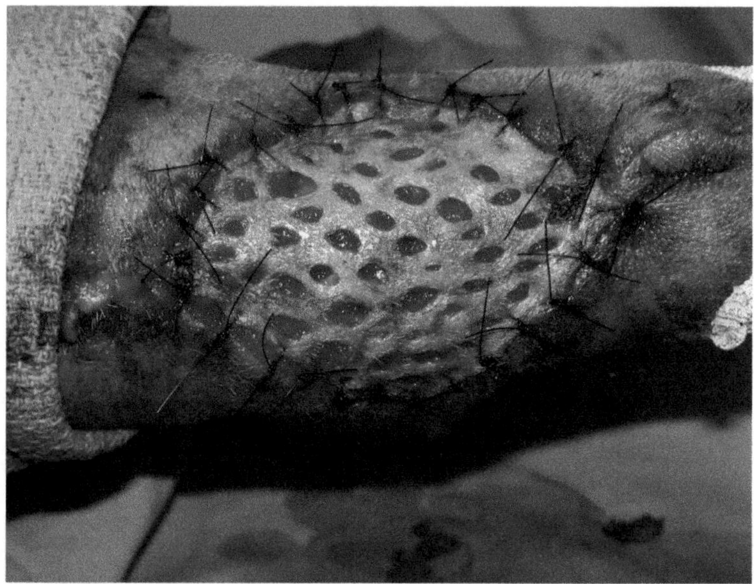

Figure 5-5 Orient the graft so that the hair growth corresponds to that surrounding the recipient bed, and appose the skin margins with sutures or staples.

iv. Remove the subcutaneous fat with tenotomy or Metzenbaum scissors or a no. 15 blade until the dermal surface is white and glistening and has a slightly cobblestone appearance.

8. With a scalpel blade, mesh the graft with multiple, staggered, 0.5- to 2-cm-long incisions, spaced 0.5 to 2 cm apart (fig. 5-4). The amount of meshing depends on the amount of drainage and expansion needed.
9. Lay the graft on the recipient site with the direction of hair growth properly oriented.
10. Secure the graft to the skin along one side of the wound with sutures or staples (fig. 5-5). If the skin edge along the recipient bed is thin, incise along the margin edge and include the granulation tissue and skin margin within the suture bites.
11. Expand the graft so that the mesh openings are at least 3 mm wide to allow drainage.
12. Excise excess donor skin before tacking the remaining sides with staples or suture. Complete the closures with staples or interrupted or continuous suture patterns.
13. Secure the graft to the wound bed by placing tacking sutures at multiple sites, especially at the graft center or any concavity (fig. 5-6).
    a. Pass the needle through one slit, in and out of the wound bed, and then out an adjacent slit.
    b. Tie the suture so that the bed and graft are gently apposed.
14. Close the donor site routinely.
15. Place a nonadherent dressing (e.g., a sponge or pad lightly impregnated with ointment) directly over the graft (fig. 5-7).
16. Cover the site with a conforming, nonconstricting padded bandage to immobilize the area and keep the graft pressed against the wound bed. Add a splint if the area is near a joint.

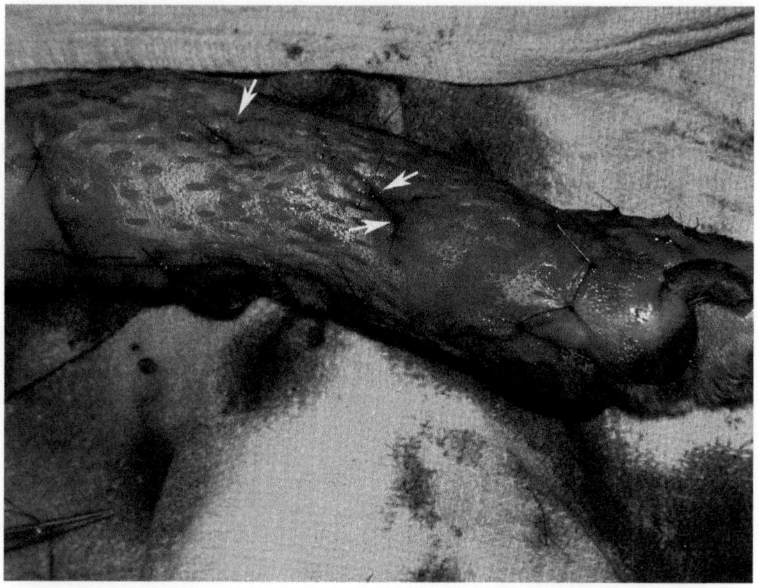

Figure 5-6 Tack the graft to the wound bed by taking suture bites through adjacent slits and tying them over the skin (arrows).

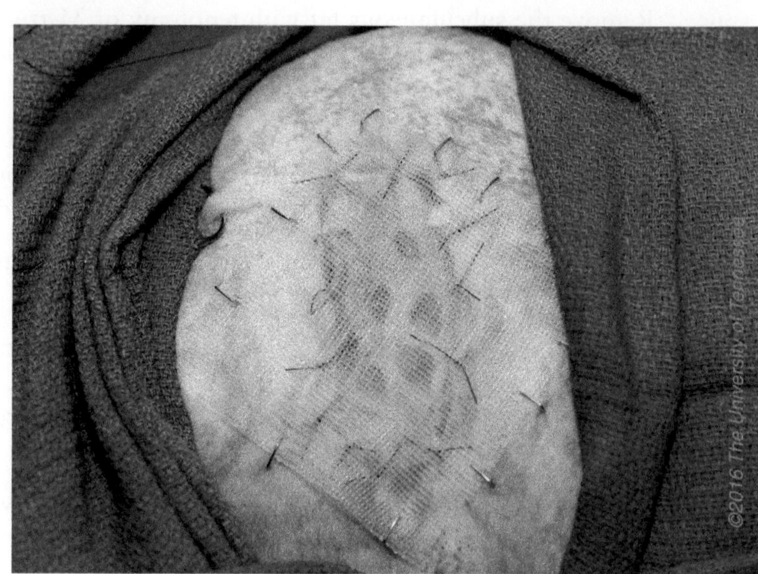

Figure 5-7 Staple a petroleum-impregnated mesh to the healthy skin around the site to help immobilize the graft during subsequent bandage changes. © 2016 The University of Tennessee.

Postoperative considerations

If possible, the initial bandage is left on for 48 hours to encourage adhesion to the wound bed. Subsequently, graft sites are rebandaged daily or every other day to keep the wounds clean and prevent skin maceration from excess moisture (fig. 5-8). Because early fibrinous graft adhesion to the bed is easily disrupted, bandages should be removed very carefully during the first 5 days. Patients may require sedation to minimize movement during bandage changes. After the first week, bandages can usually be changed every 3 to 5 days, depending on the amount of fluid and exudate produced. Animals may require Elizabethan collars for several weeks after bandage removal to prevent self-trauma. Although more expensive than bandaging, negative pressure wound therapy enhances fibroplasia, reduces graft necrosis, and results in more rapid filling of the open meshed areas.

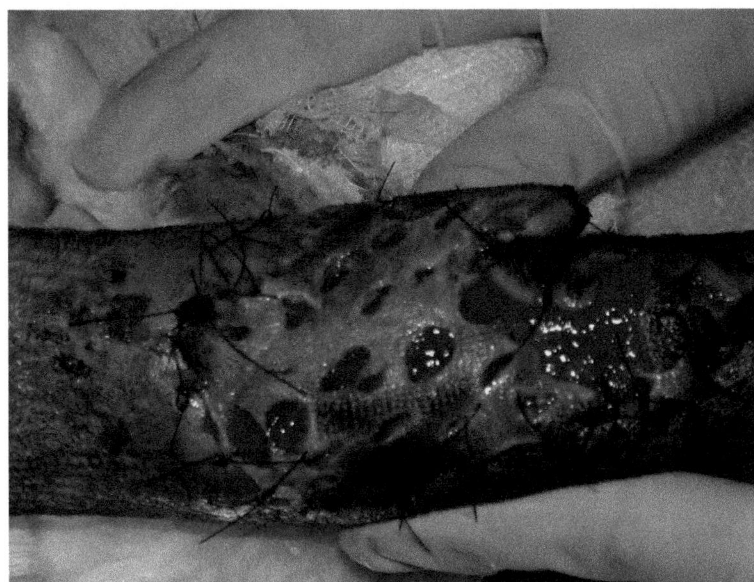

Figure 5-8 Skin maceration from over-application of a silver-based antimicrobial cream.

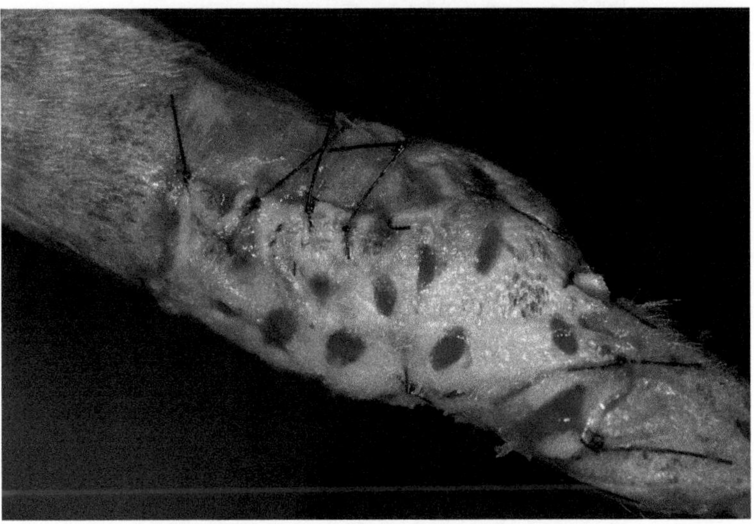

Figure 5-9 Grafts will appear pale or cyanotic before revascularization.

Mesh grafts usually appear cyanotic for the first 2 to 3 days (figs. 5-8 and 5-9). By 7 days after surgery, the amount of surviving graft should be obvious. Occasionally, the superficial layer of epidermis will slough on thicker grafts 5 to 7 days after surgery (fig. 5-10), but the remaining tissue often survives and heals. Hair growth should be evident within 2 to 3 weeks (fig. 5-11). Color and length of hair on grafted sites will usually differ from the surrounding area. Aggressive debridement of subcutaneous tissues during graft preparation can damage hair follicles, resulting in a hairless region.

The most common complication of mesh grafting is graft failure. Graft "take" is disrupted by seroma or hematoma formation, motion, trauma, infection, or overly tight bandages. Grafts that are not debrided sufficiently may be too thick to absorb nutrients during the first 48 hours. Grafts will not take over avascular fat, irradiated tissues, or exposed bone or tendon. Grafts that are black or are white and extremely thin at 7 days after surgery should be removed. The exposed bed is managed as an open wound until infection is

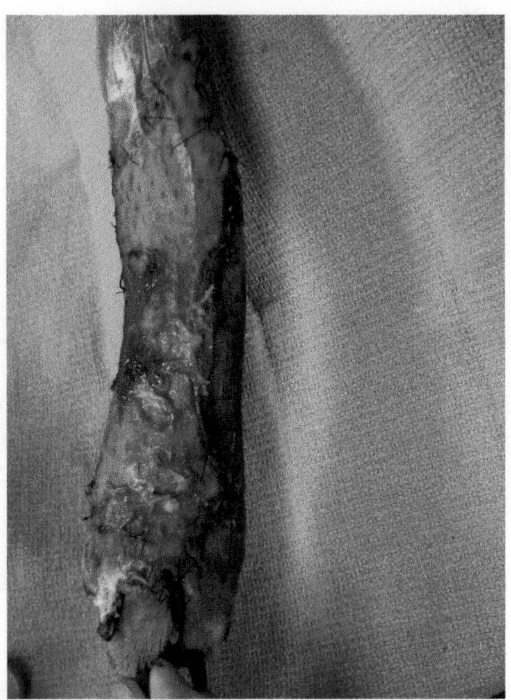

Figure 5-10 Sloughing of the superficial epithelium on a thick graft. The underlying layers of the graft are revascularized and the mesh incisions have filled in.

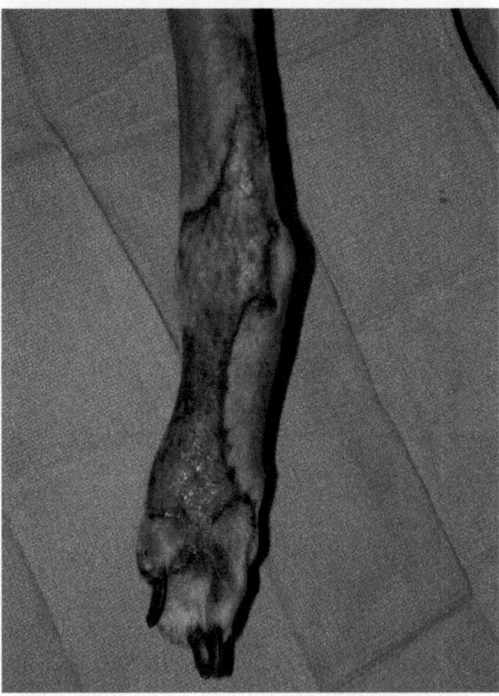

Figure 5-11 One month after grafting, hair growth is evident.

resolved and the bed has granulated. If a portion of the graft survives, the remaining wound may heal by contraction and epithelialization.

Bibliography

Fowler D: Distal limb and paw injuries. Vet Clin Small Anim 2006;36:819–845.

Gibbs A and Tobias KM: Skin reconstruction techniques: full-thickness mesh grafts. Vet Med 2004;99:882–890.

Pavletic MM: Free skin grafts. Atlas of Small Animal Wound Management, 3rd ed. Ames, Ia., Wiley-Blackwell, 2010: 404–431.

Stanley BJ, Pitt KA, Weder Cd et al: Effects of negative pressure wound therapy on healing of free full-thickness skin grafts in dogs. Vet Surg 2013;42:511–522.

Tong T, Simpson DJ: Free skin grafts for immediate wound coverage following tumor resection from the canine distal limb. J Small Anim Pract 2012;53:520–525.

Chapter 6
Caudal Superficial Epigastric Axial Pattern Flap

Axial pattern flaps are developed from skin that contains a direct cutaneous artery and vein. Because these flaps have better perfusion than random pedicle flaps (see p. 25), the transposed skin has a much better chance of surviving. Axial pattern flaps are often used to close extensive defects from tumor removal or trauma. Most flaps are rectangular; however, size and shape depend on the species of animal and the extent of the blood supply. Axial pattern flaps are usually left attached to local skin at their base; however, their skin attachments can be transected on all sides as an island of tissue (still attached to the direct cutaneous artery and vein) to make rotation easier. Flaps can be transferred immediately to a fresh surgical wound. Traumatic wounds with extensive contamination or infection, however, may require topical management for days to weeks before a flap procedure can be performed.

The caudal superficial epigastric axial pattern flap can be used for reconstruction of wounds to the upper rear legs, lateral abdominal wall, and perineum. In cats and short legged dogs, these flaps can often reach the tarsus. Development of a caudal superficial epigastric axial pattern flap is similar to unilateral chain mastectomy (p. 67), except that the major blood supply is left intact caudally. Mammary glands remain functional after flap rotation.

Preoperative management

On animals with chronic wounds, axial pattern flaps can be performed once the recipient site is healthy and free of infection. This can be confirmed by culture of a punch biopsy from the wound bed; however, presence of a thin rim of new epithelium is often a good indicator that infection is under control. In trauma patients, presence of flow within caudal superficial epigastric vessels should be verified with a Doppler flow probe or colorflow Doppler ultrasonographic imaging.

Manual of Small Animal Soft Tissue Surgery, Second Edition. Karen Tobias.
© 2017 John Wiley & Sons, Inc. Published 2017 by John Wiley & Sons, Inc.

In most animals, the donor site has enough laxity to allow for immediate primary closure. Once incised, however, the surrounding skin retracts, making the wound at the donor site appear much larger. Animals should be clipped widely around the donor site and positioned and prepped so that the surgeon can take full advantage of lateral thoracic, abdominal, and flank skin for closure (see fig. 7-1, p. 62).

For open wounds, the recipient bed should be filled with a water-soluble gel before clipping. Loose hairs should be vacuumed and the wound flushed to remove the gel before prepping the bed. The bed can be scrubbed gently with antiseptic soap and gauze sponges to remove contaminants and debris. A hanging limb prep is performed if the recipient site is on the leg or perineum. The animal is positioned on the surgery table so that the donor and recipient sites can be draped in with minimal tension on both sites. In the case of chronic wounds, hypertrophic or granulation tissue can be resected during surgery before covering the site with an axial pattern flap.

Surgery

Caudal superficial epigastric flaps in female dogs can extend to a point midway between the first and second mammary glands. The flap is shorter in cats and male dogs because necrosis may occur if the flap extends to the second nipple. To determine the appropriate flap length for wound coverage, a pattern of the flap can be constructed from sterile paper, gauze, pad, or drape; manually secured to the proposed flap base; and rotated to the recipient site. If the wound is on the rear leg, flap length and wound coverage should be evaluated with the leg in extension. Before the flap is developed, the recipient site should be debrided as needed. Thin epithelial edges are excised, and the wound is covered with moistened gauze sponges until the flap is elevated. Before the flap is incised, the skin at the donor site should be grasped, lifted, and released to make sure it is normally positioned.

All axial pattern flaps are elevated below any local panniculus muscle. In female dogs, caudal superficial epigastric flaps are elevated below the mammary glands to preserve the blood supply. Dissection continues caudally to the level of the caudal superficial epigastric artery and vein. The caudal superficial epigastric artery and vein are branches of the external pudendal vessels, which exit from the superficial inguinal ring 2 to 4 cm lateral to midline and just medial to the last nipple in female dogs or caudolateral to the last nipple in male dogs (see fig. 7-13, p. 69). Flaps will appear narrower and shorter after elevation because of elastic recoil, but they can be stretched back to their original size or to a longer, narrower tongue of tissue.

Once elevated, flaps can be rotated up to 180 degrees; however, sharp turns or kinks in the flap base can cause lymphatic or vascular obstruction and subsequent swelling and necrosis. If further mobility is needed, the flap can be turned into an "island" by incising the skin across the base. The subcutaneous tissues are left intact to prevent damage to the caudal superficial epigastric artery and vein (fig. 6-1). If the recipient bed is not directly adjacent to the donor site, a bridging incision is made through the skin between the donor and recipient beds. After elevating the surrounding tissues, the flap is laid within the new gap and over the recipient bed. Subcutaneous tissues along the flap edge can be apposed to the recipient site. The center of the flap should not be tacked down to the recipient bed, however, since this could damage blood

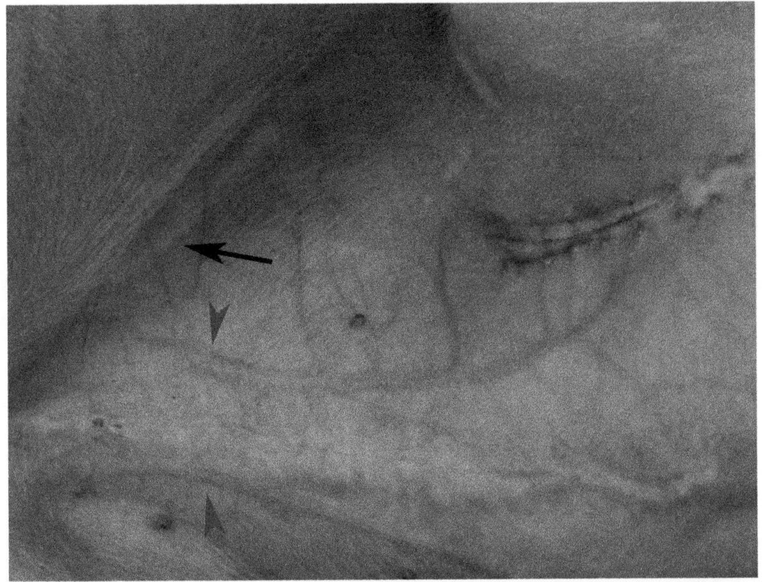

Figure 6-1 The caudal superficial epigastric vessels (arrowheads) are tributaries of the external pudendal vessels, which pass through the inguinal ring (arrow).

supply. Instead, a continuous suction drain should be placed to reduce dead space.

Surgical technique: caudal superficial epigastric flap

1. With a sterile marker, draw a line along the ventral midline from the level of the last nipple or inguinal ring to the proposed cranial flap margin. Include the base of the prepuce in male dogs (fig. 6-2).
2. Measure the distance between the nipples and the midline. Draw a second line parallel to the first, lateral to and equidistant from the nipples, and connect the lines cranially with a curvilinear incision.
3. Incise the flap borders along the predrawn lines, ligating any confluent mammary tissue or large vessels.
4. Starting cranially, elevate the flap just above the external abdominal oblique and external rectus sheath fascia, using Metzenbaum scissors (fig. 6-3).

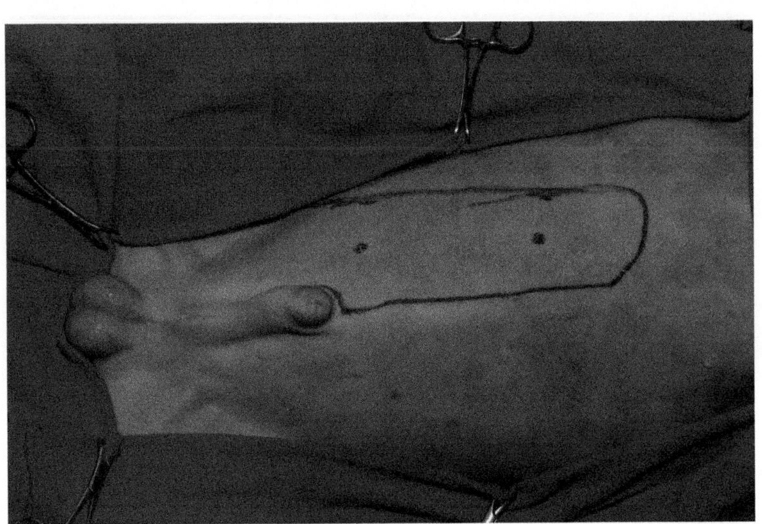

Figure 6-2 Outline the flap with a sterile marker. The distance between the nipples and the lateral border of the flap should be the same as the distance from the nipples to the midline. In female dogs, the flap can extend to a point midway between the first and second mammary glands.

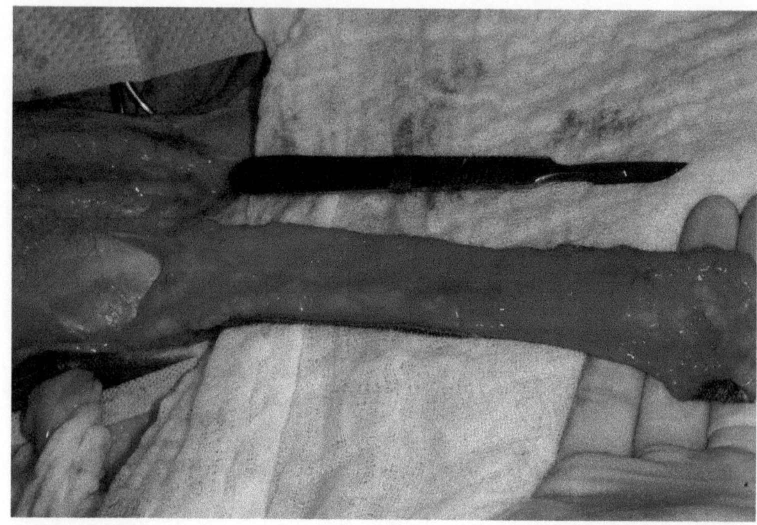

Figure 6-3 Elevate the flap from the external fascia of the abdominal wall musculature. Work caudally toward the inguinal rings, but do not damage the caudal superficial epigastric vessels.

5. Dissect caudally, gradually elevating the flap toward the inguinal ring. Avoid damaging the caudal superficial epigastric vessels (See fig. 7-13).
6. Once the flap is elevated, temporarily close the donor site with towel clamps or cover with moistened sponges.
7. Rotate the flap to the recipient site (fig. 6-4). If necessary, make a "bridging" incision through intact skin between the donor and recipient beds and undermine the tissues along either side of this incision.
    a. A "bridging incision" connects the donor and recipient beds by transecting any intervening skin.
8. Place several interrupted skin sutures or staples to hold the flap to the farthest edges of the recipient site.
9. Place a continuous suction drain under the flap, exiting the tubing through healthy skin at a site that can be bandaged easily (fig. 6-5).
    a. Do not attempt to close dead space with tacking sutures: tacking sutures could damage the blood supply to the flap.

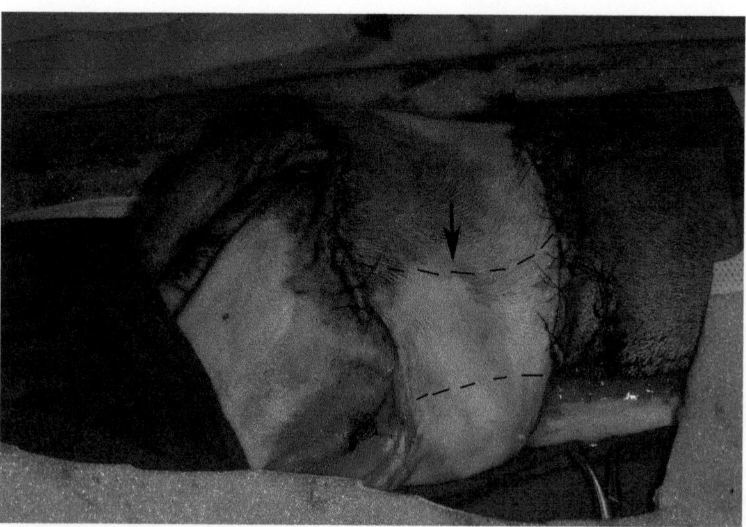

Figure 6-4 Rotate the flap to the recipient site. If the recipient and donor beds are not contiguous, incise through intact skin (dotted lines and arrow) to connect the donor and recipient beds.

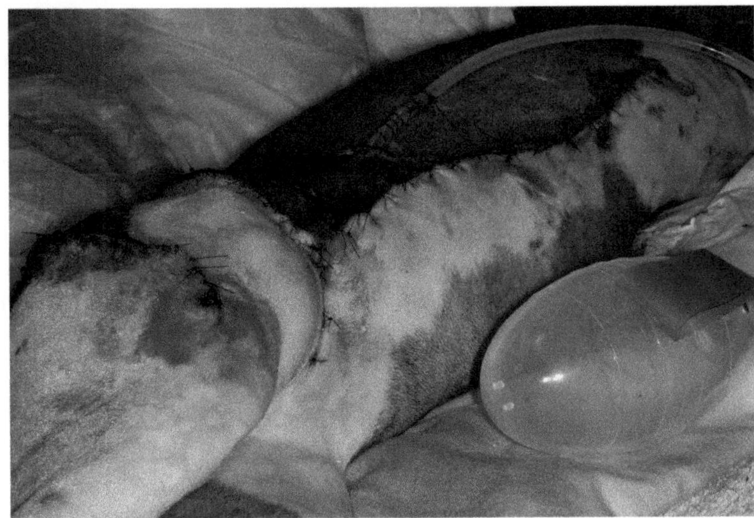

Figure 6-5 Place a suction drain and close the subcutaneous tissues and skin.

10. If possible, appose the subcutaneous fat along edges of the flap and recipient site with continuous or interrupted sutures of rapidly absorbable monofilament material. Appose skin edges of the flap and recipient bed with an interrupted or continuous suture pattern or staples.
11. If necessary, place a second continuous suction drain under the donor site. Close the subcutaneous and skin layers of the donor site routinely.

Postoperative considerations

Drain exit sites should be covered with a sterile, noncompressive adhesive dressing or bandage to reduce the risk of contamination. In most animals, drains can be removed in 16 to 72 hours. Elizabethan collars should be placed to prevent self-trauma.

Complications are very common in animals undergoing axial pattern flaps and include dehiscence, flap swelling, necrosis, infection, drainage, and

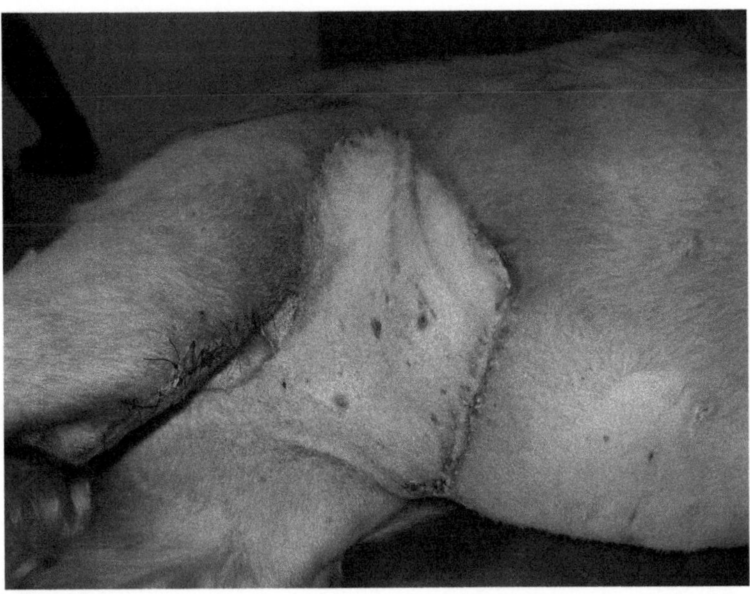

Figure 6-6 Appearance of a caudal superficial epigastric flap 2 weeks after placement.

seroma formation. Despite this, outcome is usually good to excellent. Complications can often be prevented or diminished by careful planning and placement of the flap, avoidance of tension, and use of continuous suction drains under the flap or donor site or both. Bruising and distal edema of the flap are often seen within 1 to 2 days after surgery but usually resolve without treatment. Flap integrity and vascularity should be re-evaluated at 3 days, 6 days, and 2 weeks (fig. 6-6). If necrosis occurs, the affected tissues are debrided and the remaining defect is closed primarily over a drain or left to heal by second intention. Dehiscence can often be managed conservatively with debridement, wound care, and bandage changes.

Bibliography

Aper RL and Smeak DD: Clinical evaluation of caudal superficial epigastric axial pattern flap reconstruction of skin defects in 10 dogs (1989–2001). J Am Anim Hosp Assoc 2005;41:185–192.

Bauer MS and Salisbury SK: Reconstruction of distal hind limb injuries in cats using the caudal superficial epigastric skin flap. Vet Comp Orthop Traumatol 1995;8:98–101.

Field EJ, Kelly G, Pleuvry D, et al: Indications, outcome and complications with axial pattern skin flaps in dogs and cats: 73 cases. J Small Anim Pract 2015;56:698–706.

Leonatti S and Tobias KM: Skin reconstruction techniques: axial pattern flaps. Vet Med 2004;99:862–881.

Reetz JA et al: Ultrasonographic and color-flow Dopper ultrasonographic assessment of direct cutaneous arteries used for axial pattern skin flaps in dogs. J Am Vet Med Assoc 2006;228:1361–1365.

Chapter 7
Mastectomy

Mammary neoplasia is the most common type of tumor in female dogs and is rare in male dogs. Incidence of mammary tumors in bitches ranges from 2 to >20% and depends on the regional frequency of ovariohysterectomy. Incidence is only 1% in 6-year-old female dogs but increases to 13% by 10 years of age. Risk can be decreased based on the time of ovariectomy/ovariohysterectomy: for dogs spayed before the first estrus cycle, second estrus cycle, or two years of age, respectively, risk of mammary neoplasia is 0.5%, 8%, or 26% of that in intact females. Mammary tumors are much less common in cats (25/100,000 queens or 0.025%). Spaying cats before 6 months, 12 months, and 24 months of age results in 91%, 86%, and 11% risk reduction in mammary tumor development, respectively. Spaying cats after 2 years of age or dogs after 2.5 years of age has minimal effect on incidence.

Most animals with mammary tumors have nonpainful masses that may be incidental findings on annual physical exams. Dogs with inflammatory mammary carcinomas often have anorexia, weight loss, weakness, rapid tumor growth, swelling, redness, pain, and diffuse involvement of multiple glands.

Surgical resection is the treatment of choice for noninflammatory mammary tumors. In dogs, recurrence rates and survival duration are not influenced by the type or extent of surgery performed, as long as the tumor is completely removed. However, 58% of dogs with single mammary tumors develop an ipsilateral tumor after regional mastectomy. Intact dogs should be spayed at the time of surgery. In some studies, dogs that are spayed at the time of surgery live longer or are less likely to have a relapse than those left intact. This is particularly true if the tumor contains estrogen receptors.

For dogs with inflammatory carcinoma, treatment includes supportive care for any systemic illness and daily administration of piroxicam (0.3 mg/kg per os). Duration of survival for dogs with inflammatory carcinoma is 2 to 6 months with piroxicam therapy and less than 1 month with other treatments. Mastectomy usually does not increase life span of these dogs.

Bilateral or unilateral radical mastectomy (based on lymphatic drainage) is recommended in cats with mammary carcinoma, since radical resection increases disease-free intervals (range, 575 to 1,300 days) compared with more conservative surgery (range, 300 to 325 days).

Manual of Small Animal Soft Tissue Surgery, Second Edition. Karen Tobias.
© 2017 John Wiley & Sons, Inc. Published 2017 by John Wiley & Sons, Inc.

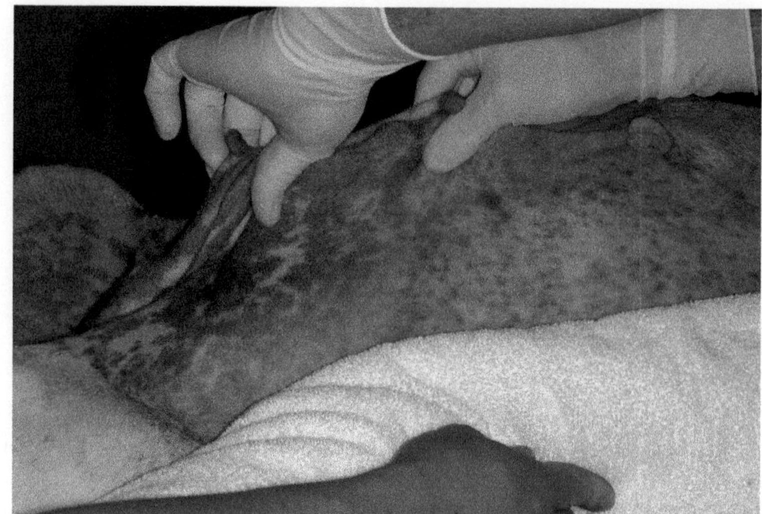

Figure 7-1 When prepping and positioning the patient, grasp and lift the skin away from the body wall and place rolled towels along the dorsal flanks to reduce tension.

Preoperative management

Because animals with mammary tumors are usually older, they should be evaluated for other systemic diseases. Half of mammary tumors in bitches and the majority of mammary tumors in cats and male dogs are malignant; therefore, diagnostics should include three-view thoracic radiographs to check for metastases. If caudal glands are affected, abdominal ultrasound should be performed to evaluate the animals for lymph node enlargement or other evidence of metastasis. Cytology of the mammary masses may be insensitive for well-differentiated masses and is therefore primarily performed to identify poorly differentiated tumors. Lymph node cytology is highly sensitive for metastases, however. Inflammatory carcinomas are associated with disseminated intravascular coagulation; therefore, coagulation panels and platelet counts should be evaluated in affected animals. Biopsies should be obtained if inflammatory carcinoma is suspected, since mastectomy is usually contraindicated in these dogs. Biopsies are also recommended in young intact cats to rule out fibroadenomatous hyperplasia, which is treated with flank ovariohysterectomy.

Under anesthesia, all mammary glands should be palpated carefully for masses, since multiple nodules are common. Cats usually have four pairs of glands and dogs usually have five, though they may have four to six pairs. Animals should be clipped and prepped very widely, particularly if masses are to be removed bilaterally. During clipping, the skin should be grasped and lifted away from the body wall to determine how much it will shift with closure (fig. 7-1). With this maneuver, the veterinarian will often find that more hair must be clipped to prevent intraoperative contamination.

Surgery

Surgical techniques for mammary gland resection include lumpectomy (removal of the mass only), simple or regional mastectomy (removal of the gland or glands containing the mass), en bloc dissection (removal of the gland containing the mass, the intervening lymphatics, and regional lymph nodes), and unilateral or "chain" mastectomy (removal of all glands on one side and the associated inguinal lymph node). Lumpectomies are often performed for encapsulated masses less than 1 cm in diameter or those along the lateral margins of the gland. Bilateral chain mastectomies are usually performed as staged procedures 1 month apart, particularly in dogs, to prevent excess tension on the wound closure.

If animals are intact, an ovariohysterectomy should be performed through a midline ventral celiotomy before mastectomy. After the linea alba is closed, the affected mammary glands are removed. If the tumor crosses over midline and is adherent to the rectus fascia, the body wall and mammary tissue can be removed en bloc before ovariohysterectomy.

For wide excisions, sterile rulers and skin markers are used to outline the skin incision. After the skin and subcutaneous tissues are incised, the glands are elevated from the body wall. In dogs, thoracic glands closely adhere to underlying pectoral muscle and are more difficult to remove than abdominal glands. Cats occasionally require abdominal wall resection because of adhesions between the mammary mass and the external rectus sheath.

Cautery, radiofrequency scalpels, and vessel sealing devices (e.g., Ligasure, Covidien) are useful for reducing hemorrhage and swelling. Lasers, monopolar cautery, and radiofrequency scalpels produce a char that penetrates >0.15 mm, however, which can interfere with histologic evaluation of margins.

Once the masses are removed, they should be marked with sutures to identify cranial and lateral margins. The cut edges and all exposed subcutaneous surfaces can be painted with a blue or green tissue stain to facilitate histologic evaluation of margins. The tissues are placed in formalin once the stain is dry.

Rotational flaps or Z-plasty (p. 36) may be needed for closure of large cranial wounds. Walking sutures reduce tension on closure. Continuous suction or Penrose drains should be placed when dead space cannot be closed. For lumpectomies and simple mastectomy, subcutaneous closure may be sufficient to reduce seroma formation. Rapidly absorbable monofilament is recommended for subcutaneous closure, since fibrous tissue around long-lasting suture material may be palpable for months, making postoperative assessment of recurrence more challenging.

Surgical technique: lumpectomy

1. If the skin is freely movable over the mass, make a 3- to 4-cm incision through the skin (fig. 7-2). Dissect the skin away from underlying subcutaneous tissues with Metzenbaum scissors.

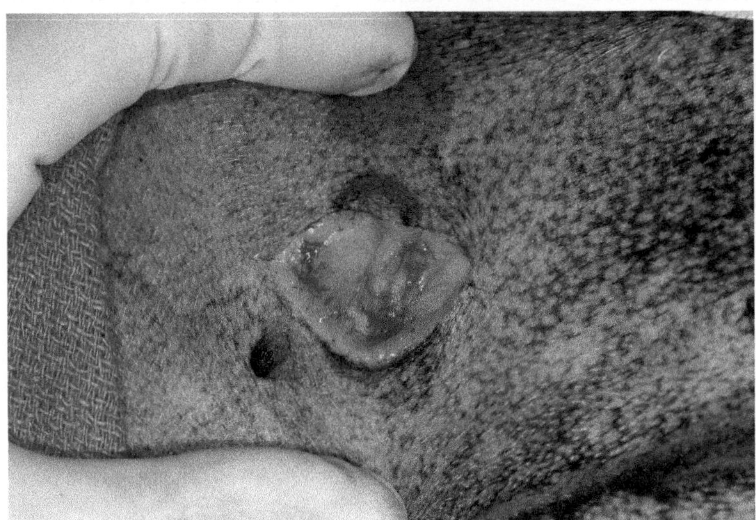

Figure 7-2 Simple lumpectomy. If the skin is freely movable over the mass, make a 3- to 4-cm incision through the skin over the lump.

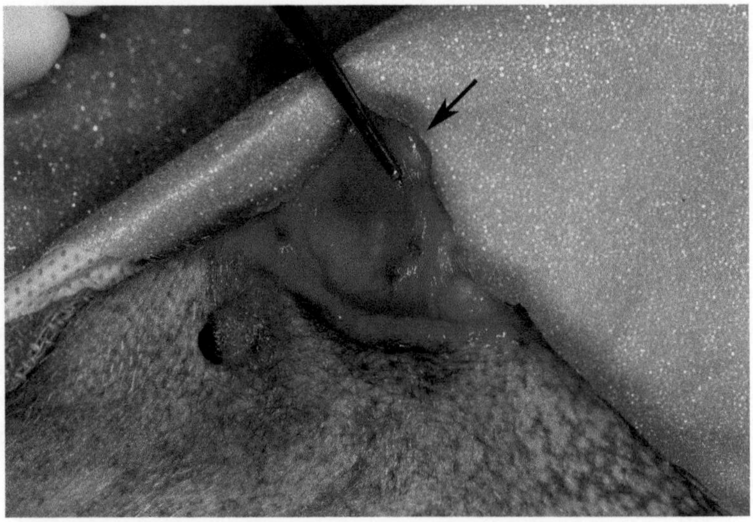

Figure 7-3 Elevate the mass (arrow) and expose 1 to 2 cm of subcutaneous and glandular tissues around the mass.

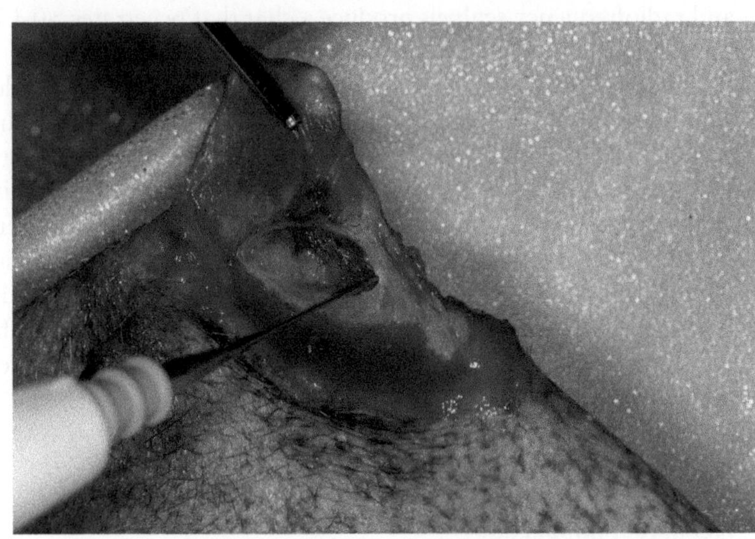

Figure 7-4 Transect subcutaneous and glandular attachments with a radiosurgical scalpel or monopolar cautery, or ligate the tissues before sharply transecting them with scissors.

2. If the skin is not freely movable, incise the skin 1 to 2 cm around the tumor.
3. Elevate the mass from the wound (fig. 7-3); if needed, bluntly free the surrounding tissues 1 to 2 cm from the mass.
4. Provide hemostasis with monopolar or bipolar cautery (fig. 7-4), a radiofrequency scalpel, laser, or en bloc suture ligation.
5. Close deep and superficial subcutaneous tissues with simple interrupted sutures of 3-0 or 4-0 rapidly absorbable monofilament material.
6. Close the skin routinely.

Surgical technique: simple or regional mastectomy

1. Make an elliptical incision through the skin around the gland(s) to be removed (fig. 7-5), starting on midline.
2. Incise through the midline subcutaneous tissues with a blade or scissors (fig. 7-6).

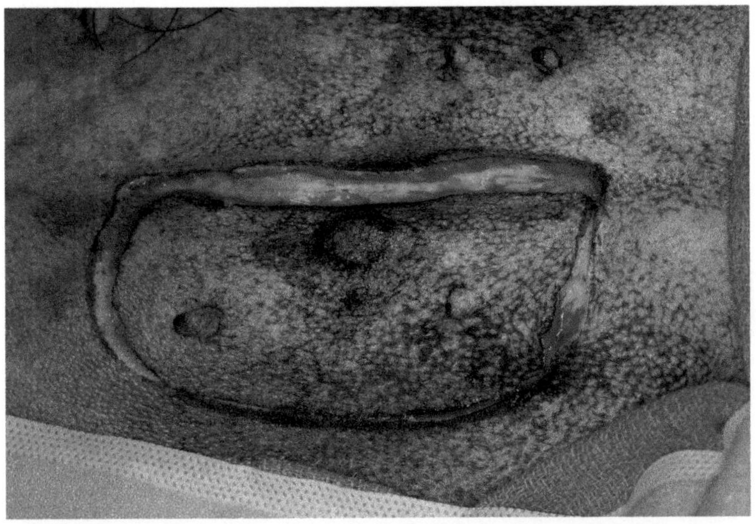

Figure 7-5 Regional mastectomy. Incise the skin around the glands, starting on ventral midline.

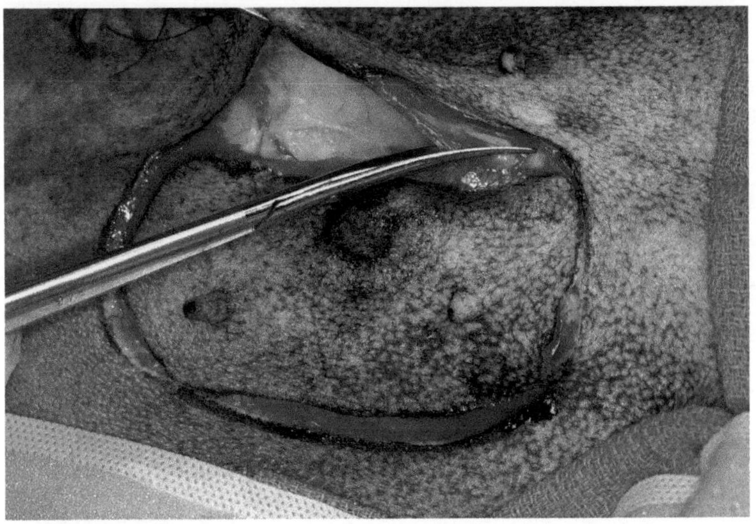

Figure 7-6 Transect the subcutaneous tissue attachments to the linea.

3. Continue subcutaneous tissue dissection and transection cranially. Ligate or cauterize any blood vessels.
4. Incise the subcutaneous tissues along the lateral margins of the gland (fig. 7-7).
5. At the cranial extent of the incision, identify any junctions between the mammary tissue to be removed and the adjacent gland(s) (fig. 7-8).
6. With 2-0 or 3-0 rapidly absorbable suture material, double ligate or transfix the confluent tissue and associated blood vessels between the glands (fig. 7-9) and transect the tissue junction.
7. Starting cranially or medially, dissect between the external abdominal fascial sheath and the mammary glands caudally and laterally (fig. 7-10). Ligate and transect any anastomosing vessels or confluent glandular tissue.
8. If the caudal mammary gland is to be removed, identify the caudal superficial epigastric artery and vein in the inguinal fat pad and ligate and transect the vessels before completing the mastectomy.

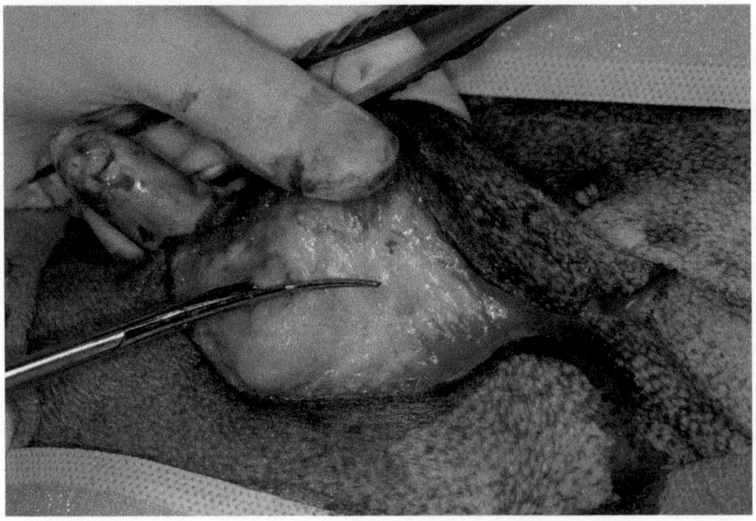

Figure 7-7 Transect the lateral subcutaneous tissues to the level of the external abdominal fascial sheath.

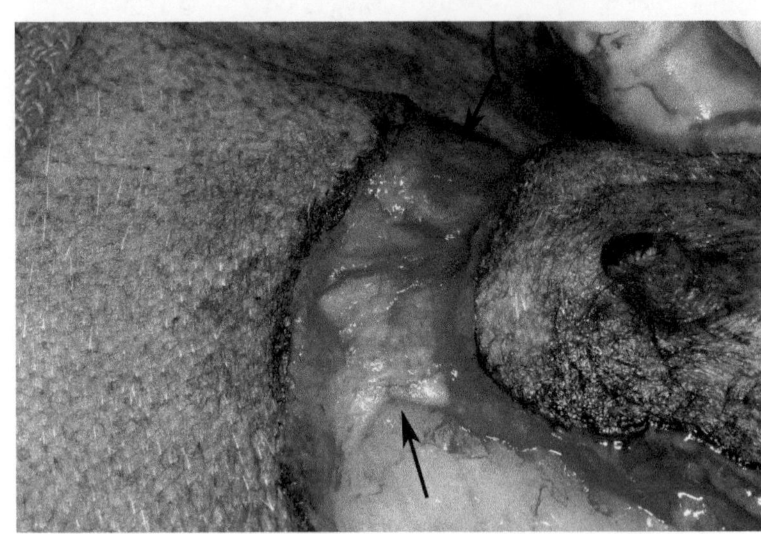

Figure 7-8 Identify the vessels and confluent mammary tissue (between arrows) between glands.

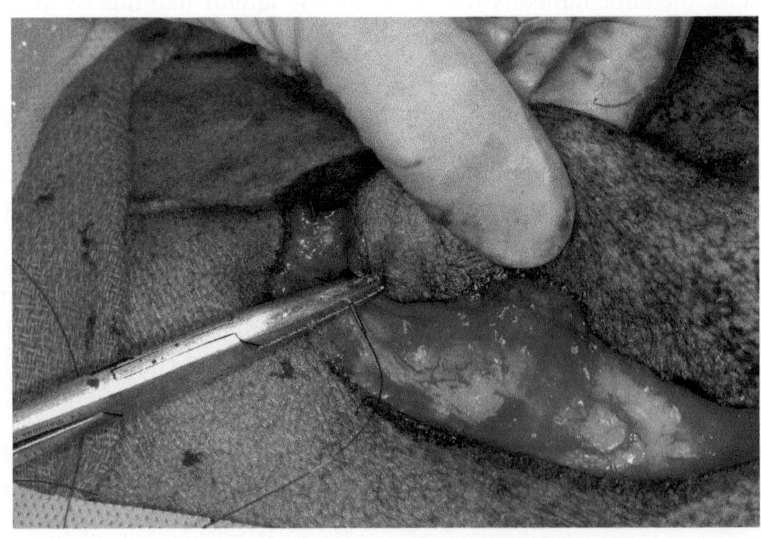

Figure 7-9 Ligate the vessels and confluent mammary tissue between the glands with transfixing or encircling ligatures before transecting.

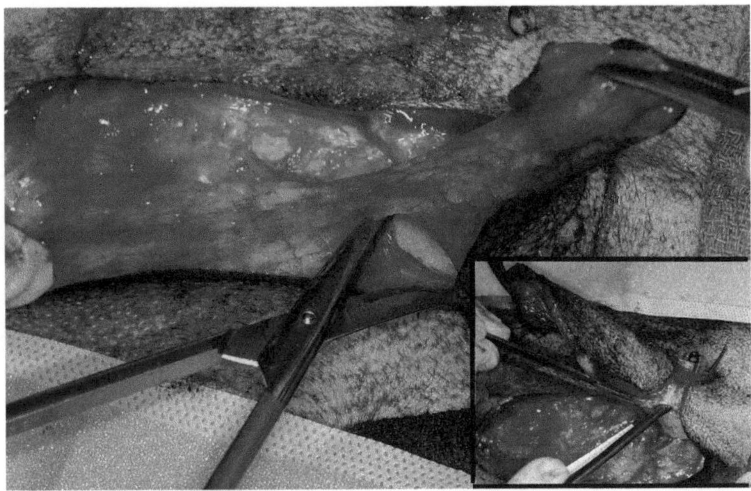

Figure 7-10 Working caudally, use blunt and sharp dissection to elevate the glands from the abdominal wall. Ligate and transect any confluent mammary tissue (inset) and blood vessels.

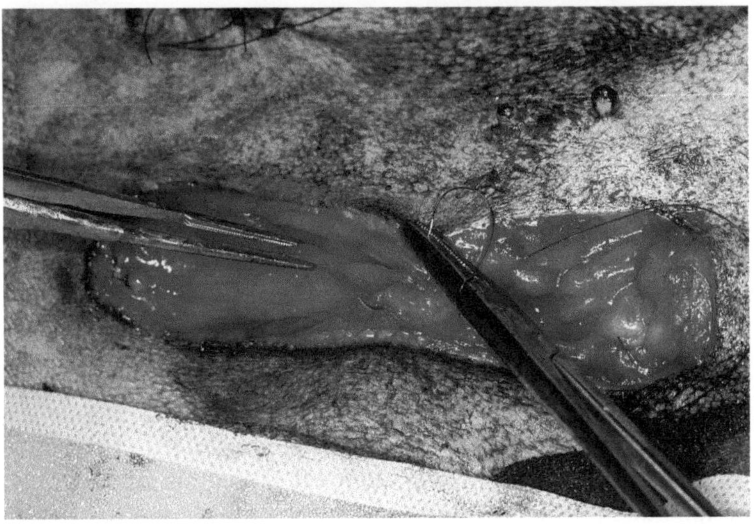

Figure 7-11 To close dead space, tack subcutaneous tissues to abdominal wall fascia or place a drain.

9. Reduce the subcutaneous dead space by placing interrupted sutures (fig. 7-11), walking sutures (p. 21), or a continuous suction drain (p. 125).
10. Close the skin routinely.

Surgical technique: unilateral (chain) mastectomy

1. Incise the skin and subcutaneous tissues medial to the glands. The incision along the caudal three glands in dogs will be centered on the ventral midline.
2. Incise the skin along the cranial, lateral, and caudal borders of the mammary glands.
    a. For a rough estimate of resection width, measure the distance from the 3rd nipple to the midline; measure this same distance lateral to the nipple. These measurements will provide a guide to a resection margin that includes the mammary glands and some surrounding subcutis. Narrower margins are often possible, however, especially cranially.

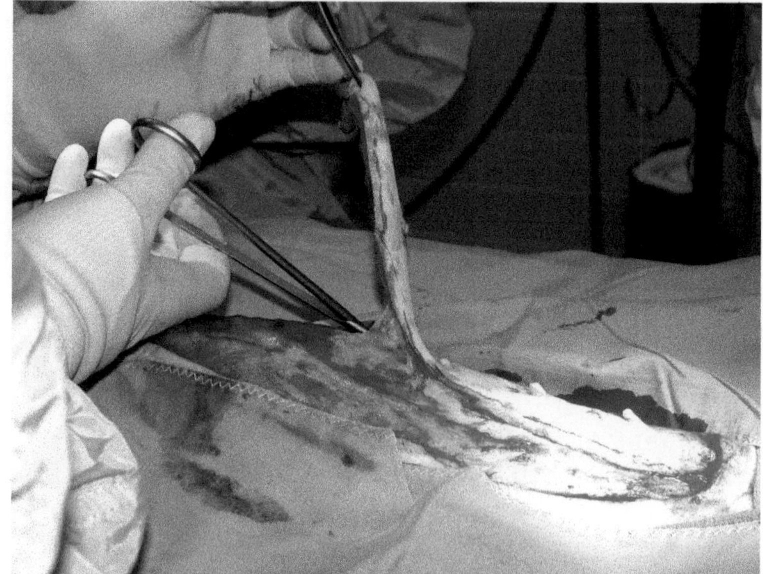

Figure 7-12 After incising the skin and subcutaneous tissues, elevate the mammary chain between the glands and the external abdominal fascia from cranial to caudal.

3. With scissors, use blunt and sharp dissection to separate the subcutaneous tissues and elevate the mammary chain along the cranial and lateral borders. Ligate large vessels and transect small vessels with cautery or a radiofrequency scalpel.
4. Expose, ligate, and transect the branches of the internal thoracic, lateral thoracic, and intercostal vessels and the cranial superficial epigastric artery and vein as they appear during dissection.
5. From cranial to caudal, dissect the mammary gland tissue from the pectorals and the external abdominal fascial sheath (fig. 7-12). The peripheral skin margins will retract laterally during dissection, giving the appearance that the resection site has doubled in size.
6. If the mammary tissue is adhered to the abdominal fascia, resect the fascia and underlying muscle and close the defect with absorbable monofilament suture.
7. Dissect cautiously at the level of the superficial inguinal ring to avoid damaging the external pudendal artery and vein.
8. Identify the caudal superficial epigastric artery and vein in the inguinal fat pad (fig. 7-13) and double ligate and transect them.
9. Bluntly dissect through any remaining subcutaneous tissues caudally and remove the mammary chain.
10. Place a continuous suction drain, exiting the tubing at a site that will be easy to cover with a bandage.
11. Using penetrating towel clamps or stay sutures, temporarily appose the skin edges (fig. 7-14). If the skin edges will not appose easily, undermine between the subcutaneous tissues and abdominal or pectoral fascia to reduce tension. Pull the clamps that attach the drapes to the skin toward midline to further reduce tension.

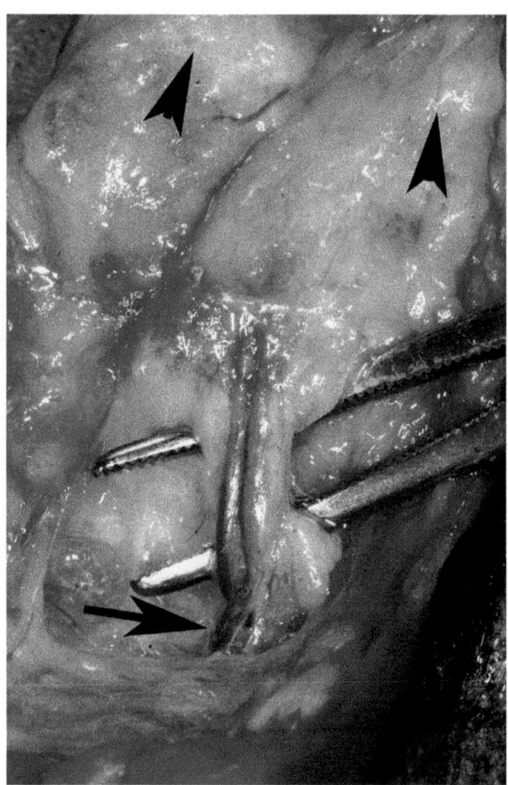

Figure 7-13 Identify the caudal superficial epigastric vessels (on forceps) at the bifurcation from the external pudendal vessels (arrow). In this photo, the elevated mammary chain (arrowheads) is flapped up away from the surgeon.

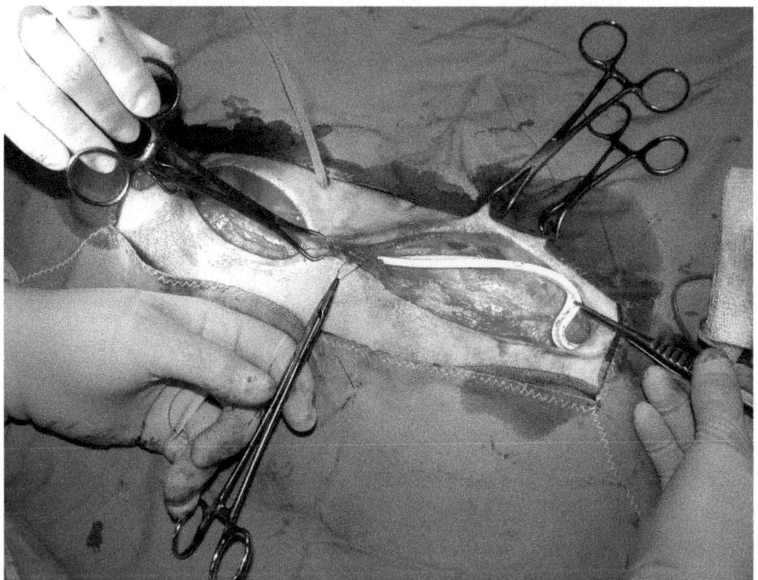

Figure 7-14 Place a continuous suction drain and use a towel clamp to appose the incision edges while closing the subcutaneous tissues and skin. In this animal, additional towel clamps were added between the drape and skin to prevent hair exposure.

12. Close the subcutaneous tissues with interrupted sutures of 2-0 or 3-0 rapidly absorbable monofilament. If desired, use walking or tacking sutures to close dead space.
13. Remove the towel clamps and close the skin routinely (fig. 7-15).
14. Close the drain exit site with a purse-string suture and secure the tubing to the skin.

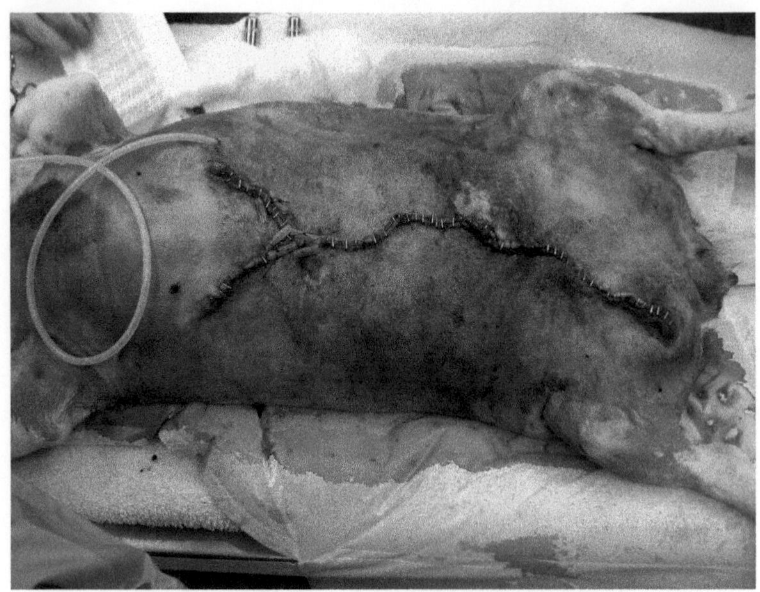

Figure 7-15 Final appearance after unilateral mastectomy plus removal of a cranial mammary mass on opposite side. Stent sutures were placed at the confluence of the Y-shaped closure to reduce tension. These sutures should be removed 1 to 3 days after placement.

Postoperative considerations

All masses should be submitted for histologic evaluation, since animals may have several histologic types of tumors within each gland or chain. Bandages, Elizabethan collars, and exercise restriction may reduce the risk of swelling. Drains can be removed in most animals within 24 to 48 hours after surgery. Animals undergoing extensive resection will usually require postoperative analgesics for 2 to 5 days.

Complications include pain, swelling, hemorrhage, seroma formation, infection, dehiscence, limb edema, tumor recurrence, and metastatic disease. Prognosis is poorer in animals with metastases, poorly differentiated or invasive tumors, inflammatory carcinomas, or tumors greater than 2 to 3 cm in diameter.

Bibliography

Alenza MDP et al: Inflammatory mammary carcinoma in dogs: 33 cases (1995–1999). J Am Vet Med Assoc 2001;219:1110–1114.

Allen SW and Mahaffey EA: Canine mammary neoplasia: prognostic indicators and response to surgical therapy. J Am Anim Hosp Assoc 1989;25:540–546.

Chang SC et al: Prognostic factors associated with survival two years after surgery in dogs with malignant mammary tumors: 79 cases (1998–2002). J Am Vet Med Assoc 2005;227:1625–1629.

Kristiansen VM, Pena L, Diez Cordova L, et al: Efect of ovariohysterectomy at the time of tumor removal in dogs with mammary carcinomas: a randomized controlled trial. J Vet Intern Med 2016;30:230–241.

Marconato L, Monaelli G, Stefanello D, et al: Prognostic factors for dogs with mammary inflammatory carcinoma: 43 cases (2003–2008). J Am Vet Med Assoc 2009;235:967–972.

Sorenmo KU et al: Effect of spaying and timing of spaying on survival of dogs with mammary carcinoma. J Vet Intern Med 2000;14:266–270.

Souza C et al: Inflammatory mammary carcinoma in 12 dogs: clinical features, cyclooxygenase-2 expression, and response to piroxicam treatment. Can Vet J 2009;50:506–510.

Stratmann N et al: Mammary tumor recurrence in bitches after regional mastectomy. Vet Surg 2008;37:82–86.

Van Nimwegen S, Kirpensteijn J: Specific disorders. In Johnston SA, Tobias KM: Veterinary Surgery: Small Animal. Elsevier, In press 2017.

Wypij J: Malignant mammary tumors: biologic behavior, prognostic factors, and therapeutic approach in cats. Vet Med 2006;101:352–366.

Chapter 8

Open Wound Management with a Tie-Over Bandage

Open wound management is often necessary for infected or dirty wounds, areas with necrosis or questionable blood supply, or for patients too unstable to undergo wound debridement and primary closure. Closure of open wounds falls under 4 categories. Immediate suturing (*primary closure*) is performed soon after a wound has occurred or if the entire wound can be resected and turned into a "fresh," clean wound. When a wound is infected or has excessive drainage or questionable circulation, closure can be delayed (*delayed primary closure*) for 3 to 5 days to allow daily evaluation, cleansing, and bandaging. In some cases, closure is delayed until after healthy granulation tissue has developed (*secondary closure*) because of persistent infection, inflammation, or necrosis. *Second intention healing* occurs when a wound is allowed to heal by contraction and epithelialization.

For delayed primary closure, secondary closure, and second intention healing, the wound is covered with a topical dressing to reduce or treat infection and keep it moist, and the area is covered with a bandage to secure the dressing, protect the wound, and prevent contamination. For wounds in the caudal half of the body, encircling bandages are difficult to place and maintain because of the risk of urine and fecal contamination. To reduce contamination and slippage, bandages can be secured locally over a wound with adhesive drapes, skin staples, or a tie-over technique. Alternatively, the dressing can be held in place with a tensioning suture (p. 40).

In animals, a tie-over bandage is usually constructed by placing suture loops in the skin. Dressings and absorptive materials are placed over the wound and secured with umbilical tape or shoelaces threaded through the suture loops and crisscrossed over the bandage. Tie-over bandages are less likely to slip or to obstruct lymphatic or venous drainage than encircling bandages. They also provide a method for stretching and lengthening the local skin to facilitate wound closure. The amount of skin relaxation obtained depends on the location of the wound and the local skin character.

Manual of Small Animal Soft Tissue Surgery, Second Edition. Karen Tobias.
© 2017 John Wiley & Sons, Inc. Published 2017 by John Wiley & Sons, Inc.

Maximal stretch is usually noted within 2 to 3 days after placement of tension on the skin.

Wound dressings for open wound management

Selection of a contact layer can be overwhelming because of the myriad of dressings available and the lack of standardized research documenting or comparing their efficacy. In general, dressing selection should be based on the character of the wound and the desired local effect (e.g., nonadherent, antimicrobial, absorptive, moisturizing, etc). Dressings should protect the wound, keep it moist without permitting maceration, treat infection when present, and promote (or at least not interfere with) healing. Some of the author's favorite dressings are listed in the table below.

Wound character	Dressing type	Brand
Fresh, hemorrhaging wound	Nonadherent pad, or Petroleum-impregnated mesh and absorptive layer (e.g., cast padding)	Telfa pad (Kendall) Adaptic (Systagenix)
Copious thick drainage and infection	Antimicrobial-impregnated gauze	Kerlix AMD roll gauze (Kendall)
Copious thin drainage	Superabsorptive polymer pad	Xtrasorb Classic pad (Dermasciences)
Infected and unhealthy wound bed with minimal to mild drainage	Honey	Grocery store honey, or Medihoney gel, paste, or pads (Dermasciences)
Infected but improving wound bed with minimal to mild drainage	Silver-impregnated absorptive pad with dextrans and alginate	Algidex pad (DeRoyal)
Dry and necrotic	Maggot therapy (or debridement with surgery or honey)	Medical maggots (Monarch Labs)
Granulating wound with infection present but clearing	Antimicrobial ointment or cream	Silver sulfadiazine cream 1% or Triple antibiotic ointment (multiple vendors)
Healthy granulation bed	Antimicrobial ointment on a nonadherent pad	Triple antibiotic ointment (multiple vendors)

Preoperative management

Suture loops for tie-over bandages can be placed under anesthesia or sedation and local blocks. To reduce hair contamination, wound beds should be filled with a water-soluble gel before clipping. After cleaning and prepping, tissue samples for culture should be obtained by punch or incisional biopsy from the beds of chronic, nonhealing, or effusive wounds.

If skin stretching is desired, the local skin should be undermined before suture loop placement. Necrotic or unhealthy tissue should be debrided with scissors or a blade. Nonabsorbable 0 monofilament material is often used to make suture loops for tie-over bandages. This type of suture is difficult to tie because it tends to hitch. If hitching is a problem, the suture loop can be formed over the narrow end of a syringe case, which is slid out of the loop once the final knots are secured. Because suture loops may pull through skin or be accidentally cut during bandage changes, extra loops should be placed.

Surgical technique: tie-over bandage

1. With 0 or 2-0 nonabsorbable monofilament suture on a cutting needle, take a full-thickness bite of skin 2 to 3cm away from and perpendicular to the wound edge.
2. Tie one or two knots in the suture close to the skin. Do not plicate or compress the skin when tying.
3. Leave a 1- to 1.5-cm loop and tie two more knots (four throws; fig. 8-1). Cut the suture ends.
    a. To facilitate loop formation, form the loop over a syringe case or syringe and tie two knots (fig. 8-2), then slip the loop off.
4. Place at least eight suture loops around and beyond the margins of the wound, spacing them 4 to 8 cm apart.
5. Place a sterile dressing on the wound bed to keep it moist. Cover the dressing and surrounding skin with a secondary layer of sterile absorptive material.
6. Lace sterile umbilical tape, shoelaces, or heavy suture through the suture loops in a crisscross fashion over bandage (fig. 8-3) and tie to secure.
    a. On large wounds, place at least two separate laces.
    b. Overtightening will cause immediate compression (fig. 8-4) and palor of the skin around the suture, and eventually skin necrosis.

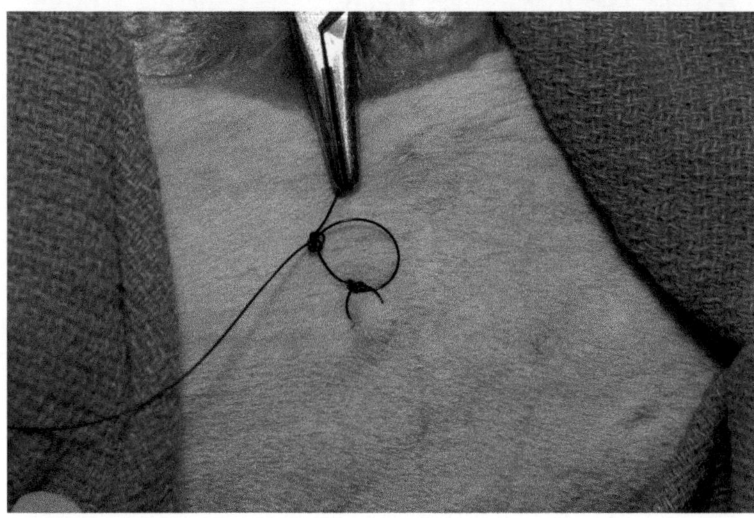

Figure 8-1 To make a suture loop for a tie-over bandage, tie one knot close to the skin. Leave a 1.5-cm loop and place two more knots.

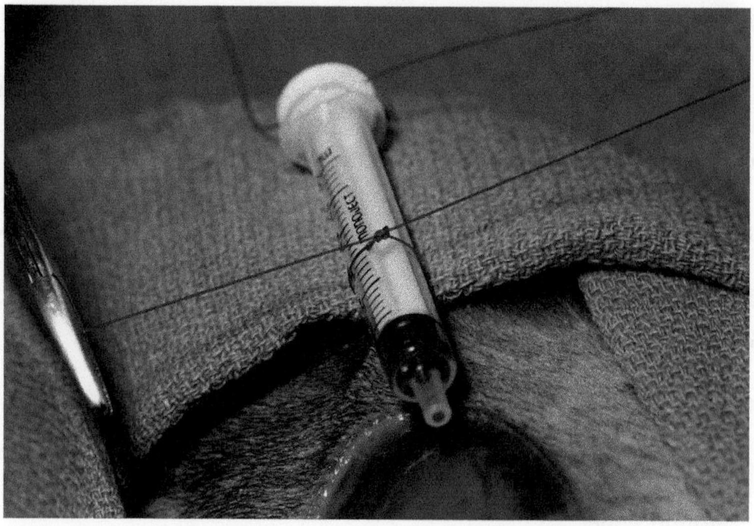

Figure 8-2 Loops can be formed and tied over a syringe or syringe case.

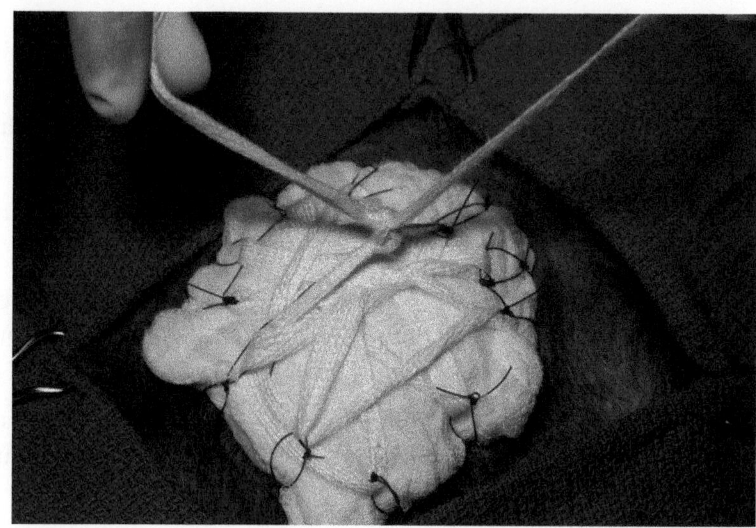

Figure 8-3 Secure the primary and secondary layers of the bandage with umbilical tape laced through the suture loops.

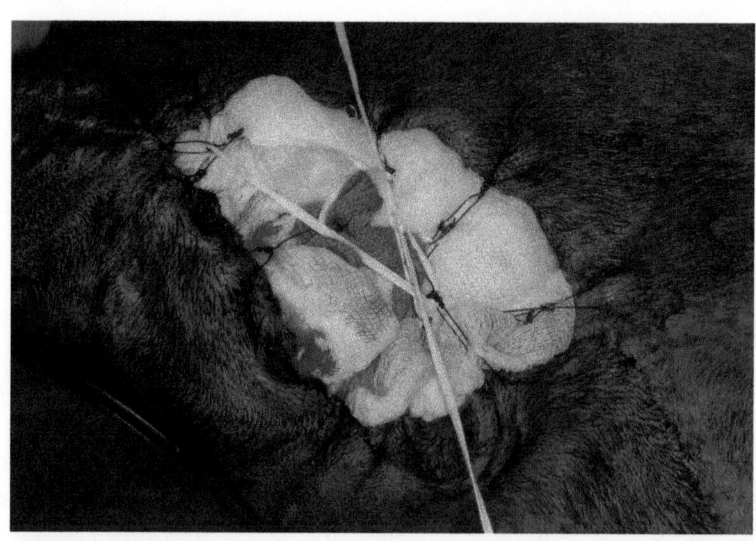

Figure 8-4 In this dog, the umbilical tape is tied too tightly, resulting in compression -of the skin. Tension should be gradually increased over several days to prevent skin damage.

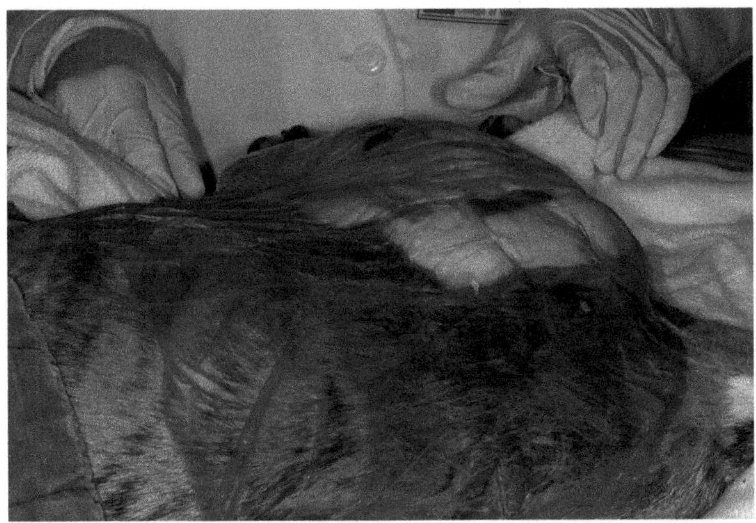

Figure 8-5 To keep the wound moist or prevent contamination or leakage, cover the bandage with an occlusive tertiary layer such as an antimicrobial-impregnated adhesive drape.

7. If desired, cover the tie-over bandage with an antimicrobial-impregnated translucent adhesive drape (fig. 8-5). Alternatively, cover the absorptive pad or sponge with a tertiary waterproof layer before tying on the bandage.

Postoperative considerations

Animals should wear Elizabethan collars until the wound is healed. Use of systemic antibiotics depends on results of the wound bed tissue culture. Topical antimicrobial dressings may be sufficient for animals with contaminated wounds or those with infection limited to the wound bed. Frequency of bandage changes depends on the amount of wound drainage. If skin stretching is desired, the umbilical tape laces should be tied in a bow or secured with an adjustable fastener. The laces are tightened two to three times a day to gradually increase tension on the skin. Most animals require sedation and analgesics during bandage changes for the first 3 to 5 days. If wounds are effusive or the laces are tight, the lacing material usually must be cut to change the bandage.

Open wounds may take weeks to months to heal by second intention, depending on wound size, infection, blood supply, and patient's health. In some patients, tie-over bandages are used until the wound is no longer infected and can be closed without tension.

Complications include suture loop failure or skin necrosis. Suture loops may pull out if they are placed too close to the edge of the tissues; occasionally they may need to be replaced as the distance between the skin edges decreases. Loops may turn into slipknots under tension. If the knots closest to the skin hitch, the underlying skin may necrose when the laces are tightened. Skin may also necrose if placed under too much tension.

Bibliography

Campbell BG: Dressings, bandages, and splints for wound management in dogs and cats. Vet Clin N Am 2006;36:759–791.

Pavletic MM: Use of an external skin-stretching device for wound closure in dogs and cats. J Am Vet Med Assoc 2000;217:350–354.

Pavletic MM: Wound care products and their use. Atlas of Small Animal Wound Management and Reconstructive Surgery, 3rd ed. Ames IA, Wiley-Blackwell, 2010, pp. 52–77.

Tobias J, Tobias KM: Tie-over bandage: it's a stretch! NAVC Clinician's Brief, August 2012, pp 34–37.

Section 2 Abdominal Procedures

Chapter 9
Abdominal Incisions

Surgical approach to the abdomen is commonly performed in veterinary practice. A few critical changes in the procedure have occurred over the last 3 decades. Suture apposition of the peritoneum is no longer performed since the peritoneum heals rapidly without closure. The abdominal musculature is often apposed with a simple continuous pattern, which is faster than interrupted closure and leaves less suture material in the wound, reducing foreign body reaction. Continuous closure has sufficient strength for uncomplicated healing as long as the external rectus sheath is included in each suture bite. If surgical technique is appropriate, use of a continuous closure does not increase the risk of incisional dehiscence.

Preoperative management

Postoperative pain is expected in any animal undergoing celiotomy and should be prevented. Pre-emptive analgesics may include opioids, nonsteroidal anti-inflammatory drugs, or a local or regional nerve block. The surgery site should be clipped, prepped, and draped widely to facilitate thorough exploration of the abdomen and allow incision extension as needed. In male dogs, the prepuce can be retracted to one side with a towel clamp and draped out of the surgical field. If the prepuce is left within the surgical field, it should be flushed with an antiseptic solution before the final prep. Balfour retractors, suction, and electrocautery should be available.

Surgery

Before the abdomen is opened, surgical sponges should be counted. Sponges should be recounted before abdominal closure to verify that none remain in the abdomen. Most frequently, the abdomen is opened along its ventral midline to avoid large vessels in the subcutis and muscle. In cats, the linea can be easily visualized once the subcutaneous fat has been incised. In dogs, subcutaneous fat attaches to the abdominal wall along the midline, obscuring the linea. Subcutaneous fat attachments to the linea can be transected sharply with a "push-cut" technique (described below) to reduce the risk of tissue trauma and seroma formation that can occur with extensive undermining. In patients that have previously undergone laparotomy, the initial linea perforation should be

Manual of Small Animal Soft Tissue Surgery, Second Edition. Karen Tobias.
© 2017 John Wiley & Sons, Inc. Published 2017 by John Wiley & Sons, Inc.

made in an unscarred area. Before extending the incision, the peritoneal surface of the linea should be palpated with an index finger or blunt instrument to verify that there are no visceral adhesions. The incision can be extended cranially superficial to the xiphoid to improve exposure of the diaphragm, liver, and stomach without inadvertently entering the chest (see fig. 20-10).

Once the abdomen is open, the falciform ligament can be torn along midline or freed from its lateral attachements, ligated at its base, and transected. In cats, the falciform ligament adheres to the peritoneal surface below the linea, making insertion of spay hooks more difficult. Exposure of abdominal organs can be maintained with appropriate retractors (e.g., Balfour retractors). If laparotomy pads are placed under the retractors along the incised margins of the abdominal wall edges, the portion of the pad contacting the viscera should be moistened with saline. Soaking the entire pad, however, will increase heat loss and risk of bacterial wicking from underlying skin surfaces.

The abdominal incision is usually closed in two or three layers. Abdominal musculature is apposed with monofilament, synthetic, absorbable material. Suture size depends on the thickness of the abdominal wall. Usually, cats are closed with 3-0 suture and giant breed dogs are closed with 0 suture. Strength of the closure is more dependent on bite size and location than suture size, however. Suture bites should include the external rectus fascia and should be at least 0.5 to 1 cm wide, depending on the animal's size. In very thin animals, sutures are often placed full thickness; including muscle fibers or peritoneum, however, does not increase the strength of the closure. The subcutaneous tissues should be apposed if there is dead space, persistent hemorrhage, or tension on the skin closure. Subcutaneous apposition will also provide an extra layer of protection if skin sutures are removed prematurely, and improves wound healing in cats.

Surgical technique: midline abdominal incision

1. Incise the skin.
   a. Stabilize the skin with the thumb and middle finger of your nondominant hand (fig. 9-1).
      i. If you are right-handed, stretch the skin at the left end of the proposed incision line with your left thumb and middle finger.

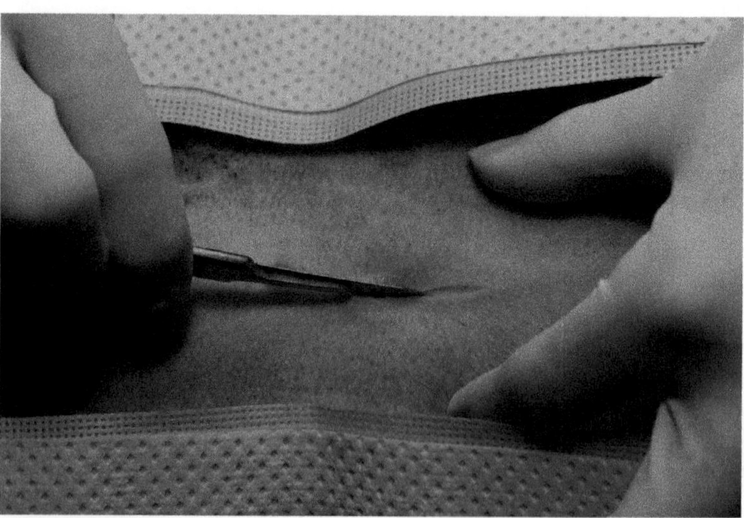

Figure 9-1 Stabilize and stretch the skin with the thumb and index finger of your nondominant hand while making the skin incision.

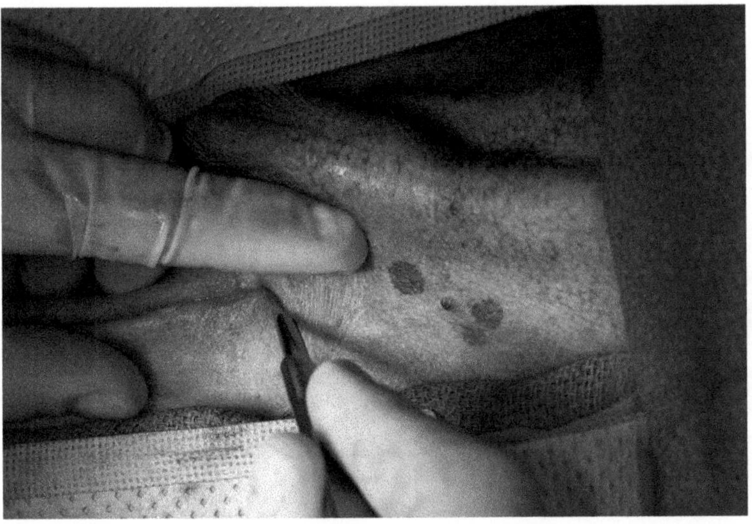

Figure 9-2 For caudal incisions in male dogs, continue incising the skin around the prepuce and lateral to the last nipple, staying superficial to the branches of the external pudendal vessels.

ii. Make sure your fingers stay within the sterile field and do not slip under the drape.

b. Hold the scalpel handle in your dominant hand to incise the skin.

i. For short incisions, use a pencil grip and cut with the tip of the blade.

ii. For long incisions, hold the scalpel handle parallel to the body wall with an overhand grip. Incise through the skin with the entire flat cutting edge of the blade. Move your nondominant hand caudally to keep the skin taut as you lengthen the incision.

c. In male dogs, extend caudal incisions around the prepuce (fig. 9-2), cutting only through skin to avoid inadvertently damaging the external pudendal vessels (fig. 9-3).

2. Extend the incision through the subcutaneous fat. Continue to stretch the skin and spread the incision edges with your nondominant thumb and middle finger as you incise.

a. In male dogs, identify and transect the ipsilateral preputial muscle (fig. 9-4). These muscle ends should be reapposed during closure.

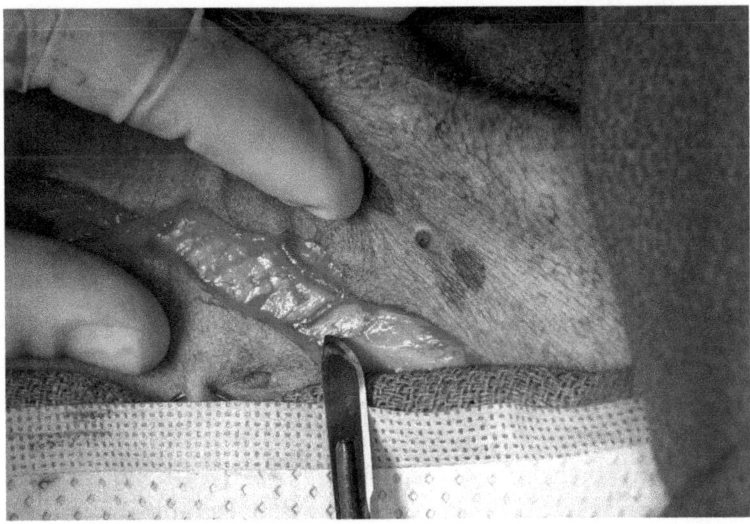

Figure 9-3 Branches of the external pudendal vessels.

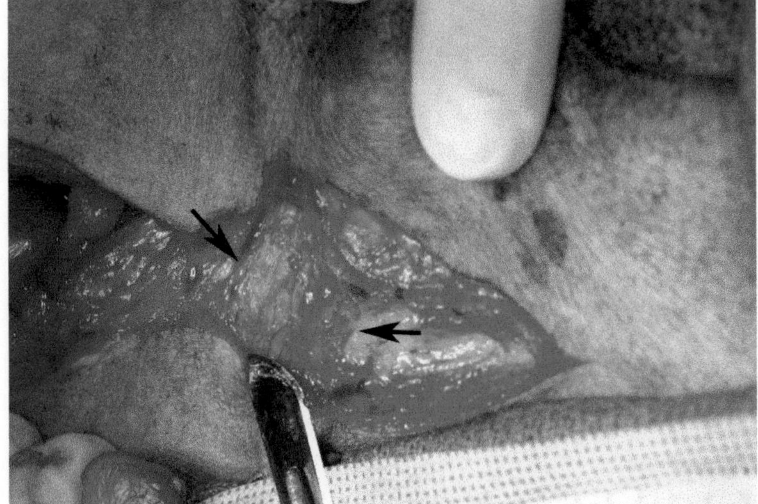

Figure 9-4 Right preputial muscle (between arrows).

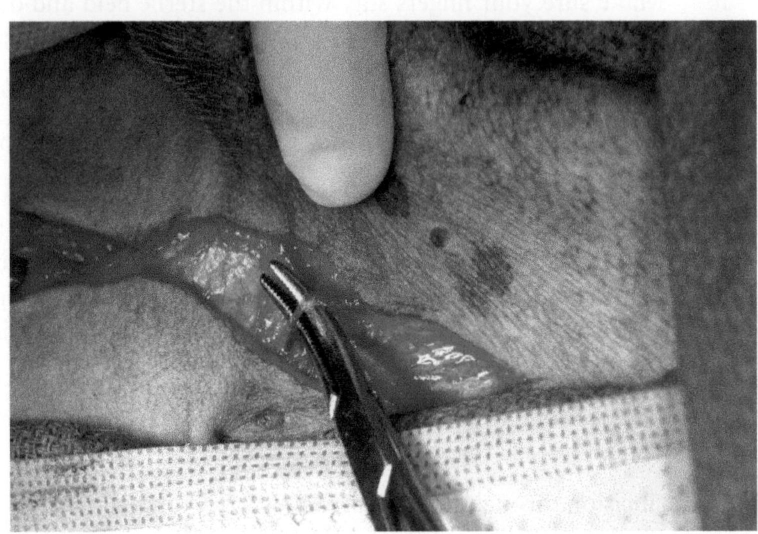

Figure 9-5 Isolate and ligate branches of the external pudendal vessels.

b. In male dogs, ligate and transect preputial branches of the external pudendal vein before deepening the peripreputial subcutaneous incision (fig. 9-5).

3. In dogs, transect the subcutaneous tissue attachments to the linea with a push-cut technique.

   a. Start the dissection at the same end of the incision line as your dominant hand.

   b. With thumb forceps, grasp the subcutaneous fat adjacent to one side of the incision line. Lift upward to elevate and tense the tissue.

   c. With scissor tips facing upwards, insert one scissor blade of a curved Metzenbaum scissors into the fat near its linea attachment (fig. 9-6).

   d. Transect the subcutaneous attachments to the linea with a push-cut technique. Slide the scissors forward, partially closed, as if you were cutting wrapping paper. Keep them against the abdominal wall so that the fat is transected close to the linea without cutting the rectus sheath.

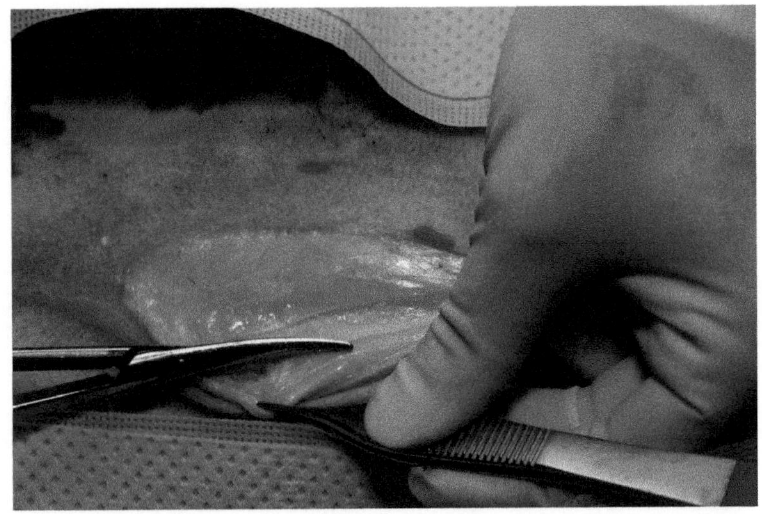

Figure 9-6 Elevate the subcutaneous fat at one end of the incision and insert one scissor blade through the subcutaneous attachment near the linea. Push-cut to transect attachments.

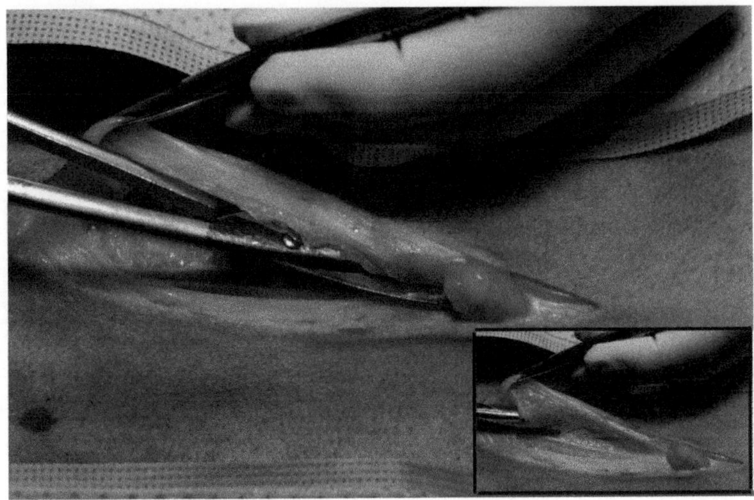

Figure 9-7 Repeat on the opposite side. Position the scissors with the tips curved up and the blades close to the base of the fat attachment and partially closed.

   e. If a push-cut technique is not sufficient, actively cut attachments, especially at the umbilicus or previous surgical sites.
   f. Repeat on the opposite side of the incision (fig. 9-7) to expose the linea (fig. 9-8).
4. Make a stab incision through the linea (fig. 9-9).
   a. Elevate the linea with thumb forceps. Tent the abdominal wall away from underlying viscera.
   b. Hold the scalpel handle in an overhand grip with the blade's cutting edge facing up. Angle the handle so that it is parallel with the body wall.
   c. Sharply and firmly penetrate the tented linea 1 cm away from the thumb forceps (fig. 9-9). Keep the blade parallel to and above the abdominal wall.
      i. If the blade is inserted too close to the thumb forceps, it will hit the thumb forceps and will not fully penetrate into the abdomen.

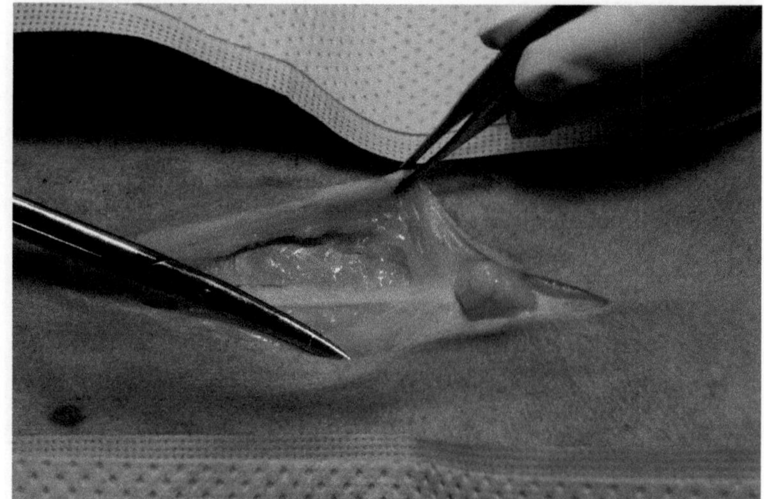

Figure 9-8 Exposed linea. This dog has an umbilical hernia.

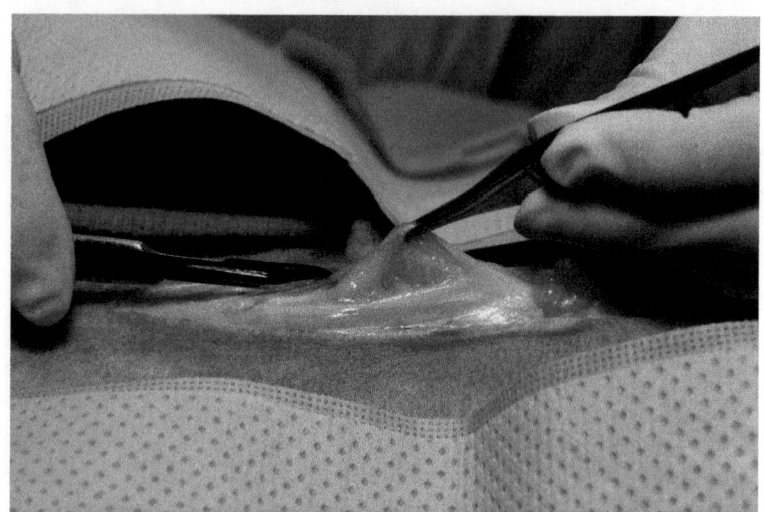

Figure 9-9 Elevate the linea with thumb forceps and perforate it with a blade.

ii. If the blade is inserted off midline, it will cut along the muscle planes, leaving the peritoneum intact.

iii. If the blade is angled down toward the abdominal cavity, it may inadvertently penetrate viscera.

d. Insert an index finger or closed, blunt tip scissors into the incision and palpate or sweep cranially and caudally to verify there are no visceral adhesions at the linea.

5. Extend the linea incision cranially with curved Mayo scissors or a blade.

a. Extend the incision with curved Mayo scissors (fig. 9-10).

i. Hold the scissors so that the concave surface faces the surgeon and the tips are directed cranially.

ii. Extend the incision cranially with several short cuts.

iii. Reposition the scissors in your dominant hand so that the tips are directed caudally and the concave surface faces the surgeon,

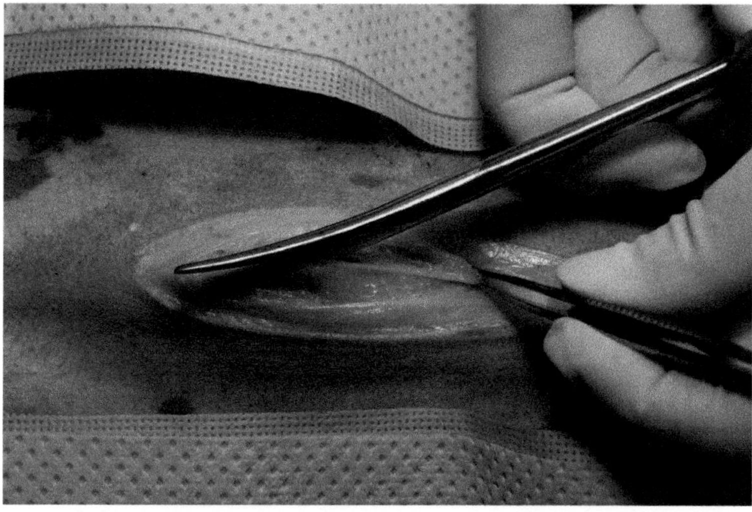

Figure 9-10 Extend the linea incision with Mayo scissors.

and cut the linea caudally. Note: to cut in the caudal direction, the scissors are held in a normal grip but with the wrist extended instead of mildly flexed.

b. Alternatively, extend the incision with a blade.
   i. Grasp a pair of thumb forceps in the fist of one hand.
   ii. Insert the apposed tips of the thumb forceps through the linea incision, and lift up the abdominal wall.
   iii. Place the cutting edge of the scalpel blade between the arms of the forceps and against the edge of the incision.
   iv. Cut the tissues between the arms of the forceps with the blade while advancing the forceps simultaneously. The forceps will keep the abdominal wall elevated and protect any underlying viscera from inadvertent incision.

6. Remove the falciform ligament as needed.
   a. Cut or cauterize the lateral attachments (fig. 9-11).
   b. Ligate the ligament at its cranial base with 2-0 or 3-0 suture (fig. 9-12).

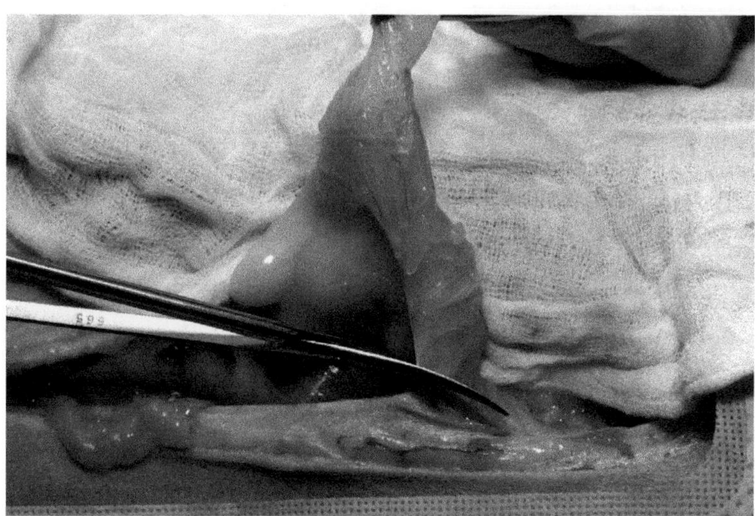

Figure 9-11 Transect lateral attachments of the falciform ligament with scissors or electrocautery.

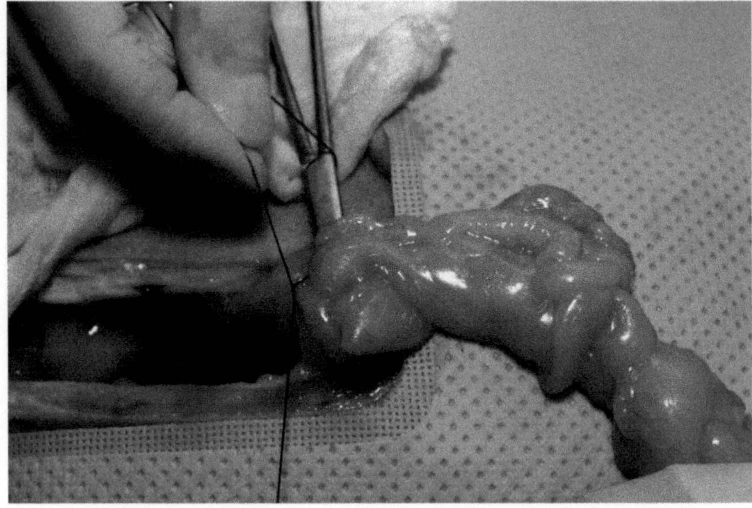

Figure 9-12 Ligate the base of the falciform ligament before transecting.

7. Place abdominal wall retractors. Make sure the incision is long enough to prevent trauma near its ends from excessive tension during retraction. In small animals, baby Balfour retractors can be secured to the abdominal wall muscle with towel clamps to prevent them from shifting.

Surgical technique: abdominal wall closure

1. Use 0, 2-0, or 3-0 synthetic absorbable monofilament suture on a taper needle in large, medium, or small animals, respectively.
2. Take a bite across one end of the incision line and tie two or three knots.
    a. To expose the external rectus sheath on the far side of the incision, use your needle temporarily as a retractor (fig. 9-13).
        i. Take a bite of the skin and subcutaneous tissues with your suture needle and retract the tissues laterally with the needle.
        ii. Grasp the edge of the external rectus sheath with thumb forceps. Pull the external rectus sheath across midline and away from the retracted subcutaneous tissues.

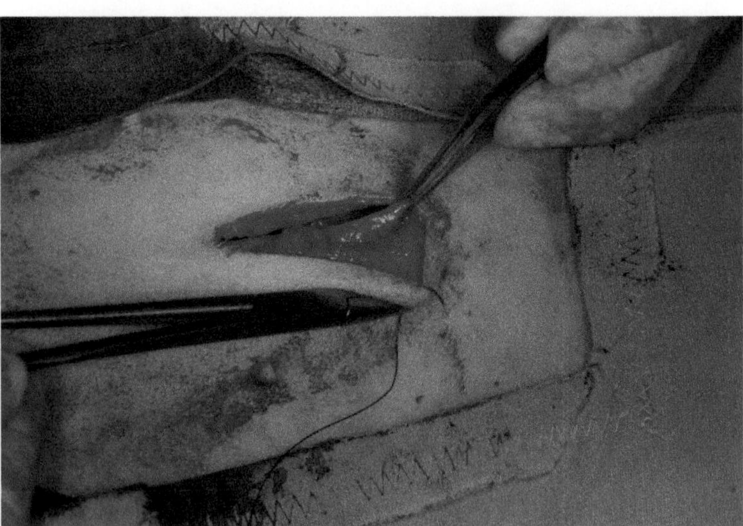

Figure 9-13 To expose the rectus sheath, retract the skin and subcutaneous tissues temporarily with the needle.

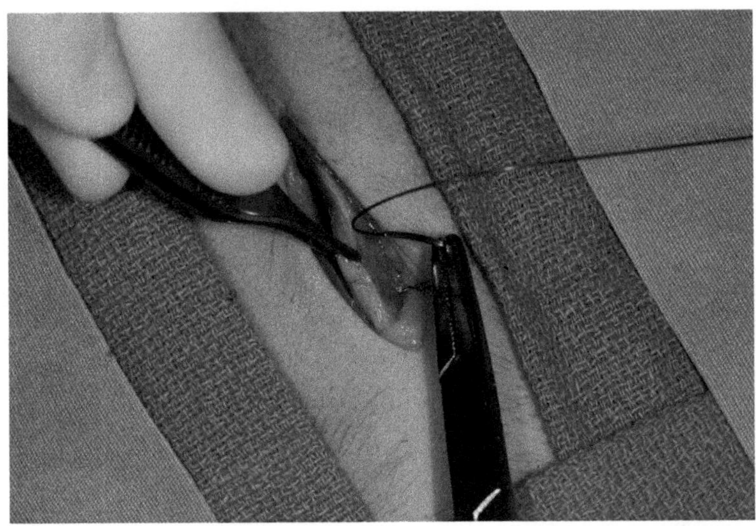

Figure 9-14 Grasp the external rectus muscle with thumb forceps and pull it toward the contralateral side as you take bites of the white fascial sheath.

  iii. Release the skin and subcutis from the needle and take a 5- to 10-mm-wide bite of the fibrous external rectus sheath (fig. 9-14). Pull the needle through the tissues and reposition it on the needle holder.

b. Take a 5- to 10-mm bite of the external rectus sheath on the near (contralateral) side of the incision.
  i. If the external rectus sheath is visible on the near side, grasp it with thumb forceps. Pull the external rectus sheath toward midline while taking bites of the ventral (external) fascial layer.
  ii. If the external rectus sheath is obscured by overlying tissues, push the skin and subcutis away from the external rectus sheath with closed thumb forceps to expose the fascia, and take a bite of the fascia.
  iii. If the fascial bite is poorly placed, grasp the rectus sheath edge with thumb forceps before releasing the tissue off of the needle, and pull the rectus sheath toward midline before taking a better bite.
c. Tie a surgeon's throw and tighten to appose the rectus sheath without crushing it.
d. Add an additional four or five simple throws to form several knots.
  i. To tie square knots, pull on the suture ends in a horizontal plane perpendicular to the incision line. As you tighten the suture, watch each throw to make sure it remains horizontal and drops directly over the incision line.
  ii. If the short end of the suture sticks straight up ("hitches") during knot tying, pull harder on the long (needle) end with your nondominant hand while slightly relaxing your dominant hand to resolve the hitching.

3. Continue the closure in a simple continuous pattern with bites 5 to 10 mm apart and 5 to 10 mm wide, depending on the size of the animal.

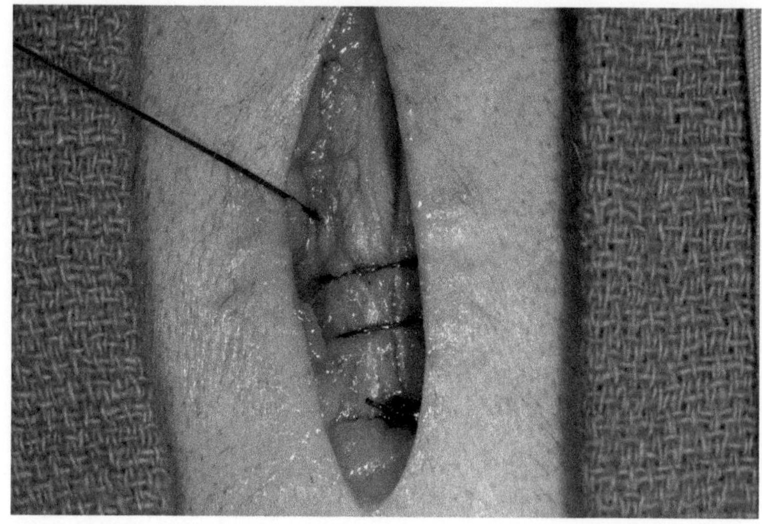

Figure 9-15 Take bites of fascia at least 5 mm wide on each side. If bites are taken correctly, the fascia will appose on the midline and no muscle fibers will be visible.

Gently tighten the suture after each set of bites to appose the rectus fascia (fig. 9-15).

4. One-third and two-thirds of the way through the closure, insert an index finger into the abdominal cavity and palpate the peritoneal surface of the closed incision. If the external rectus sheath was not included in the suture bites, palpable gaps will be present.
5. Tie off the suture pattern to a final loop with three knots (fig 9-16).
   a. Leave the loop at least 2 cm long to facilitate placement of square throws.
   b. Tighten each throw with the needle holder jaws open on the loop so that both sides of the loop tighten.
   c. When tightening, keep hands and suture low and close to the incision (especially the dominant hand) and pull so that the throw remains

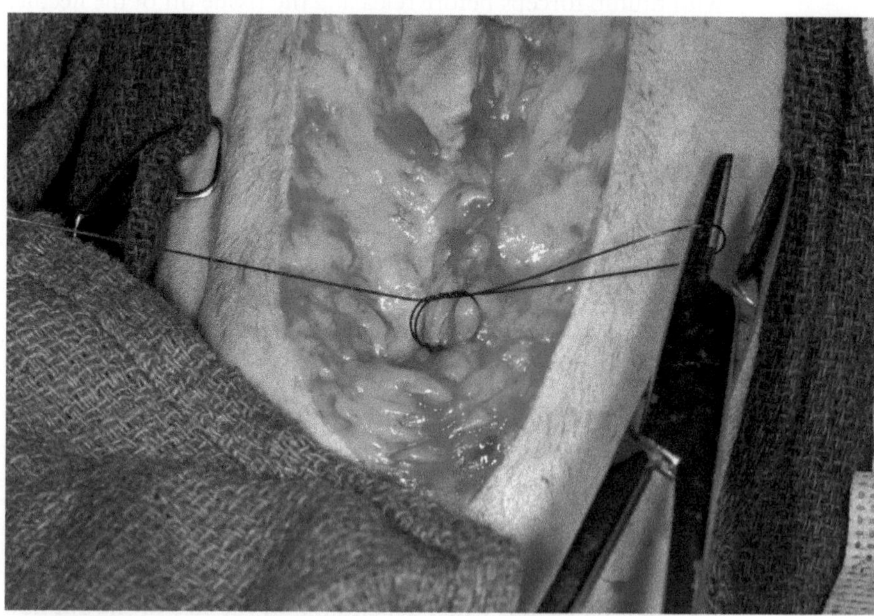

Figure 9-16 To form square knots, make sure each throw maintains a position that is horizontally oriented and directly over the incision line.

horizontally oriented and directly over the incision. This usually requires pulling harder with the nondominant hand.

6. Cut suture ends 3 to 5 mm away from the knots.
7. In male dogs, appose the preputial muscle ends and close peripreputial dead space with interrupted sutures of absorbable monofilament.
8. Close subcutaneous tissues and skin routinely.

Postoperative considerations

Some swelling is expected along the incision line after celiotomy. Cats, however, can develop significant tissue reaction and thickening that can be confused with herniation. Unlike hernias, this swelling is firm, nonpainful, and irreducible and usually extends the entire length of the incision line. Tissue reaction is more severe with traumatic surgical technique, excessive dissection, suture material reaction, excessive postoperative activity, or incisional trauma. Tissue reaction in cats usually resolves within a month after surgery.

Abdominal hernias may occur from musculofascial weakness secondary to underlying disease or, more commonly, because of poor surgical technique. The external rectus sheath can be easily missed if the overlying subcutaneous fat has not been elevated or if the external rectus sheath is everted during closure. Eversion of the sheath reduces the amount of exposed rectus fascia, increasing the chance that it will be inadvertently excluded during suture placement. Pullout force of suture is primarily related to bite size and fascial thickness; therefore, wide bites of the external rectus sheath will strengthen the closure. Knots can fail if half-hitched. Half-hitching occurs easily with monofilament, synthetic suture material. It can be avoided by pulling harder on the long (needle) end of the suture with the nondominant hand and relaxing the dominant hand so that the throw remains horizontally oriented as it is tightened.

Other potential complications include seroma formation, incisional infection, dehiscence, ileus, peritonitis, and seeding of tumor cells. If the incision site is extended too far cranially, the diaphragm may be inadvertently perforated, resulting in a pneumothorax. Deep penetration during linea incision could damage underlying viscera, resulting in peritonitis (see chapter 15). Incisional infection rates are positively correlated with duration of anesthesia and surgery. Infection rates for surgeries lasting 90 minutes are doubled compared with those lasting 60 minutes. Clipping the surgery site 4 or more hours before surgery also increases the risk of infection. Incisional infections that do not respond to systemic antibiotics may require open drainage. Dogs with suture reaction may develop firm, red, swollen incision lines and draining tracts. If tissue cultures are negative, dogs with severe suture reaction may require glucocorticoid treatment or aggressive body wall resection to resolve the condition.

Bibliography

Campbell JA et al: A biomechanical study of suture pullout in linea alba. Surgery 1989;106:888–892.

Freeman LJ et al: Tissue reaction to suture material in the feline linea alba: a retrospective, prospective, and histologic study. Vet Surg 1987;16:440–445.

Mayhew PD, Freeman L, Kwan T, et al: Comparison of surgical site infection rates in clean and clean-contaminated wounds in dogs and cats after minimally invasive versus open surgery: 179 cases (2007–2008). J Am Vet Med Assoc 2012;240:193–198.

Muir P et al: Incisional swelling following celiotomy in cats. Vet Rec 1993;132:189–190.

Probst CW et al: Duration of pneumoperitoneum in the dog. Am J Vet Res 1986;47:176–178.

Rosin E: Single layer, simple continuous suture pattern for closure of abdominal incisions. J Am Anim Hosp Assoc 1985;6:751–756.

Tobias KM: Laparotomy: complications. NAVC Clinician's Brief 2005;3:13–18.

Chapter 10
Umbilical Hernia

In the fetus, the umbilical aperture provides passage for umbilical blood vessels, the vitelline duct, and the stalk of the allantois. After these structures are disrupted at birth, the umbilical opening closes rapidly. Congenital persistence of the umbilical aperture may allow herniation of abdominal contents—usually fat or omentum. Occasionally, the umbilical ring will scar down around herniated omentum or fat, resulting in a nonreducible button of tissue at the umbilicus. Animals with umbilical hernias are usually asymptomatic, except for a small, soft, nonpainful swelling. Rarely, intestines or other structures may herniate. In most animals, umbilical hernias are clinically insignificant and repair is performed for cosmetic reasons. Umbilical hernias may close spontaneously as late as 6 months of age.

Preoperative management

Unless hernia contents are incarcerated or strangulated, umbilical hernias are usually repaired at the time of ovariohysterectomy or castration. Minimal preoperative diagnostics are required in healthy animals. A thorough physical examination should be performed, since animals with umbilical hernias may have other congenital anomalies such as cryptorchidism, ventricular septal defects, or inguinal or peritoneopericardial diaphragmatic hernias. The ventral abdomen should be clipped and prepped routinely, as for an ovariohysterectomy.

Surgery

Some clinicians will "freshen" the edges of hernia rings by excising a few mm of the muscular or fascial margin. In most animals, the abdominal wall will heal if the edges of the hernia ring are directly apposed without marginal resection.

Surgical technique

1. Make a ventral midline incision through the skin.
    a. If the hernia is small and contains only fat, incise directly over the contents (See fig. 9-8 p. 86).

Manual of Small Animal Soft Tissue Surgery, Second Edition. Karen Tobias.
© 2017 John Wiley & Sons, Inc. Published 2017 by John Wiley & Sons, Inc.

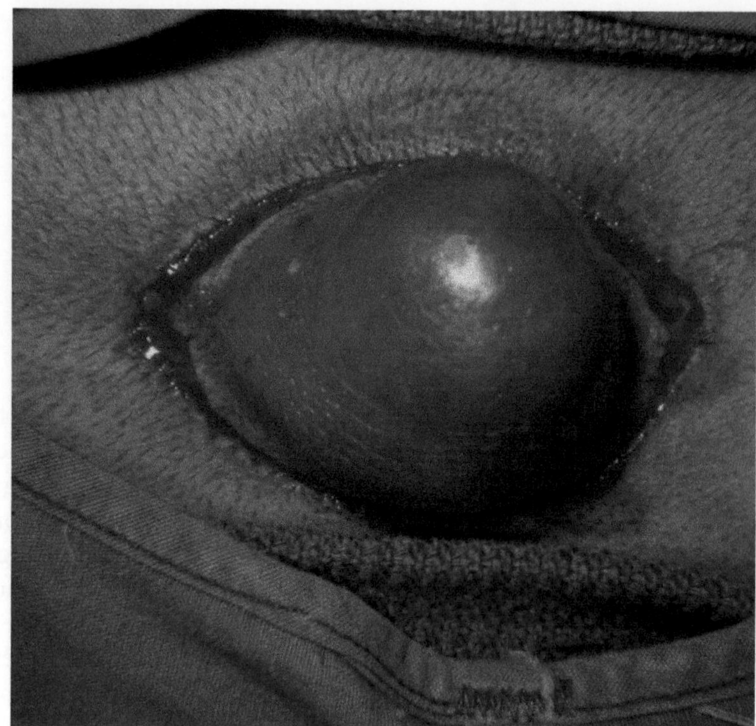

Figure 10-1 Incise the skin around the hernia if it is thin, inflamed, or necrotic.

b. If the hernia contains incarcerated or necrotic tissue, begin the skin incision caudal to the hernia. Elevate the skin over the hernia with blunt dissection and carefully extend the incision cranially to avoid damaging entrapped viscera.

c. If the hernia skin is thin, inflamed, or necrotic, incise around the hernia (fig. 10-1).

2. Dissect the subcutaneous tissues away from the hernia contents (fig. 10-2).
3. Reduce or remove the hernial contents (fig. 10-3).

a. If the hernia contents are healthy and easily reducible, return them to the abdominal cavity.

b. If the hernia contains entrapped fat or omentum that is adhered to the external abdominal fascia, amputate the protruding tissue. Ligation of fat or omentum may be necessary in some animals.

c. If the hernia contains incarcerated or devitalized intestine, or the animal is concurrently undergoing ovariohysterectomy, enlarge the hernial ring.

i. Make a midline incision through the linea 1 to 3 cm caudal to the hernia.

ii. Insert an index finger to identify the location of the hernial ring internally (fig. 10-4).

iii. Cautiously extend the linea incision cranially until the hernial ring has been transected.

iv. Resect any devitalized contents.

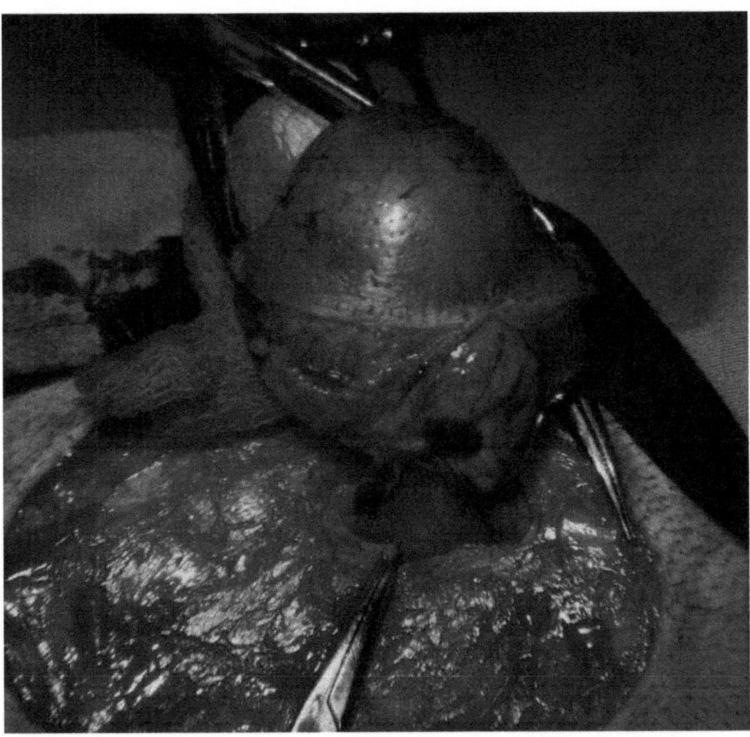

Figure 10-2 Dissect the subcutaneous tissues away from the hernia contents.

4. Reappose the external rectus sheath with simple interrupted or simple continuous sutures of absorbable monofilament material.
   a. Include the hernia site as part of the routine abdominal wall closure in animals undergoing ovariohysterectomy or laparotomy.
   b. Use interrupted sutures in dogs with excessive tension or hernia recurrence.

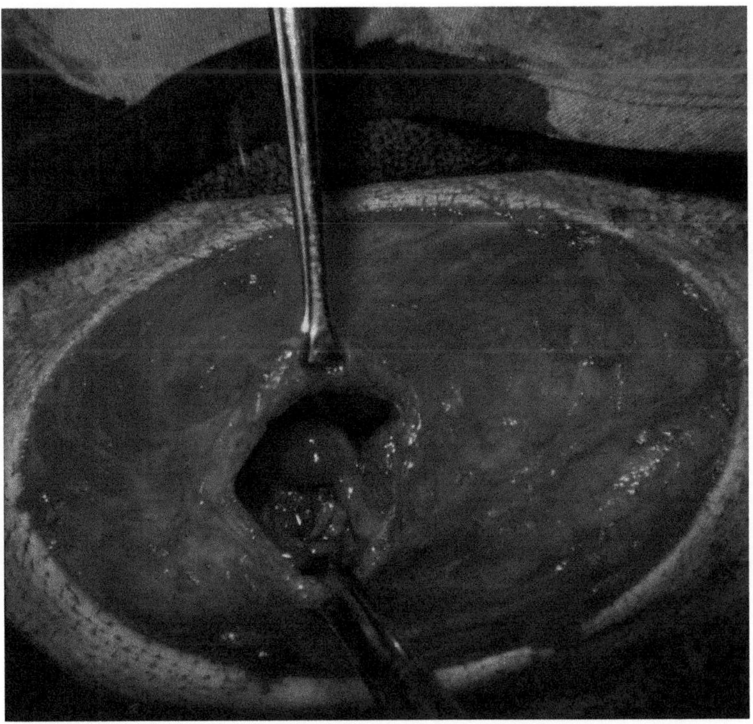

Figure 10-3 Expose rectus edges along the hernia opening.

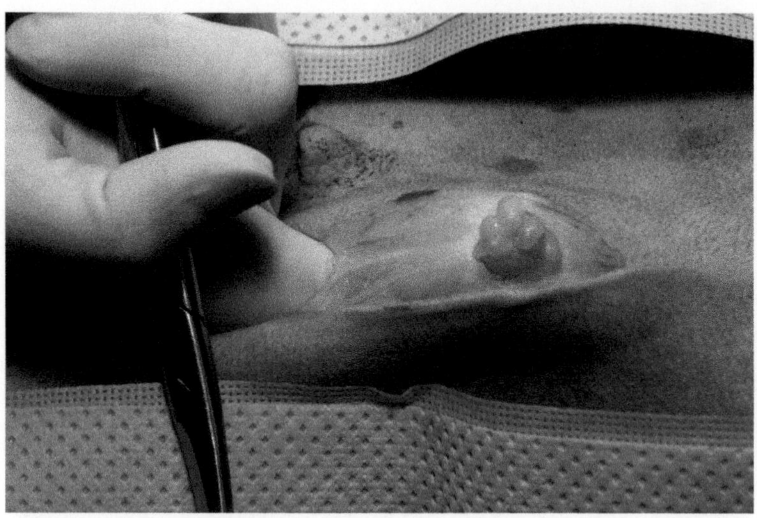

Figure 10-4 For a more cautious approach, incise the linea caudal to the hernia and locate the ring by digital palpation before extending the incision cranially.

5. If redundant skin is present, resect a portion before closing the subcutaneous tissues and skin routinely.

Postoperative considerations

Activity should be restricted for 1 to 2 weeks. Complications are uncommon after umbilical hernia repair. Hernias may reoccur if external rectus suture bites are too small, spaced too widely, or do not contain rectus fascia. Occasionally, hernias will reoccur in animals with abnormal fibrous tissue development. These animals may require placement of a synthetic mesh over the hernia site to strengthen additional repairs.

Bibliography

Pratschke K: Management of hernias and ruptures in small animals. In Practice 2002; Nov/Dec: 570–581.

Chapter 11

Inguinal Hernia

The inguinal canal, which is located about 1 cm craniomedial to the femoral ring, is a fissure or potential space between the abdominal muscles and their aponeuroses. In the male dog, the inguinal canal provides a passageway for testicular descent and contains the spermatic cord contents, including the ductus deferens and testicular artery, vein, and nerve. The cremaster muscle originates from the deeper, cranial border of the canal. The genitofemoral nerve, external pudendal artery and vein, and vaginal process—a peritoneal outpouching—pass through the canal in male and female dogs (fig. 11-1). In female dogs, the round ligament of the uterus extends from the uterine horn through the ipsilateral inguinal canal to the vulva. The inguinal canal and rings are bounded cranially by the transversus abdominus and internal abdominal oblique muscles, medially by the rectus abdominus muscle, and caudolaterally by the inguinal ligament. The superficial inguinal ring (fig. 11-1), a slit in the external abdominal oblique aponeurosis, is located 2 to 4 cm lateral to the linea alba.

Congenital or traumatic enlargement of the inguinal canal may permit herniation of abdominal contents. The most common contents within inguinal hernias are fat and omentum; however, intestinal herniation is reported in 35% of affected dogs. Bladder or uterus may also be herniated (fig. 11-2). Organs may herniate alongside or within the vaginal process (direct and indirect hernias, respectively). In male dogs, herniation within the vaginal process may extend caudally to become a scrotal hernia.

Inguinal hernias are most frequently reported in female dogs. Clinical signs depend on hernia size and contents and may vary from nonpainful swelling to visceral obstruction, shock, and death. Hernias most commonly occur on the left side. Bilateral hernias are reported in 17% of dogs. Diagnosis is based on palpation, radiographs, and ultrasonography. In male dogs, scrotal hernias must be differentiated from testicular torsion, infection, or neoplasia.

Preoperative management

Depending on the severity of clinical signs, affected patients should be evaluated for sepsis, disseminated intravascular coagulation, electrolyte- and acid-based abnormalities, hypoglycemia, and renal dysfunction. If possible, patients should be stabilized before surgery. Digital rectal examination should be performed, since some dogs may have concurrent perineal hernias.

Manual of Small Animal Soft Tissue Surgery, Second Edition. Karen Tobias.
© 2017 John Wiley & Sons, Inc. Published 2017 by John Wiley & Sons, Inc.

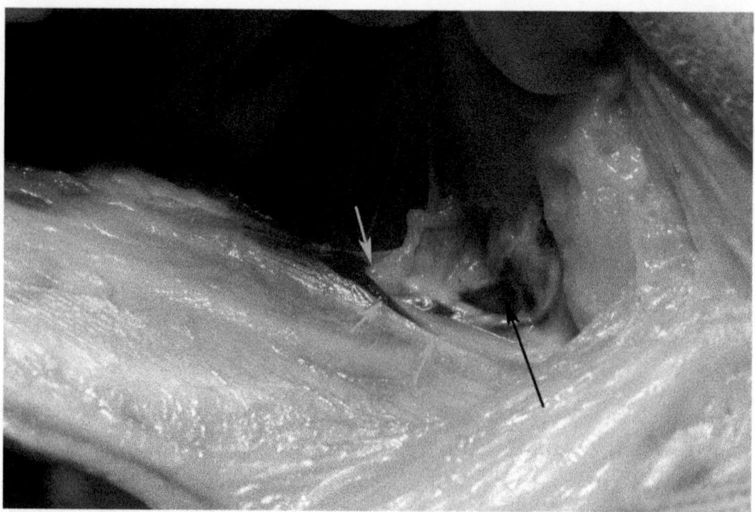

Figure 11-1 The superficial inguinal ring (green arrows) is a slit in the external abdominal oblique aponeurosis. The external pudendal artery and vein (black arrow), genitofemoral nerve, vaginal process, and spermatic cord or round ligament of the uterus exit the abdomen from this site.

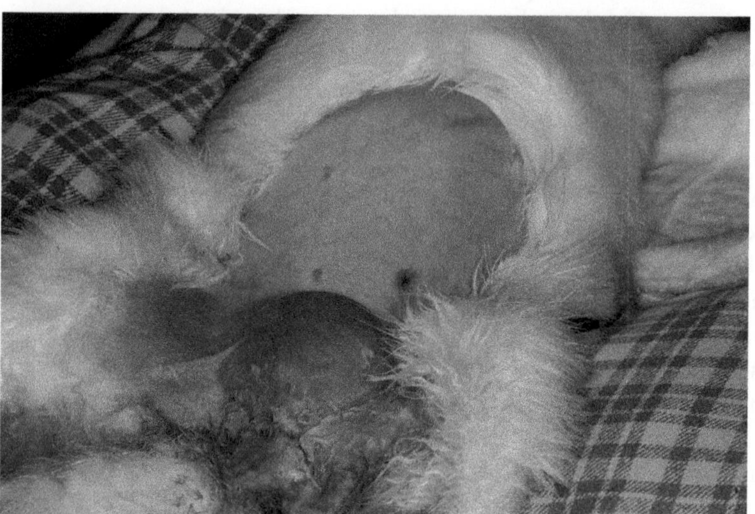

Figure 11-2 Inguinal hernia with incarcerated bladder.

Emergency surgery should be performed in animals with evidence of visceral obstruction or ischemia or herniation of a gravid uterus that is infected or contains dead fetuses. Dogs with intestinal herniation that have been vomiting for 2 to 6 days before diagnosis are more likely to have nonviable intestines at surgery.

Surgery

Unilateral hernias can be approached through an incision directly over the superficial inguinal ring. Bilateral hernias are approached through two separate inguinal incisions or through a larger ventral midline incision that is retracted toward the hernia being repaired (fig. 11-3). A ventral midline celiotomy is also performed in animals with obstructed or devitalized organs (fig. 11-2) or that require ovariohysterectomy.

Organs that are distended or necrotic may be difficult to return to the abdomen. In this case, the inguinal canal should be enlarged cranially to permit

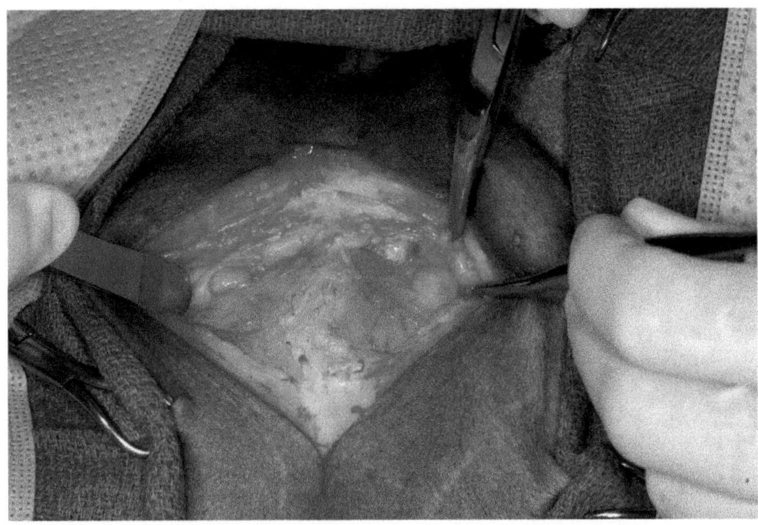

Figure 11-3 Midline approach for bilateral inguinal hernias. In this dog most of the herniated fat on the left side has been reduced into the abdomen.

reduction of viscera. Damaged viscera are resected once they have been returned to the abdomen. Neutering of affected intact animals is recommended, since the defect may be heritable in some breeds. Fetuses can be successfully carried to term when a herniated gravid uterus is returned to the abdomen by the seventh week of pregnancy.

Surgical technique: inguinal herniorrhaphy

1. Palpate both inguinal rings under anesthesia to determine if the condition is unilateral or bilateral.
2. Make a caudal ventral midline skin incision (fig. 11-3) or, for small unilateral hernias, incise directly over the inguinal hernia or superficial inguinal ring.
3. With Metzenbaum scissors, bluntly and sharply dissect the subcutaneous tissues away from external abdominal fascia and reflect them away from the external rectus sheath and hernial sac.
4. Return the hernial contents to the abdomen.
   a. If hernia contents are freely movable and not swollen, gently milk the contents and the hernia sac back into the abdominal cavity.
   b. If hernia contents are trapped but viable, enlarge the inguinal canal cranially by incising the hernial sac (fig. 11-4), external abdominal oblique aponeurosis (figs. 11-5 and 11-6), and, if necessary, the transversus abdominus and internal abdominal oblique muscles.
   c. If hernia contents are swollen or ischemic, perform a midline celiotomy. Incise the hernial sac and enlarge the inguinal canal (fig. 11-7), as described above, and excise devitalized tissues as needed.
5. Transect the hernial sac at its fascial attachments and remove it. Alternatively, if the sac is easily reducible and does not interfere with visualization of abdominal wall fascia, invert the sac into the abdominal cavity.
6. Close any inguinal muscle incision from side to side with interrupted sutures of 2-0 or 3-0 absorbable monofilament material.

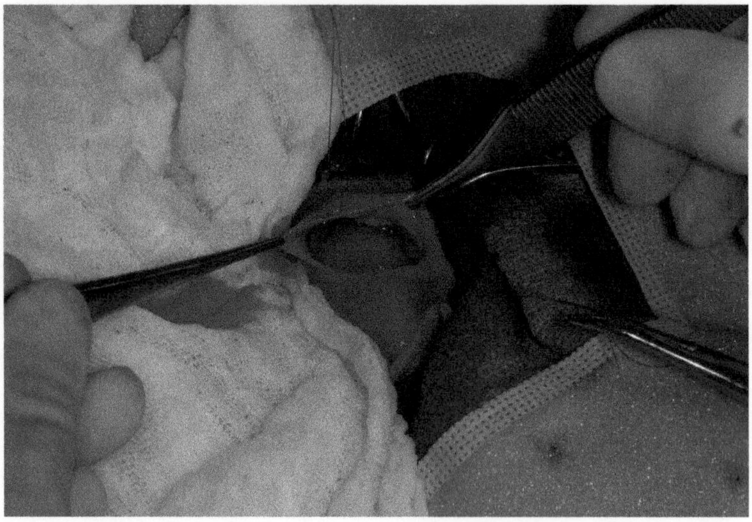

Figure 11-4 The hernia sac has been incised to expose the contents.

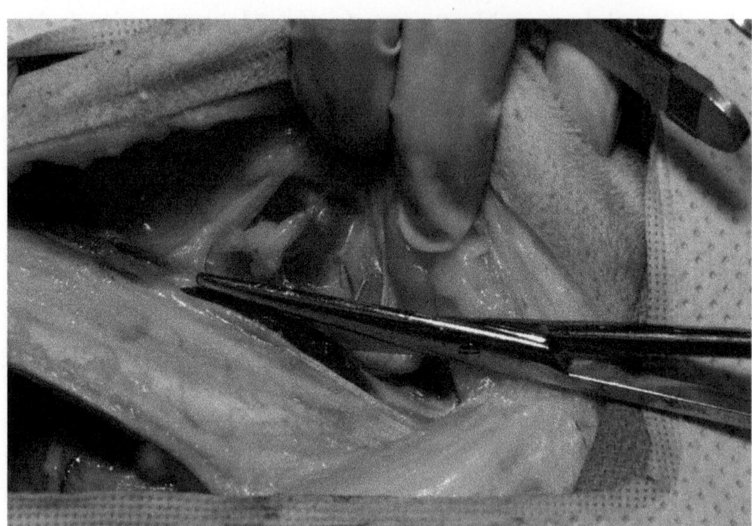

Figure 11-5 To enlarge the hernia ring, incise the external abdominal oblique aponeurosis cranially with scissors.

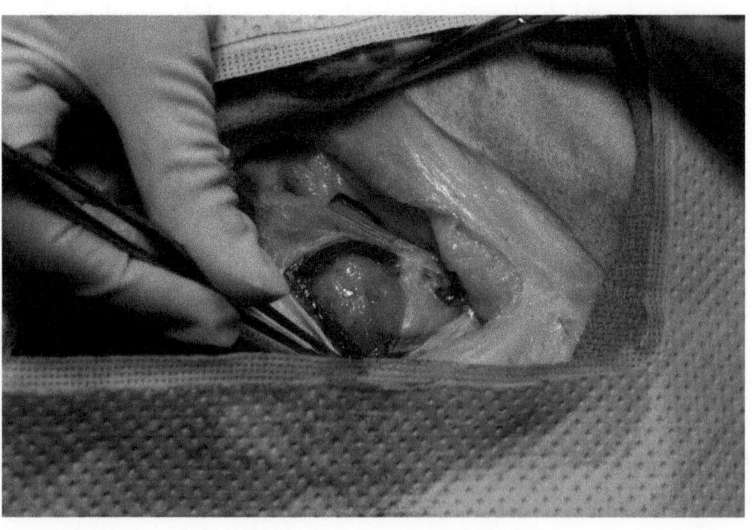

Figure 11-6 Enlarged ring.

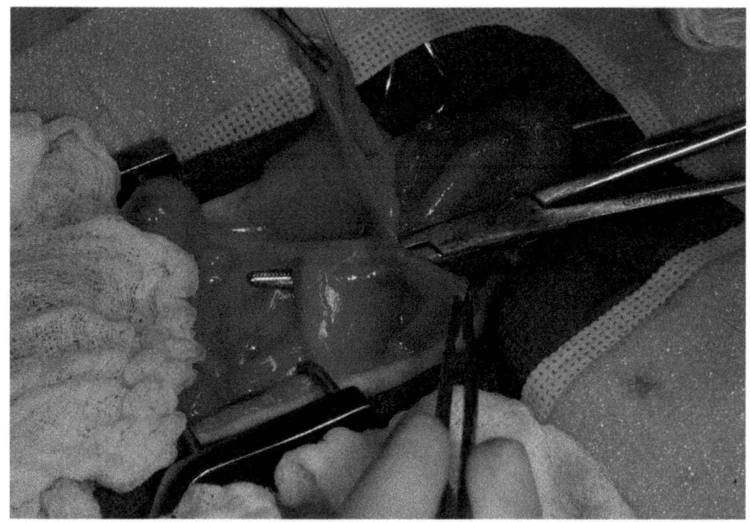

Figure 11-7 To reduce the incarcerated bladder in the animal in fig. 11-2, a combined abdominal and inguinal approach was used. A Carmalt forceps was passed between the entrapped bladder and the abdominal wall to protect the viscera during ring enlargement.

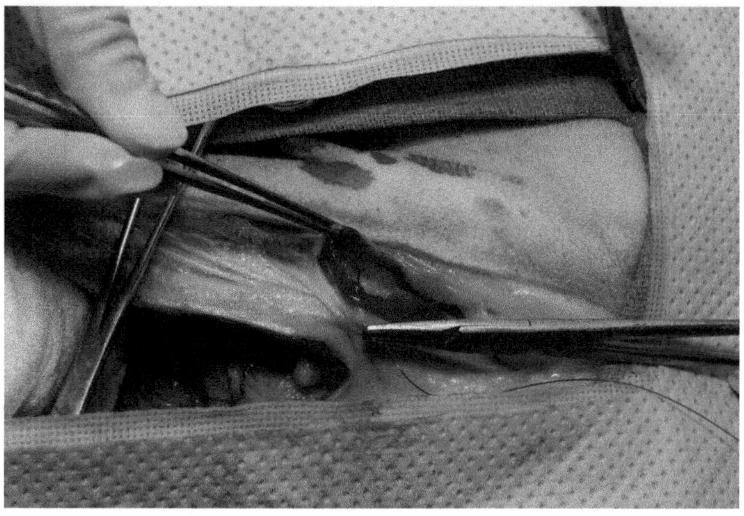

Figure 11-8 Appose the muscle with interrupted sutures, taking wide bites. Include external fascia in all suture bites.

7. Appose the external abdominal oblique aponeurosis from side to side with simple interrupted sutures of 2-0 or 3-0 absorbable monofilament (fig. 11-8), leaving a gap caudally for passage of any vessels and nerves and, in intact males, the spermatic cord (fig. 11-9).

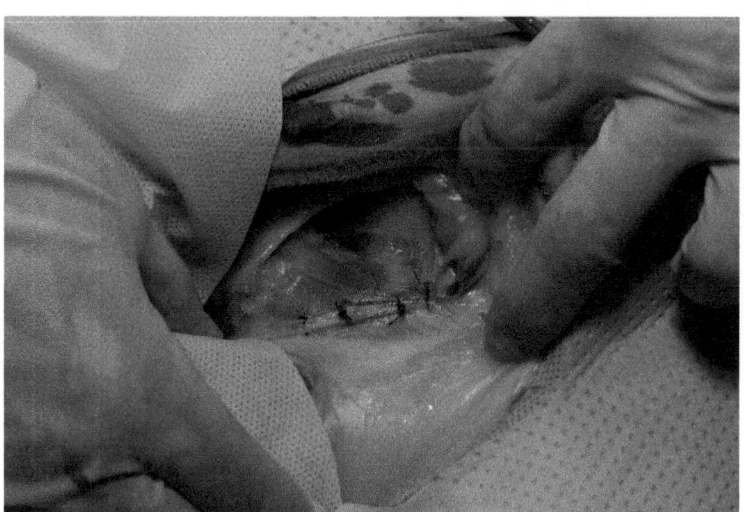

Figure 11-9 Leave a gap in the inguinal ring caudally to prevent compression of vessels and nerves.

8. Obliterate subcutaneous dead space by closing the subcutis in multiple layers with monofilament absorbable suture, tacking the deepest layer to the external abdominal oblique aponeurosis.
9. Close the skin routinely.

Postoperative considerations

Exercise should be limited during recovery, and analgesics are usually administered for several days. Animals that have undergone intestinal resection and anastomosis should be monitored for intestinal leakage (see p. 121). Postoperative complications are reported in 17% of animals and include swelling, incisional infection, dehiscence, peritonitis, sepsis, vomiting, and recurrence. Recurrence is uncommon.

Bibliography

Pratschke K: Management of hernias and ruptures in small animals. In Practice 2002; Nov/Dec:570–581.

Shahar R: A possible association between acquired nontraumatic inguinal and perineal hernia in adult male dogs. Can Vet J 1996;37:614–616.

Waters DJ et al: A retrospective study of inguinal hernia in 35 dogs. Vet Surg 1993;22:44–49.

Chapter 12
Diaphragmatic Hernia

Diaphragmatic hernia can occur as a congenital defect or secondary to trauma. In animals with congenital hernias, most often the hernia is classified as peritoneopericardial, with continuity of the peritoneal cavity and pericardial sac. Peritoneopericardial diaphragmatic hernia (PPDH) can be an incidental finding or can cause gastrointestinal or respiratory signs. Fat, liver, or other abdominal contents herniate into the pericardial sac, reducing intrathoracic volume. Affected animals may have concurrent skeletal defects, such as pectus excavatum, vertebral anomalies, umbilical or supraumbilical hernias, and cardiovascular defects.

Traumatic muscular rupture or avulsion of the diaphragm permits abdominal contents to enter the pleural cavity, resulting in reduced lung volume and subsequent dyspnea. The liver is the most common organ to herniate and further compromises lung expansion by producing significant pleural effusion. Entrapped intestines or stomach may become gas distended, obstructed, or ischemic, resulting in metabolic disturbances, decreased cardiac return, and sepsis. Animals with acute traumatic diaphragmatic hernias can present in severe respiratory distress and shock and may require emergency surgery. Clinical signs in animals with chronic diaphragmatic hernias may be nonspecific, such as vomiting or weight loss.

Diagnosis is often made on plain thoracic films. Animals with PPDH will have an enlarged cardiac silhouette and abnormal soft tissue densities overlying the heart (fig. 12-1). Animals with traumatic diaphragmatic hernia may have an indistinct diaphragmatic line, pleural effusion, dorsal displacement of the lungs, and abnormal soft tissue densities within the pleural space (fig. 12-2). Ultrasonography, computed tomography, or gastrointestinal contrast studies can be useful when pleural effusion or silhouetting of structures obscures the diagnosis.

Most traumatic diaphragmatic hernias require surgical repair. Animals with chronic traumatic hernias are often referred to experienced surgeons for repair, particularly when the liver is involved, because of extensive adhesions. In some of these patients, a prosthetic implant, transversus abdominal muscle flap, or diaphragmatic advancement may be required to close the hernia. The decision to surgically correct congenital hernias depends on the clinical signs. In cats with PPDH, 75% of those that are asymptomatic or mildly affected do well long term with conservative treatment.

Manual of Small Animal Soft Tissue Surgery, Second Edition. Karen Tobias.
© 2017 John Wiley & Sons, Inc. Published 2017 by John Wiley & Sons, Inc.

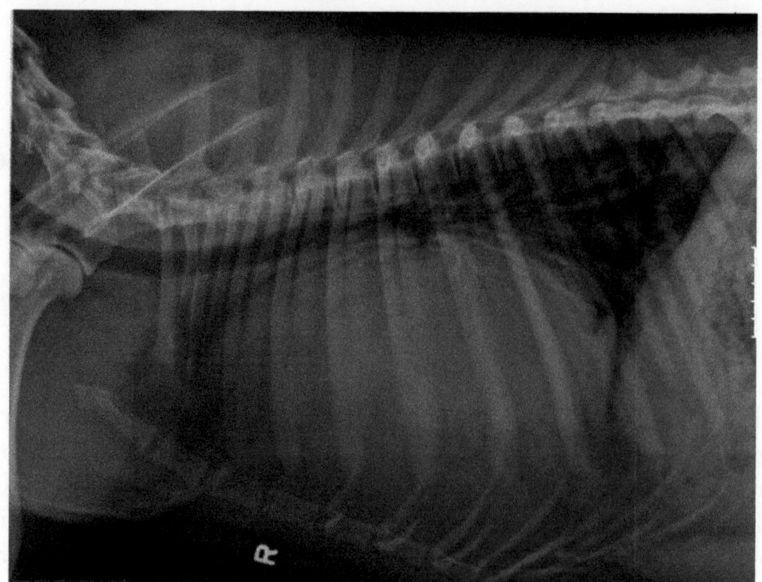

Figure 12-1 Peritoneopericardial diaphragmatic hernia with liver herniation.

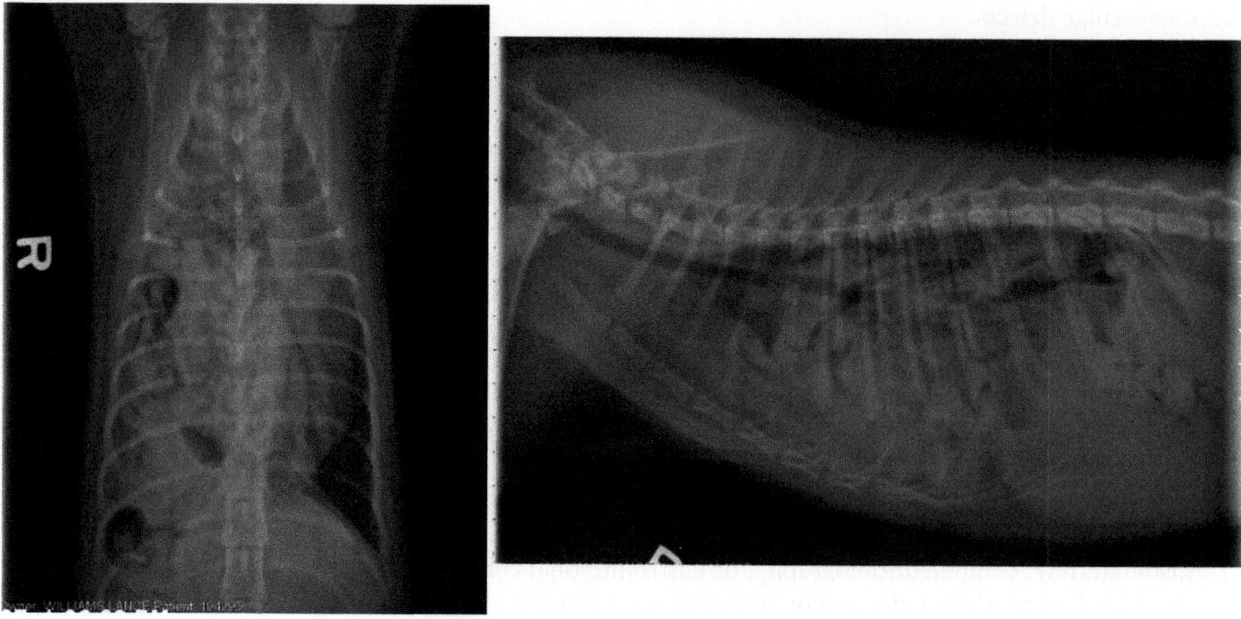

Figure 12-2 Traumatic right-sided diaphragmatic hernia with intestinal herniation.

Preoperative management

Thoracocentesis should be performed in animals with significant pleural effusion. If gastric entrapment and distension are present, the stomach should be decompressed by passage of an orogastric tube under sedation or by percutaneous transthoracic gastrocentesis. Supportive care (oxygen, fluids, analgesics, etc.) should be provided based on the animal's clinical condition. A traumatized animal that is in shock but has no significant respiratory compromise should be completely stabilized before considering surgery. A thorough physical and neurologic examination should be performed, and blood work should be evaluated for abnormalities. If respiratory compromise from

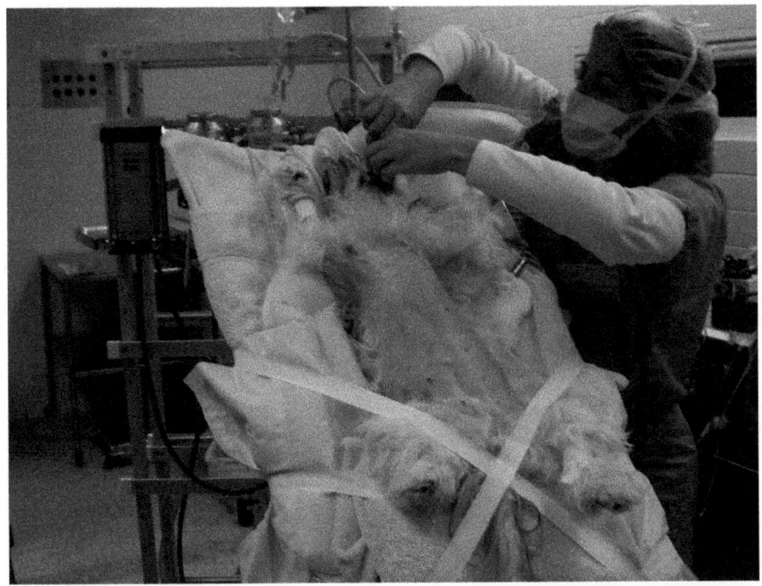

Figure 12-3 Because of severe positional hypoxia, this dog was placed in an upright position for prep and surgery. The table was returned to a horizontal positon once the organs were removed from the thoracic cavity.

organ entrapment is severe enough to prevent stabilization, emergency surgery may be required.

Before and during induction, oxygen should be administered by face mask. Induction should be rapid so that ventilation can be assisted as soon as possible. During anesthesia, animals will need to be ventilated manually or mechanically. A wide prep from midsternum to pubis is performed. In severely compromised animals, the table can be tilted during prep and surgery (fig. 12-3) to elevate the head and reduce pressure on the diaphragm until the hernia contents are reduced.

Surgery

Diaphragmatic hernias are approached through a midline abdominal incision. If necessary, the incision can be extended through the sternum to increase exposure. Herniated organs may swell, distend, or adhere to surrounding tissues. If organ reduction is difficult, the diaphragm should be incised to enlarge the hernial ring. Adhesions to lung or liver lobes may require partial lobectomy. In animals with PPDH, the pericardial peritoneal connection can often be left intact during surgery, preventing pneumothorax during and after the procedure. Once the organs have been removed from the chest, the lungs must be inflated carefully (<20 cm H_2O) to reduce the risk of pulmonary edema. Amount of lung inflation should be based on SPO_2.

Hernia edges are apposed with a simple continuous closure of 2-0 or 3-0 monofilament absorbable suture. Muscle edges do not require debridement before closure. The suture pattern is usually started at the dorsal aspect of the hernia, which is most difficult to reach. Closure should not constrict the caudal vena cava or esophagus. If the diaphragm has avulsed off of the body wall, it can be sutured directly back to the avulsion site by taking wide deep bites of the body wall musculature or going around a rib.

In animals with traumatic diaphragmatic hernias, a chest tube can be placed during surgery through the lateral chest wall or transdiaphragmatically, as described below. Complete, rapid lung expansion could result in pulmonary edema; therefore, many surgeons do not remove residual air from the thorax unless the pneumothorax is significantly collapsing the lung lobes. In animals with PPDH that have no pneumothorax, a chest tube is unnecessary. If needed, air can be removed from the pericardial sac with a catheter and syringe before abdominal closure.

The abdomen may be difficult to close in animals with chronic diaphragmatic hernias. Primary closure of a tight abdomen can result in abdominal compartment syndrome, with increased abdominal pressure causing oliguria and eventually renal failure. If the abdomen is very tight, the spleen should be removed. Alternatively, the abdominal wall diameter can be extended several centimeters by suturing fascia or a synthetic material (i.e., porcine small intestinal submucosa or polypropylene mesh) to connect the rectus sheath from each side, covering the gap in the incision, or by making a unilateral or bilateral releasing incision in the rectus fascia several cm lateral to the linea.

Surgical procedure: traumatic diaphragmatic hernia repair

1. With the animal ventilated and the head of the table elevated, make a midline abdominal incision from xiphoid to caudal abdomen. Check with the anesthetist to verify that the animal is being ventilated once the abdomen is open.
2. Ligate and excise the falciform ligament (see figs. 9-11 and 9-12).
3. Identify the hernia site (fig. 12-4); if necessary, extend the abdominal wall incision through the sternum cranially and to the pubis caudally to improve exposure.
4. Place abdominal wall retractors.
5. Retract the hernia contents into the abdomen (fig. 12-5), and examine them for ischemia or other damage.
    a. Gently break down adhesions with blind digital dissection. If adhesions are not easily broken, extend the abdominal wall incision or perform a median sternotomy to improve access.
    b. If needed, transect the diaphragm across one edge of the hernia with scissors to enlarge the hernia opening and facilitate reduction of

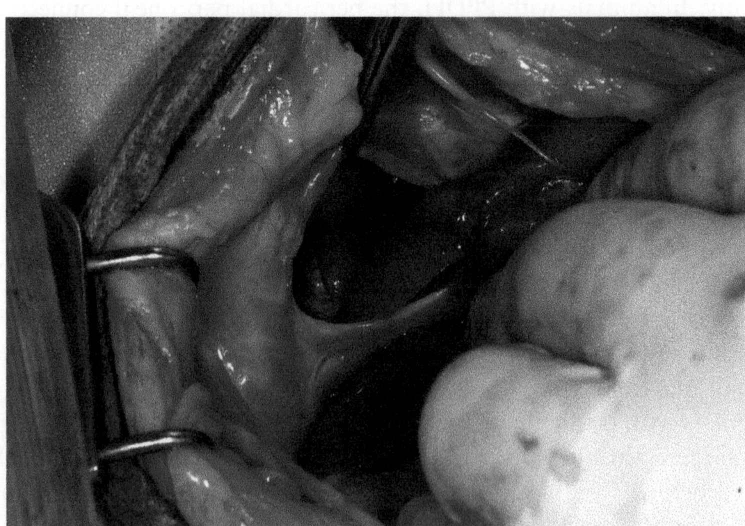

Figure 12-4 Traumatic diaphragmatic hernia with adhesions between the spleen and pericardium. If necessary, enlarge the hernial ring ventrally or laterally or split the sternum to improve exposure.

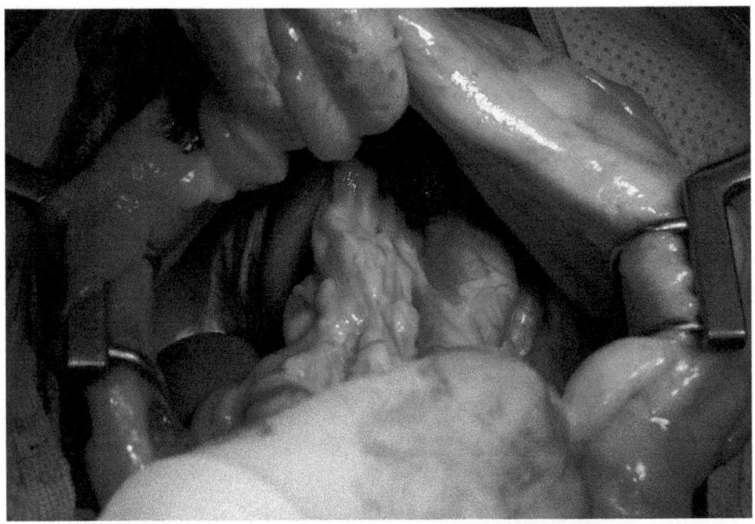

Figure 12-5 If contents are freely movable, retract them gently into the abdomen.

hernial contents. Extend the hernia opening outward toward the ventral or lateral body wall, away from the caudal vena cava, esophagus, or aorta.

6. Resect any compromised viscera.
7. Prepare a chest tube by cutting extra holes in a 12 to 20 French red rubber catheter (fold the catheter over and cut off one corner of the fold to make each hole; see fig. 60-7).
8. Identify the torn/cut muscle edges of the hernia (fig. 12-6). If they have rolled up into the pleural cavity, unroll them before suturing.
9. Start a simple continuous closure at the end of the hernia that is most difficult to reach or to close (usually the dorsal-most aspect). Leave a hemostat attached to the initial suture end to provide traction on the diaphragm as needed. Take wide (0.5 to 1 cm) bites of the muscle edges.
    a. If the hernia is difficult to close, place Allis tissue or Babcock forceps or stay sutures on each side of the hernia to pull the muscle edges together (fig. 12-7).

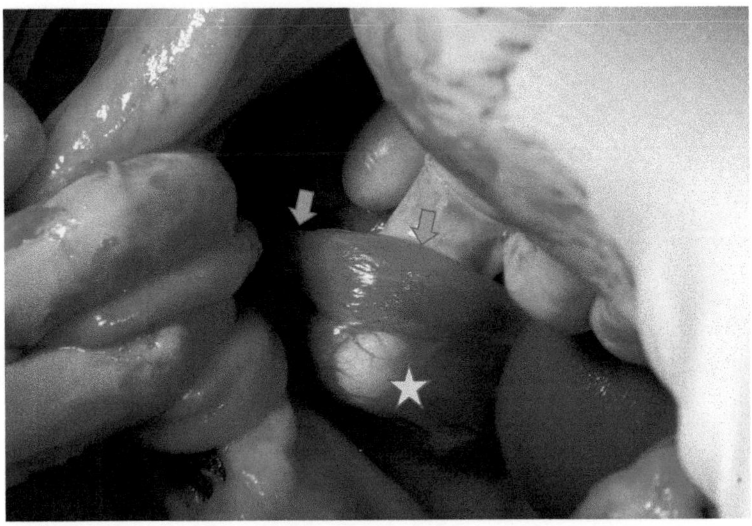

Figure 12-6 Left-sided traumatic diaphragmatic hernia. The torn muscle edges are not visible because they have rolled craniodorsally (arrows) into the thoracic cavity . The central tendon is indicated by the star.

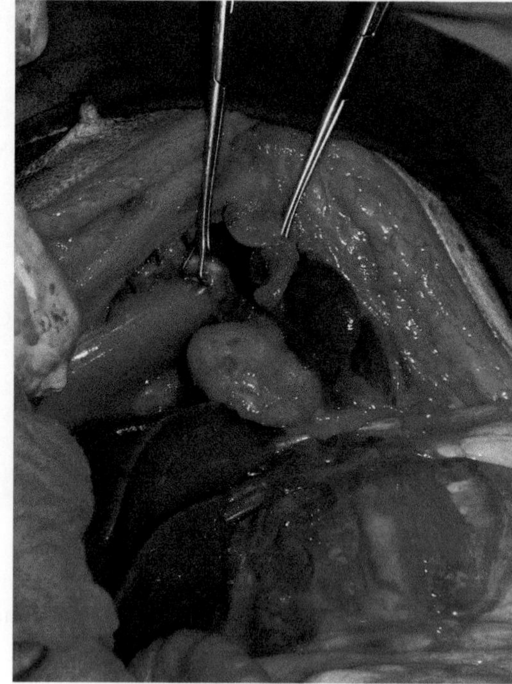

Figure 12-7 Grasp hernia edges with Babcock forceps or stay sutures to facilitate manipulation.

b. If the hernia is T- or L-shaped, preplace a suture to align the corner(s) before apposing the remaining edges. Remaining muscle edges may be easier to identify during suturing if the sutures that align the corners of the T or L are secured with a hemostat and left untied.

10. When the hernia is two-thirds closed, slide the fenestrated end of the red rubber catheter through the midline abdominal incision and diaphragmatic rent (fig. 12-8) and into the pleural cavity. Alternatively, place a transthoracic thoracotomy tube before hernia closure.
11. Finish the hernia closure. Remove the hemostat from the dorsal suture and cut the suture end short.
12. If the hernia site has gaps, add interrupted sutures. If caudal vena cava flow might be compromised with additional hernia closure, tack the omentum over the gap instead.

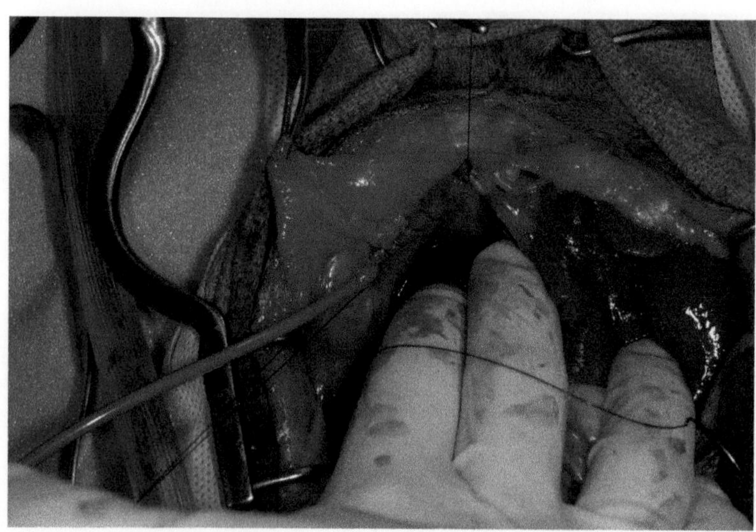

Figure 12-8 Incorporate the transdiaphragmatic thoracic tube within the herniorrhaphy closure.

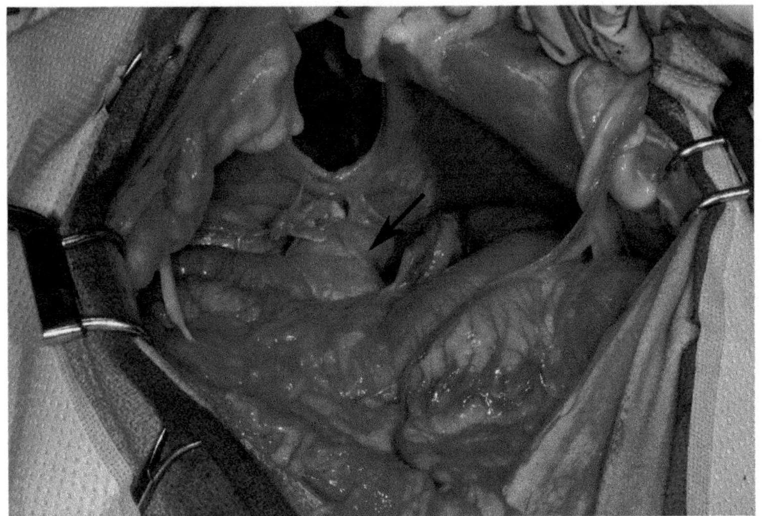

Figure 12-9 Peritoneopericardial diaphragmatic hernia. The left liver lobes were pale and atrophied (arrow). The pericardium remained contiguous with the diaphragm during hernia reduction and closure; therefore, no thoracotomy tube was placed in this patient.

13. Attach a connector and three-way stopcock to the red rubber catheter. If the diaphragm is billowing caudally, remove some of the excess air from the pleural space. Do not re-establish negative pressure. Cap off the stopcock ends.
14. Check the diaphragmatic surface and abdominal cavity wall and contents for other defects or injuries.
15. Close the abdominal incision routinely, exiting the transdiaphragmatic red rubber catheter through the incision line. Median sternotomy can be closed with orthopedic wire or encircling sutures.
16. Secure the chest tube to the skin. Place a bandage over the tube exit site and recover the animal on oxygen.

Surgical procedure: peritoneopericardial diaphragmatic hernia repair

1. Make a midline abdominal incision.
2. Gently retract the hernia contents into the abdomen, using digital dissection around them to disrupt adhesions (fig. 12-9). If possible, leave the hernial sac intact to prevent pneumothorax.
3. If the hernia contents are adherent to the sac, extend the midline incision cranially into the thoracic cavity and free the organs with sharp and blunt dissection, or transect the pericardium and leave the adherent portions attached to the abdominal organs.
4. Proceed as for a traumatic diaphragmatic hernia.

Postoperative management

Oxygen should be provided by mask or nasal catheter after surgery. Animals will usually require analgesics for 48 to 96 hours. Further removal of air from the chest may not be required unless the animal is dyspneic or the SPO_2 is less than 95%. Alternatively, 10 to 20 mL of air can be removed every 1 to 2 hours. Thoracic radiographs and blood gases should be evaluated in dyspneic animals. The chest tube can usually be removed within 12 to 24 hours; residual pneumothorax will gradually resolve without treatment. To remove a transabdominal or transthoracic tube, cut the finger trap suture; clamp the tube and gently pull it out.

Potential complications include cardiac or respiratory arrest, pulmonary edema, persistent pneumothorax, and organ failure. Animals with liver adhesions occasionally go into shock during surgery when the liver is flipped back into position. Rapid reinflation of the lungs during or after surgery may cause re-expansion pulmonary edema. Prognosis for this condition is grave, and affected animals may require mechanical ventilation for 1 to 3 days to recover. Abdominal compartment syndrome may occur if the organs are compressed after abdominal closure. Abdominal pressures can be monitored by inserting a urinary catheter into the bladder. The bladder is emptied and then distended with 0.5 to 1 mL/kg of sterile saline, and the catheter is attached to a manometer. Renal damage may occur if intra-abdominal pressure is ≥12 mm Hg (16.3 cm H_2O).

Mortality rates after surgical repair of traumatic diaphragmatic hernias are 10% to 18%. Prognosis is worse for unstable animals, older cats, dogs with gastric entrapment and dilatation, and animals with concurrent injuries. Postoperative mortality rate for peritoneopericardial diaphragmatic hernia is 9% to 14%; the most common causes of death are re-expansion pulmonary edema and hemorrhage.

Bibliography

Burns CG, Bergh MS, McLoughlin MA: Surgical and nonsurgical treatment of peritoneopericardial diaphragmatic hernia in dogs and cats: 58 cases (1999–2008). J Am Vet Med Assoc 2013;242:643–650.

Drelich S: Intraabdominal pressure and abdominal compartment syndrome. Compend Contin Educ Pract Vet 2000;22:764–769.

Gibson TWG et al: Perioperative survival rates after surgery for diaphragmatic hernia in dogs and cats: 92 cases (1990–2002). J Am Vet Med Assoc 2005;227:105–109.

Minihan AC et al: Chronic diaphragmatic hernias in 34 dogs and 16 cats. J Am Anim Hosp Assoc 2004;40:51–63.

Reimer SB et al: Long-term outcome of cats treated conservatively or surgically for peritoneopericardial diaphragmatic hernia: 66 cases (1987–2002). J Am Vet Med Assoc 2004;224:728–732.

Schmiedt C et al: Traumatic diaphragmatic hernias in cats: 34 cases (1991–2001). J Am Vet Med Assoc 2003;222:1237–1240.

Chapter 13
Splenectomy

Splenectomy is commonly performed for palliation of clinical signs and hemorrhage in dogs with splenic neoplasia such as hemangiosarcoma (fig. 13-1). Other indications include masses, trauma, torsion (fig. 13-2), abscess, or ruptured hematoma. Animals with immune mediated thrombocytopenia or anemia refractory to medical management may also benefit from splenic removal. Cats most often undergo splenectomy for splenic mast cell tumor.

Animals with splenic masses may be asymptomatic or present with signs of shock, anemia, or sepsis. German shepherds and Great Danes are at an increased risk for splenic torsion, which may cause acute cardiovascular collapse or prolonged malaise, intermittent vomiting, abdominal distension, weight loss, and discolored urine. Dogs with splenic torsions may have a previous history of gastric dilatation and volvulus. Splenic enlargement is often detected on abdominal palpation and plain radiographs. Ultrasonography is useful for confirmation of splenic enlargement and detection of specific etiologies such as torsion or abscessation.

Preoperative management

If neoplasia is suspected, thoracic and abdominal radiographs and abdominal ultrasound should be performed for staging purposes. Hemangiosarcoma frequently metastasizes to liver, lungs, and other organs and can occur primarily in the atria. Animals should be evaluated for anemia, thrombocytopenia, hypoglycemia, and prolonged clotting times. Packed red cell transfusions are recommended before surgery in animals with packed cell volume ≤20%. Fresh frozen plasma should be administered prior to surgery in animals with prolonged clotting times. In animals that are unstable or severely anemic, a jugular catheter should be placed for fluid administration and measurement of central venous pressures. Hypotensive animals may require colloids such as hetastarch. Broad spectrum antibiotics are administered in septic patients.

Splenectomy is performed as an emergency procedure in patients that have uncontrollable bleeding, splenic torsion, or abscess. The abdomen is clipped from midthorax to pubis. Suction and cautery should be available during surgery, and blood pressure should be monitored during the procedure. Cardiac return may be reduced from compression of the caudal vena cava by an enlarged spleen, collapse of the portal vein during splenic retraction, or severe blood loss.

Manual of Small Animal Soft Tissue Surgery, Second Edition. Karen Tobias.
© 2017 John Wiley & Sons, Inc. Published 2017 by John Wiley & Sons, Inc.

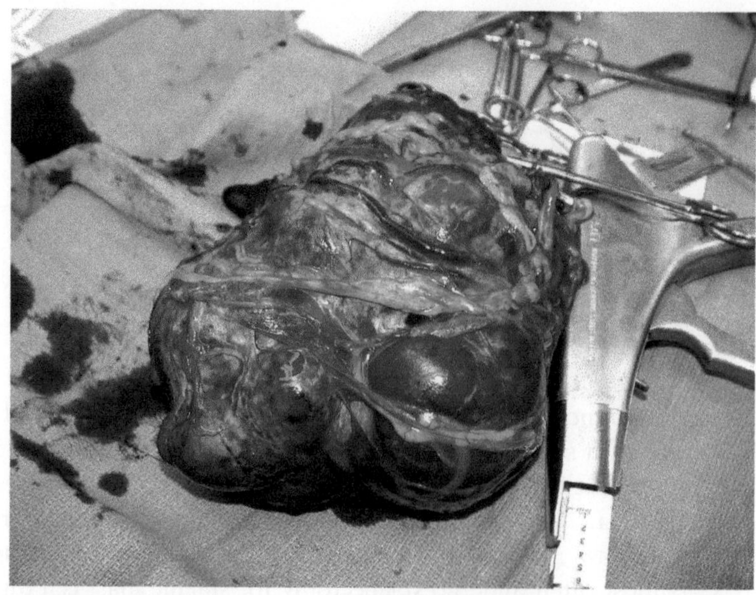

Figure 13-1 Splenic hemangiosarcoma. Because of omental adhesions and mass size, individual splenic branches were sealed and transected with a ligating dividing stapler. Larger vessels were ligated with multiple sutures.

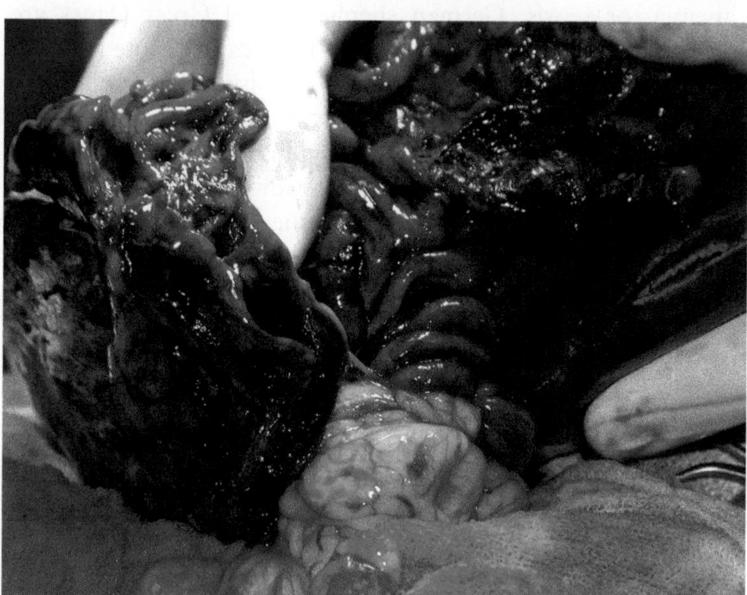

Figure 13-2 Splenic torsion. Leave the vascular pedicle torsed and ligate it with multiple encircling and transfixing sutures or a vascular stapling device.

Surgery

Splenectomy can be performed by ligation and transection of individual splenic branches or by ligation of the splenic artery and vein and the short gastric vessels (fig. 13-3) and any anastomosing gastroepiploic vessels that may provide backflow to the transected tissues. This technique is fast because it requires fewer ligatures, and it does not result in gastric wall necrosis. It may not be possible in animals with large, asymmetrical masses or omental adhesions, however, because the splenic artery and vein are often hard to expose in these animals. Ligations are often performed with free-tie silk (2-0 or 3-0) strands because of its low cost and excellent handling characteristics. During splenectomy, the splenic vessels can be double or triple ligated and transected. Leaving one ligature on the splenic side, or the proximal ends can be ligated and the distal end clamped with hemostats before transection. The

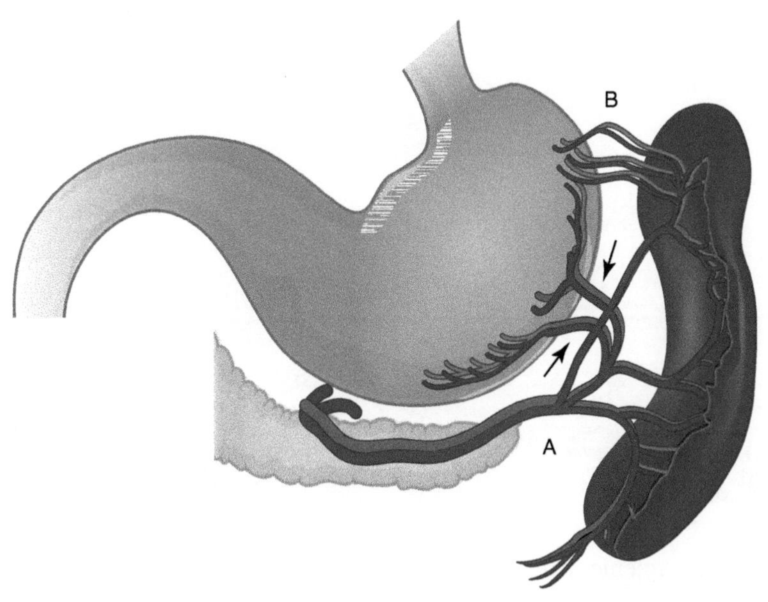

Figure 13-3 Blood supply to the spleen. If larger vessels are readily visible, remove the spleen by ligating the splenic artery and vein (A), short gastric vessels (B), and anastomosing gastroepiploic branches (arrows).

latter technique reduces surgery time but requires more hemostatic forceps. Use of ligating-dividing staplers, hemostatic clips, or vessel-sealing devices (e.g., Ligasure, Covidien) dramatically reduces surgery time, which offsets the increase in cost of equipment. Some surgeons will ligate the short gastric vessels first to release the tension on the head of the spleen, making the entire organ more mobile.

In animals with splenic torsion (fig. 13-2), the vascular pedicle is ligated with multiple encircling and transfixing sutures or sealed with a stapler or vessel-sealing device. The spleen should not be detorsed before ligation and removal, since this could release toxins and inflammatory mediators from ischemic tissue. Dogs with splenic torsion may have ischemia of the left limb of the pancreas, requiring resection via a guillotine technique. Reports conflict as to whether splenectomy increases the future risk of gastric dilatation-volvulus; in deep-chested dogs, concurrent gastropexy may be performed to prevent the condition.

Surgical technique: splenectomy

1. Make a midline incision from xiphoid to the caudal abdomen and insert Balfour retractors. If hemoperitoneum is present, insert a Poole suction tip through a small linea incision first and remove as much fluid as possible before extending the incision.
2. Ligate the splenic vessels.
   a. If the spleen is torsed:
      i. Ligate the torsed pedicle in multiple sections with transfixing and encircling sutures of 2-0 monofilament absorbable suture.
      ii. To avoid damaging the vessels, pass the suture through the pedicle by inserting the swaged-on needle backwards through the tissues. Alternatively, insert a closed hemostat bluntly through the pedicle; grasp the suture end with the hemostat and pull it through, then tie around a portion of the pedicle.

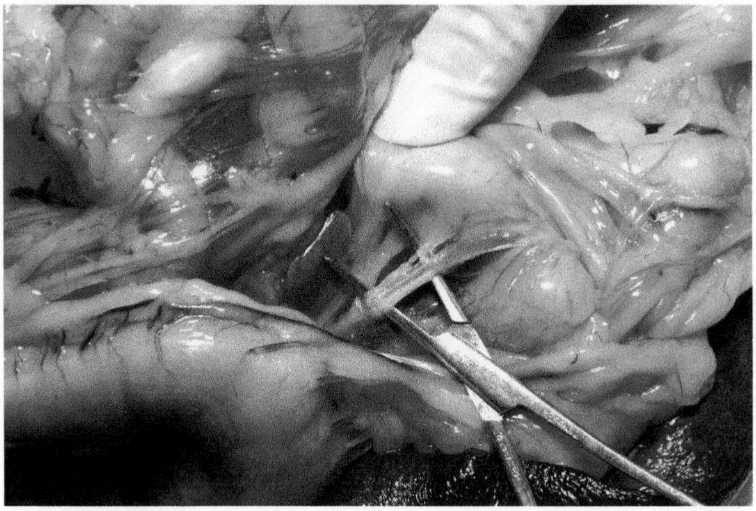

Figure 13-4 Isolate the splenic artery from the vein just beyond the tip of the pancreas.

b. If the splenic artery and vein are visible:

   i. Identify the splenic artery and vein at the tip of the left pancreatic lobe, proximal to the origin of the left gastroepiploic artery (fig. 13-3).

   ii. Isolate the splenic artery and vein between the tip of the pancreas and the gastroepiploic vessels by dissecting parallel to the vessels through the surrounding mesentery (fig. 13-4).

   iii. Triple ligate each vessel separately and transect between the distal two ligatures.

   iv. Ligate and transect the short gastric arteries and veins en masse in one to three blocks of tissue.

   v. Ligate any anastomosing gastroepiploic vessels that might provide backflow to the transected tissues.

c. If the splenic artery and vein cannot be exposed:

   i. Ligate individual hilar vessels 1 to 2 cm from their entrance into the splenic parenchyma, starting at the most mobile end of the spleen (figs. 13-5 and 13-6) (often the tail). Ligate larger vessels individually and small vessels in groups (fig. 13-7).

   ii. Expose adjacent vessels by tearing the intervening omentum.

   iii. Ligate with one or two encircling ligatures around each vessel, depending on pedicle size.

3. Ligate and transect any attached omentum, and remove the spleen from the surgery area.

4. Examine the liver for metastatic disease and biopsy any questionable areas (see Chapter 16) before closing the abdomen.

Postoperative considerations

Supportive care should be continued as needed. Intermittent or persistent ventricular arrhythmias are common in dogs after splenectomy; therefore,

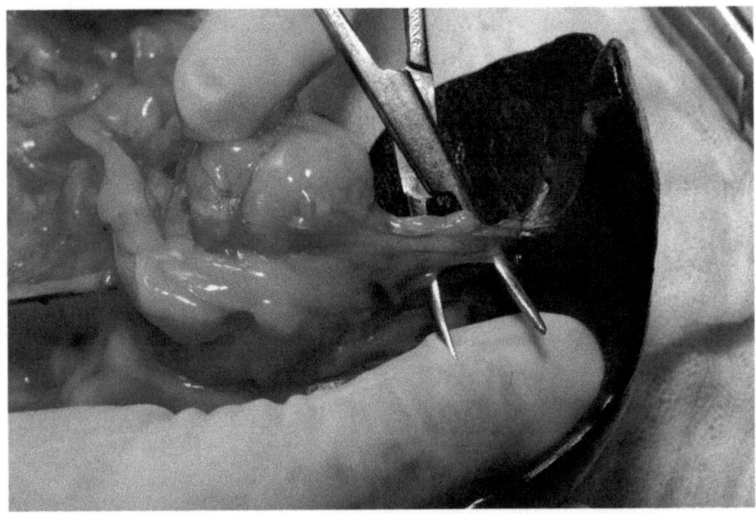

Figure 13-5 To ligate hilar vessels, make a window parallel to the blood vessel with hemostats.

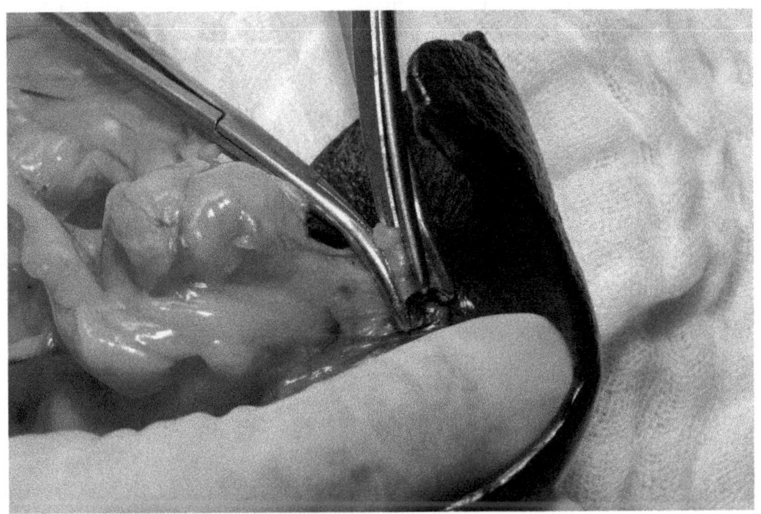

Figure 13-6 Double clamp each vessel. Transect before or after ligation.

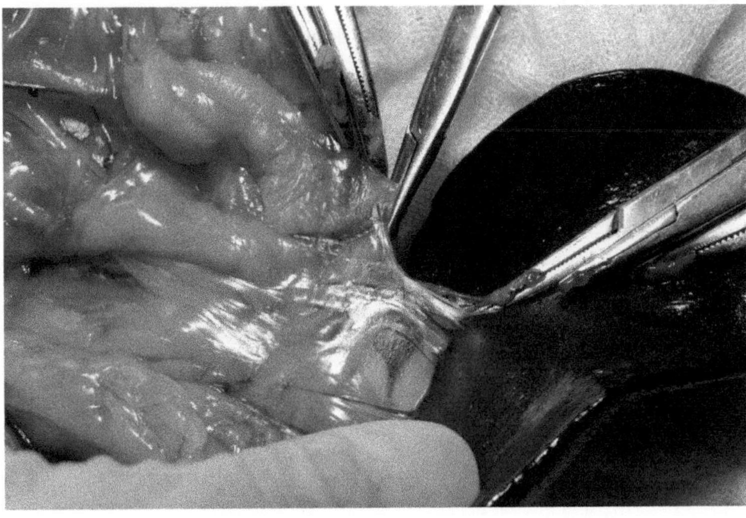

Figure 13-7 Small vessels can be ligated or clamped in groups.

continuous electrocardiographic monitoring is recommended for up to 36 hours after surgery. Hematocrit should be measured immediately after surgery to obtain a baseline, since intraoperative fluid administration may produce significant dilution.

The most frequent complications after splenectomy are hemorrhage, arrhythmias, or problems associated with the underlying condition. Unlike people, dogs and cats do not have an increased risk of overwhelming septicemia after splenectomy. Hemorrhage may occur with improper or inadequate ligation or development of disseminated intravascular coagulation. Packed cell volume and clotting times should be re-evaluated if significant hemorrhage is suspected. Postsplenectomy arrhythmias are usually ventricular in origin. Treatment should be considered in animals with tachycardia, pulse deficits, or multifocal premature ventricular contractions. Lidocaine boluses (2 mg/kg IV; maximum 8 mg/kg) and continuous rate infusion (25–80 µg/kg/min) are antiarrhythmic and provide analgesia.

An unusual complication of splenectomy is emergence of blood-borne infections. The spleen plays an important role in erythrophagocytosis; and pre-existing subclinical infections with Ehrlichia, Babesia, or Mycoplasma (formerly known as Haemobartonella) species may become evident after its removal.

Perioperative death is approximately 8% in dogs undergoing splenectomy for mass removal; death is most commonly associated with uncontrolled hemorrhage or portal or pulmonary thrombosis. Prognosis is excellent after splenectomy for torsion or hematoma but guarded for animals with hemangiosarcoma. Dogs with splenic hemangiosarcoma that have no gross evidence of metastasis have a median survival time of 2 months if treated with splenectomy alone. Chemotherapy can increase survival to a median of 4 to 6 months.

Bibliography

Gordon SSN, McClaran JK, Bergman PJ, et al.: Outcome following splenectomy in cats. J Feline Med Surg 2010;12:256–261.

Grange AM, Clough W, Casale SA: Evaluation of splenectomy as a risk factor for gastric dilatation-volvulus. J Am Vet Med Assoc 2012;241:461–466.

Hosgood G: Splenectomy in the dog by ligation of the splenic and short gastric arteries. Vet Surg 1989;18:110–113.

Marino DJ et al: Ventricular arrhythmias in dogs undergoing splenectomy: a prospective study. Vet Surg 1994;23:101–106.

Neath PJ et al: Retrospective analysis of 19 cases of isolated torsion of the splenic pedicle in dogs. J Small Anim Pract 1997;38:387–392.

Sartor AJ, Bentley AM, Brown DC: Association between previous splenectomy and gastric dilatation-volvulus in dogs: 453 cases (2004–2009). J Am Vet Med Assoc 2013;242:1381–1384.

Wendelburg KM, O'Toole TE, McCobb E, et al: Risk factors for perioperative death in dogs undergoing splenectomy for splenic masses: 539 cases (2001–2012). J Am Vet Med Assoc 2014;245:1382–1390.

Wendleburg KM, Price LL, Burgess KE, et al: Survival time of dogs with splenic hemangiosarcoma treated by splenectomy with or without adjuvant chemotherapy: 208 cases (2001–2012). J Am Vet Med Assoc 2015;247:393–403.

Chapter 14
Abdominal Lymph Node Biopsy

During exploratory celiotomy, lymph nodes that are enlarged or receive lymphatic drainage from tumors and other masses should be biopsied for diagnostic and staging purposes. Some lymph nodes, such as the ileocecal colic, are easily found. Sublumbar lymph nodes can be difficult to find or expose, unless they are grossly enlarged, because of surrounding tissues. Sublumbar lymph nodes and those along the portal vein or in the root of the mesentery are closely associated with major vascular structures (fig. 14-1). Biopsying these nodes can be particularly intimidating because of the risk of severe complications.

Preoperative management

Formalin, slides, and sterile syringes and needles should be available for histopathology and cytology. Intraoperative aspiration of vascular lymph nodes may be safer than biopsy. If lymphoma is suspected and cytologic evaluation is available, slide samples can be made from lymph node aspirates or tissue impressions to provide a more immediate diagnosis. Immunohistochemistry stains of histologic sections will provide definitive diagnosis and phenotyping, however.

Surgery

Abdominal lymph nodes are exposed through a ventral midline celiotomy. Lymph node aspirates are performed with a sterile 6- or 12-cc syringe and a 20- or 22-gauge needle. The needle is inserted into the node parenchyma at an angle parallel to the surface of the lymph node, and suction is applied. If the lymph node is large enough, the needle is moved forward and backward within the node while applying suction. The needle tip must remain within the nodal parenchyma during aspiration. Suction is released and the needle is retracted from the tissues. The needle is detached from the syringe, which is then filled with air. The needle is reattached, and the syringe plunger is depressed rapidly to expel cells onto a slide for cytology or into a vial of sterile saline for flow

Manual of Small Animal Soft Tissue Surgery, Second Edition. Karen Tobias.
© 2017 John Wiley & Sons, Inc. Published 2017 by John Wiley & Sons, Inc.

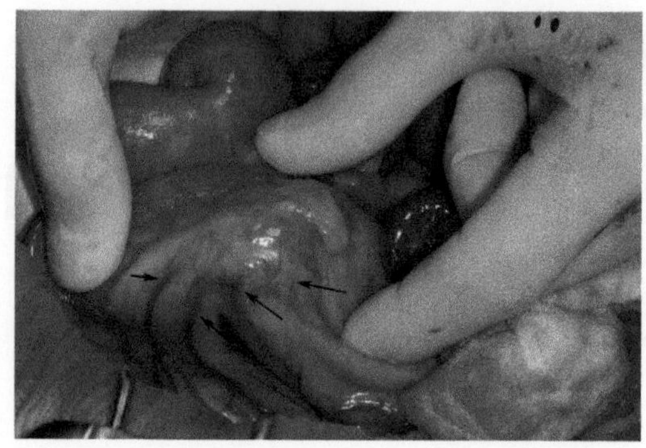

Figure 14-1 Enlarged lymph node near the root of the mesentery. The lymph node is closely associated with the intestinal blood supply (arrows).

cytometry. Three to six samples should be obtained to ensure sufficient cellularity.

Techniques for lymph node biopsy include excision, incision, guillotine, "shaving," and tru-cut. Technique selection is based on the size and shape of the lymph node and its proximity to large vessels and other structures. With most techniques, local hemorrhage can be controlled by closing mesentery over the site or applying digital pressure. If enlarged lymph nodes have necrotic, cystic, or friable centers, the nodal interior can be gently suctioned or digitally evacuated. The free edge of the omentum is then inserted into the cavity and tacked to the edges of the node with multiple interrupted sutures of absorbable material. This will decrease node size, provide drainage, and improve blood supply.

Surgical technique: abdominal lymph node biopsy

1. With a hemostat or Metzenbaum scissors, gently spread the overlying peritoneum or mesentery away to expose the surface of the node. To avoid damaging vessels, use sharp transection only on tissues that are transparent (fig. 14-2).
2. If the node is easily freed from its surrounding tissue, perform an excisional biopsy.
    a. Using hemostats, bluntly dissect around the node to its vascular pedicle.

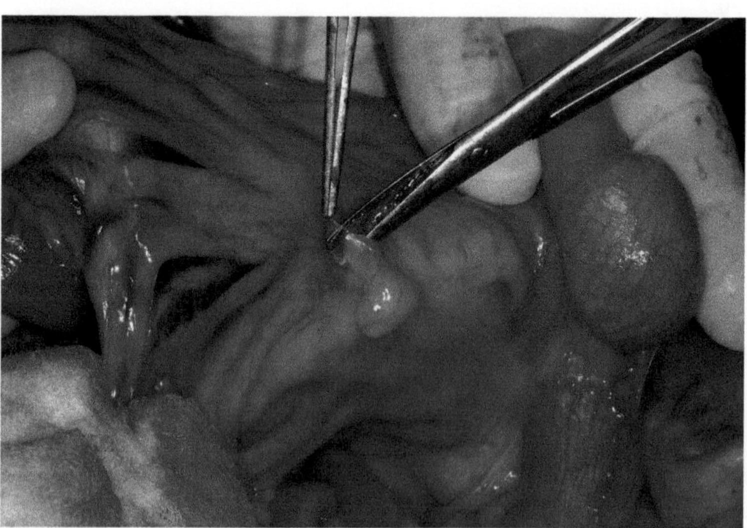

Figure 14-2 Bluntly elevate the mesentery over the lymph node. To avoid damaging the intestinal blood supply, transect only transparent tissues.

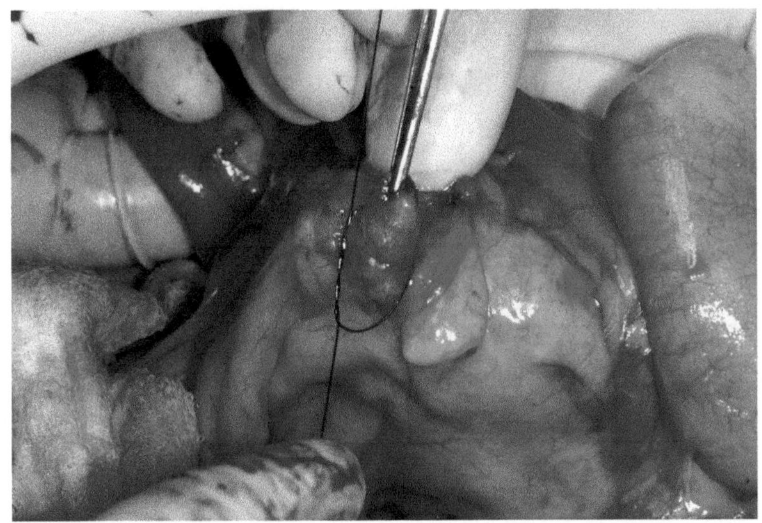

Figure 14-3 Guillotine technique. Ligate the base of the exposed tissue with an absorbable suture. If possible, use forceps only on mesenteric attachments to avoid producing a crush artifact in the sample.

b. Ligate the pedicle at its base with absorbable suture.

c. Transect the pedicle between the ligature and lymph node.

3. If the node is oblong and one end can be freed, perform a guillotine technique (fig. 14-3).

   a. With hemostats, bluntly dissect the mesentery from one end of the node.

   b. If necessary, grasp the end of the node with Babcock or Allis tissue forceps at least 1 cm from the edge to maintain traction on the node. Crushing artifact will occur around the instrument and ligation sites.

   c. Tilt the exposed end of the node upward and pass a loop of absorbable suture around the end. If a tissue forceps was placed, pass the suture beyond the instrument tips to include the crushed area and undamaged tissue in the biopsy sample.

   d. Tighten the suture with one surgeon's throw so that the suture crushes the tissues. Additional throws can be added if they can be tied without pulling the suture through the tissue.

   e. Transect the end of the lymph node distal to the ligature with scissors or blade. Cut the suture ends short.

4. If the lymph node is small and embedded in local tissues, sample by aspiration or tru-cut biopsy, or by shaving a small piece of the rounded surface off.

   a. Select a site away from the lymph node hilus and critical surrounding structures. Expose the wall of the lymph node by dissecting away any overlying mesentery.

   b. Stabilize the lymph node gently with thumb forceps or between your thumb and middle finger.

   c. With Metzenbaum scissors or a sharp blade, shave a thin (1 to 2 mm) layer of lymph node off of the outer surface of the node.

d. Appose the mesentery or peritoneum overlying the node with an interrupted or cruciate suture of 3-0 or 4-0 absorbable material, avoiding any important blood vessels. Because the tissue is friable, use a single knot (two throws). Appose the tissues gently and do not lift up on the suture ends when tying. Cut the suture ends short.

5. If the lymph node is large and away from major blood vessels but not removable in its entirety, perform a wedge biopsy.

   a. With a #15 blade, make a curvilinear incision 0.5 to 1 cm long by 2 to 3 mm deep into the outer parenchyma of the exposed node, angling toward the node's midline.

   b. Make a second, apposing, curvilinear incision of similar proportions, angling inward, to produce an elliptical wedge of tissue. Gently lift the wedge out of the incision with the blade tip.

   c. Appose the incised edges of the node with a cruciate suture of 3-0 or 4-0 absorbable material, using a surgeon's throw and second throw to form a single knot. Cut the suture ends short.

Postoperative considerations

The most common complication of abdominal lymph node biopsy or excision is intraoperative hemorrhage, which can be avoided by carefully selecting lymph nodes in avascular and noncritical areas. If hemorrhage continues after apposition of the node edges or the overlying tissue, digital pressure should be applied. The omentum can also be sewn over any bleeding area to reduce hemorrhage.

Bibliography

Amores-Fuster I, Cripps P, Graham P, et al: The diagnostic utility of lymph node cytology samples in dogs and cats. J Small Anim Pract 2015;56:125–129.

Gibson D et al: Flow cytometric immunophenotype of canine lymph node aspirates. J Vet Intern Med 2004;18:710–717.

Hoelzler MG et al: Omentalization of cystic sublumbar lymph node metastases for long-term palliation of tenesmus and dysuria in a dog with anal sac adenocarcinoma. J Am Vet Med Assoc 2001;219:1729–1731.

Sözmen M et al: Use of fine needle aspirates and flow cytometry for the diagnosis, classification, and immunophenotyping of canine lymphomas. J Vet Diag Invest 2005;17:323–329.

Chapter 15
Peritonitis

Septic peritonitis is commonly caused by dehiscence of gastrointestinal surgical wounds. Other common etiologies include penetrating or blunt trauma; gastrointestinal perforation from foreign bodies, neoplasia, or use of non-steroidal anti-inflammatory drugs; intestinal ischemia; rupture of infected or abscessed organs (e.g., prostatic abscess or pyometra); leakage around feeding tubes; abdominal wall dehiscence; or intraoperative contamination. With few exceptions (e.g., feline infectious peritonitis), peritonitis requires emergency surgical treatment, and therefore diagnosis must be swift and accurate.

Clinical signs of peritonitis may include depression, anorexia, vomiting, abdominal pain, unusual posturing ("praying position"), abdominal distension, and signs of sepsis or shock (pale or injected mucous membranes, prolonged capillary refill time, tachycardia, tachypnea, weakness, collapse, depressed mentation, dehydration, pyrexia or hypothermia). Septic cats may be bradycardic and hypothermic and are less likely to exhibit abdominal pain.

Diagnosis of peritonitis is based on historical findings, radiographic and ultrasonographic evaluation, and abdominal fluid analysis. Hemogram, chemistry, and coagulation panels should be evaluated for evidence of sepsis (neutropenia, hypoglycemia, and toxic cells or a degenerative left shift), disseminated intravascular coagulation (DIC), or organ dysfunction. On abdominal radiographs, loss of serosal detail, ground glass appearance, gas distended intestines, and free gas may be seen. Presence of free air in the abdomen on radiographs (pneumoperitoneum) in an animal that has not had surgery or penetrating trauma in the last 2 to 3 weeks is an indication for exploratory laparotomy. A horizontal radiographic view may assist in determining the presence of free air in equivocal cases.

The most important diagnostic test for peritonitis is cytologic analysis and culture of fluid obtained by abdominocentesis or diagnostic peritoneal lavage. Surgery is indicated if microbes, degenerative neutrophils, or foreign material are present. Initially, needle abdominocentesis can be attempted; aspiration under ultrasound guidance is recommended to improve yield. Peritonitis is present if fluid from abdominocentesis has degenerate neutrophils, intracellular bacteria, or >10,000 white blood cells/μL of fluid. In animals without peritonitis, peritoneal fluid may contain up to 100,000 white blood cells/μL 1 to 3 days after abdominal surgery, but these cells should not be degenerate or contain bacteria. Peritonitis can also be diagnosed by biochemical comparison of abdominal fluid and blood samples that have been collected simultaneously. In animals with septic peritonitis, peritoneal fluid glucose is more than

Manual of Small Animal Soft Tissue Surgery, Second Edition. Karen Tobias.
© 2017 John Wiley & Sons, Inc. Published 2017 by John Wiley & Sons, Inc.

20 mg/dL lower than that of peripheral blood when measured with a laboratory chemistry analyzer. In addition, dogs with septic effusions may have a peritoneal fluid lactate concentration at least 2 mmol/L greater than peripheral blood lactate. Peritoneal fluid lactate concentration is not an accurate test for detecting septic peritonitis in cats. In animals with uroabdomen, creatinine concentrations of peritoneal fluid will be at least twice serum concentrations, and peritoneal fluid potassium concentrations will be at least 1.9 and 1.4 times that of serum in cats and dogs, respectively. Concentration of bilirubin in peritoneal fluid is at least twice that of blood in animals with biliary tract rupture.

Abdominocentesis is not always diagnostic, since fluid can be pocketed away from the aspiration site. Diagnostic peritoneal lavage (DPL) is more sensitive, particularly if fluid is not easily obtained by needle aspirate. To perform DPL, position the animal in right lateral recumbency. Make a small abdominal incision, and insert a multifenestrated catheter 1 to 2 cm caudal to and to the right of the umbilicus into the peritoneal cavity. Remove the stylette and place an EDTA tube below the catheter to collect any free fluid. If no fluid is obtained from the catheter, attach a warm bag of 0.9% saline with a fluid set to the catheter and infuse 22 mL/kg of fluid into the abdominal cavity. Gently roll the animal side to side several times. After a 10-minute dwell time, remove as much fluid as possible (at least 10 mL/kg) by dropping the bag and allowing gravitational flow or by aspiration of the catheter. Analyze the fluid and submit a sample for Gram stain and culture/sensitivity. Peritonitis is present if fluid from lavage contains degenerate cells or bacteria or has more than 1,000 (mild to moderate inflammation) to 2,000 (marked peritonitis) white blood cells/µL of fluid. In animals that have recently undergone abdominal surgery, peritonitis is present if the white blood cell count is >10,000/µL of fluid on DPL samples.

Preoperative management

Treatment for animals with peritonitis should include stabilization, administration of appropriate antimicrobials, correction of the underlying problem, and drainage of the abdominal cavity as needed. Preoperative treatment is outlined as follows:

1. Place a large-bore peripheral catheter and a triple lumen central venous catheter.
2. Collect blood for a hemogram, platelet count, biochemistry panel, electrolytes (including magnesium), antithrombin III, and coagulation panel or activated clotting time. Evaluate packed cell volume, total protein, electrolytes, blood lactate, and blood glucose immediately.
3. Measure central venous pressure (CVP) to help determine fluid needs. Normal CVP is 2 to 5 cmH_2O for cats and 3 to 8 cmH_2O for dogs.
4. Administer crystalloids, basing the rate on clinical response and CVP; add colloids if CVP is low. A bolus of 5 to 10 mL/kg (cats) or 10 to 20 mL/kg (dogs) of crystalloids can be given over 15 to 20 minutes. This may be repeated 4 to 5 times. Animals may need 1 to 10 mLs of crystalloids/kg/hour thereafter, depending on physiologic status, ongoing fluid loss, and volume of other fluids administered. Cats can be easily overhydrated.

5. If CVP remains <2 cmH_2O, administer hetastarch (10 and 20 mL/kg IV total dose in cats and dogs, respectively) over 2 to 24 hours. A bolus of 5 to 20 mL/kg can be given rapidly in animals with shock. Cats are more likely to become volume overloaded; therefore, smaller volumes should be used.
6. Measure indirect peripheral blood pressures frequently. For animals with mean arterial pressure <60 mmHg or systolic blood pressure <90 mmHg that do not respond to appropriate fluid administration, provide sympathomimetic support.
   a. If hypotension is present, administer dopamine (2.5–20 µg/kg/minute) IV.
   b. If cardiac output is poor, administer dobutamine (2–20 µg/kg/minute in dogs and 1–5 µg/kg/minute in cats). Cats are more susceptible to the adverse effects of dobutamine and may develop tremors, seizures, or arrhythmias.
   c. If blood pressure does not respond to dopamine or dobutamine, administer norepinephrine (0.05–3 µg/kg/min), phenylephrine (1–10 µg/kg/min), or vasopressin (0.01–0.1 units/kg as a bolus, followed by 0.001–0.1 units/kg/hr). Use the lowest dose possible to reduce the risk of ischemia secondary to vasoconstriction.
   d. Titrate the drug doses according to blood pressure measurements. An arterial catheter may need to be placed for direct blood pressure monitoring and arterial blood gas measurements in critical patients.
7. Measure blood lactate concentration before and during treatment to monitor response to fluid therapy.
   a. Normal blood lactate is <2 mmol/L. Blood lactate is normally higher in puppies (approximately 4 mmol/L).
   b. If high blood lactate does not decrease with treatment, prognosis is poor.
8. Measure SPO_2 with a pulse oximeter. If <95%, administer oxygen through a nasal catheter, mask, or other system.
9. Administer intravenous cefoxitin (22–30 mg/kg IV q6–8h), ampicillin-sulbactam (15–30 mg/kg IV q6-8h), or other broad spectrum antibiotic combinations (e.g., enrofloxacin/ampicillin or amikacin/ampicillin; add metronidazole for anaerobic contamination).
   a. If possible, obtain an abdominal fluid sample for culture before initiating antibiotics, but start antibiotic therapy as early as possible.
   b. In dogs the most common bacteria in peritonitis are *E. coli and Enterococcus spp.*
10. Provide analgesia with opioids given as intermittent boluses (e.g., buprenorphine, hydromorphone, or methadone) or by constant rate infusion (e.g., fentanyl CRI).
    a. Cats can be treated with a fentanyl CRI (2 to 6 micrograms/kg/h). Lidocaine IV is often avoided in cats because of cardiovascular depression.

b. Dogs can be treated with a fentanyl CRI (2 to 10 micrograms/kg/h); lidocaine can be delivered concurrently as a CRI at 1.5 to 3 mg/kg/h.

11. If coagulation times are prolonged or if other evidence is suggestive of DIC, administer fresh frozen plasma at 10 mL/kg IV over 3 to 4 hours.
12. If hematocrit is <25%, crossmatch and administer packed red cells (cats, 5 mL/kg; dogs, 10 mL/kg) IV over 1 to 4 hours.
13. If hypoglycemia is present, give a bolus of 50% dextrose (0.5 g/kg IV, diluted 1 : 1 with sterile water for injection), and supplement dextrose in the IV crystalloid solution.
14. If hypomagnesemia is present, administer 1 to 2 mEq/kg IV over 2 or more hours.
15. Administer physiologic doses of glucocorticoids (e.g., prednisone, 0.1–0.3 mg/kg q12–24h; or dexamethasone, 0.01–0.04 mg/kg q12–24h IV) if hypotenstion or hypoglycema is nonresponsive to treatment. Use of steroids is controversial.
16. For patients with severe hypoalbuminemia and clinical edema that have failed to respond to colloidal support, consider 25% human serum albumin supplementation (3–10 ml/kg). Human serum albumin has been associated with serious delayed side effects in healthy dogs and should only be used in patients that have not responded to other treatments.
17. Administer unfractionated or low molecular weight (dalteparin) heparin at 100 U/kg SQ q8h for patients in DIC. Use of heparin is controversial and varies with clinician preference.
18. Place a urinary catheter to measure urine output (normal, 1–2 mL/kg/hour) and to maintain good hygiene.
19. Correct acid base and electrolyte imbalances.
20. Administer gastrointestinal protectants and antiemetic drugs in animals with nausea, emesis, or suspected gastrointestinal ulcerations.
21. Correct the underlying etiology of peritonitis as soon as possible.

Surgery

The animal should be clipped and prepped widely, including the lateral aspect of the left or right abdomen, respectively, if a gastrostomy or enterostomy tube is going to be placed. Suction and copious quantities of warm lavage solution should be available. After the primary problem is corrected, the abdominal cavity should be evaluated for inflammation and contamination. If the abdomen can be flushed out well and the peritoneum is only mildly inflamed, the abdomen can be closed primarily. Patients that have extensive fibrin tags, debris, or severe inflammation should be treated with abdominal drainage. Multifenestrated closed-suction drains (fig. 15-1) provide excellent post-operative drainage in most patients and are easier to manage than open abdominal drainage. Because of the one-way valve in the suction bulb, fluid and contaminants from the bulb cannot be accidentally flushed back into the abdomen.

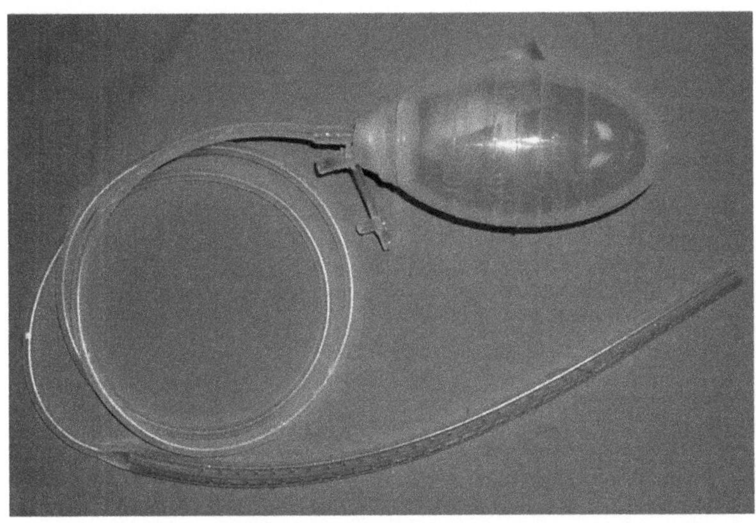

Figure 15-1 Multifenestrated closed suction drain with suction bulb. The one-way valve in the suction bulb prevents backflow into the abdomen.

Surgical technique: abdominal exploratory and drain placement

1. Make a long midline incision and remove abdominal effusion with suction using a Poole tip.
2. If not yet submitted, take an abdominal fluid sample for Gram stain, culture, and sensitivity. Some clinicians prefer to take fluid samples after the abdomen has been flushed.
3. Explore the abdomen and correct the primary problem.
4. Place a gastrostomy, duodenostomy, or jejunostomy tube as needed (see Chapters 19 and 24). Alternatively, have a nonsterile assistant place a nasogastric tube; the surgeon can manipulate the tube through the pylorus and into the duodenum if gastric bypass is desired.
5. Flush the abdomen with 3 to 15 liters of warm saline and remove the fluid completely. Volume of lavage fluid depends on the amount of debris.
6. Provide abdominal drainage in patients with fibrin tags, foreign material, necrotic debris, or moderate to severe peritoneal inflammation.
    a. To place a closed-suction (e.g., Jackson Pratt) drain, force a closed Kelly or Carmalt hemostatic forceps through the body wall musculature and subcutaneous fat lateral to the midline incision. In male dogs, exit the forceps far enough cranially so that the prepuce will not be included in postoperative bandages. In female dogs, exit the mid-abdomen so that bandage slippage will not be a problem.
    b. Incise over the forceps tips with a blade, and push the tips through (fig. 15-2).
    c. Grasp the fenestrated end of the drain with the forceps and pull the drain through the abdominal wall (fig. 15-3) into the peritoneal cavity.
        i. If the drain is hard to pull through the skin and body wall, cut the end of the drain at an angle.
    d. Place a purse-string suture of 3-0 nylon in the skin around the drain exit site (fig. 15-4). Tie the suture to appose the skin around the tube without necrosing it.

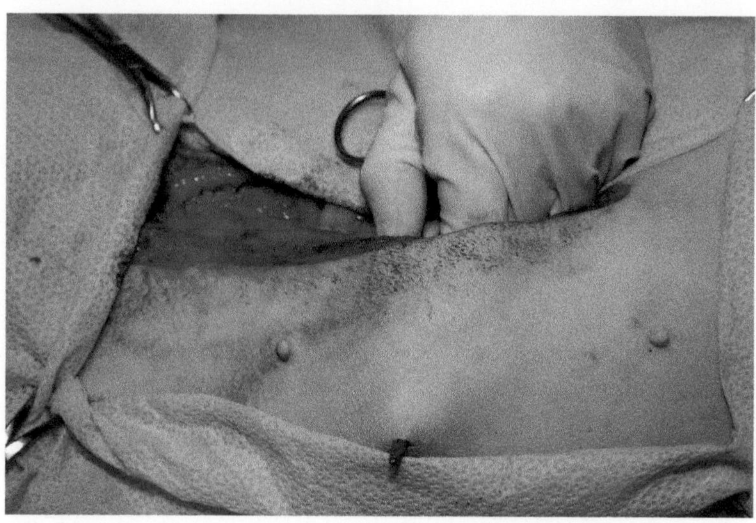

Figure 15-2 Force a Kelly or Carmalt hemostatic forceps through the abdominal wall musculature and incise over the tip to expose.

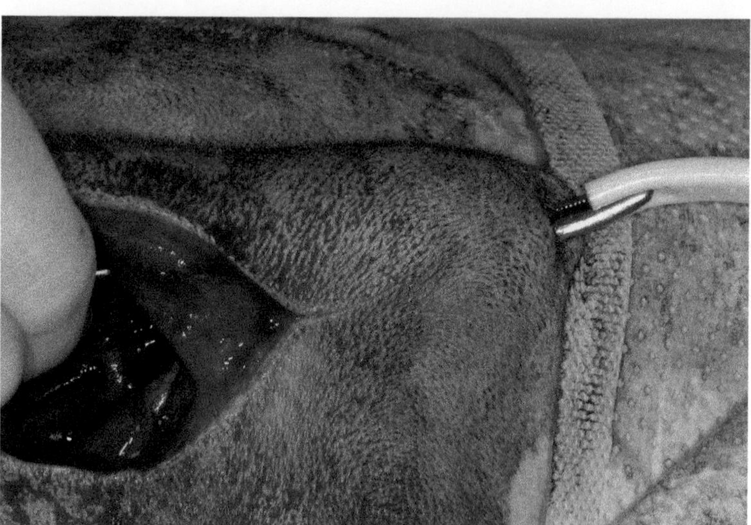

Figure 15-3 Pull the multifenestrated portion of the drain into the abdomen.

e. Secure the external tubing to the skin with a separate finger trap pattern (see Ch. 61).

f. Place 2 to 5 continuous suction (e.g., Jackson Pratt) drains in dependent positions, with each exiting the abdomen from a separate incision (fig. 15-5). Drains should be spread cranially and caudally throughout the abdomen. In medium-sized dogs with generalized peritonitis, 2 drains are placed cranially between the liver and diaphragm and 1 or 2 drains are placed caudally.

7. Close the abdomen routinely.
8. Attach the suction bulb reservoirs to the tubing. Empty the air from each reservoir and cap it to provide continuous suction.
9. Place an abdominal bandage to cover all drain exit sites. Secure the reservoirs to the bandage or a collar (fig. 15-6).

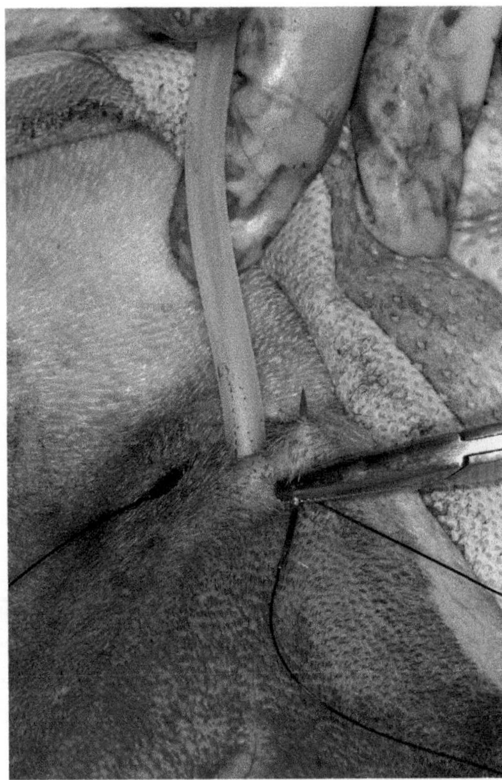

Figure 15-4 To prevent fluid or air leakage around tube exit site, place a purse-string suture.

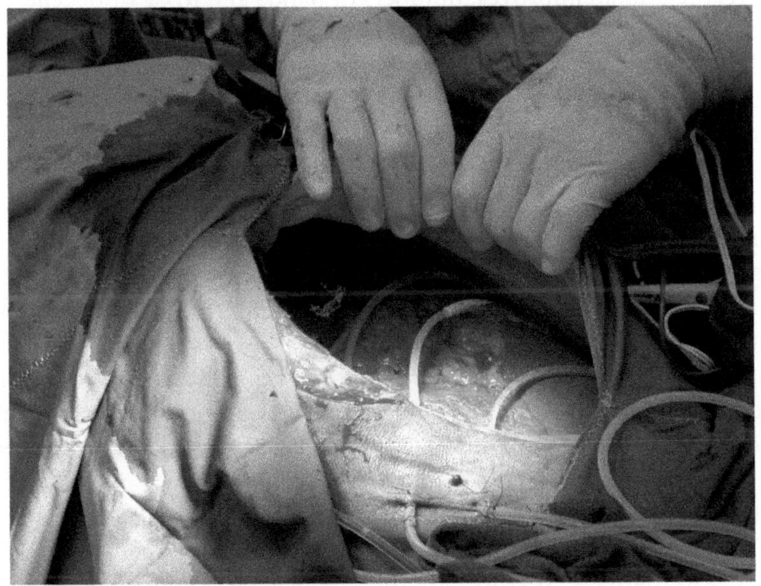

Figure 15-5 Final placement. Drains exit from separate sites and are evenly spaced throughout the abdomen.

Postoperative considerations

Postoperatively CVP, arterial blood pressure, weight, and urine output should be monitored frequently to determine appropriate fluid therapy. Fluid replacement volume should include maintenance requirements (40–60 mL/kg/day), amount collected from the drains, and replacement for other ongoing losses. Opioids are administered for analgesia. Antibiotics should be selected based on culture and sensitivity results and continued for at least 7 days. Nutrition is

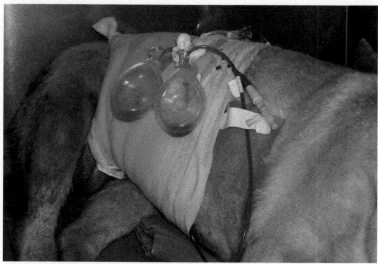

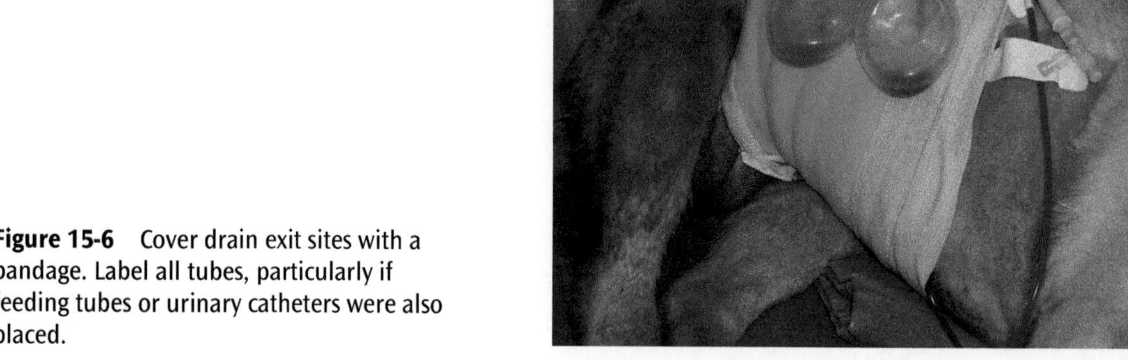

Figure 15-6 Cover drain exit sites with a bandage. Label all tubes, particularly if feeding tubes or urinary catheters were also placed.

critical for recovery and resolution of ileus (particularly enteral feeding); affected animals may need 20–60 Kcal/kg/day. If not vomiting, animals can be fed the day after surgery, even if gastrointestinal surgery has been performed. Maintenance of comfort and hygiene is important in recumbent animals and should include periodic rotation, comfortable bedding, wound care, and skin protectants to avoid urine or fecal scalding.

Abdominal drainage may result in anemia, hypoproteinemia, electrolyte disturbances, and dehydration, so these parameters must be checked at least daily. As the animal improves, numbers of bands and toxic or degenerate cells in the peripheral blood should decrease. Colloid-osmotic pressure measurements are helpful for guiding colloidal fluid therapy in hypoproteinemic animals.

Drain reservoirs are emptied and recharged every 4 hours as needed. Fluid production is usually dramatic for the first 16 hours (up to 20 mL/kg/day), especially if lavage fluid was not completely removed. Fluid production will gradually decrease over the next 2 to 3 days to 8 mL/kg/day, as long as the primary cause has been corrected and appropriate antimicrobials are being given. Usually one or two drains will become nonproductive as omentum surrounds them.

Because peritoneal effusion is normal, drain removal is based on changes in fluid character. Abdominal fluid white blood cell counts may increase one day after surgery, but cells should not appear more toxic or degenerate. Cells that have been sitting in the reservoir or drain tubing may look unhealthy. To obtain a fresh sample of fluid, empty the reservoir to recharge the drain; empty it again after 5 to 10 mL of fluid have been collected, and then sample the next effluent. Alternatively, perform an abdominocentesis under ultrasound guidance to get the most accurate idea of fluid character. Drains can be pulled without anesthesia: simply cut the finger trap and purse string sutures and pull gently but firmly.

Reported mortality rates for peritonitis range from 15% to 73%. Prognosis is worse for very young or very old animals or in the presence of delayed diagnosis, greater or more virulent contamination (e.g., contamination from the large intestines), decreased immune function, or poor nutrition. Presence of organ failure, shock, refractory hypotension, cardiovascular collapse, respiratory dysfunction, disseminated intravascular coagulation, or septic bile peritonitis increases mortality rates.

Bibliography

Adams RJ, Doyle RS, Bray JP, et al: Closed suction drainage for treatment of septic peritonitis of confirmed gastrointestinal origin in 20 dogs. Vet Surg 2014;43:843–851.

Bonczynski JJ et al: Comparison of peritoneal fluid and peripheral blood pH, bicarbonate, glucose, and lactate concentration as a diagnostic tool for septic peritonitis in dogs and cats. Vet Surg 2003;32:161–166.

Costello MF et al: Underlying cause, pathophysiologic abnormalities, and response to treatment in cats with septic peritonitis: 51 cases (1990–2001). J Am Vet Med Assoc 2004;225:897–902.

Dickinson AE, Summers JF, Wignal J, et al: Impact of appropriate empirical antimicrobial therapy on outcome of dogs with septic peritonitis. J Vet Emerg Crit Care 2015;25:152–159.

Levin GM et al: Lactate as a diagnostic test for septic peritoneal effusions in dogs and cats. J Am Anim Hosp Assoc 2004;40:364–371.

Mueller MG et al: Use of closed-suction drains to treat generalized peritonitis in dogs and cats: 40 cases (1997–1999). J Am Vet Med Assoc 2001;219:789–794.

Schmiedt C et al: Evaluation of abdominal and peripheral potassium and creatinine concentrations for diagnosis of uroperitoneum in dogs. J Vet Emerg Crit Care 2001;11:275–280.

Staatz AJ et al: Open peritoneal drainage versus primary closure for the treatment of septic peritonitis in dogs and cats: 42 cases (1993–99). Vet Surg 2002;31:174–180.

Section 3 Surgery of the Digestive System

Chapter 16
Liver Biopsy

Indications for liver biopsy include hepatic masses or nodules, hepatic hyperbilirubinemia, or persistent increase in liver enzyme, serum bile acid, or plasma ammonia concentration. Liver biopsies are also recommended in patients with unexplained generalized hepatomegaly or altered hepatic echogenicity on ultrasound. Liver samples can be obtained percutaneously or by open or laparoscopic surgical biopsy. Samples obtained by surgical biopsy are larger and more likely to be of diagnostic quality than those obtained percutaneously. Surgical approaches also reduce the risk of inadvertent damage to the gallbladder or other organs in patients with small livers.

Preoperative management

Preoperative diagnostics and treatment depend on the underlying disease process. Coagulation panels and buccal mucosal bleeding times should be performed in patients with thrombocytopenia, significant hypoalbuminemia, biliary obstruction, severe liver disease, or sepsis. If prolonged clotting times are detected, the patient should receive fresh frozen plasma or fresh whole blood before surgery. Vitamin K1, which is necessary for production of clotting factors II, VII, IX, and X, should be administered in patients with biliary obstruction (1–5 mg/kg SC with a small needle). For surgical preparation, animals should be clipped to midthorax, since the abdominal incision often extends to the xiphoid cartilage.

Surgery

In animals undergoing liver biopsy, ventral midline incisions should start caudal to the xiphoid process to avoid perforation of the diaphragm. Ligation and amputation of falciform fat may be necessary to expose small livers. The incision can be extended superficial to the xiphoid process to increase exposure (see p. 170). If a celiotomy is to be performed, the entire abdomen should be explored for abnormalities. To improve exposure, a moistened laparotomy pad can be placed between the diaphragm and liver lobes. One corner of the pad can be secured to the drape with a hemostat so that it can't be accidently left in the abdomen. In animals with diffuse disease that do not require

Manual of Small Animal Soft Tissue Surgery, Second Edition. Karen Tobias.
© 2017 John Wiley & Sons, Inc. Published 2017 by John Wiley & Sons, Inc.

exploration, the liver can be biopsied through a 2- to 4-cm midline keyhole incision.

Livers with diffuse disease can be sampled with a clamshell biopsy forceps or a guillotine suture ligation technique. A box stitch may be needed in animals with rounded lobes. Suture ligations are usually performed with 3-0 rapidly absorbable monofilament material. Samples from central lesions can be obtained with clamshell biopsy forceps or a skin punch. A 6-mm punch biopsy instrument is preferred in animals with microvascular disease, since the 4-mm instruments are less likely to provide an adequate number of portal triads for evaluation. Because hepatic veins are located closer to the caudodorsal (visceral) surface of the liver, punch biopsies are taken from the convex, diaphragmatic surface. Punch biopsy depth should not exceed 50% of the liver lobe thickness.

If focal lesions are present, the junction between normal and abnormal tissue should be included in the biopsy sample. Multiple lobes are usually biopsied when congenital microvascular anomalies are suspected (e.g., microvascular dysplasia secondary to congenital portal hypoplasia).

Surgical technique: guillotine biopsy

1. Using 3-0 rapidly absorbable monofilament material, fashion a 3- to 4-cm suture loop that has a surgeon's throw.
2. Encircle the tip of a liver lobe with the suture loop. Include at least 1 cm of tissue in the suture loop.
    a. If a natural fissure is present near the tip of the lobe, drop the suture into the fissure (fig. 16-1).
    b. If the liver lobe cannot be easily exposed, insert an Allis tissue forceps through the suture loop. Grasp at least 1 cm of the tip of the liver with the forceps. Gently retract the liver lobe and slide the suture around the liver tissue just beyond the forceps.

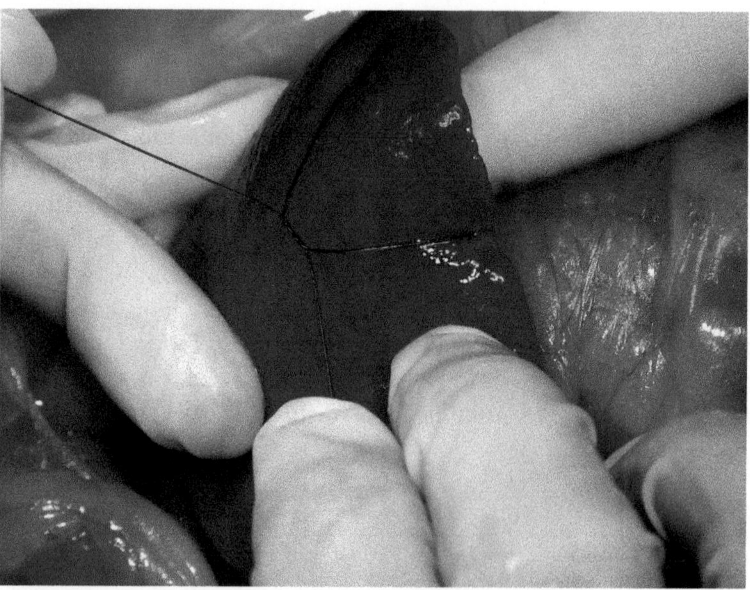

Figure 16-1 Drop the suture loop over the liver tip into natural fissures along the margins.

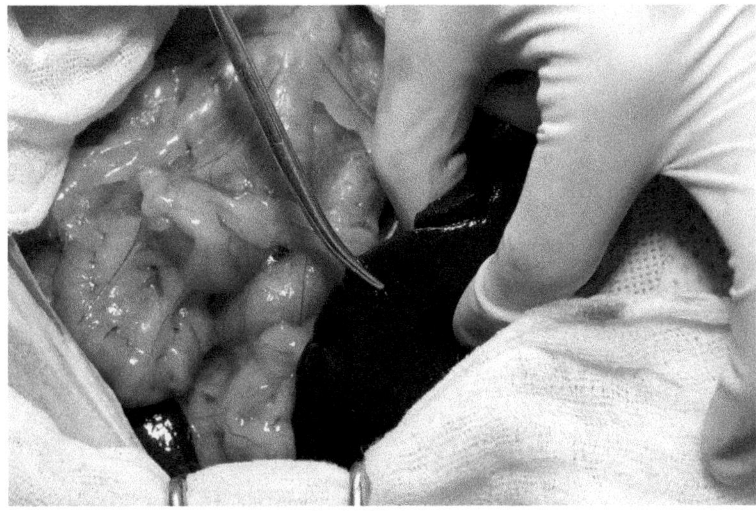

Figure 16-2 If the margin is rounded, crush the edge of the liver margin with hemostats to make a fissure.

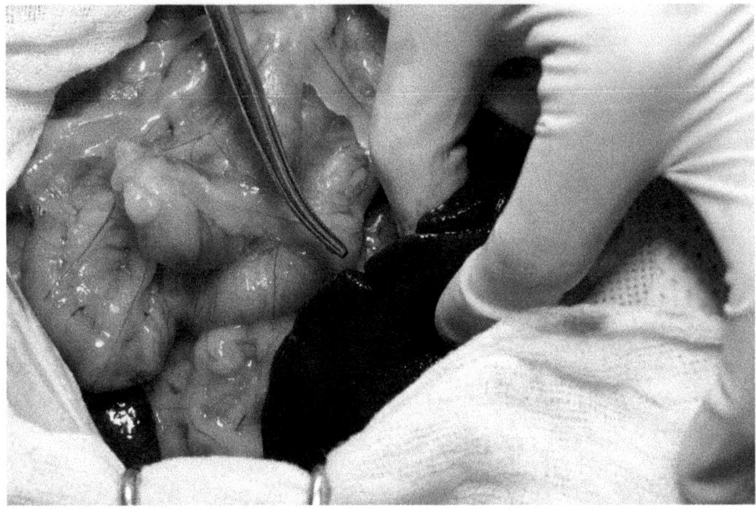

Figure 16-3 Pull the closed hemostat gently away from the edge to make a fissure.

c. If the liver margin is rounded, crush the edge of the liver lobe tip on one or both sides of the desired sample site with a hemostatic forceps to make fissures (figs. 16-2 and 16-3) that angle inward toward the base of the desired tissue sample. Drop the suture into the fissures.

3. Tighten the suture loop until it crushes through all the liver tissue, leaving the vessels and ducts intact (figs. 16-4 and 16-5). Do not lift up on the suture when tightening or you will pull the ligature off and tear the vessels. A single throw is sufficient for hemostasis.
4. With scissors or a blade, transect the tissue distal to the ligature (fig. 16-6), leaving the ligature and a small stump of tissue on the liver lobe. Do not grasp the liver sample with forceps.

Surgical technique: box suture biopsy

1. With 3-0 absorbable suture material on a taper needle, take a full-thickness bite through the liver tissue adjacent to the desired biopsy site (fig. 16-7).

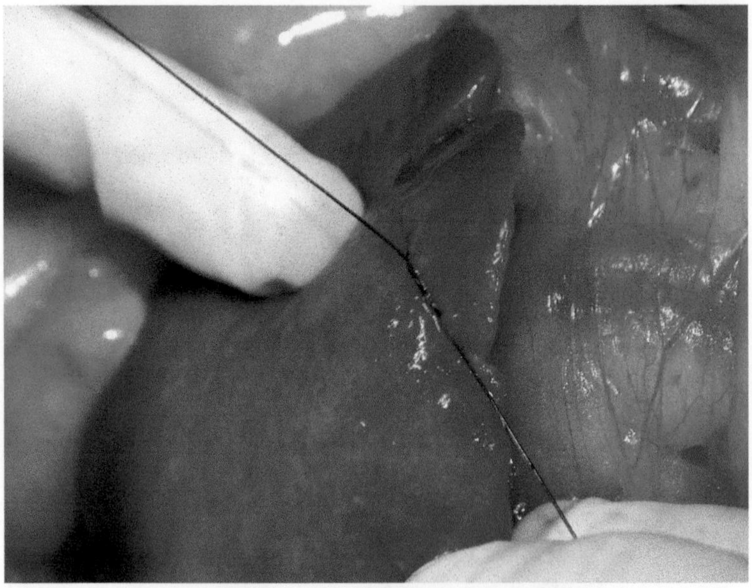

Figure 16-4 Tighten the suture loop around the base of the tissue, keeping hands low and suture ends oriented horizontally.

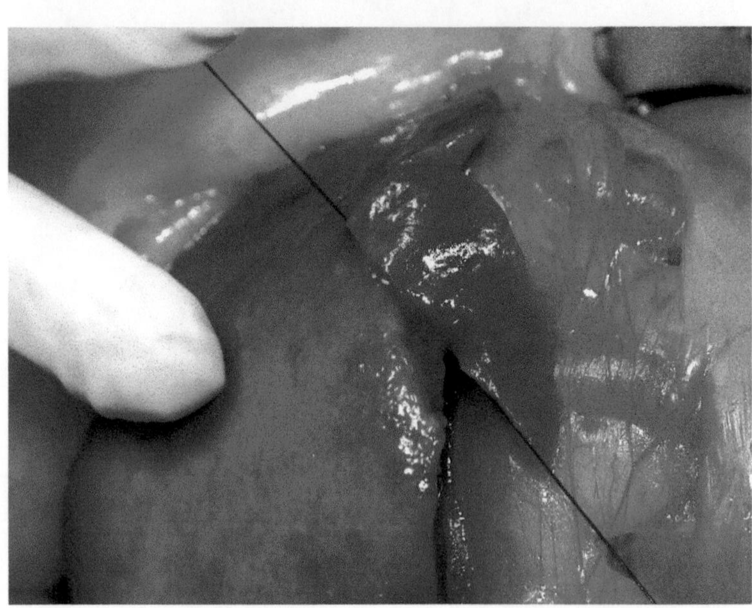

Figure 16-5 Tighten the suture until it crushes through all the enclosed parenchyma. A single surgeon's throw is sufficient for hemostasis.

2. Tie a surgeon's throw and tighten it to crush through the hepatic margin and encircled tissue (fig. 16-8). Keep hands low and level when tightening the throw. If desired, tie a second throw. Cut the suture ends.
3. Place a second full-thickness suture bite on the opposite side of the tissue to be biopsied: angle this bite toward the base of the original bite. The second suture bite should be 1.5 to 2 cm away from the first suture. Tie a surgeon's throw and crush the encircled tissue. If desired, tie a second throw. Cut the suture ends.
4. If the two sutures meet at the base of the tissue, the tissue sample can now be harvested with scissors. If the two sutures do not meet at the base of the tissue, use an additional encircling suture, as with the guillotine technique, to ligate the remaining tissue at the base, then harvest the tissue sample with scissors (fig 16-9).

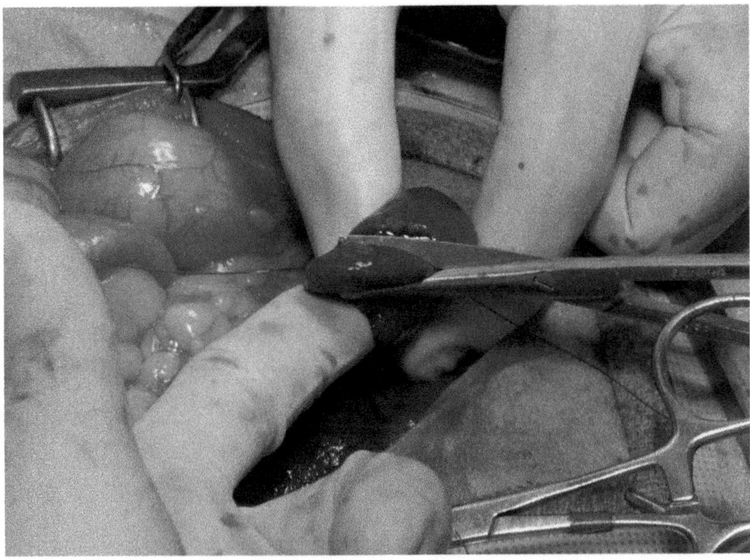

Figure 16-6 Transect the tissue distal to the ligature, leaving the ligature and a small stump of tissue in place.

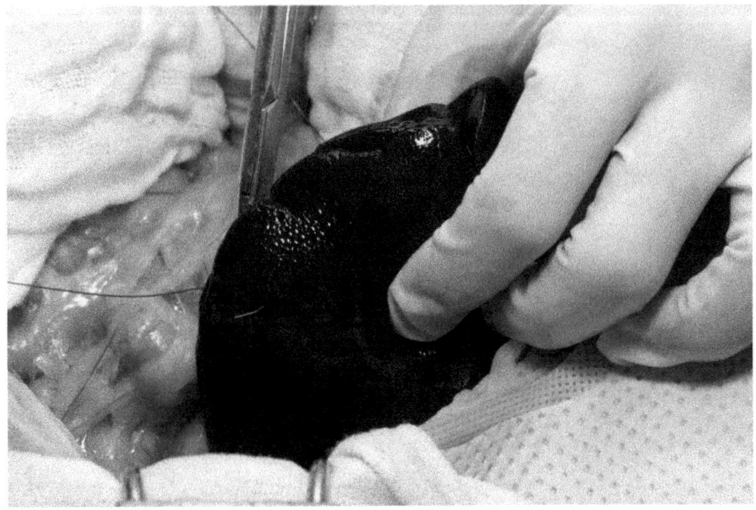

Figure 16-7 Take a bite through the liver perpendicular to the margin.

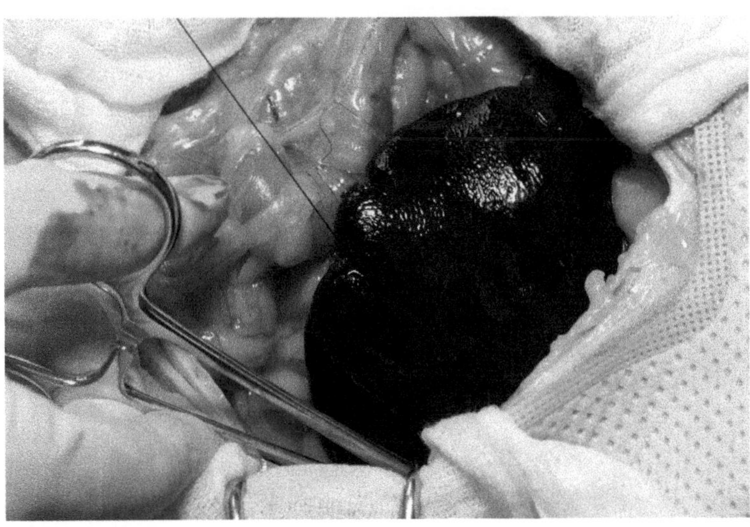

Figure 16-8 Tie one or two throws, tightening to cut through the parenchyma. Cut the suture ends short.

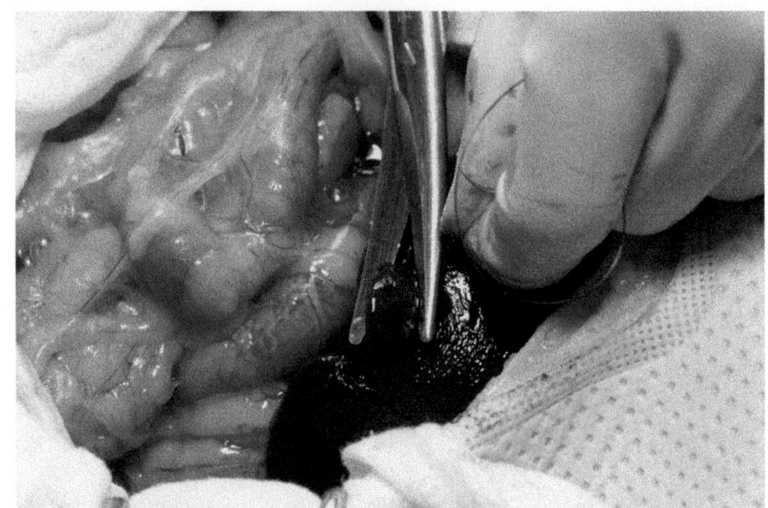

Figure 16-9 The base of tissue has been crushed with a guillotine suture. The tissue sample is transected such that the sutures and a small stump of tissue remain in place.

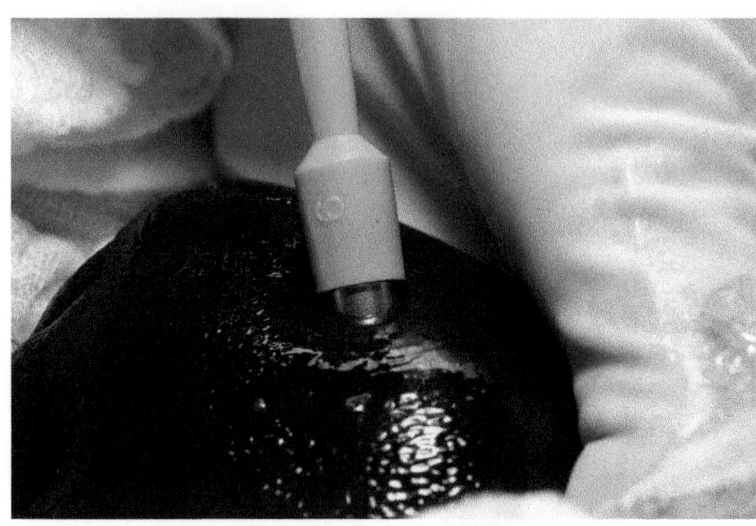

Figure 16-10 Rotate the punch into the hepatic parenchyma, then tilt the punch slightly while advancing further to sever the tissue base.

Surgical technique: skin punch liver biopsy

1. Position a 6-mm skin punch perpendicular to the diaphragmatic (convex) surface of the liver.
2. Press downward while rotating the punch clockwise and counterclockwise to twist it into the liver tissue. Do not penetrate more than halfway through the liver thickness.
3. Tilt the punch 45 degrees and rotate while advancing slightly to sever any remaining tissue attachments (fig. 16-10).
4. Withdraw the punch at an angle to retain the sample within the instrument (fig. 16-11). If the sample remains in the liver, use Metzenbaum scissors to transect its base and retrieve the sample. Do not handle the sample with thumb forceps.
5. If the biopsy site is bleeding, insert a plug of hemostatic material (e.g., gelatin foam) into the defect, or apply direct pressure for several minutes. Alternatively, carefully place a wide mattress or cruciate suture of

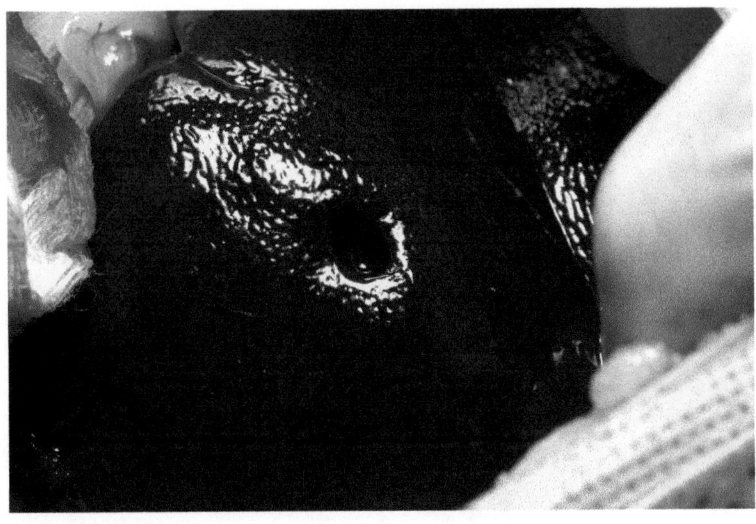

Figure 16-11 Resultant punch hole.

absorbable material across the site. Tie with 1 or 2 knots, using a surgeon's throw for the first throw; tighten gently so that the suture material does not tear the liver parenchyma.

Surgical technique: keyhole incision

1. Make a 2- to 4-cm ventral midline skin incision just caudal to the xiphoid process (fig. 16-12).
2. Extend the incision through the subcutaneous fat and linea.
3. Insert a finger gently through the incision to separate the falciform fat.
4. Reach forward with your index or pinkie finger and hook the lesser curvature of the stomach. With downward digital pressure, pull the stomach caudally and then withdraw your finger. This will allow the liver lobes to move caudally so they are under the incision.
5. Lift one side of the abdominal wall with thumb forceps to expose the underlying liver. If the liver is not visible, extend the linea incision or retract the abdominal wall cranially.

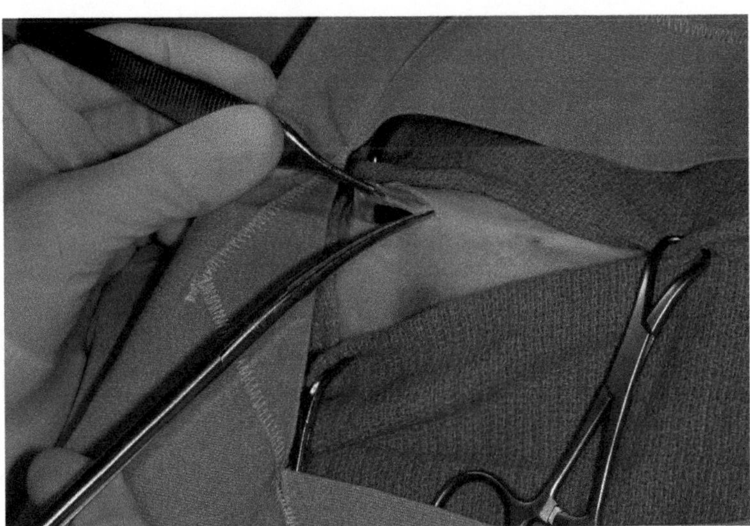

Figure 16-12 Make a 2- to 4-cm incision through the skin, subcutaneous tissues, and linea just caudal to the xiphoid. Cranial is to the left in this photo.

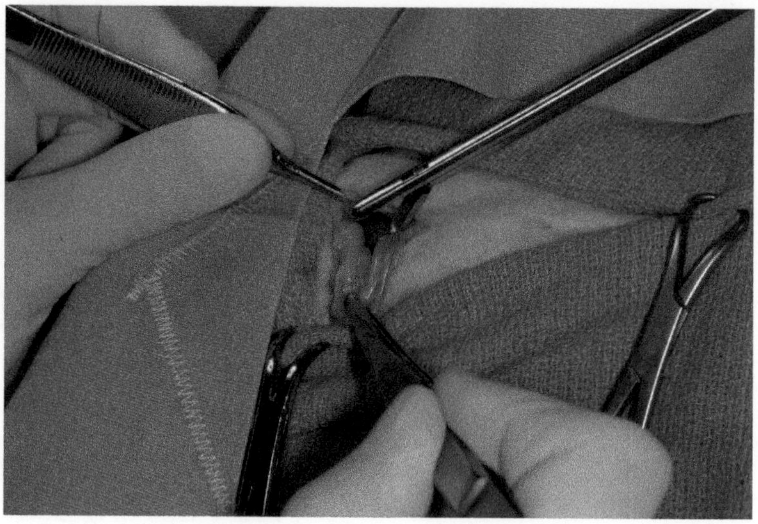

Figure 16-13 Grasp the exposed liver margin with clamshell biopsy forceps; hold the jaws closed for 10 to 20 seconds before pulling the forceps away from the liver.

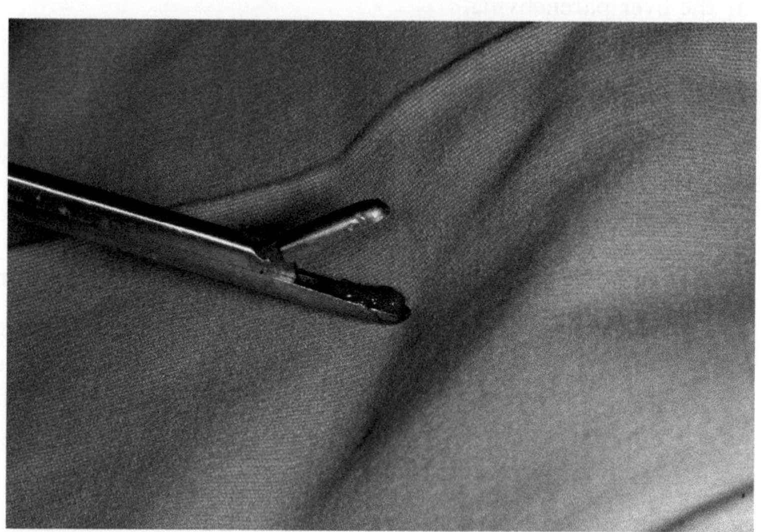

Figure 16-14 Final sample.

6. Grasp a large bite of the edge of the liver with clamshell biopsy forceps (fig. 16-13). Insert the forceps over the parenchymal edge so that the liver tissue reaches the angle of the jaws. Make sure the forceps jaws contain only liver.
7. Close the jaws firmly and hold them apposed for 10 to 20 seconds.
8. Twist the forceps while pulling back gently until the piece of liver tissue is freed (fig. 16-14).
9. If the tissue is trapped within the jaws of the instrument, use a needle to gently tease it out. Do not handle the sample with thumb forceps.
10. If possible, sample additional liver lobes.
11. Close the external rectus sheath with a continuous or interrupted pattern. Close the subcutis and skin routinely.

Postoperative considerations

Since complications of surgical liver biopsy are rare, postoperative care is primarily focused on treatment of the underlying condition. Liver biopsy sites rarely bleed, even when a clamshell or "grab and twist" method is used. If hemorrhage is a concern, hematocrit should be measured immediately after surgery and then several hours later to evaluate the animal for progressive anemia. Punch biopsies cause significantly more hemorrhage than guillotine or clamshell techniques.

Bibliography

Cole TL et al: Diagnostic comparison of needle and wedge biopsy specimens of the liver in dogs and cats. J Am Vet Med Assoc 2002;220:1483–1490.

Kemp SD, Zimmerman KL, Panciera DL, et al: A comparison of liver sampling techniques in dogs. J Vet Intern Med 2015;29:51–57.

Kemp SD, Zimmerman KL, Panciera DL, et al: Histopathologic variation between liver lobes in dogs. J Vet Inter Med 2015;29:58–62.

McDevitt HL, Mayhew PD, Giuffrida MA, et al: Short-term clinical outcome of laparoscopic liver biopsy in dogs: 106 cases (2003–2013). J Am Vet Med Assoc 2016;248:83–90.

Roth L: Comparison of liver cytology and biopsy diagnoses in dogs and cats: 56 cases. Vet Clin Pathol 2001;30:35–38.

Vasanjee SC et al: Evaluation of hemorrhage, sample size, and collateral damage for five hepatic biopsy methods in dogs. Vet Surg 2006;35:86–93.

Chapter 17
Pancreatic Biopsy

Histologic evaluation of the pancreas is useful for diagnosis of inflammation, atrophy, subclinical exocrine pancreatic insufficiency, or neoplasia. Many clinicians avoid routine pancreatic biopsy, however, because of the potential for intestinal vascular compromise. The cranial pancreaticoduodenal artery travels within the body and right lobe of the pancreas, anastomosing with the caudal pancreaticoduodenal artery at the caudal end of the right pancreatic limb (fig. 17-1). Segmental branches from these arteries traverse the pancreatic parenchyma to supply the descending duodenum. Inadvertent damage to the cranial or caudal pancreaticoduodenal artery could result in duodenal ischemia. The pancreatic ducts travel within the center of the parenchyma and can also be damaged during biopsy.

Preoperative management

Preoperative diagnostics and supportive care depend on the underlying condition. Most patients undergo abdominal ultrasound to evaluate the pancreas for focal or generalized disease. Pancreatitis can be diagnosed by measuring pancreatic lipase immunoreactivity. Serum trypsin-like immunoreactivity is the preferred test for exocrine pancreatic insufficiency. If neoplasia is suspected, thoracic and abdominal radiographs and abdominal ultrasound should be evaluated for metastases.

Surgery

When pancreatic disease is diffuse, the distal lateral aspect of the right or left limb of the pancreas is usually biopsied to avoid organ or vessel damage (fig. 17-2). Unfortunately, a single biopsy may be insufficient to exclude pancreatitis, since pancreatic inflammation can occur in discrete areas within the pancreas, rather than diffusely. Biopsy samples can be obtained by guillotine ("suture fracture") technique, interlobular dissection and vessel/duct ligation, or cup biopsy forceps retrieval (similar to a liver biopsy; see p. 140). When the pancreas is firm, a sample can be trimmed off the pancreatic surface or margin with a blade or fine scissors.

Manual of Small Animal Soft Tissue Surgery, Second Edition. Karen Tobias.
© 2017 John Wiley & Sons, Inc. Published 2017 by John Wiley & Sons, Inc.

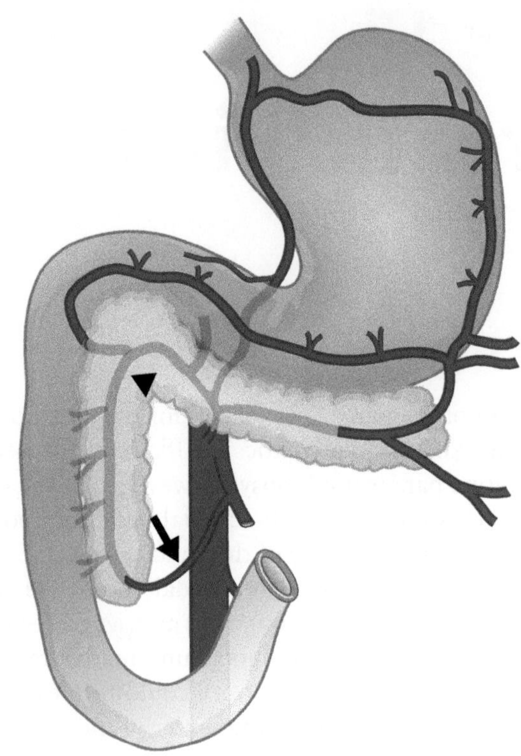

Figure 17-1 Illustration of the pancreatic blood supply. The cranial pancreaticoduodenal artery (arrowhead) travels within the pancreatic parenchyma and anastomoses with the caudal pancreaticoduodenal artery (arrow). These vessels provide critical blood supply to the descending duodenum.

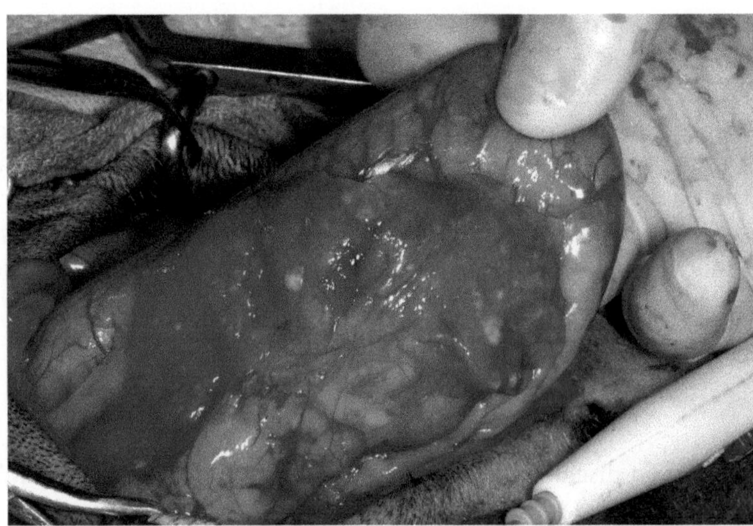

Figure 17-2 Diffuse pancreatic disease with multiple nodules. In this dog, the pancreaticoduodenal vessels were obscured by the overlying pancreas.

Surgical technique: guillotine biopsy of the pancreas

1. Expose the distal limb of the pancreas.
    a. Expose the right limb of the pancreas along the descending duodenum by retracting the duodenum ventrally and out of the abdominal cavity.
    b. Expose the left limb of the pancreas by tearing a hole in the ventral leaf of the omentum and retracting the stomach cranially. The splenic artery and vein are visible just beyond the tip of the pancreas (see fig. 13-4).

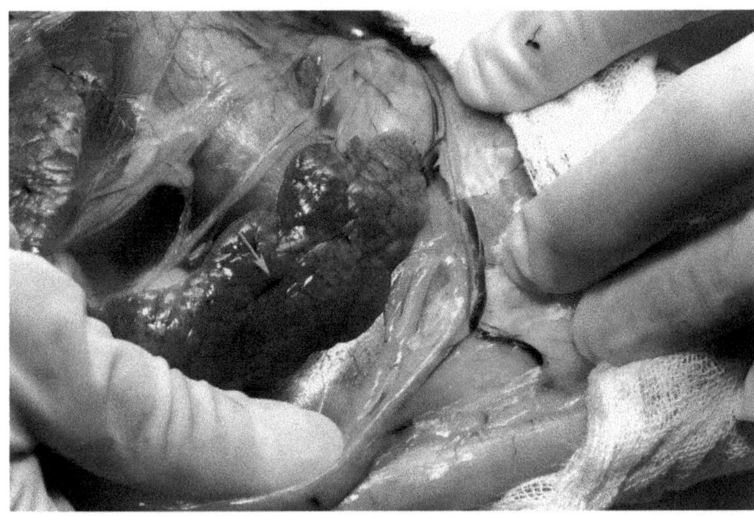

Figure 17-3 In the right limb of the pancreas, identify the pancreaticoduodenal arteries and vein (arrow); avoid damaging these vessels.

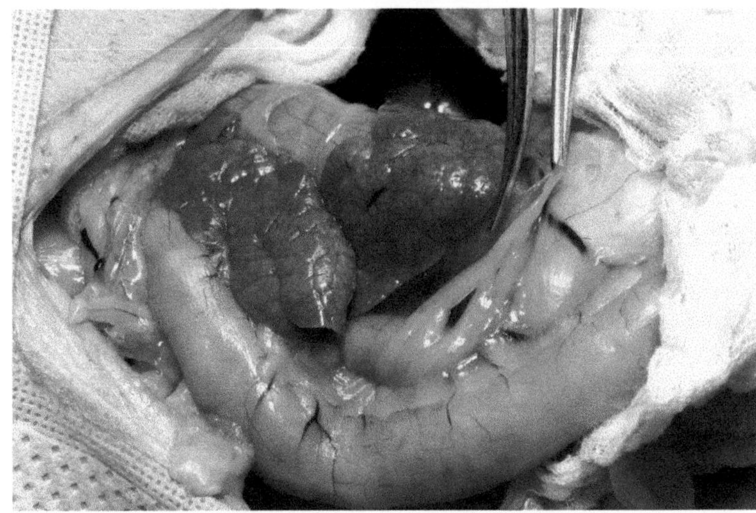

Figure 17-4 Bluntly dissect the mesoduodenum away from the pancreas.

2. Identify the cranial and caudal pancreaticoduodenal vessels and duodenal branches (fig. 17-3) or splenic artery and vein (see fig. 13-4). Select a biopsy site away from these vessels.
3. Bluntly dissect the mesentery away from the distal 1 cm of the pancreatic limb (fig. 17-4).
4. Fashion a loop of 3-0, rapidly absorbable suture with a surgeon's throw. Pass the suture loop around the free edge of the exposed pancreatic tissue to obtain a 0.5- to 1.0-cm sample. Tighten the throw to crush the tissue (fig. 17-5). Add extra throws and cut suture ends short.
5. Excise the specimen distal to the ligature with scissors (fig. 17-6) or a blade. Leave the ligature in place.
6. Examine the site for hemorrhage (fig. 17-7). If bleeding is present, apply digital pressure or a plug of hemostatic gelatin foam. Closure of small defects in the mesoduodenum is unnecessary.

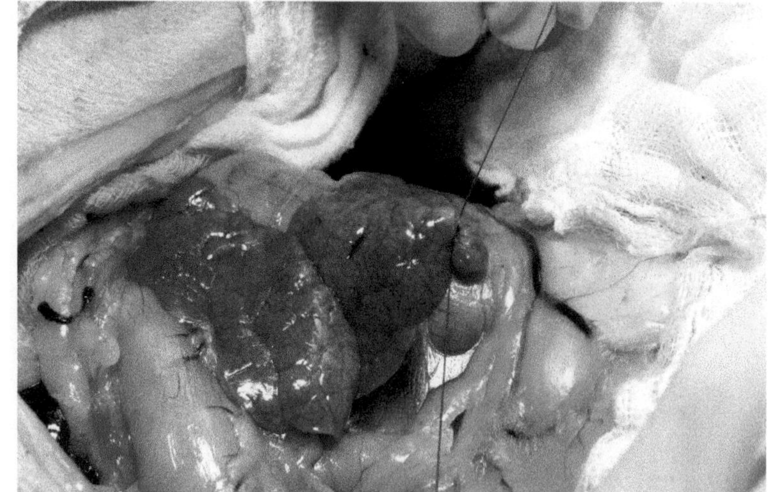

Figure 17-5 Ligate the base of the desired sample, taking care to avoid major vessels.

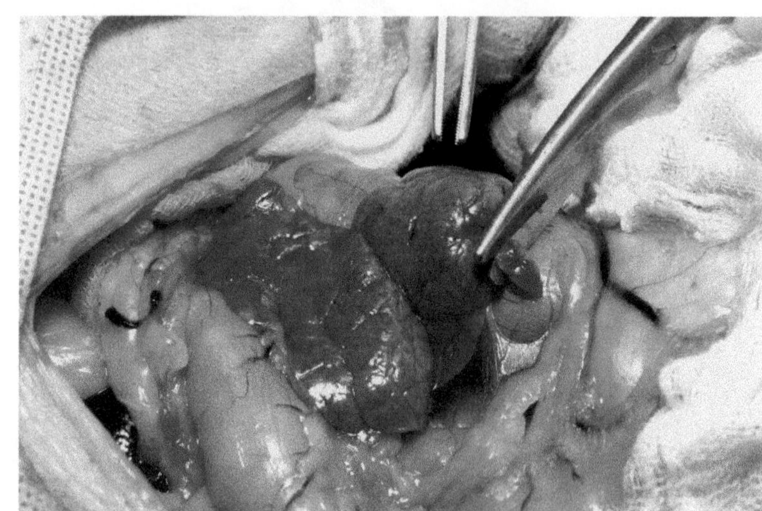

Figure 17-6 Transect the base of the tissue distal to the ligature.

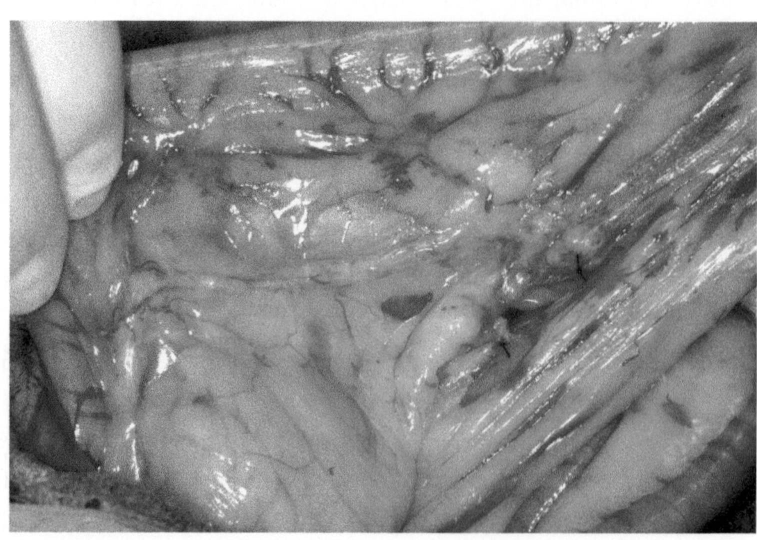

Figure 17-7 Final appearance of the biopsy site in a dog with pancreatic atrophy. In this dog, a small mesenteric branch was also ligated.

Postoperative considerations

Compared with interlobular dissection and vessel ligation, pancreatic biopsy with a guillotine or cup forceps technique may result in significant increases in lipase, amylase, or trypsin-like immunoreactivity. Histologically, the guillotine technique may also cause more local inflammation. Despite this, none of these techniques causes clinical signs of pancreatitis in healthy dogs. Pancreatitis after guillotine biopsy has been reported in dogs and cats undergoing exploratory laparotomy for other conditions, however. Patients should therefore be monitored for signs of pancreatitis (abdominal pain, nausea, lethargy, inappetance, pyrexia) after surgery. If pancreatitis is suspected, supportive care (fluids, analgesics, antiemetics, gastroprotectants, and nutritional support) should be provided and, if possible, the abdomen ultrasounded to provide diagnostic evidence of the condition and rule out other differentials.

Bibliography

Allen SW et al: A comparison of two methods of partial pancreatectomy in the dog. Vet Surg 1989;18:274–278.

Barnes RF et al: Comparison of biopsy samples obtained using standard endoscopic instruments and the harmonic scalpel during laparoscopic and laparoscopic-assisted surgery in normal dogs. Vet Surg 2006;35:243–251.

Case JB, Fox-Alvarez WA: Pancreatic biopsy (Procedures Pro). Clinician's Brief 2015;13:19–24.

Cordner AP, Armstrong PJ, Newman SJ et al: Effect of pancreatic tissue sampling on serum pancreatic enzyme levels in clinically healthy dogs. J Vet Diagn Invest 2010;22:702–707.

Harmoinen J et al: Evaluation of pancreatic forceps biopsy by laparoscopy in healthy beagles. Vet Therapeutics 2002;3:31–36.

Lutz TA et al: Pancreatic biopsy in normal cats. Austr Vet J 1994;71:223–225.

Pratschke KM, Ryan J, McAlinden A, et al: Pancreatic surgical biopsy in 24 dogs and 19 cats: postoperative complications and clinical relevance of histological findings. J Small Anim Pract 2015;56:60–66.

Chapter 18
Gastrotomy

The most common indication for gastrotomy is gastric foreign body removal. Gastrotomy also permits evaluation of the gastric mucosa for pathologic changes, such as ulceration, and digital palpation of the pyloric ostium to verify size and patency. In some animals, distal esophageal foreign bodies can be removed through a gastrotomy. Gastrotomy incisions can be converted into a partial gastrectomy for full thickness biopsy or to remove tumors or other focal lesions. A gastrotomy site can be incorporated into an incisional gastropexy if the mucosa/submucosa is closed with a continuous pattern before the gastropexy is performed.

Preoperative management

Prior to anaesthesia, dehydration, acid-base imbalances, and electrolyte disturbances should be corrected. Animals with zinc toxicity may require transfusion for hemolytic anemia. Prophylactic antibiotics may be administered intravenously at induction and 1.5 to 6 hours later; continuation of antibiotics is usually not necessary. Animals should be clipped and prepped from midthorax to prepuce or pubis. The endotracheal tube cuff should be checked for adequate inflation, since manipulation of the stomach may force gastric contents into the esophagus. Laparotomy pads, suction, and lavage solution should be available.

Surgery

As with any gastrointestinal surgery, the abdomen should be fully explored, and any clean procedures, such as liver biopsy, should be performed before opening the stomach. Abdominal incisions usually start at the xiphoid and extend caudal to the umbilicus. Extending the incision lateral to the xiphoid may result in diaphragmatic perforation and subsequent pneumothorax; if greater exposure is needed, the incision can be extended superficial (ventral) to the xiphoid without opening the chest (see p. 170). The falciform ligament may require ligation and resection to expose the stomach (see p. 87). Before entering contaminated viscera, the organ should be isolated with moistened laparotomy pads and sterile instruments set aside for closure.

Manual of Small Animal Soft Tissue Surgery, Second Edition. Karen Tobias.
© 2017 John Wiley & Sons, Inc. Published 2017 by John Wiley & Sons, Inc.

Gastrotomies for foreign body removal are usually made in the body of the stomach so that the pyloric region will not be obstructed by an inverting closure. If possible, the stomach is incised midway between the greater and lesser curvatures in the least vascular region of the serosa. Stay sutures can be placed along the edges of the incision to facilitate retraction and exposure, and gastric contents can be removed by suction to reduce contamination. Gastric foreign bodies are usually removed by grasping them with Allis tissue, Carmalt, or Kelly forceps. If a distal esophageal foreign body is present, blunt-tipped forceps (e.g., Carmalt or sponge forceps) are inserted through the gastrotomy incision and lower esophageal sphincter and advanced into the esophagus. If the foreign body cannot be grasped easily, the animal is manually ventilated and the diaphragm is incised so that the surgeon's free hand can be used to stabilize or manipulate the esophagus while attempting to grasp the foreign body with the instrument. Once the esophageal foreign body is removed and the stomach is closed, the diaphragmatic incision is apposed around a red rubber catheter; the pleural cavity is evacuated before catheter removal and abdominal closure.

A variety of methods have been recommended for closure of gastrotomy incisions, which heal quickly and rarely dehisce. Some surgeons will close the gastric mucosa with a continuous pattern to reduce intragastric hemorrhage, then close the seromuscular layers of the stomach with a Cushing or Lembert inverting pattern. Other surgeons will perform a two-layer inverting closure that extends only to the submucosa, since the gastric mucosa will eventually seal itself. Gastrotomy near the pylorus should be closed with a single-layer, appositional interrupted or continuous pattern to prevent outflow obstruction. Gastric closure is usually performed with 2-0 or 3-0 absorbable monofilament suture on a taper needle, depending on stomach thickness and needle size. Absorbable, knotless barbed suture may be equally as effective.

After the gastrotomy is completed, contaminated gloves and instruments are replaced, and the abdomen is flushed and suctioned to remove any contaminants.

Surgical technique: gastrotomy

1. To provide retraction, place stay sutures in the stomach, making sure to include submucosa in each suture bite. (fig. 18-1). Stay sutures can be attached to the abdominal wall retractors to keep the stomach retracted from the abdomen (fig. 18-2).
2. Isolate the stomach with moistened laparotomy pads to reduce contamination.
3. Incise the gastric body parallel to the long axis of the stomach and midway between the greater and lesser curvatures (fig. 18-3).
    a. With a scalpel blade, make a stab incision full thickness into the stomach. The mucosa may fall away from the blade during the initial incision. If still intact, grasp the mucosa with atraumatic thumb forceps and perforate it with the scalpel blade.
    b. Extend the incision as needed with scissors.
    c. Proceed with foreign body removal, biopsy, or lumenal exploration.
        i. To obtain a biopsy, resect a full-thickness sample from the incision edge with scissors.

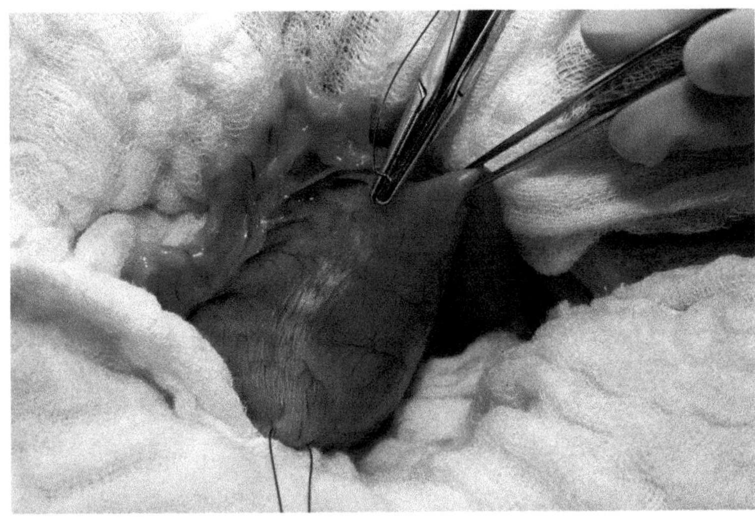

Figure 18-1 Isolate the stomach with moistened laparotomy pads and place stay sutures to provide retraction.

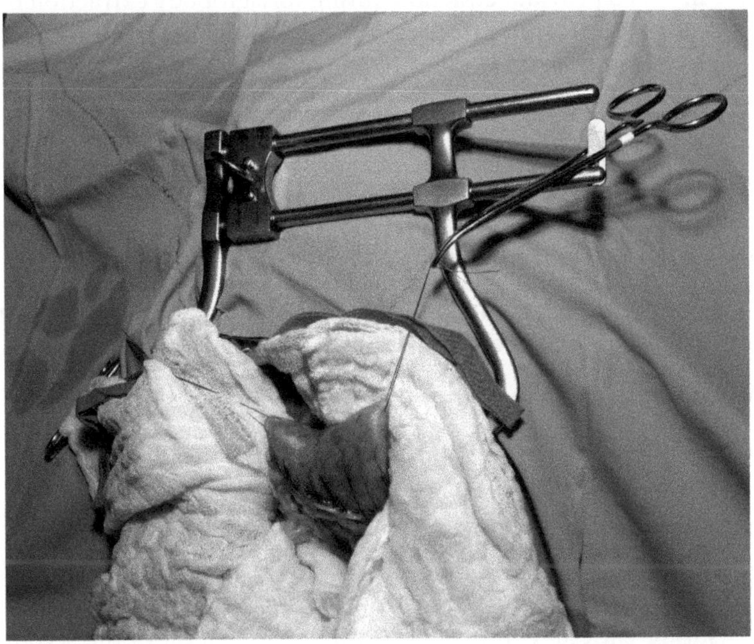

Figure 18-2 If desired, hook the stay sutures over the abdominal wall retractors to keep the stomach exposed.

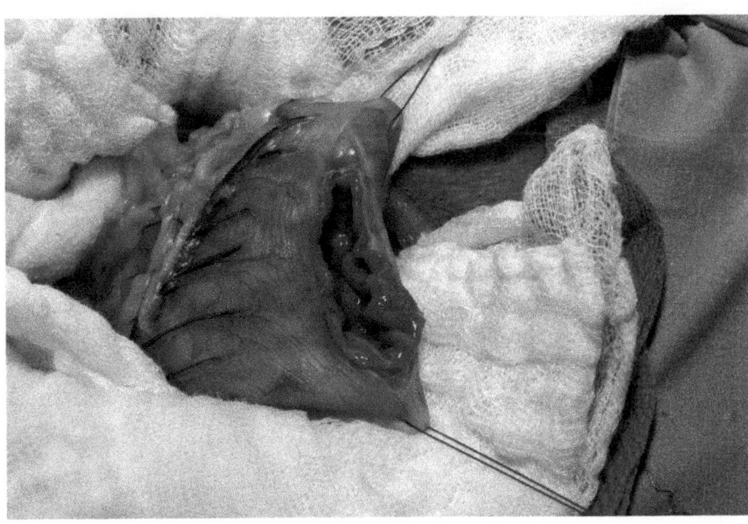

Figure 18-3 Make the gastric incision parallel to the long axis of the stomach, midway between the greater and lesser curvatures.

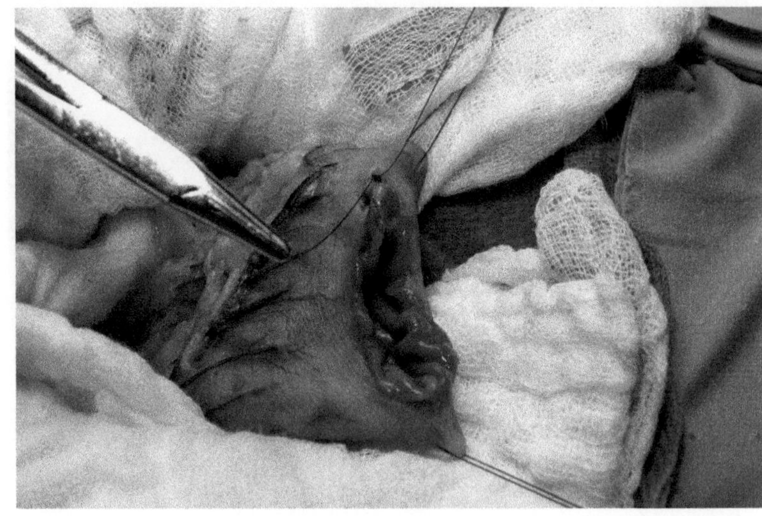

Figure 18-4 Begin the closure by taking a suture bite in the mucosa adjacent to the end of the seromuscular incision. Tie two knots and leave the suture end long and secured in a hemostat.

   ii. To provide retraction during foreign-body extraction or lumen examination, place stay sutures at the midpoint of each side of the gastric incision, and retract the stay sutures to open the incision.

4. If postoperative nutritional supplementation is desired, have the anaesthetist pass a nasogastric feeding tube. Through the gastrotomy incision, manipulate the tube through the pylorus and into the duodenum to provide nasoenteral feeding.
5. Close the mucosa in a simple continuous pattern and the seromuscular layer in an inverting pattern with absorbable monofilament suture.
6. Alternatively, close the incision with a rapid 2-layer closure:
   a. Take a suture bite through the gastric mucosa/submucosa at the end of the seromuscular incision and tie two knots, leaving the free end of the suture long so you can tie back to it (fig. 18-4). Attach a hemostat to the free end to keep it visible.
   b. Close the mucosa/submucosa with a simple continuous or Cushing suture pattern; continue the pattern to the level of the seromuscular incision (fig. 18-5).

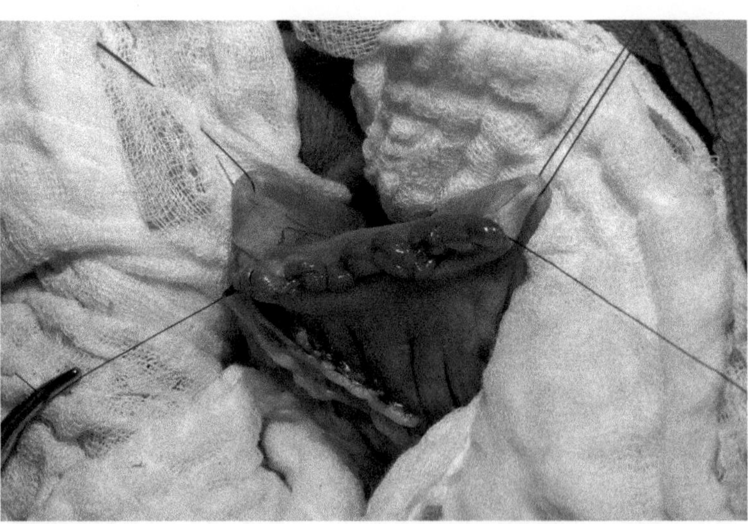

Figure 18-5 Close the mucosa with a simple continuous or Cushing pattern.

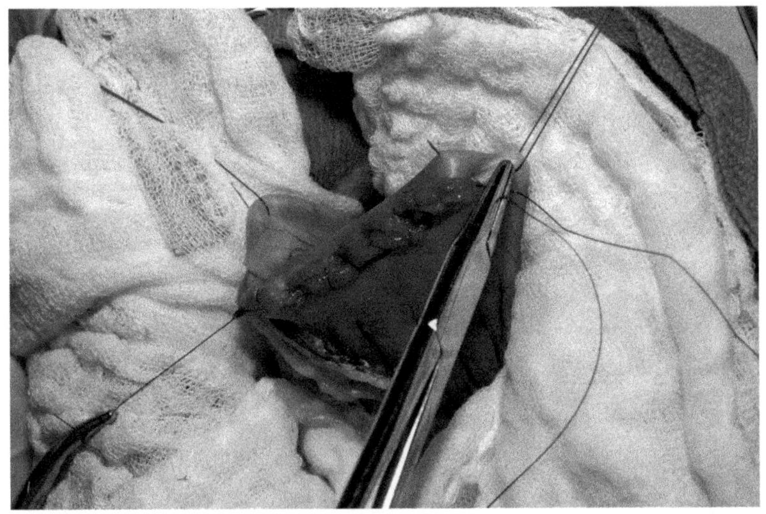

Figure 18-6 Once the mucosa is closed, close the remaining layers with a Cushing pattern. Angle bites outward and overlap each successive bite slightly with the previous one on the opposite side to promote inversion.

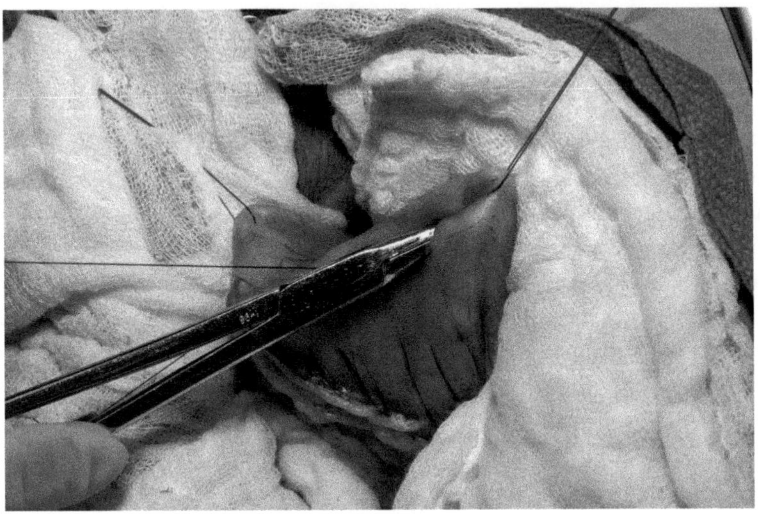

Figure 18-7 Invert the gastric wall each time you tighten the Cushing pattern.

c. Without tying a knot, begin a Cushing pattern in the outer, seromuscular layer of the stomach, taking bites roughly parallel to the incision edge (fig. 18-6).
   i. To help invert the tissues, make sure the level of each subsequent bite overlaps slightly with the previous bite on the opposite side, and angle bites slightly away from the incision.
   ii. Use the needle holder tips to help invert the gastric wall each time you tighten the suture (fig. 18-7).
d. Take the final suture bite beyond the end of the incision and tie off to the free suture end (fig. 18-8).

Postoperative considerations

During recovery, keep the animal's head elevated to reduce gastric reflux. A baseline hematocrit should be measured; serial hematocrits are evaluated if hematomesis, pallor, or significant anemia or melena occurs. Food can be

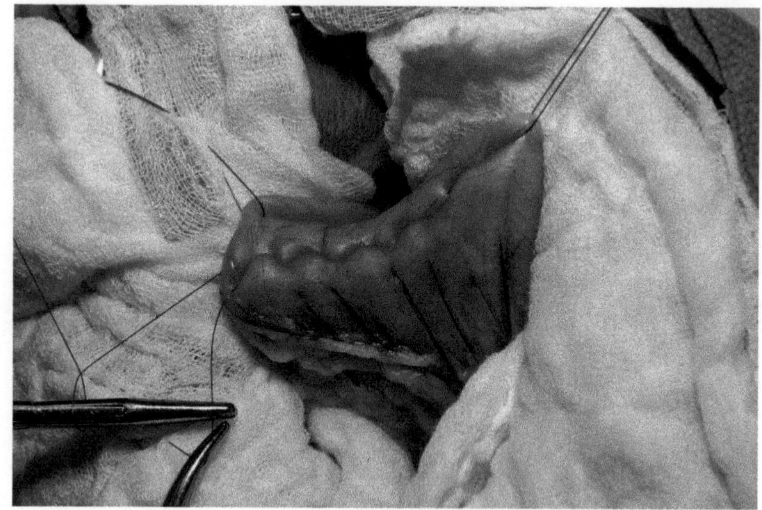

Figure 18-8 Continue the pattern to a point just beyond the end of the incision. Tie off the suture to the original suture end.

offered within 12 after surgery if the animal is not vomiting, nauseated, or sedate. Postoperative vomiting or nausea may result from ileus, electrolyte abnormalities (especially hypomagnesemia), pain, gastric irritation, or the underlying condition. Treatment may include intravenous fluids, gastroprotectants (sucralfate), gastric acid inhibitors (e.g., omeprazole), motility-enhancing drugs for ileus (e.g., metoclopramide, ranitidine), or antiemetics (e.g., maropitant, dolasetron). Toxicity from lead or zinc gastric foreign bodies may require chelation therapy.

The most common complication of gastrotomy is vomiting, which could lead to aspiration pneumonia. If the mucosa has not been sutured closed, animals may vomit partially digested blood, which looks like coffee grounds. Animals that persistently vomit should be evaluated with plain or contrast radiographs, ultrasound, or endoscopy for potential obstruction. Dehiscence of gastrotomy closure is rare since the stomach heals rapidly and has extensive blood supply. Gastric dehiscence could occur with violent vomiting or in animals with ischemic, neoplastic, or markedly diseased stomachs. Closure of antral gastrotomies with nonabsorbable suture (e.g., polypropylene) can result in inflammatory pyloric obstruction. Pyloric obstruction can also occur from excessive tissue inversion or distortion of the antrum during incision closure.

Bibliography

Bright RM et al: Pyloric obstruction in a dog related to a gastrotomy incision closed with polypropylene. J Small Anim Pract 1994;35:629–632.

Ehrhart NP, Kaminskaya K, Miller JA, et al: In vivo assessment of absorbable knotless barbed suture for single layer gastrostomy and enterotomy closure. Vet Surg 2013;42:210–210.

Fossum TS et al: Presumptive, iatrogenic gastric outflow obstruction associated with prior gastric surgery. J Am Anim Hosp Assoc 1995;31:391–395.

Round S, Popovitch C: Prophylactic gastropexy incorporating a gastrotomy incision in dogs: a retrospective study of 21 cases (2011–2013). J Am Anim Hosp Assoc 2016;52:115–118.

Shuler E and Tobias KM: Gastrotomy. Veterinary Medicine 2006;101:207–210.

Chapter 19
Gastrostomy Tube Placement

Gastrostomy tubes are used for enteral supplementation in animals that require long-term nutritional support or have esophageal disorders. Less commonly, they are used as a method for creating a permanent gastropexy to prevent recurrence of gastric dilatation-volvulus (see p. 165).

Gastric feeding tubes can be placed percutaneously with the aid of an endoscope or placed surgically or laparoscopically through a midline or paracostal incision. Surgical placement is required when animals have a condition that would prevent percutaneous placement, such as an esophageal stricture or vascular ring anomaly. Animals with intermittent vomiting often can still be fed through a gastrostomy tube, as long as vomiting is not associated with feeding and the pylorus is not obstructed. Enterostomy feeding is preferred in animals with gastroesophageal reflux, gastric disease, or frequent or persistent vomiting. A gastrostomy tube can be turned into an intestinal feeding tube during surgery by inserting a smaller feeding tube through the gastrostomy tube into the stomach and advancing it through the pylorus and into the duodenum or proximal jejunum.

Preoperative management

When placed for feeding, gastrostomy tubes are inserted through the left ventrolateral body wall. If the animal is undergoing simultaneous exploratory laparotomy, the ventral skin is clipped and prepped from midthorax to pubis. The lateral margin of the prep should continue halfway up the animal's left side, particularly around the paracostal region. Prophylactic antibiotics are optional; when used, they often are administered intravenously at induction and discontinued after surgery.

Surgery

Standard and low-profile versions of gastrostomy feeding tubes are available. Standard gastrostomy tubes (e.g., Malecot or Pezzar tube) can be purchased with a flexible dome or mushroom tip that acts as a flange, reducing the risk of

Manual of Small Animal Soft Tissue Surgery, Second Edition. Karen Tobias.
© 2017 John Wiley & Sons, Inc. Published 2017 by John Wiley & Sons, Inc.

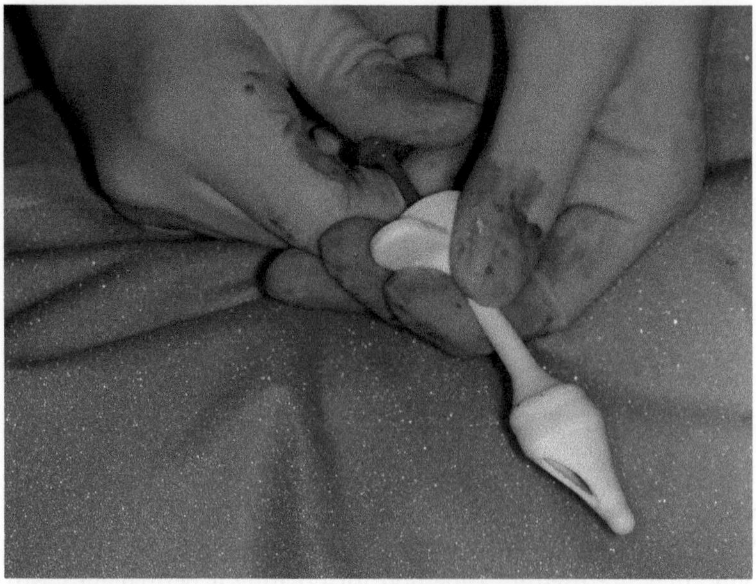

Figure 19-1 Straighten the low-profile tube by pressing the stylet into the mushroom tip.

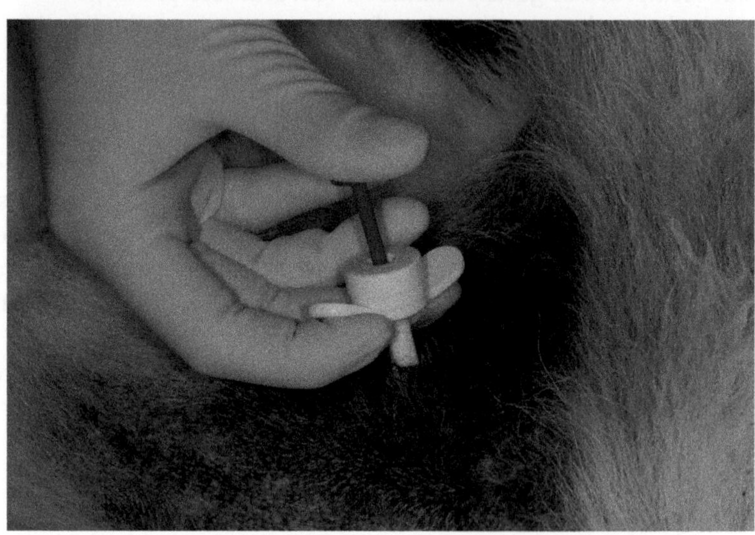

Figure 19-2 Insert the low-profile tube through the original tube stoma, then remove the stylet.

tube pull-out. Foley catheters should be avoided for long-term use since the balloon deteriorates when exposed to gastric secretions. Low-profile gastrostomy tubes have a one-way valve to prevent egress of gastric contents. Because of their short length, they are more comfortable for the patient long term and less likely to be dislodged than standard tubes. Low-profile tubes can be difficult to place surgically; thus, most clinicians use standard gastrostomy tubes at the initial placement. Once the standard tube has been in place for 3 to 4 weeks, it can be pulled and immediately replaced with a low-profile tube inserted through the same fistula (figs. 19-1, 19-2). A small amount of contrast can be inserted through the tube so that placement can be verified radiographically. Selection of tube diameter depends on the size of the animal. A 20 French tube is commonly placed in cats and small dogs; a 24 French tube is often used in medium to large dogs.

When gastrostomy tubes are placed during exploratory laparotomy, the abdominal midline is incised from the xiphoid to caudal abdomen. The abdomen should be thoroughly explored and any clean procedures performed before gastrostomy tube placement. The stomach should be isolated with moistened laparotomy pads to minimize peritoneal contamination, and clean instruments are set aside for abdominal closure. If gross spillage occurs during the gastrostomy tube placement, the abdomen is thoroughly lavaged with warm saline and suctioned.

Surgical technique: standard mushroom-tip gastrostomy tube for enteral feeding

1. Select the site for gastric wall penetration. Gastrostomy feeding tubes are usually placed through the midbody of the stomach halfway between the greater and lesser curvatures.
2. Select a location for body wall penetration caudal to the last rib in the left ventrolateral abdominal wall. This site should match the proposed site of gastric penetration so that the stomach will rest in a natural position once the animal is sternal.
3. Insert the gastrostomy tube through the ventrolateral body wall and into the abdominal cavity.
    a. Force the tips of a closed Carmalt or Kelly forceps through the peritoneum, body wall musculature, and subcutis.
    b. Incise the skin over the tips of the forceps (fig. 19-3).
    c. Grasp the tube end with the forceps to flatten the mushroom tip and pull the tube into the abdomen (fig. 19-4).
4. If the stomach is difficult to keep retracted out of the abdomen, place full-thickness stay sutures in the gastric wall or grasp the wall with Babcock forceps.
5. Place a purse-string suture in the gastric wall with 2-0 or 3-0 monofilament absorbable suture, penetrating the submucosa (fig. 19-5). Secure the free ends of the suture with a hemostat, but do not tighten the purse string.
6. Make a full thickness stab incision into the stomach in the center of the purse-stringed area without cutting the purse-string suture. The mucosa

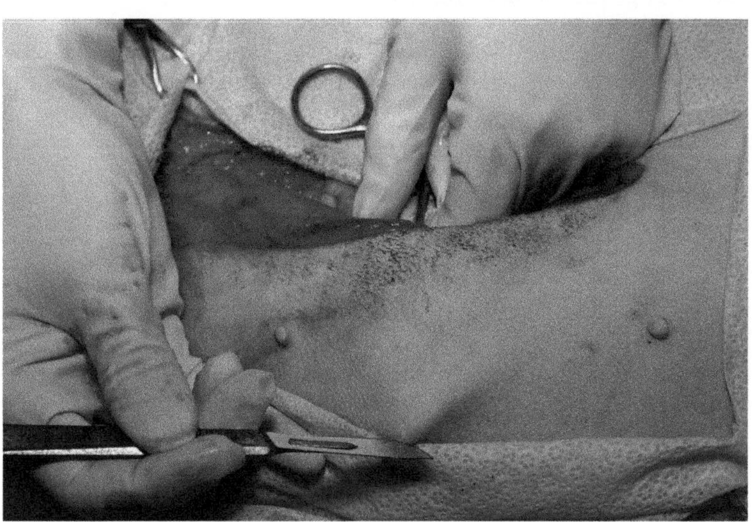

Figure 19-3 Force the tips of closed forceps through the abdominal wall musculature and subcutis, and incise the skin over the tips.

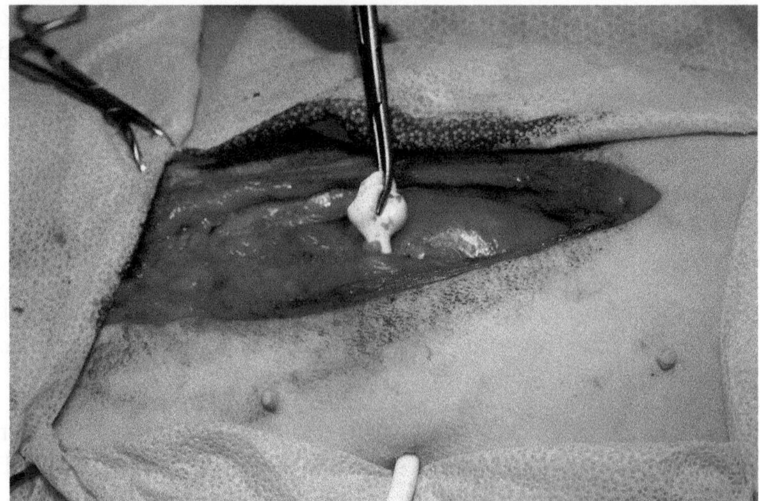

Figure 19-4 Flatten the mushroom tip of the tube and pull it into the abdominal cavity.

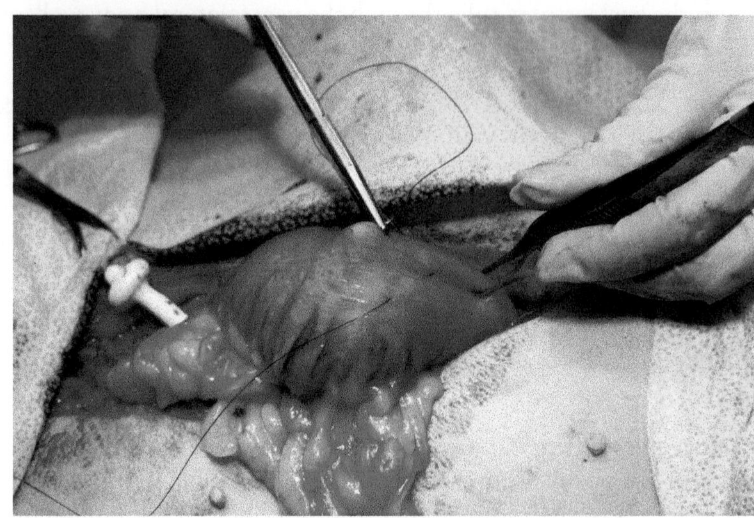

Figure 19-5 Place a purse-string suture in the body of the stomach, penetrating the submucosa with each suture bite.

may separate from the muscularis during incision. If the mucosa is still intact, pick it up with thumb forceps and cut it with a blade or scissors to enter the gastric lumen (fig. 19-6).

7. Flatten the mushroom tip of the tube with Kelly or Carmalt forceps. Insert the forceps with enclosed tube tip through the incision and into the gastric lumen (fig. 19-7). If necessary, spread the gastrotomy site open with a second pair of forceps to facilitate tube insertion.

8. Invert the mucosa into the gastric lumen while tightening the purse-string suture (fig. 19-8). Tie the suture to appose, but not necrose, the gastric wall, and cut the suture ends.

9. Pexy the stomach to the abdominal wall (fig. 19-9).

    a. If the left abdominal wall is difficult to expose, grasp the muscle across the edge of the body wall incision with a towel clamp. Press inward with your fingers dorsal to the towel clamp while rolling the muscle edge outward with the clamp and your thumb to expose the peritoneal surface around the gastrostomy tube (fig. 19-9).

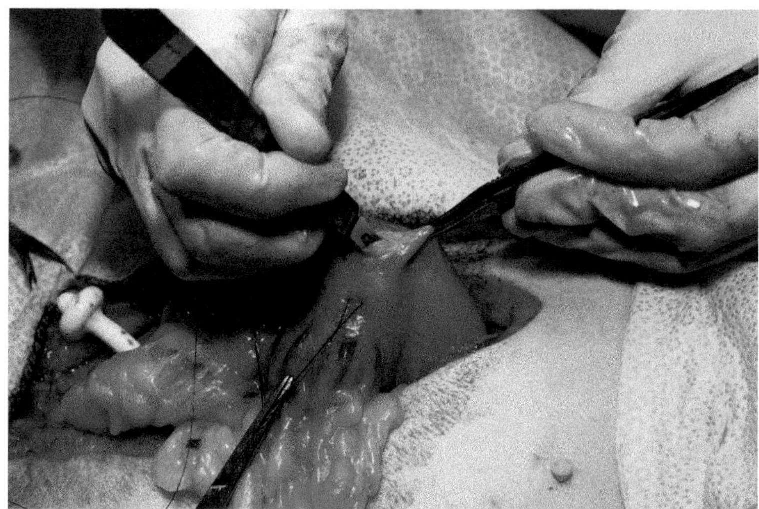

Figure 19-6 Make a full-thickness stab incision through the gastric wall within the purse-string suture. In this dog, the mucosa was incised with a second stab incision.

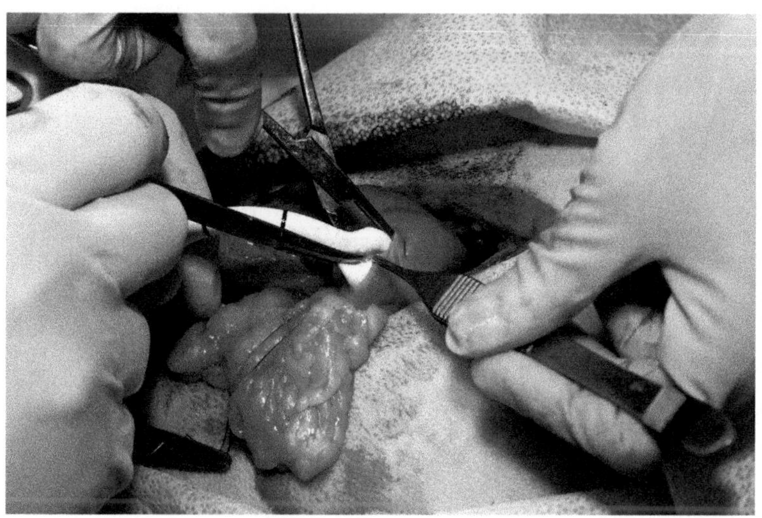

Figure 19-7 Flatten the mushroom tip of the tube and insert it through the gastric perforation.

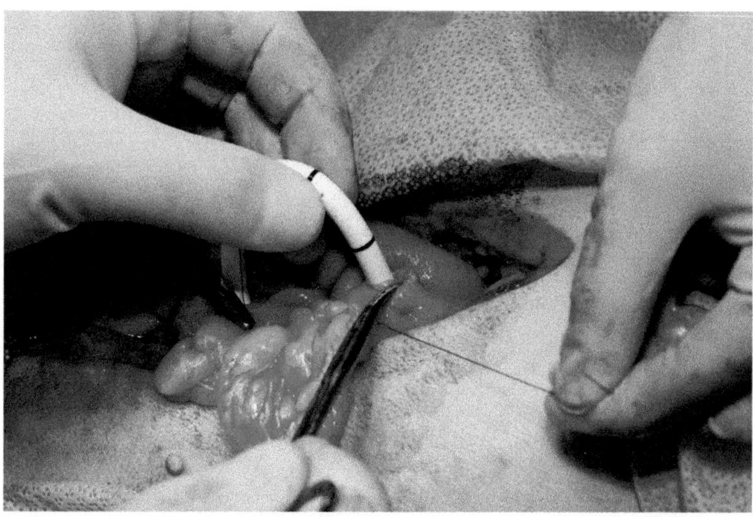

Figure 19-8 Invert the gastric mucosa as the purse string is tightened.

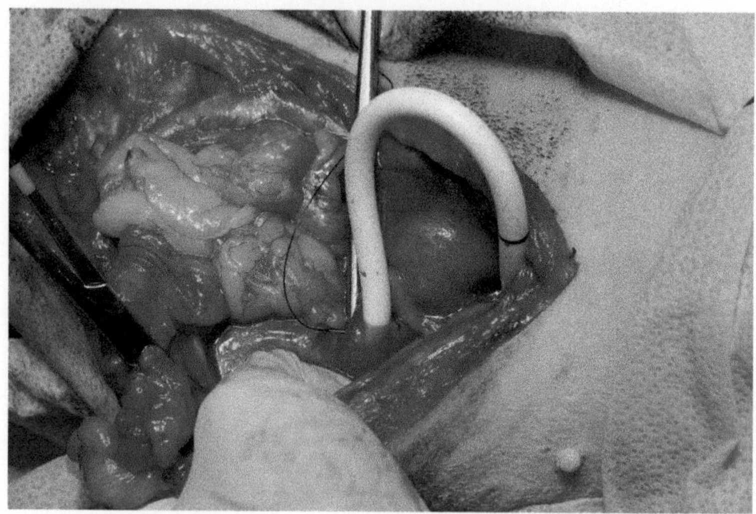

Figure 19-9 Pexy the gastric wall to the abdominal wall with simple interrupted sutures. Grasp the abdominal wall with a towel clamp and rotate the tube perforation site upward with thumb and forefingers to improve exposure.

   b. Start the pexy on the dorsal side of the tube (the side most difficult to expose.
   c. With 2-0 or 3-0 monofilament absorbable suture, take a bite of abdominal wall musculature and a bite of gastric wall (including submucosa). Tie the suture to appose, but not necrose, the enclosed tissues.
   d. Place 3 to 5 additional sutures between the body wall and stomach, working ventrally, so that the stomach is secured to the body all the way around the tube exit site.

10. If desired, wrap omentum around the pexy site and tack it back to itself with a simple interrupted suture of absorbable material (fig. 19-10).
11. Secure the tube to the body wall externally with a finger trap pattern (see Chapter 61).
    a. Do not place a purse-string suture around the stoma site, since this traps contaminants under the skin in animals with stomal leakage.
    b. In most dogs, the finger trap suture is attached only to the skin.

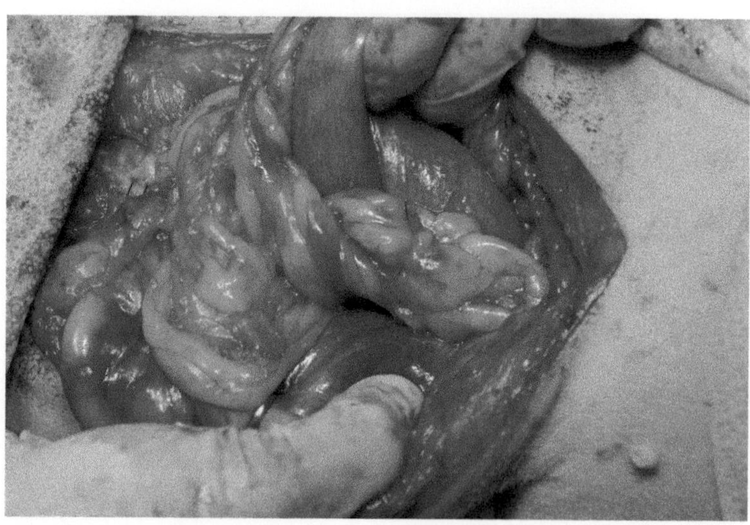

Figure 19-10 If desired, wrap omentum around the pexy site and tack it back to itself.

   c. In cats or dogs with loose or very mobile skin, take a bite of skin and underlying muscle when starting the finger trap suture to reduce tube motion.

12. Close the abdomen routinely.

Surgical technique: low-profile gastrostomy tube (see Chapter 41)

1. Place a purse-string suture in the gastric wall, as described above.
2. Make a stab incision in the skin at the proposed site of body wall penetration.
3. Perforate the body wall by inserting Carmalt or Kelly hemostats through the skin incision.
4. Perform the dorsal portion of the pexy.
   a. Place one or two interrupted sutures of 2-0 or 3-0 monofilament absorbable material between the stomach and abdominal wall. Include abdominal musculature and gastric submucosa in each suture, as described for a standard gastrostomy tube.
   b. Tie the pexy sutures and cut the ends short.
5. Select a tube that is slightly longer than the combined thickness of the gastric and body wall.
   a. To estimate tube length:
      i. Measure the thickness of the abdominal wall near the incision edge.
      ii. Grasp a full thickness fold of stomach. Measure the thickness and divide the number by two to estimate gastric wall thickness.
      iii. Add the gastric and body wall measurements together to determine total thickness.
   b. For a more accurate measurement, use the L-shaped measuring device included in some low-profile tube kits. Once the stomach has been incised:
      i. Insert the device through the skin and body wall perforation. Pull the end of the device against the peritoneum and measure the total thickness of the abdominal wall.
      ii. Insert the device through the gastric stab incision and measure the gastric wall thickness.
      iii. Set the contaminated device aside.
      iv. Add the gastric and body wall measurements together to determine total thickness.
6. Insert the low-profile tube through the body wall.
   a. Insert the accompanying stylet ("obturator") into the tube to straighten the tip (fig. 19-1).
   b. Insert the tube through the skin incision and body wall perforation. If necessary, insert a Kelly or Carmalt hemostat from the peritoneal

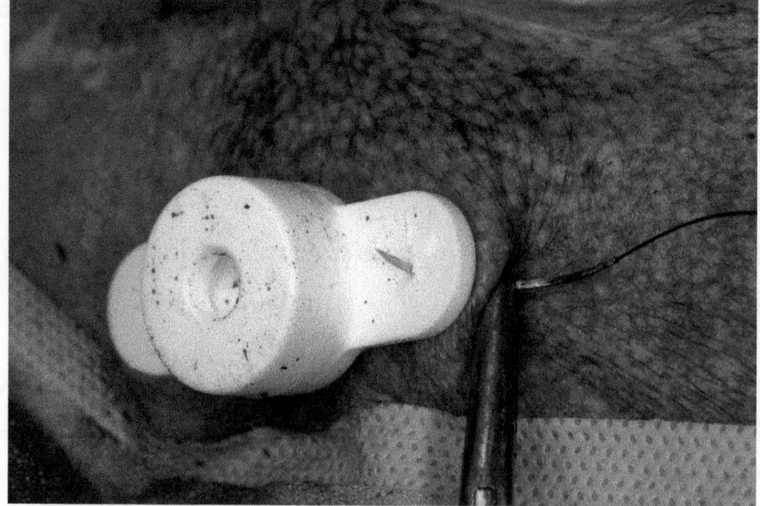

Figure 19-11 Secure the low-profile tube to the skin with interrupted sutures.

surface and through the body wall to spread the body wall incision and assist tube passage.

c. Once the tube tip is in the abdominal cavity, relax pressure on the stylet.

7. Make a stab incision through the gastric wall inside the purse-string suture and into the gastric lumen.
8. Using the stylet to straighten the tip, insert the tube tip into the gastric lumen. Remove the stylet.
9. Tighten the gastric wall purse-string suture securely around the tube. Tie the suture and cut the ends.
10. Add additional pexy sutures lateral and ventral to the tube as described for a standard gastrostomy tube.
11. Secure the tube to the skin with interrupted sutures (fig. 19-11).

Postoperative considerations

Animals can be fed once they are awake and sternal. Initial feedings should be small and frequent (e.g., every 2 to 4 hours), or delivered continuously via a trickle feed of liquid diet to reduce the likelihood of vomiting and diarrhea.

> **Calculating Caloric Requirements**
>
> Caloric resting energy requirements (RER; kcal/day) can be calculated using the formula $RER = 70 \times (\text{current body weight in kg})^{0.75}$ or, for animals between 2 and 45 kg, with the formula $RER = (30 \times \text{current body weight in kg}) + 70$.

Feeding is usually started at a third of resting energy requirements for the first day and gradually increased to full resting energy requirements by the third or fourth day. Canned recovery diets are useful because they are blenderized and therefore pass easily through feeding tubes.

Once intermittent feeding has begun, tubes should be flushed with water and capped after each use. The skin around the stoma often needs to be cleaned daily and covered with a nonadherent dressing. A thin layer of antibiotic ointment can be applied around the tube; excessive amounts of ointment, however, may cause local skin maceration.

The tubes themselves are often kept under a bandage or body suit to prevent trauma or inadvertent pull-out.

Once gastrostomy tube feedings are initiated, animals should be monitored for severe electrolyte disturbances that can result in "refeeding syndrome." In animals that are severely malnourished or have been anorexic for prolonged periods, intracellular cations can be depleted, even though plasma levels are normal before surgery. When feeding resumes, plasma cations rapidly shift into the cells, resulting in hypokalemia, hypophosphatemia, and hypomagnesemia. In animals with refeeding syndrome, changes in electrolytes are usually noted within the first 4 days of food reintroduction. Animals with severe electrolyte depletion (e.g., phosphorus <1.5 mg/dL) may show weakness, fluid retention, electrocardiographic abnormalities, dyspnea, vomiting, diarrhea, ileus, renal dysfunction, and tetany. If refeeding syndrome is suspected, electrolyte and acid-base imbalances should be corrected and the feeding rate should be reduced to 50% of resting energy requirements until the animal is stable.

Gastrostomy tubes should be left in place for a minimum of 7 days to allow fibrous fistula formation around the tube. Tubes may be left in longer in immunosuppressed animals or cats with renal disease, since fibrous tissue formation can be delayed in these patients. Peritonitis may occur if the tube is removed prematurely. Low-profile tubes are removed by straightening the tip with the stylet before pulling them out. Standard mushroom-tip tubes can be removed in most animals by pulling steadily and firmly to collapse the tip. If poor fibrous tissue production is expected, the mushroom tip can be straightened with a stylet during removal. Alternatively, the tube tip can be visualized with an endoscope and secured with graspers; the tube is then transected and the tip retrieved from the stomach. After tube removal, the stoma is covered with a bandage. Gastrocutaneous stomas typically close by contraction within 1 to 2 days after tube removal.

Tube obstruction frequently occurs if food administered through the tube contains large particles or dessicates inside the tube. Risk of tube blockage can be reduced by placing large diameter tubes, feeding commercial pureed recovery diets, and flushing the tube with water after each use. Animals may develop cellulitis from peristomal leakage around or under the skin. Because the skin in cats is extremely mobile, movement during normal activity can cause long tubes to slide in and out. This will pull gastric contents out into the subcutaneous space or onto the skin. Occasionally, animals will form abscesses around the stoma that require local drainage or tube removal. Other complications include fungal colonization of the tube and metastasis of gastric neoplasia to the abdominal wall around the tube.

Bibliography

Campbell SJ et al: Complications and outcomes of one-step low-profile gastrostomy devices for long-term enteral feeding in dogs and cats. J Am Anim Hosp Assoc 2006;42:197–206.

Mesich ML et al: Gastrostomy feeding tubes: surgical placement. Vet Med 2004;99:604–610.

Salinardi BJ et al: Comparison of complications of percutaneous endoscopic versus surgically placed gastrostomy tubes in 42 dogs and 52 cats. J Am Anim Hosp Assoc 2006;42:51–56.

Chapter 20
Incisional Gastropexy

Rotation of a distended stomach on its mesenteric axis is called gastric dilatation-volvulus (GDV). GDV is a life-threatening condition that results in gastric obstruction, visceral ischemia, hypotension, arrhythmias, shock, and death. Affected animals usually require intensive stabilization and emergency surgery to detorse the stomach. Recurrence of GDV can be prevented by permanent fixation of the pyloric antrum to the right ventrolateral abdominal wall (gastropexy). "Prophylactic" gastropexy is recommended in any large- or giant-breed dog that has a history of gastric bloating or a first degree relative with GDV, or that is undergoing splenectomy. Gastropexy is also performed as part of the surgical repair for dogs with hiatal hernias. In those dogs, the stomach is returned to the abdominal cavity, the esophageal hiatus is narrowed with sutures, and the body of the stomach is pexied to the left abdominal wall.

To form a permanent adhesion, exposed muscle of the abdominal wall is sutured to a partial-thickness gastric wall incision. A variety of techniques are available for permanent gastropexy, including circumcostal, belt loop, tube, incorporational, incisional (muscular), and laparoscopic assisted. Incorporation of the gastric wall into the midline abdominal incision closure ("incorporational gastropexy") is rapid and produces a permanent adhesion but may increase the risk of inadvertent gastric perforation during subsequent celiotomy. Tube gastropexy requires intensive postoperative management, compared with other techniques. Incisional (muscular) gastropexy produces a strong adhesion without the risk of pneumothorax reported with circumcostal or belt loop techniques.

Preoperative management

Animals with gastric dilatation and volvulus require extensive supportive care, including intravenous fluids; hetastarch or hypertonic 7% saline, analgesics, gastric decompression via orogastric tube or percutaneous gastrocentesis, oxygen, electrocardiography, antibiotics, and correction of acid-base, electrolyte, and coagulation disturbances. Lidocaine constant rate infusion (CRI; 25–50 μg/kg/min) can be administered in dogs for analgesic, antiarrhythmic, and anti-inflammatory effects. Prophylactic antibiotics are not required in stable animals undergoing elective gastropexy, since the surgery duration is short and the gastric lumen is not penetrated.

Manual of Small Animal Soft Tissue Surgery, Second Edition. Karen Tobias.
© 2017 John Wiley & Sons, Inc. Published 2017 by John Wiley & Sons, Inc.

For a midline approach, the abdominal clip and prep should extend to midthorax. A right-sided grid approach can also be performed caudal to the thirteenth rib for prophylactic gastropexy. In animals with GDV, suction, cautery, and laparotomy sponges should be available since partial gastrectomy may be required, and ventilation should be assisted because of compression on the diaphragm by the dilated stomach.

Surgery

In dogs with GDV, an orogastric tube can be passed by a nonsterile assistant during surgery to facilitate gastric decompression and repositioning. The surgeon can help guide the tube into the stomach by gently manipulating the abdominal portion of the distal esophagus. To reposition the stomach, the surgeon stands on the dog's right, grasps the pylorus near the left dorsolateral abdominal wall, and pulls it ventrally and back to the right. The gastric wall is examined for damage before the pexy is performed. In most dogs with GDV, the pylorus is normal and does not need to be enlarged or removed. The spleen is often engorged but is usually not torsed.

The traditional incisional gastropexy technique involves apposition of partial thickness incisions in the pyloric antrum and right ventrolateral body wall (fig. 20-1). This is the author's preferred technique because it is quick and easy; additionally, when a towel clamp is used to evert the abdominal wall, the exposure is reasonable for a solo surgeon. The surgeon will need to release the abdominal wall hold, however, when tying knots. Another option developed by Dr. Dan Smeak is a subcostal incisional gastropexy that uses two towel clamps around the 12th rib to provide "hands free" exposure of the abdominal wall. The latter technique has been used clinically for over a decade but has not been objectively evaluated.

Surgical technique: traditional incisional (muscular) gastropexy

1. Position yourself on the animal's right side, with the dog in dorsal recumbancy.

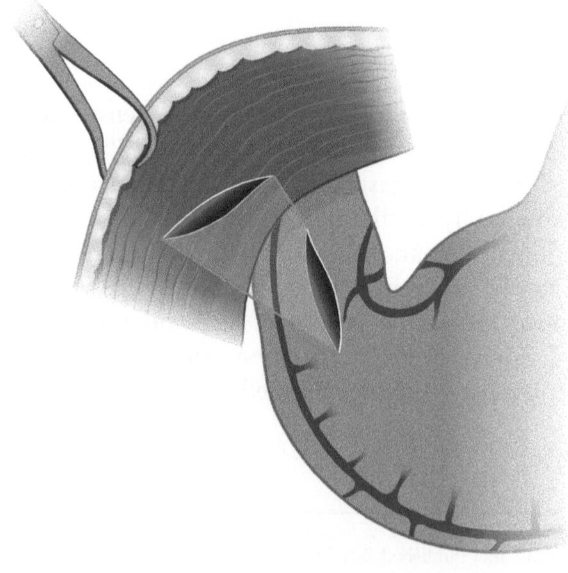

Figure 20-1 An incisional gastropexy apposes the edges of a partial thickness (seromuscular) gastrotomy incision to the edges of a partial thickness abdominal wall (transversus abdominus) incision. Courtesy of Samantha Elmurst.

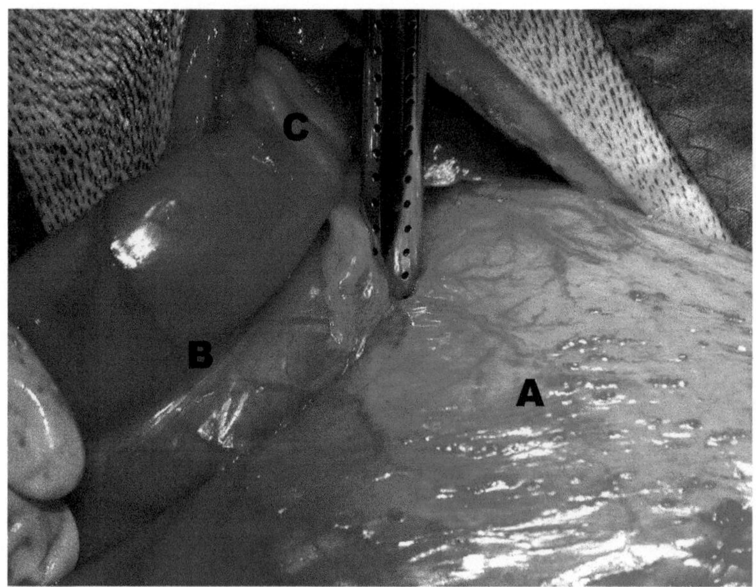

Figure 20-2 Identify the gastric body (A), pyloric antrum (B), and pylorus (C). The antrum is located between the level of the incisure and the pylorus. In this dog the Poole suction tip is resting in the incisure and the fingers are holding a portion of the antrum.

2. Identify the pyloric antrum, which extends from the incisure (the notch of the lesser curvature) to the pylorus (fig. 20-2). The gastric incision will be located along the center of the antrum.
3. To test the thickness of the seromuscular layer, grasp the full thickness gastric wall between your thumb and fingers and allow the mucosal layer to slip out of your grasp as you slowly pull your hand backwards. The partial thickness gastric incision will go through everything that remains within your fingers.
4. Make a 5- to 8-cm partial-thickness incision through the seromuscular layers of the stomach, parallel to the long axis of the antrum and midway between the greater and lesser curvatures (fig. 20-3). If depth of the cut is appropriate, the incision edges will gape open, revealing the bulging mucosa.
5. Place a towel clamp around the muscle of the right edge of the abdominal wall incision and evert the tissues to expose the peritoneal surface (fig. 20-4).
    a. Grasp the towel clamp in your left fist, thumb downward, and rotate your wrist outward ("supinate") to evert the abdominal wall muscle edge over your fist and expose the peritoneum.
6. Match the gastric wall incision to the right body wall to determine the location and length of the body wall incision at the pexy site. The body wall incision will be caudal to the last rib and in the ventral half of the right abdominal wall, 6 to 10 cm lateral to the ventral midline incision.
7. Make an incision through the peritoneum and into the transversus abdominus muscle, angling from craniodorsal to caudoventral (fig. 20-5). The incision should be the same length as the gastric wall incision.
8. Appose the peritoneal and gastric wall incision edges with a simple continuous pattern of 2-0 monofilament absorbable suture.

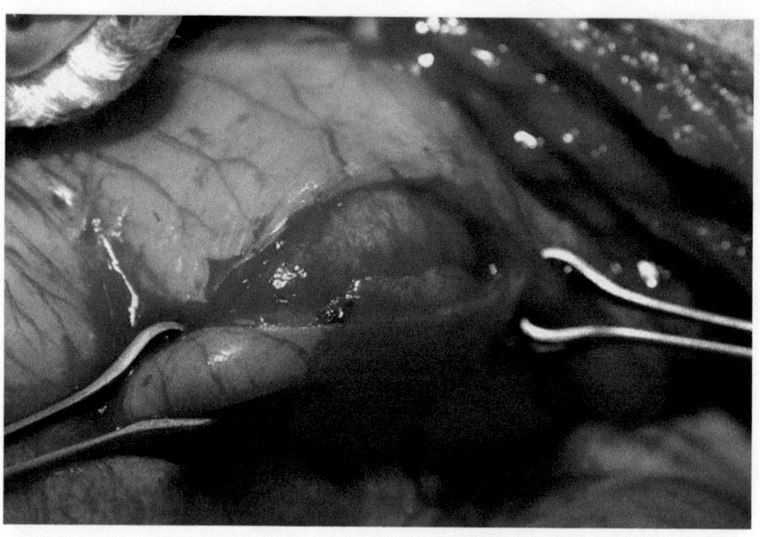

Figure 20-3 Make a 5- to 8-cm incision through the seromuscular layer of the antrum, midway between the greater and lesser curvatures of the stomach. The mucosa will bulge through the incision. This stomach is being stabilized with Babcock forceps.

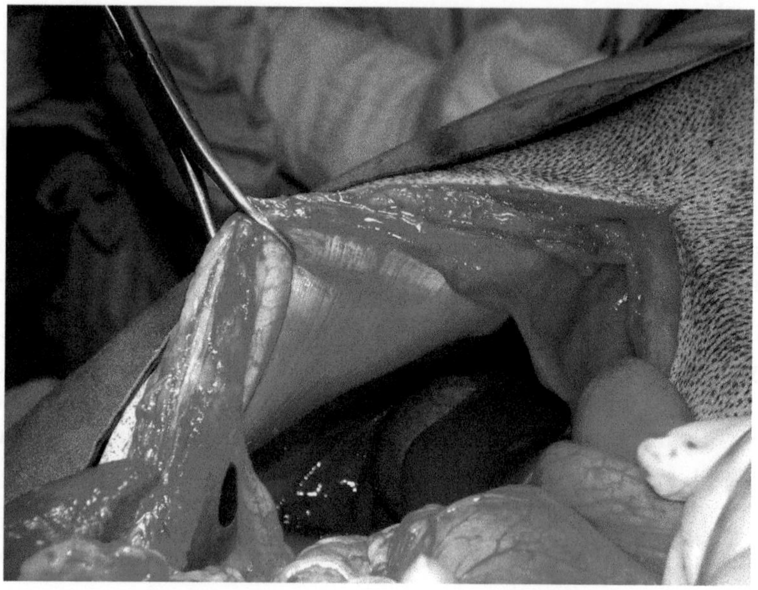

Figure 20-4 Evert the body wall with a towel clamp to expose the peritoneal surface.

a. Take the first suture bite at the craniodorsal ends of the incisions; tie two knots, leaving the free end long, and attach a hemostat to the free end so you can find it later (fig. 20-6).

b. Appose the dorsal edges of both incisions with a continuous pattern, taking 1- to 1.5-cm wide bites around the seromuscular edge of the gastric wall incision and the incised edge peritoneum and underlying transversus abdominus muscle (fig. 20-7).

c. Once the caudal extent of the pexy site is reached, continue cranially, apposing the ventral edges of the incisions.

d. Tie off to the original suture end (figs. 20-8, 20-9).

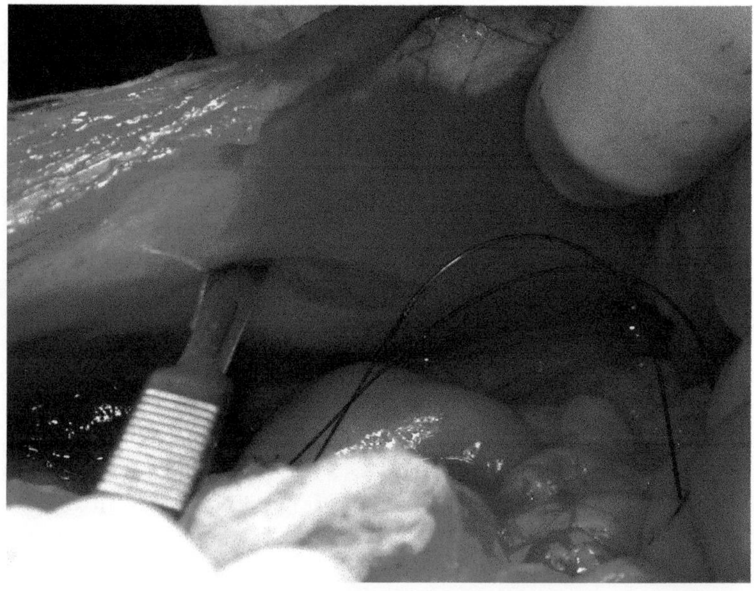

Figure 20-5 Make an angled incision through the peritoneum caudal to the last rib.

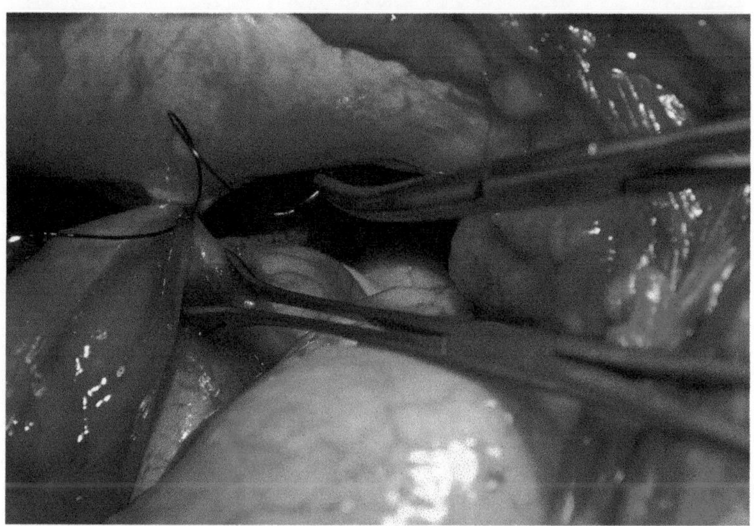

Figure 20-6 Take a bite of the craniodorsal edges of the gastric and peritoneal incisions. Tie two knots, and tag the suture end with a hemostat.

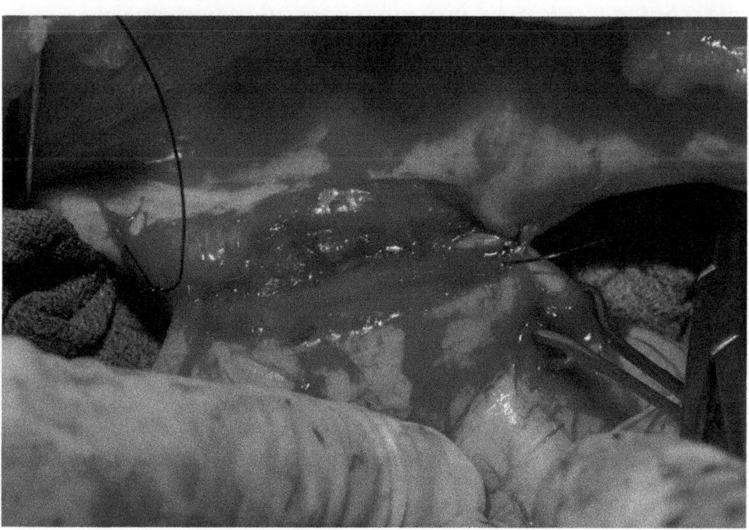

Figure 20-7 Suture the dorsal edges of the gastric and abdominal wall incisions together in a continuous pattern from cranial to caudal.

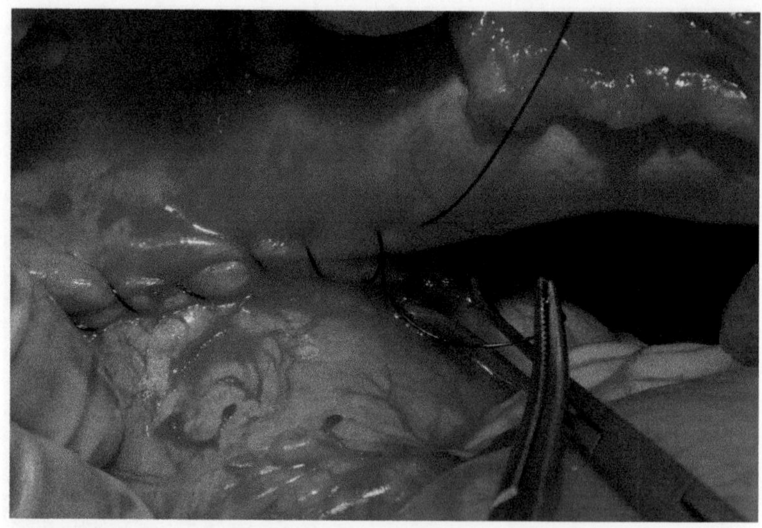

Figure 20-8 Continue the pattern from caudal to cranial to appose the ventral edges of the gastric and abdominal wall incisions, then tie the suture off to the original suture end.

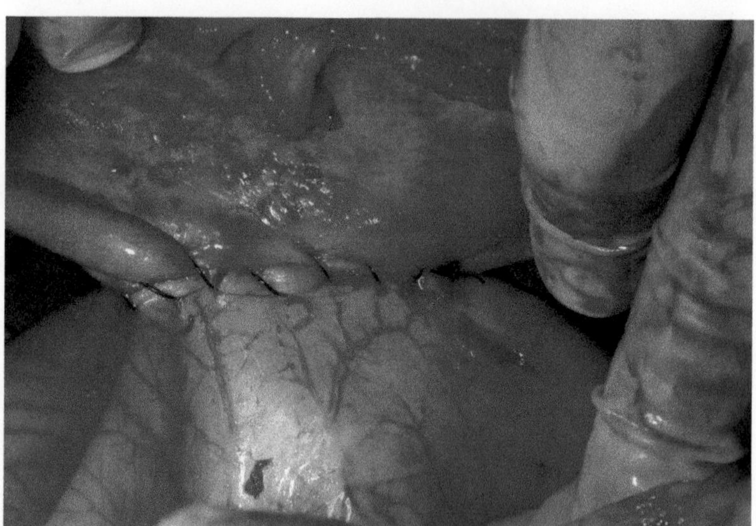

Figure 20-9 Completed gastropexy.

Surgical technique: subcostal incisional (muscular) gastropexy

1. Stand on the animal's left side.
2. Make a midline abdominal incision, and remove the falciform ligament if it is in the way (p. 87).
3. To extend the incision cranially,
    a. Incise the skin over the xiphoid process.
    b. Insert closed scissors superficial to the xiphoid process and spread the tissues (fig. 20-10A).
    c. Transect the subcutaneous tissues overlying the xiphoid process with scissors (fig. 20-10B).
4. Grasp the right side of the cranial abdominal wall incision and roll it outward (evert it) to expose the abdominal wall muscle.

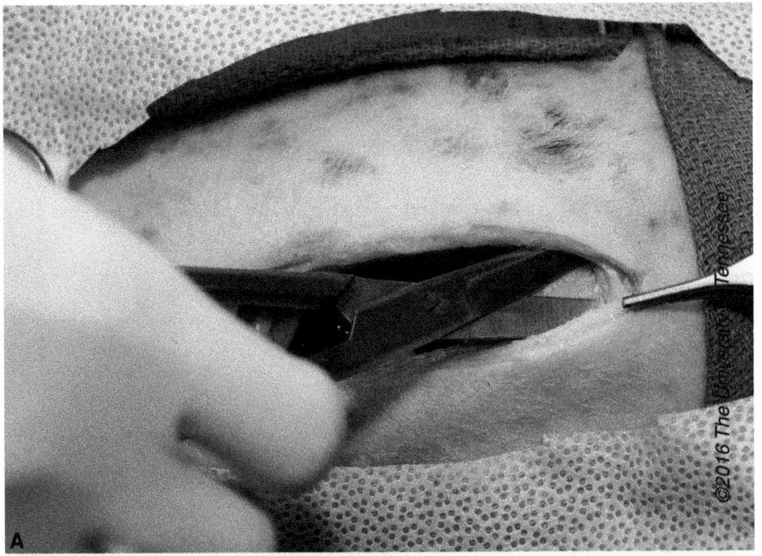

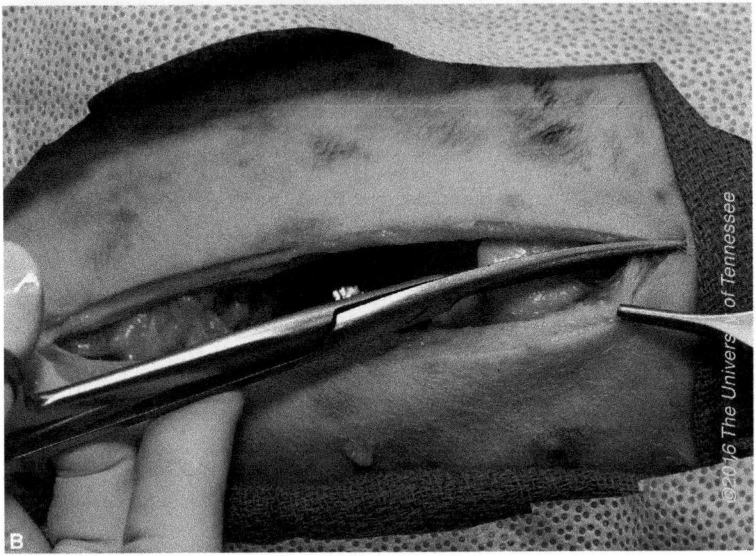

Figure 20-10 To extend an abdominal incision cranially without penetrating the diaphragm, insert closed scissors superficial (ventral) to the xiphoid process, and separate the overlying tissues from the xiphoid process (**A**). Transect the subcutaneous tissues overlying the xiphoid process with scissors (**B**). © 2016 The University of Tennessee.

5. Find the cartilaginous portion of the 12th rib, which should end several cm caudal to the xiphoid process, and grasp it between thumb and index finger of your left hand.
6. Pull the cartilagenous portion of the 12th rib away from the deeper structures, and place 2 towel clamps around it (fig. 20-11).
   a. The cranial clamp should be positioned several cm caudal to the xiphoid.
   b. The caudal clamp should be 5 to 6 cm away from the cranial clamp.
7. Make an incision through the muscle directly overlying the cartilaginous portion of the rib between the towel clamps (fig. 20-11).
8. Make the partial thickness gastric antrum incision.
   a. Identify the pyloric antrum and the portion of the antral wall midway between the greater and lesser curvatures.

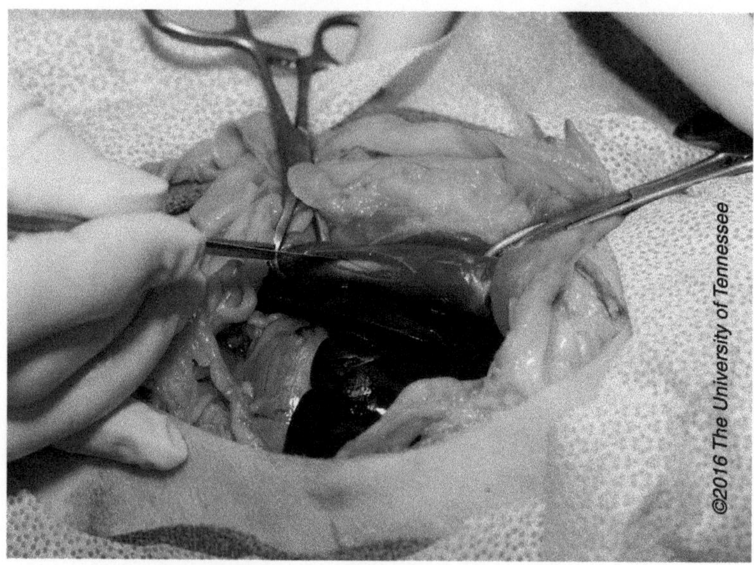

Figure 20-11 Evert the body wall and place towel clamps around the cartilaginous portion of the 12th rib. The cranial towel clamp should be several cm caudal to the xiphoid, and the caudal clamp should be 5 to 6 cm away from the cranial clamp. © 2016 The University of Tennessee.

b. Pinch about 4 cm of the antral wall along its long axis between thumb and fingers, then lift up to let the mucosa slip out of your grasp (fig. 20-12).

c. With Metzenbaum scissors, cut through the remaining tissue within your grasp. This will produce a partial thickness (seromuscular) incision that is oriented along the long axis of the antrum (fig. 20-13).

d. If the antral incision is too short, separate the mucosa/submucosa from the seromuscular layer at one end of the incision with blunt dissection (fig. 20-14A), then transect the seromuscular layer with scissors (fig. 20-14B).

9. Bring the antral incision adjacent to the subcostal abdominal wall incision, making sure the stomach maintains its normal U-shaped bend with the pylorus oriented cranially. If desired, secure the incisions together at each end with stay sutures.

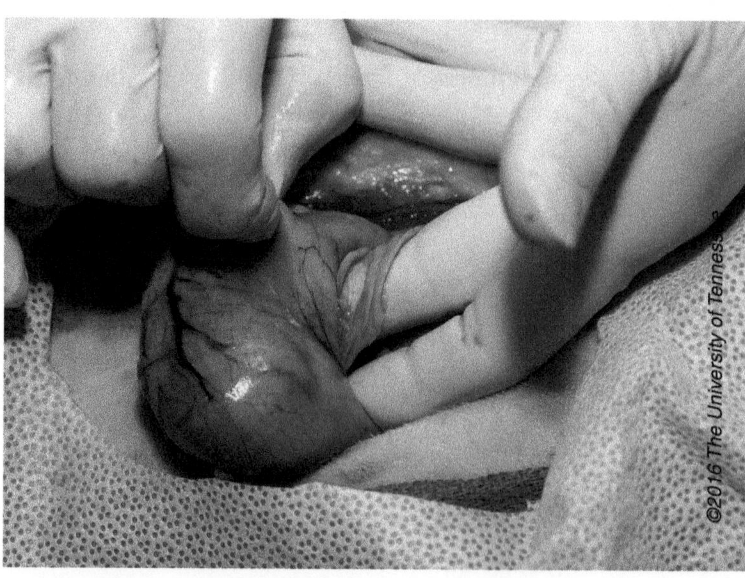

Figure 20-12 Pinch the antral wall midway between the greater and lesser curvatures, and let the mucosa slide out of your fingers. The tissue remaining in your grasp will be transected with scissors to make the partial thickness antral incision. © 2016 The University of Tennessee.

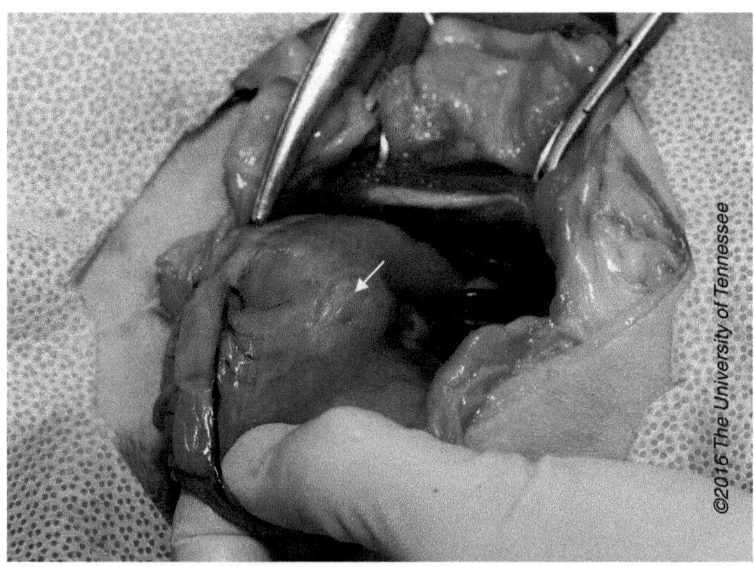

Figure 20-13 The antral incision should be partial thickness, oriented longitudinally, and midway between the greater and lesser curvatures. © 2016 The University of Tennessee.

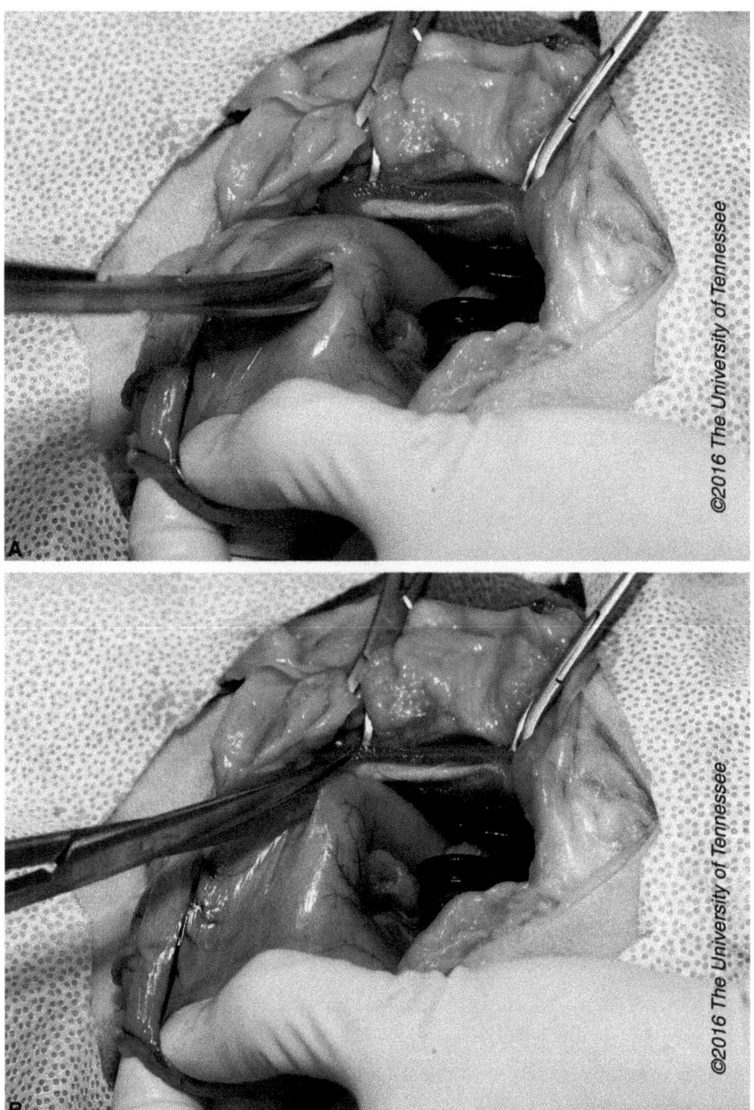

Figure 20-14 If the antral incision is too short, separate the seromuscular layer from the mucosa with blunt dissection (**A**) and transect the seromuscular layer with scissors (**B**). © 2016 The University of Tennessee.

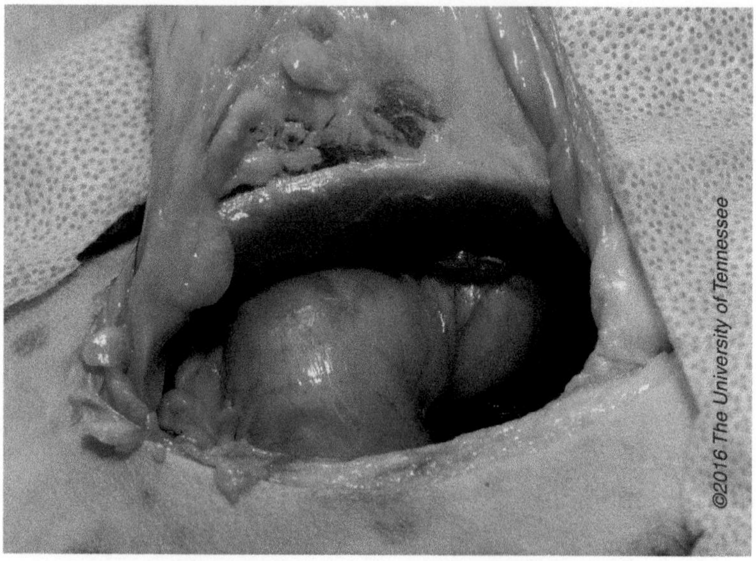

Figure 20-15 Final appearance after release of towel clamps. © 2016 The University of Tennessee.

10. Using 2-0 monofilament absorbable suture in a simple continuous pattern, suture the caudal edge of the gastric incision (the edge closest to the greater curvature of the stomach) to the dorsal edge of the abdominal incision (the edge farthest from the surgeon), then suture the cranial edge of the gastric incision to the ventral (near) edge of the abdominal incision. The sutures can be tied off to the previous stay sutures.
11. Release the towel clamps, if you have not already done so, and evaluate the final position of the stomach. Once the muscle is relaxed, the pexy should be several cm from midline and the stomach should lie in a natural. U-shaped position (fig. 20-15).
12. Check for evidence of pneumothorax. Normally the diaphragm is domed and the pink lung parenchyma will be visible against the pleural surface of the central tendon. The diaphragm will billow and lose its concavity with severe pneumothorax.

Postoperative considerations

Animals with GDV are continued on fluid therapy, analgesics, antibiotics, gastroprotectants, gastric acid inhibitors, and lidocaine CRI and are monitored for disseminated intravascular coagulation and electrocardiographic abnormalities. Arrhythmias are common and can be exacerbated by pain, hypokalemia, and hypomagnesemia. Motility-enhancing agents (e.g., metoclopramide, ranitidine, or low dose erythromycin) may be required in animals with gastric atony. Water and food can be offered 12 hours after surgery if no vomiting has occurred.

Although perioperative death occurs in 10% to 27% of dogs with GDV, gastropexy itself has few complications. Gastric dilataion can still occur after incisional gastropexy; it is reported in 5% to 11% of dogs and is most often secondary to functional ileus or primary gastric disease. It does not signify a recurrence of the volvulus, however. Occurrence of GDV after incisional gastropexy is not expected, as long as surgical technique is good. Accidental perforation of the mucosa during flap elevation does not cause problems as long as the mucosa is sutured closed before the gastropexy is performed. Rarely, gastric obstruction will occur from improper location of the pexy. This may be of greater concern when gastropexy is performed in an immature dog. Contrast radiographs may be useful for diagnosis of a mechanical obstruction secondary to surgery. Fistula formation has been reported with use of polypropylene (nonabsorbable) sutures for laparoscopic-assisted incisional gastropexy.

Bibliography

Benitez ME, Schmiedt CW, Radlinsky MAG, et al: Efficacy of incisional gastropexy for prevention of GDV in dogs. J Am Anim Hosp Assoc 2013;49:185–189.

Hammel SP and Novo RE: Recurrence of gastric dilatation-volvulus after incisional gastropexy in a Rottweiler. J Am Anim Hosp Assoc 2006;42:147–150.

Mackenzie G, Barnhart M, Kennedy S, et al: A retrospective study of factors influencing survival following surgery for gastric dilatation-volvulus syndrome in 306 dogs. J Am Anim Hosp Assoc 2010;46:97–102.

Przywara JF, Abel SB, Peacock JT, et al: Occurrence and recurrence of gastric dilatation with or without volvulus after incisional gastropexy. Can Vet J 2014;55:981–984.

Round S, Popovitch C: Prophylactic gastropexy incorporating a gastrotomy incision in dogs: a retrospective study of 21 cases (2011–2013). J Am Anim Hosp Assoc 2016;52:115–118.

Smeak DD: Quick and simple incisional gastropexy. Western Veterinary Conference Proceedings: WVC 2006.

Ward MP et al: Benefits of prophylactic gastropexy for dogs at risk of gastric dilatation-volvulus. Prev Vet Med 2003;60:319–329.

Chapter 21
Intestinal Biopsy

Intestinal biopsies can be obtained by endoscopy or laparotomy. Endoscopy allows thorough examination of the duodenal and colonic mucosa and avoids the potential complications of laparotomy. In some patients, however, full-thickness biopsies may be required if pathologic changes do not penetrate the mucosa, such as with lymphoma, feline infectious peritonitis, or lymphangiectasia. A surgical approach is also required for biopsy of intestines that cannot be reached endoscopically.

Preoperative management

Prophylactic antibiotics (e.g., first generation cephalosporins) can be administered intravenously at induction and again 1.5 to 6 hours later. Laparotomy sponges, warm lavage solution, and suction should be available during the procedure.

Surgery

Before entering the gastrointestinal tract, clean instruments should be set aside for closure. Clean procedures such as liver biopsy should be performed before intestinal biopsy. Intestine samples can be obtained with a scalpel blade, fine scissors, or skin biopsy punch (fig. 21-1). A skin biopsy punch produces a small, uniform intestinal perforation (fig. 21-2). With a skin punch, the mucosa may need to be transected with scissors to completely free the sample, especially if the biopsy instrument is dull. If the punch is very sharp, it is possible to damage or even perforate the opposite wall of the intestine. The hole left by the punch is closed transversely in small diameter intestines. When scissors are used, an antimesenteric enterotomy is performed. A narrow, full-thickness sample is cut from one edge of the incision using sharp Metzenbaum or tenotomy scissors. When the enterotomy is oriented sagitally (along the long axis of the intestine), closure can result in significant narrowing of the intestine. When the scalpel blade technique is used, a stay suture, oriented transversely (perpendicular to the long axis of the intestine), can be placed full thickness through the proposed biopsy site. The stay suture allows manipulation of the sample without damage, and the perpendicular orientation of the biopsy prevents luminal narrowing. The intestinal wall incisions should be made

Manual of Small Animal Soft Tissue Surgery, Second Edition. Karen Tobias.
© 2017 John Wiley & Sons, Inc. Published 2017 by John Wiley & Sons, Inc.

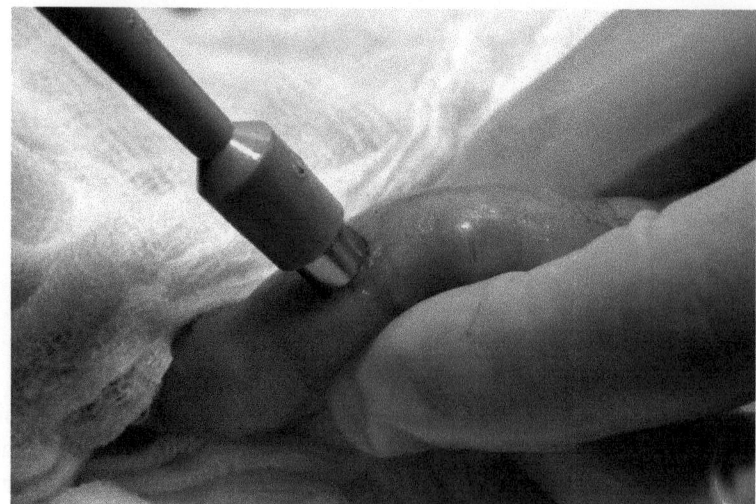

Figure 21-1 Use a 4- or 6-mm punch to remove a small core of intestinal wall.

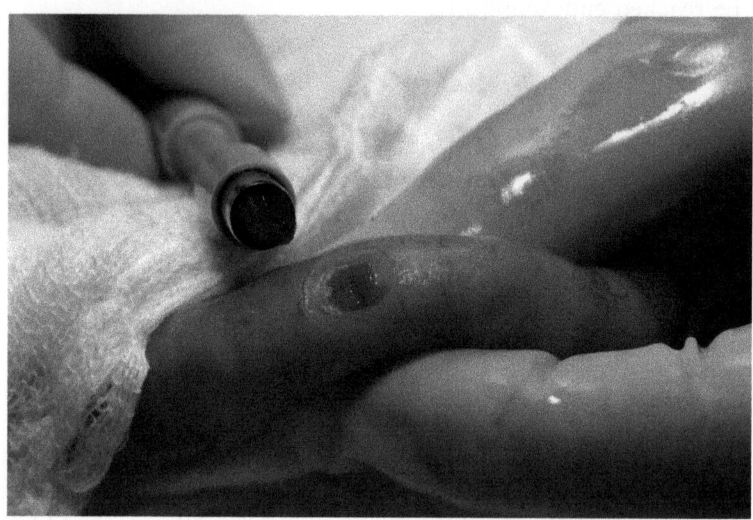

Figure 21-2 Biopsy site and sample. Close the resultant wound transversely with interrupted sutures placed parallel to the long axis of the intestines.

near the stay suture to limit the size of the resulting surgical wound. The sample and attached stay suture can be placed directly in formalin; the suture will not interfere with processing.

Biopsy sites can be closed with a simple interrupted, simple continuous, or Gambee pattern using 3-0 or 4-0 absorbable monofilament suture on a taper or tapercut needle. The Gambee pattern inverts the mucosa, which usually protrudes from the biopsy site, and apposes the remaining intestinal layers. If a simple continuous or interrupted pattern is used, everted mucosa may need to be trimmed from the incision site before closure. If intestinal integrity is questionable, interrupted closure of biopsy sites should be performed to reduce the risk of dehiscence.

Surgery technique: incisional biopsy of the intestine using a stay suture method

1. Isolate the intestine with moistened laparotomy pads. Include all potential biopsy sites in the isolated area.

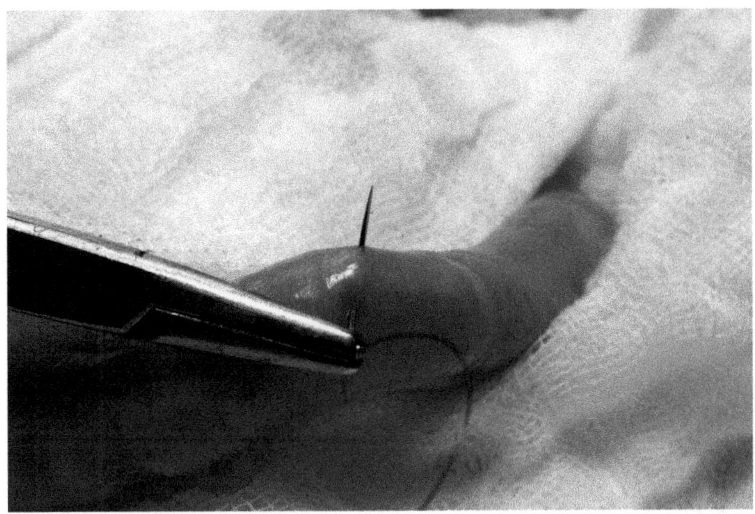

Figure 21-3 Place a full-thickness stay suture through the antimesenteric wall of the intestine.

2. Gently milk intestinal contents away from the site.
3. Place a full-thickness stay suture through the antimesenteric border of the intestinal wall, taking a bite that is 4 to 5 mm wide and perpendicular to the long axis of the intestine (fig. 21-3). Attach a hemostatic forceps to the suture ends.
4. Lift up gently on the stay suture and, with a no. 15 blade placed to one side of the suture, cut the intestinal wall, angling inward to a point below the suture (fig. 21-4).
5. Repeat the angled cut on the opposite side to remove a full-thickness wedge of tissue attached to the stay suture (fig. 21-4). The final sample should be about 3 to 4 mm wide and 5 to 6 mm long. Mucosa usually bulges from the incision site (fig. 21-5), blocking the surgeon's view of the outer tissue layers.

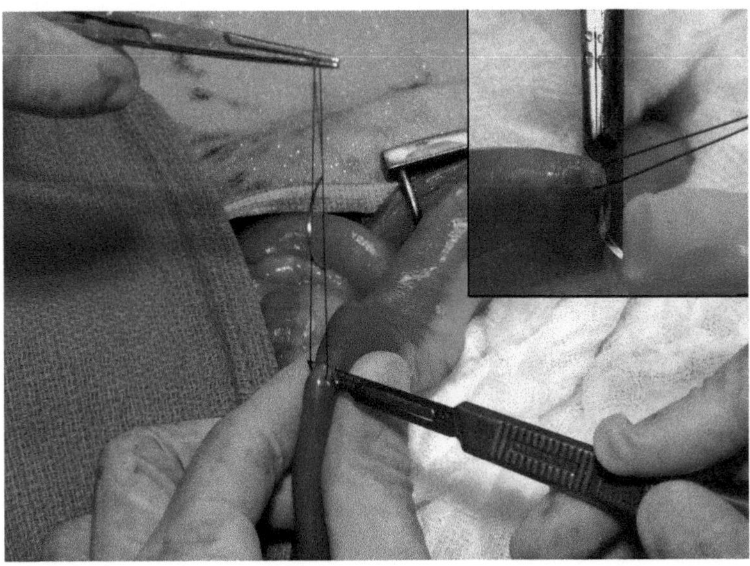

Figure 21-4 Incise the wall on both sides of the stay suture, angling downward and inward to remove a wedge of tissue.

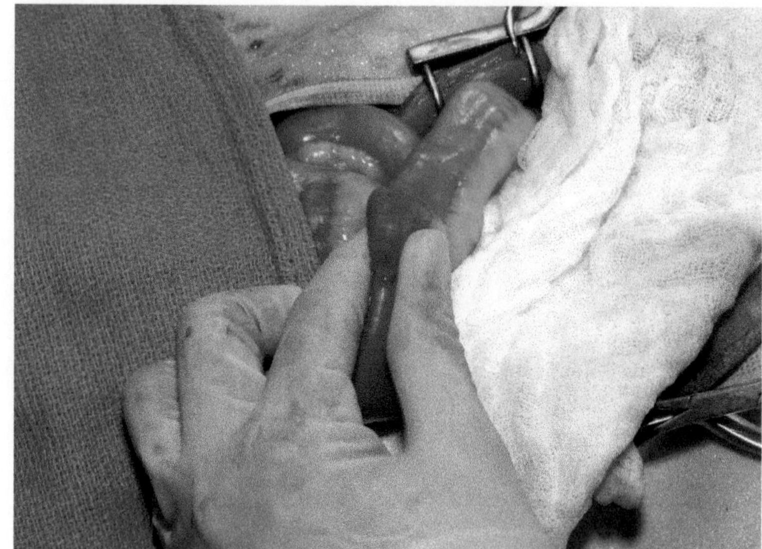

Figure 21-5 Wedge biopsy site. In live animals, the mucosa will bulge out of the incision site.

6. Close the defect with a simple interrupted pattern or interrupted Gambee pattern, placing the first suture across the center of the defect. Space sutures 2 to 4 mm apart. To place a Gambee suture:
    a. Take a full-thickness bite, 2 to 4 mm wide, through one side of the intestinal incision (fig. 21-6).
    b. To exclude mucosa from the bite, back the needle out as you lift it gently upwards, so that the everted intestinal mucosa rolls over the needle tip and back into the intestinal lumen. Next, advance the needle tip through the white mucosa-submucosa junction (fig. 21-7). Rotate your wrist (supinate) to follow the curve of the needle as you advance it. This will limit tissue damage. Pull the needle and suture through.

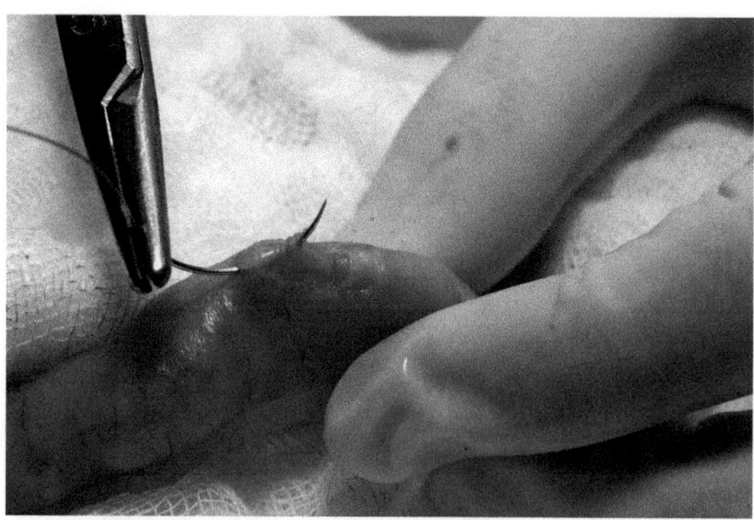

Figure 21-6 Take a full-thickness bite to include mucosa.

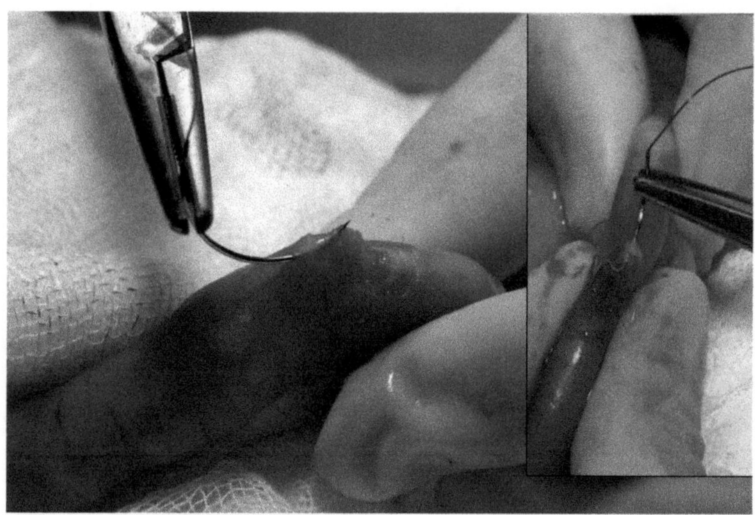

Figure 21-7 Lift the tissue up gently with the needle and slowly back out the needle until the mucosa rolls over the tip of the needle; then advance the needle through the mucosa-submucosa junction.

c. On the contralateral side, use the needle tip to force the mucosa down and into the lumen, and take a bite of the intestinal wall with the needle, starting at the mucosa-submucosa junction (fig. 21-8).

d. Tie four throws, starting with a surgeon's throw or simple throw. Appose the tissues without cutting, crushing, or indenting (fig. 21-9).

7. Test enterotomy closures by compressing the intestinal lumen on both sides of the biopsy site and distending the isolated segment with sterile saline injected through the intestinal wall (see p. 198). Add additional sutures if leakage is noted.

8. If desired, tack omentum over the site with simple interrupted absorbable sutures that engage the submucosa (fig. 21-10).

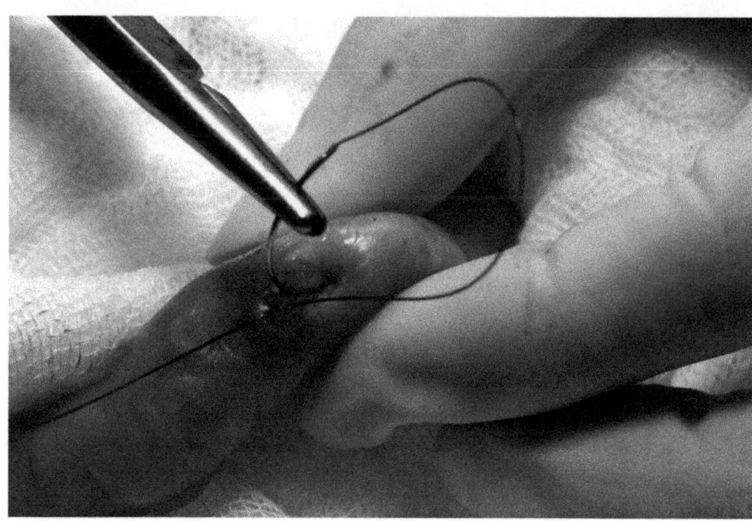

Figure 21-8 Invert the mucosa on the contralateral side with the needle tip before taking a bite through the white mucosal-submucosal junction.

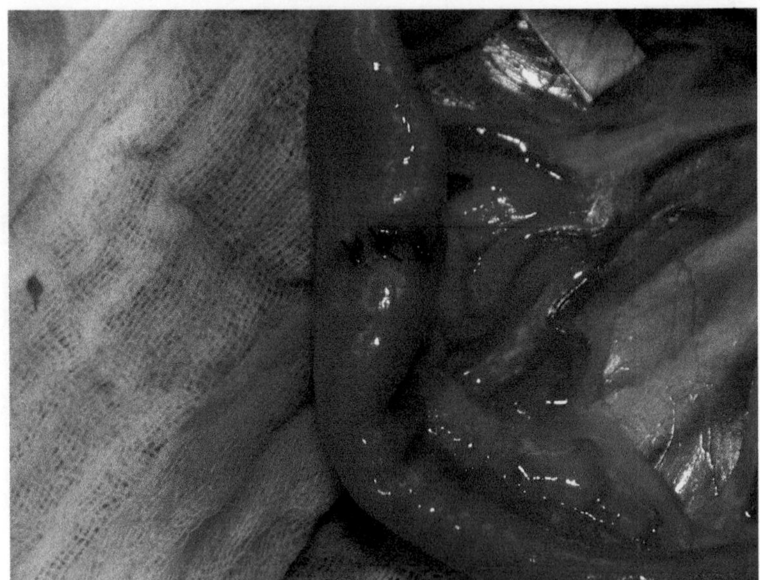

Figure 21-9 Final appearance. The mucosa should be inverted into the lumen.

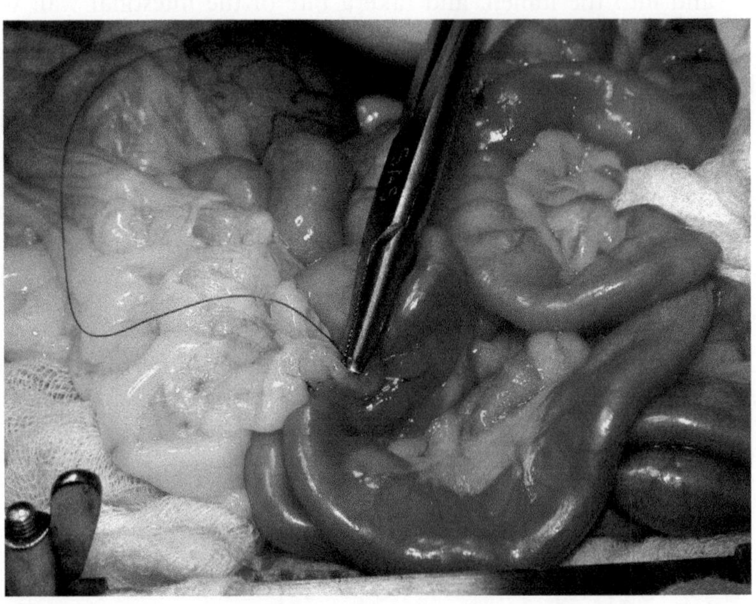

Figure 21-10 Tack omentum over the site with interrupted sutures.

Postoperative considerations

Animals can be fed within 12 hours after surgery if they are not vomiting. If minimal contamination has occurred, antibiotics do not need to be continued. Analgesics are administered for several days.

Major complications are reported in 5% to 12% of animals undergoing intestinal biopsy and include dehiscence, peritonitis, and hemorrhage. While hypoalbuminemia and glucocorticoids have deleterious effects on intestinal wound healing, dehiscence rates of intestinal biopsy have not been statistically correlated with systemic albumin concentrations or use of anti-inflammatory doses of corticosteroids. Clinical signs of intestinal leakage usually occur within 3–5 days of surgery but may become apparent as late as 9 days after surgery. Abdominocentesis or diagnostic peritoneal lavage may be required to diagnose peritonitis secondary to dehiscence, since radiographic evidence of free air is usually present as a result of the original surgery. Diagnosis and treatment of peritonitis are discussed in Chapter 15.

Bibliography

Evans SE et al: Comparison of endoscopic and full-thickness biopsy specimens for diagnosis of inflammatory bowel disease and alimentary tract lymphoma in cats. J Am Vet Med Assoc 2006;229:1447–1450.

Keats MM et al: Investigation of Keyes skin biopsy instrument for intestinal biopsy versus a standard biopsy technique. J Am Anim Hosp Assoc 2004;40:405–410.

Kleinschmidt S et al: Retrospective study on the diagnostic value of full-thickness biopsies from the stomach and intestines of dogs with chronic gastrointestinal disease symptoms. Vet Pathol 2006;43:1000–1003.

Matz BM, Boothe HW, Wright JC, et al: Effect of the enteric biopsy closure orientation on enteric circumference and volume of saline needed for leak testing. Can Vet J 2014;55:1255–1257.

Shales CJ et al: Complications following full-thickness small intestinal biopsy in 66 dogs: a retrospective study. J Small Anim Pract 2005;46:317–321.

Chapter 22
Intestinal Foreign Bodies

Intestinal foreign bodies in dogs and cats most frequently lodge in the jejunum. Common foreign bodies include latex bottle nipples, plastic or rubber objects, and various types of linear foreign bodies such as string or fishing line. Focal foreign bodies cause dilation of the intestines aboral to the obstruction and narrowing of the intestines distally (fig. 22-1). Local intestinal ischemia may occur from pressure on the wall overlying the object. Linear foreign bodies cause plication of the small intestines and may lead to extensive necrosis from ischemia or direct mechanical damage (fig. 22-2). Severity of clinical signs and metabolic abnormalities in affected animals depends on the degree, duration, and location of the obstruction. Common clinical signs include vomiting, anorexia, lethargy, and abdominal pain, but some dogs are asyptomatic or only have vague signs.

Diagnosis is sometimes made on abdominal palpation but is often based on detection of a foreign body or persistent obstructive pattern on survey or contrast radiographs or abdominal ultrasound. Radiographic findings associated with linear foreign bodies include clumped or pleated intestine and multiple small, eccentrically located intraluminal gas bubbles. Presence of free air on abdominal radiographs is indicative of peritonitis, which requires immediate surgical intervention after patient stabilization (see Chapter 15). Results of ultrasonography are more accurate for detecting foreign bodies than survey radiographs. In general, early surgery reduces mortality rates in animals with intestinal foreign bodies.

Preoperative management

Regardless of the level of obstruction, the most common electrolyte and acid-base abnormalities in animals with gastrointestinal foreign bodies are hypochloremia and metabolic alkalosis. Hypokalemia, hyponatremia, and hypomagnesemia may also occur.

Hydration, electrolyte, and acid-base abnormalities should be treated before anesthesia when possible. Analgesics such as hydromorphine, methadone, buprenorphine, or fentanyl are administered before and after surgery. Animals with chronic partial obstruction may be anemic or hypoproteinemic and

Manual of Small Animal Soft Tissue Surgery, Second Edition. Karen Tobias.
© 2017 John Wiley & Sons, Inc. Published 2017 by John Wiley & Sons, Inc.

Figure 22-1 Jejunal foreign body. The proximal intestine is dilated and the intestinal wall over the foreign body has been stretched thin.

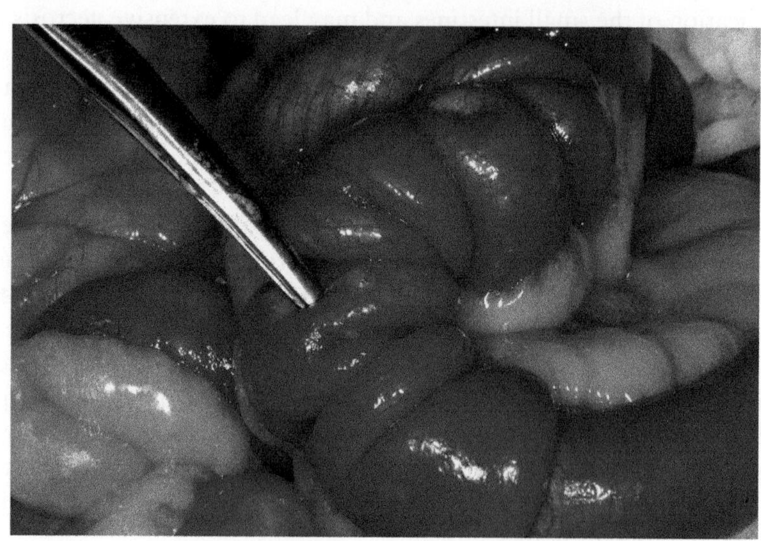

Figure 22-2 The intestines have plicated along the linear foreign body in this dog. Areas of necrosis and leakage are noted within the folds and near the scissor tips.

require transfusions or oncotic support. Coagulation panels should be evaluated in animals with severe hypoproteinemia, evidence of sepsis (e.g., degenerative left shift or toxic neutrophils), or peritonitis. If possible, free abdominal fluid detected on ultrasonography should be aspirated and submitted for culture and sensitivity before antibiotics are administered. In patients with sepsis or peritonitis, a broad-spectrum intravenous antibiotic (e.g., cefoxitin or ampicillin-sulbactam) or antibiotic combination should be administered. Animals with severe vomiting or increased lung sounds should be evaluated for evidence of aspiration pneumonia.

In dogs, linear intestinal foreign bodies usually anchor at the pylorus. In cats, linear foreign bodies may be fixed around the tongue. If a linear foreign body is suspected in a cat, the sublingual region should be examined carefully under anesthesia and, if located, the foreign body should be transected. Occasionally, thread or line will become embedded in the tongue and hidden by overlying tissues. Cats that present early after ingestion of a linear foreign body and that have no or mild clinical signs can sometimes be managed conservatively with transection of the foreign body from around the tongue and supportive care. If the foreign body does not pass within 3 days or the cat develops vomiting, abdominal pain, pyrexia, or a degenerative left shift at any time, surgery should be performed.

Surgery

The animal should be prepped from midthorax to pubis, since many animals with linear foreign bodies require gastrotomy and multiple enterotomies. During surgery, the entire abdomen should be explored for perforations or multiple foreign bodies. The affected intestine is isolated with moistened laparotomy pads to reduce contamination, and clean instruments are set aside for abdominal closure.

Focal intestinal foreign bodies are removed through a longitudinal antimesenteric enterotomy (fig. 22-3). If possible, enterotomy incisions should be made through healthy tissue aboral to the foreign body. The foreign body is gently milked toward the incision or grasped through the enterotomy with hemostatic or Allis tissue forceps and carefully extracted. If the aboral intestinal segment is narrow, the incision may need to be extended orally over the foreign body with Metzenbaum scissors or a blade to permit extraction. Severely compromised intestines should be resected (see Chapter 23). Enterotomy sites are closed with a continuous or interrupted appositional or Gambee (pp. 180–181) pattern, using 3-0 or 4-0 absorbable monofilament suture on a taper or tapercut needle. Suture bites are usually 2 to 4 mm wide and placed 2 to 4 mm apart, depending on the thickness of the intestine, and should always include submucosa. Mucosa that has everted out of the enterotomy site can be trimmed with scissors to improve visualization of

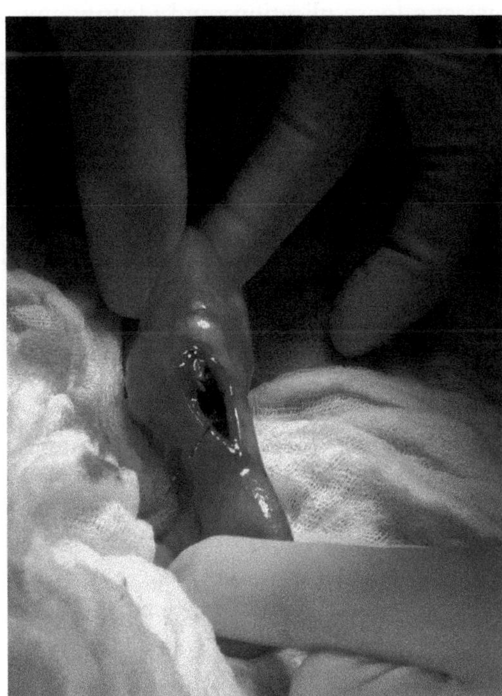

Figure 22-3 If possible, make the enterotomy through healthy intestinal wall distal (aboral) to the focal foreign body.

the tissue layers during suture placement. Omentum can be tacked over the closed site with interrupted, absorbable sutures. The abdomen should be flushed and suctioned after enterotomy, particularly if contamination has occurred. Gloves and instruments are changed before abdominal closure.

Linear foreign bodies are usually removed through a gastrotomy and one or more enterotomies. Some surgeons prefer to make the proximal enterotomy before gastrotomy so that they can grasp the enteral portion of the string with a hemostat and transect its oral end. This facilitates removal of the gastric portion of the foreign body and allows the surgeon to maintain control of the intestinal portion of the foreign body so it won't be "lost". Other surgeons will make the gastrotomy first, transecting the base of the entangled material and removing it to allow relaxation of the intestine. This usually allows the surgeon to make the first enterotomy farther distally and through intestine that is less tightly plicated. With either technique, it is important not to pull too hard on the linear foreign body as it is being retracted or removed to prevent it from sawing through the pyloric or intestinal wall. In cats with thin linear foreign bodies (e.g., floss, thread, fishing line), the foreign body sometimes can be removed by using a single enterotomy, "catheter-assisted" technique if it is not embedded in the intestinal wall, The foreign body is secured to a piece of red rubber tubing that is milked through the intestines and out the anus, gradually dislodging the foreign body from the intestinal wall. Strings that are matted, knotted, or severely embedded should not be removed with this technique.

Surgical technique: linear foreign body removal

1. If the linear foreign body is anchored around the tongue, transect the oral portion of foreign body after the animal has been intubated. If the linear foreign body is anchored in the stomach, perform a gastrotomy near the pyloric antrum (see p. 149). Cut the base of the material near the pylorus and remove the gastric portion of the foreign body, then close the gastrotomy.
2. Gently milk the proximal portion of the intestines off the linear foreign body to release any loose plications and identify any points of fixation.
3. With a no. 15 blade, perform a 1.5- to 2-cm antimesenteric longitudinal enterotomy in the proximal or middle third of the remaining plicated region.
4. Use the tips of a curved hemostatic forceps through the enterotomy to locate the linear foreign body along the mesenteric surface of the intestinal lumen. Secure the foreign body in the tips of the hemostats and gently retract the proximal end of the foreign body from the intestine.
5. If the entire linear foreign body is freed easily with gentle retraction and manual loosening of intestinal plications, retrieve the foreign body from the intestine and close the enterotomy site. If the foreign body is still fixed, remove the linear foreign body from the intestines through multiple enterotomies or using a catheter-assisted technique.
    a. Multiple enterotomy technique:
        i. Placing gentle traction on the linear foreign body. Identify the next point of aboral (distal) fixation and perform an enterotomy at that site. Locate the linear foreign body through the second enterotomy and extract it from the proximal intestinal segment.

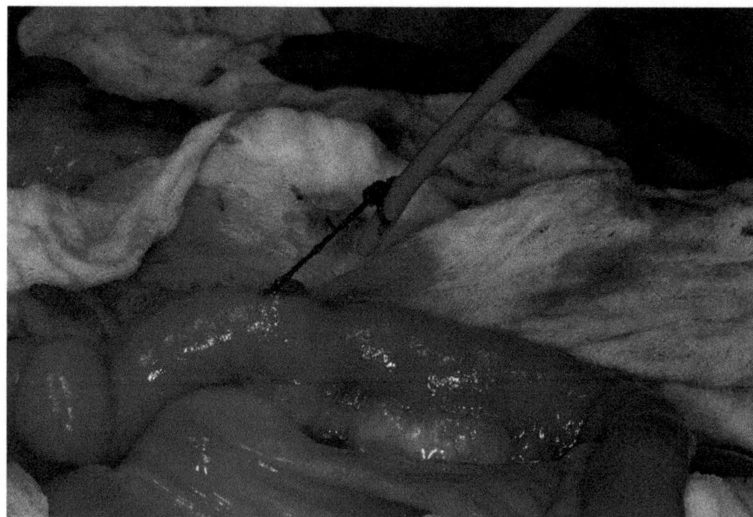

Figure 22-4 Tie the linear foreign body through the hole in the end of a red rubber catheter.

ii. If the distal end of the linear foreign body is not easily extracted from the intestines, repeat step 5.a.i. until the entire linear foreign body has been removed.

iii. Close enterotomy sites after each successive enterotomy or after the linear foreign body has been completely removed.

b. Single enterotomy (catheter-assisted) technique:

i. Cut the syringe adapter end off of a 12 or 14 French red rubber catheter, leaving a blunt-ended piece of tubing 10 to 20 cm in length. Pass the thread or string foreign body through the holes in the rounded end of the catheter and tie it back to itself (fig. 22-4). Alternatively, suture the linear foreign body to the catheter end.

ii. Insert the catheter, blunt end first, into the enterotomy site, directing it downstream (aborally).

iii. Once the entire catheter is in the intestinal lumen, close the enterotomy site.

iv. Milk the catheter gently through the intestines, gradually relieving the plication as the foreign body is pulled along with the catheter (fig. 22-5).

v. Once the catheter reaches the distal rectum, have a nonsterile assistant reach under the drape and retrieve the catheter from the anus, pulling gently to remove the linear foreign body.

vi. If the tube will not advance through the small intestines, perform a second enterotomy distal to the tube. Cut the string or thread, retrieve the tube, and remove the remaining foreign body with multiple enterotomies as described above.

6. Close enterotomy sites with 3-0 or 4-0 absorbable monofiliament suture in an interrupted or continuous appositional pattern, taking bites 2-4 mm wide and 2-4 mm apart, depending on intestinal thickness.

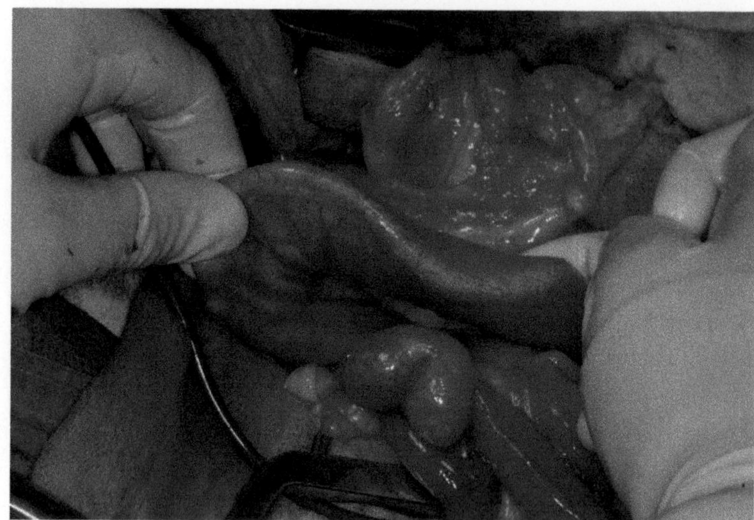

Figure 22-5 Milk the catheter aborally through the intestines to gradually remove the string foreign body and relieve the plication.

7. Test enterotomy closures by distending the intestinal lumen (see fig. 23-8).
   a. With atraumatic (e.g., Doyen) clamps or an assistant's fingers, compressing the intestinal lumen on each side of the enterotomy site.
   b. Fill a sterile 12 or 20 ml syringe with sterile saline and cap it with a 22 gauge needle.
   c. Inject the lumen of the isolated segment with sterile saline until the segment is distended and the incisional closure is under mild tension. Examine the closure site for leaks; add additional sutures if leakage is noted.
8. Check the remaining intestines for perforations or necrosis, especially along the mesenteric border, and resect or debride and close affected areas as needed. Tack omentum over any areas that have questionable blood supply (see p. 182).

Postoperative considerations

Antibiotics are continued after surgery in patients with intestinal ischemia, necrosis, peritonitis, or significant intraoperative contamination. Intravenous fluids are administered until hydration status can be maintained through oral intake. Most animals can be fed within 12 hours after surgery if they are not nauseated or sedated. Patients may experience a few bouts of vomiting, diarrhea, or nausea after surgery; however, animals with protracted vomiting or diarrhea should be evaluated for peritonitis, pancreatitis, or recurrent obstruction. Analgesics are usually required for several days. Initially, patients can be maintained on a fentanyl constant-rate infusion, with lidocaine added for dogs (see p. 124), or intermittent injections of hydromorphine, methadone, or buprenorphine. Some clinicians will administer nonsteroidal anti-inflammatory drugs within a few days after surgery.

Complications after intestinal foreign body removal include peritonitis, dehiscence of the intestinal closure, and motility disorders. Dehiscence rates range from 2% to 28%. Dehiscence is most likely to occur 2 to 5 days after surgery. Mortality rates are 1% to 22% and depend on duration of obstruction, type of foreign body, and metabolic status. Mortality rates increase when perforations and peritonitis are present or when surgery is delayed. Delaying surgery may increase the mortality rate because of bowel compromise and severe metabolic derangements.

Bibliography

Anderson S et al: Single enterotomy removal of gastrointestinal linear foreign bodies. J Am Anim Hosp Assoc 1992;28:487–490.

Basher AWP and Fowler JD: Conservative versus surgical management of gastrointestinal linear foreign bodies in the cat. Vet Surg 1987;16:135–138.

Bebchuck TN: Feline gastrointestinal foreign bodies. Vet Clin N Am Small Anim Pract 2002;32:861–880.

Boag AK et al: Acid-base and electrolyte abnormalities in dogs with gastrointestinal foreign bodies. J Vet Intern Med 2005;19:816–821.

Hayes G: Gastrointestinal foreign bodies in dogs and cats: a retrospective study of 208 cases. J Small Anim Pract 2009; 576–583.

Hobday MM, Pachtinger GE, Drobatz KJ, et al: Linear versus non-linear gastrointestinal foreign bodies in 499 dogs: clinical presentation, management, and short-term outcome. J Small Anim Pract 2014;55:560–565.

Tyrrell D and Beck C: Survey of the use of radiography vs. ultrasonography in the investigation of gastrointestinal foreign bodies in small animals. Vet Radiol Ultrasound 2006;47:404–408.

Chapter 23
Intestinal Resection and Anastomosis

Common indications for intestinal resection and anastomosis include intestinal neoplasia, intussusception, ischemia, or trauma. Perforated or ulcerated intestines and those obstructed by foreign bodies may also require resection (versus debridement and primary closure) if tissue health is questionable. In cats with megacolon, subtotal colectomy is performed when medical management fails.

Preoperative management

Animals should be evaluated for dehydration, anemia, hypoproteinemia, hypoglycemia, acid-base and electrolyte imbalances, sepsis, coagulopathy, and organ failure. If possible, patients should be metabolically stable before surgery. Intestinal perforation, complete obstruction, peritonitis (see Chapter 15), and uncontrollable hemorrhage require emergency surgery. Antibiotics are often administered prophylactically; they should be continued therapeutically in animals with infection, ischemia, sepsis, or significant intestinal wall compromise. First-generation cephalosporins are often used in patients undergoing proximal intestinal procedures. Antimicrobial drugs with good anaerobic spectrum, such as cefoxitin, are recommended for distal intestinal procedures.

Enemas are not performed before surgery because they liquefy the feces, increasing the chance of leakage during the procedure. The abdominal cavity should be clipped and prepped widely in the event that feeding tubes or peritoneal drains are required. Laparotomy sponges, retractors, lavage fluid, and suction should be available. Clean gloves and instruments should be set aside for closure.

Surgery

The amount of intestine to be resected depends on the underlying condition and intestinal viability. Neoplastic lesions are usually resected with 2.5- to 5-cm margins. In cats with idiopathic megacolon and normal ileum, resection can be limited to the colon, with anastomosis of the proximal ascending colon (just beyond the cecocolic junction) to the distal colon near its junction with the rectum (colocolectomy). If the ileum and ileocolic sphincter are also dilated, the sphincter and distal ileum are also removed, and the ileum is anastomosed to the distal colon

Manual of Small Animal Soft Tissue Surgery, Second Edition. Karen Tobias.
© 2017 John Wiley & Sons, Inc. Published 2017 by John Wiley & Sons, Inc.

(ileocolectomy). Ileocolectomy in cats may be required if tension from restraint by the vascular pedicles is too great to anastomose the colic ends together.

Determination of intestinal viability is usually based on clinical judgment. Mesenteric arteries supplying healthy intestine should have detectable pulsations. Intestinal walls that are black, green, dark red, extremely thin-walled, or friable or do not bleed when cut should be removed. Animals can tolerate removal of 50% to 70% of the intestines, depending on the health of the remaining gastrointestinal tract.

Intestinal anastomosis can be performed with staplers or suture. Sutured intestinal anastomosis is performed in a single-layer closure using a continuous or interrupted appositional pattern. Complication rates are similar for both techniques, and continuous closure is faster and provides better mucosal apposition. Absorbable suture (3-0 or 4-0) on a taper or tapercut needle is preferred. Foreign body obstruction has been reported after anastomosis with polypropylene suture using a continuous pattern; in affected animals, foreign material became entrapped by loops of nonabsorbable suture that have worked their way into the intestinal lumen.

Anastomotic sites can be supported with omentalization or serosal patching (suturing of adjacent, healthy intestines over the site). Omentalization is quick and easy to perform. A free edge of the omentum is tacked over one side of the anastomosis with interrupted sutures of 3-0 absorbable material (see p. 182). Suture bites should include submucosa. The omentum is loosely wrapped around the antimesenteric surface and then tacked over the anastomosis 180 degrees from the first sutures. The omental flap should not be wrapped 360 degrees around the intestines because it may cause stenosis.

Some surgeons recommend plication of the jejunum and ileum (placement of interrupted sutures between adjacent antimesenteric surfaces of gently looped bowel segments) to prevent recurrence after resection and anastomosis of small intestinal intussusception. Intestinal plication can predispose animals to obstruction or ischemia, particularly if the intestines are sharply folded when plicated. Plication is only recommended if intestines are hypermotile during surgery, the underlying cause of intussusception cannot be resolved, or the intussuscepted intestine has been reduced but not resected.

Surgical technique: intestinal resection and anastomosis

1. Explore the abdomen through a midline celiotomy and then isolate the affected intestinal segment with moistened laparotomy pads.
2. If an intussusception is present, attempt reduction with gentle traction.
    a. If reduction is successful, intestines are viable, and no mass is present, perform an enteroplication.
    b. If reduction is unsuccessful, vessels are thrombosed, intestinal wall integrity is questionable, or a mass is detected, perform a resection and anastomosis.
3. Milk intestinal contents away from the proposed resection site. Several centimeters of healthy tissue should be removed with the diseased segment to ensure adequate margins.
4. To reduce leakage, atraumatically clamp the intestines 3 to 5 cm beyond the proposed transection sites with Doyen forceps (fig. 23-1), Penrose drains, or an assistant's fingers.

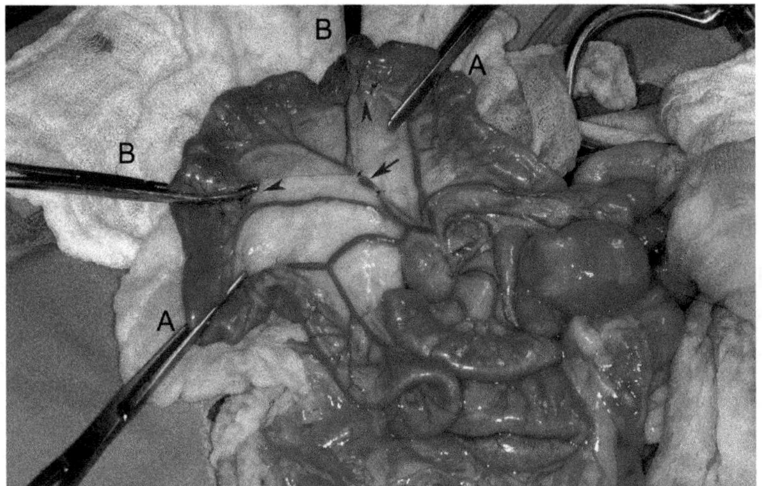

Figure 23-1 Clamp the intestine with Doyen forceps (A) or other atraumatic clamps 3 to 5 cm beyond the proposed sites of transection. Clamp the segment to be removed with Kelly or Carmalt forceps (B). Double ligate the major blood supply (arrow) in the mesentery and the terminal arcuate branches along the intestinal wall (arrowheads).

5. Ligate and transect the blood supply to the intestines.
   a. For resection of small intestines (fig. 23-1):
      i. Make windows in the mesentery around the vessels to the affected segment, and double ligate and transect the vessels.
      ii. To ligate the terminal arcuate vessels running along the mesenteric attachment to the intestines, take suture bites of the mesentery adjacent to the intestinal wall at the proposed sites of transection.
   b. For subtotal colectomy (fig. 23-2):
      i. Make windows in the mesocolon around the right colic, middle colic, and accessory middle colic arteries and veins. Ligate and transect the vessels. Leave the ileocolic artery and vein intact.

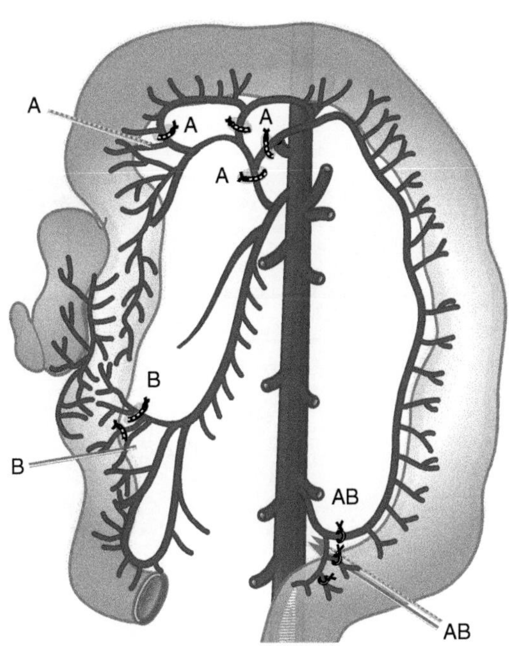

Figure 23-2 Colon resection. A indicates the locations of ligations and transections for a colocolic anastomosis, while B indicates the locatiosn for an ileocolic anastomosis. When possible, the blood supply to the proximal rectum should be left intact.

    ii. Ligate the left colic artery and vein after their bifurcations with the caudal mesenteric artery and vein, respectively.
    iii. For more distal resections, ligate individual segmental rectal branches (vasa recta). Leave the cranial rectal artery and vein intact (fig. 23-2).

6. Transect the mesentery along the segment to be removed.
7. Place Carmalt or Kelly forceps across the proposed ends of the intestinal segment to be resected.
8. Transect the intestine near the Carmalt or Kelly forceps adjacent to the arcuate ligatures.
    a. Transection can be performed perpendicular to the long axis of the intestine.
    b. Some surgeons will transect the intestine at a slight angle to reduce the length of the less vascular antimesenteric wall. Cutting both intestinal ends at a more than a slight angle makes anastomosis along the mesenteric edge more difficult, however.
9. To correct intestinal diameter disparity, incise the antimesenteric surface so that the diameter of the intestinal ends match (fig. 23-3), or cut the smaller segment at a greater angle.
10. Gently suction the intestinal ends or wipe them with a moistened gauze sponge to remove any debris.
11. Place full thickness interrupted mesenteric and antimesenteric sutures to align the intestine ends (fig. 23-4). Tie the sutures, but leave the suture ends long and grasped within hemostats to facilitate handling of the intestine. Pulling the sutures away from each other will stretch the intestinal wall edges and line them up.
12. Appose the intestine edges on the near side with an interrupted or continuous appositional pattern.
    a. If using a simple interrupted or simple continuous pattern, trim off any everted mucosa so that the remaining tissue layers can be seen.

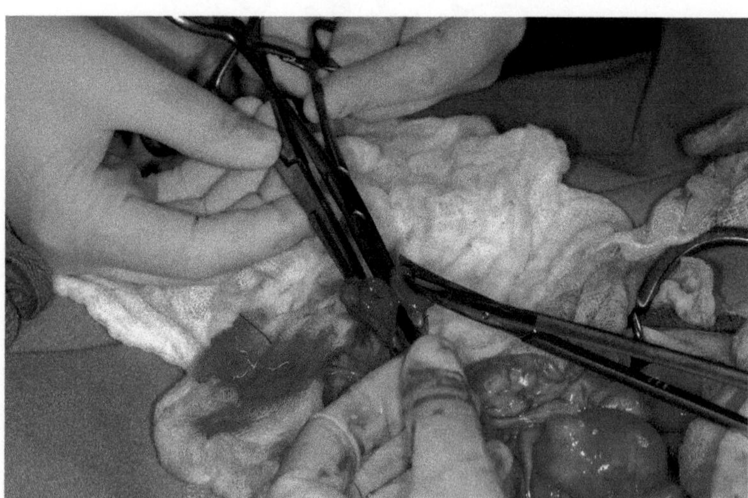

Figure 23-3 To correct for intestinal diameter disparity, incise the antimesenteric wall of the small segment with scissors.

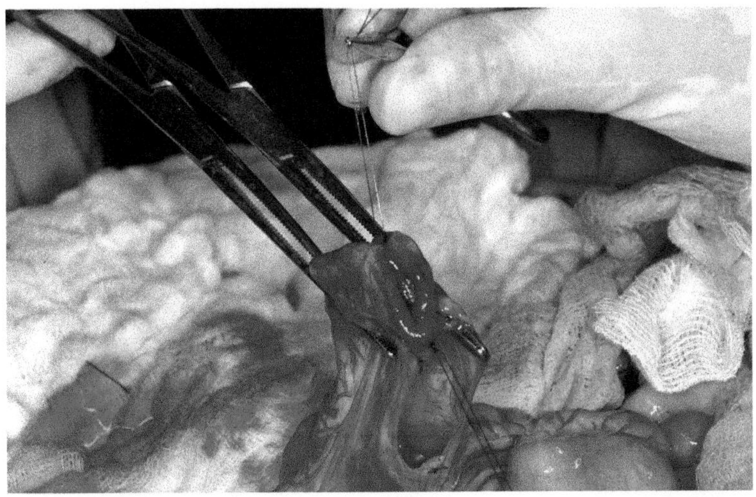

Figure 23-4 Place interrupted sutures at the mesenteric and antimesenteric borders to align intestine ends. Tie each suture and leave the ends long to facilitate intestinal handling.

b. Alternatively, invert the mucosa and appose the intestinal wall by using a continuous or interrupted Gambee or modified Gambee pattern (p. 180).

c. Start the anastomosis adjacent to the mesenteric border (the area most likely to fail) and work toward the antimesenteric border.

d. Using 3-0 or 4-0 absorbable monofilament suture, take suture bites 2 to 4 mm wide and 2 to 4 mm apart, depending on intestinal thickness and diameter. Include submucosa in each bite.

e. If using a continuous pattern, tie the suture off to the free end of the preplaced antimesenteric suture (fig. 23-5).

13. Flip the clamped intestine over to suture the edges on the opposite side.

a. Start a new suture pattern at the mesenteric border (fig. 23-6) and work toward the antimesenteric border.

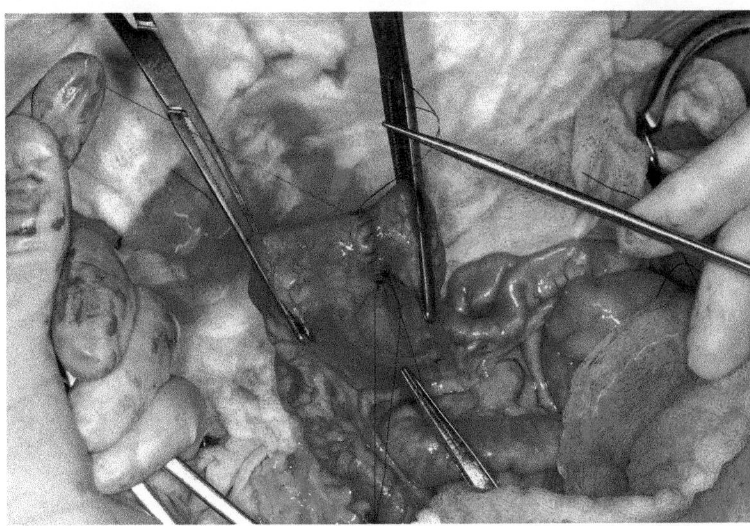

Figure 23-5 This anastomosis is being performed with a continuous Gambee pattern, which was started at the mesenteric border. When anastomosis of the near side is complete, the suture is tied off to the preplaced antimesenteric suture.

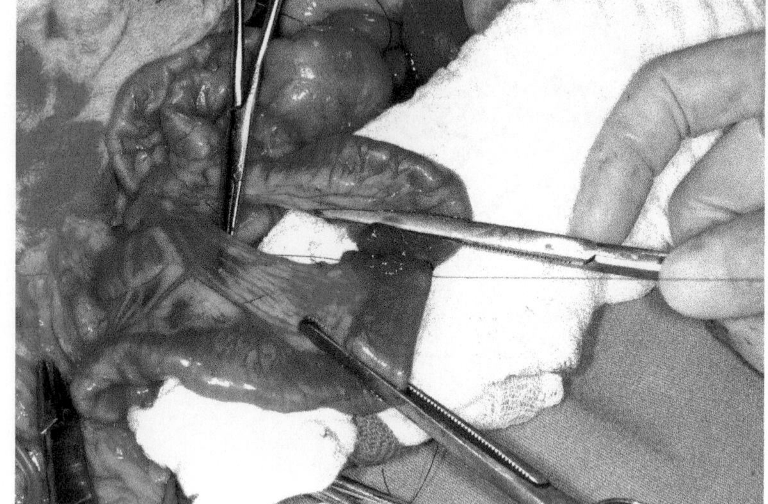

Figure 23-6 Flip the intestine and clamps over and appose the opposite side, starting at the mesenteric border.

b. If using a continuous pattern, tie the end off to the preplaced antimesenteric suture. Tie carefully to prevent a "purse-string" effect at the anastomotic site (fig. 23-7).

c. Cut all suture ends short.

14. Test the anastomotic seal by injecting saline into the lumen (fig. 23-8) or releasing the clamps and milking intestinal contents across the anastomotic site. Look for leakage, and close any gaps with interrupted sutures.

    a. With atraumatic (e.g., Doyen) clamps or an assistant's fingers, compress the intestinal lumen on each side of the anastomosis.

    b. Fill a sterile 12 or 20 ml syringe with sterile saline and cap it with a 22 gauge needle.

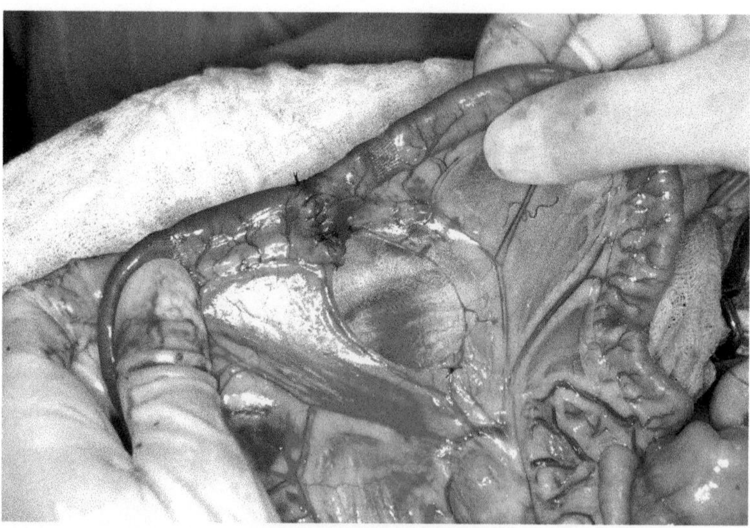

Figure 23-7 Completed anastomosis with Doyen clamps removed.

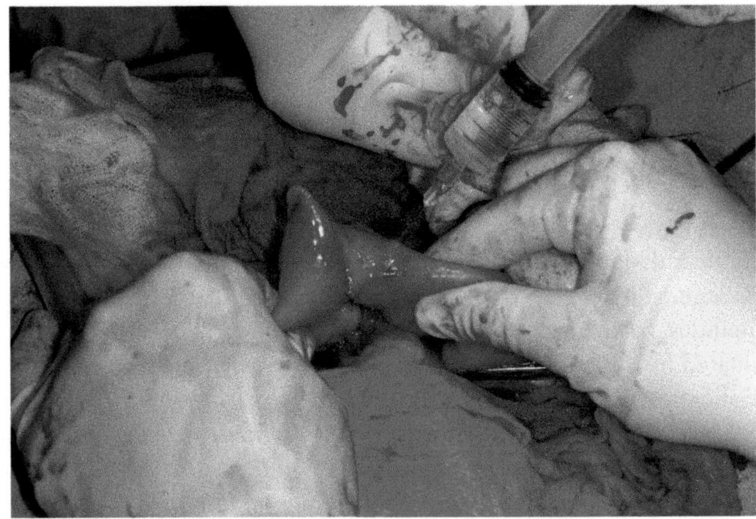

Figure 23-8 Test the anastomotic closure by distending the intestinal lumen with saline. In this dog GIA and TA staplers were used to form a functional end-to-end anastomosis.

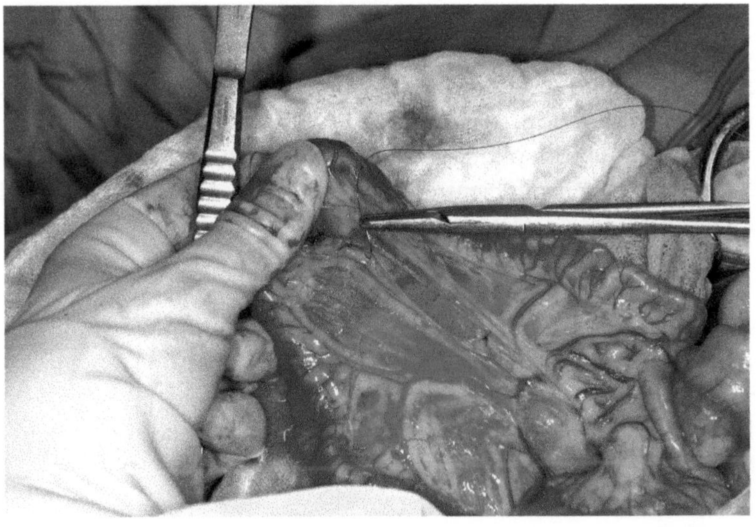

Figure 23-9 Appose the mesentery with a simple continuous pattern. Place suture bites medial to the intestinal vessels to avoid damaging the anastomotic blood supply.

c. Inject the lumen of the isolated segment with sterile saline until the segment is distended and the incisional closure is under mild tension. Examine the closure site for leaks; add additional sutures if leakage is noted.

15. Change gloves and instruments, then close the mesenteric defect with 4-0 rapidly absorbable suture, avoiding any blood vessels (fig. 23-9).
16. Tack the omentum over the anastomotic site with several interrupted sutures. Do not wrap the omentum 360 degrees around the site.
17. Lavage and suction the abdomen, then count sponges and laparotomy pads and change gloves and instruments before closing.

Postoperative considerations

Intravenous fluids are continued after surgery until the animal is drinking. Analgesics are administered for 2 to 5 days. Food and water can be offered within 12 to 24 hours, unless postoperative vomiting occurs. Malnourished animals should be monitored for refeeding syndrome (decreased phosphorus, potassium, and magnesium and fluid retention). Vomiting can be treated with an antiemetic (e.g., maropitant), metoclopramide, and correction of any electrolyte abnormalities, particularly hypomagnesemia. If vomiting persists, animals should be evaluated for peritonitis (see p. 121), pancreatitis, or mechanical obstruction.

Complications of intestinal resection and anastomosis include dehiscence, leakage, infection, ileus, and short bowel syndrome. Of greatest concern is peritonitis secondary to anastomotic leakage or dehiscence because it increases the mortality rate. Reported rates of dehiscence or anastomotic leakage range from 3% to 14%. Dehiscence rates are similar for interrupted and continuous patterns and for sutured and stapled anastomoses. Risk factors associated with dehiscence are not consistent among reports but have included hypoalbuminemia, intraoperative hypotension, pre-existing peritonitis or inflammatory bowel disease, large intestine resection in dogs, and resection and anastomosis for an intestinal foreign body removal or trauma. Dehiscence is usually detected 2 to 5 days after surgery and may result from poor surgical technique or presence of diseased tissue at the anastomotic ends. Diagnosis and treatment of peritonitis is described in Chapter 15.

Up to 45% of cats with idiopathic megacolon may have recurrence of clinical signs, particularly if insufficient colonic tissue is removed. Immediately after colocolic anastomosis, feces are usually soft but formed, and they gradually solidify over days to weeks. Cats undergoing removal of the ileocolic sphincter often have diarrhea after surgery, but feces usually become formed in 1 to 13 weeks. Frequency of defecation is increased with both procedures; however, most owners appreciate the fact that their cats are defecating regularly. Patients that have undergone ileocolectomy or extensive small bowel resection are usually started on a low residue diet; if diarrhea persists, they may benefit from addition of dietary soluble fiber, which stimulates hypertrophy of the remaining intestinal mucosa.

Bibliography

Allen DA et al: Prevalence of small intestinal dehiscence and associated clinical factors: a retrospective study of 121 dogs. J Am Anim Hosp Assoc 1992;28:70–76.

Applewhite AA et al: Complications of enteroplication for the prevention of intussusception recurrence in dogs: 35 cases (1989–1999). J Am Vet Med Assoc 2001;219: 1415–1418.

Duell JR, Thieman-Mankin KM, Rochat MC, et al: Frequency of dehiscence in hand-sutured and stapled intestinal anastomoses in dogs. Vet Surg 2016;45:100–103.

Gorman SC et al: Extensive small bowel resection in dogs and cats: 20 cases (1998–2004). J Am Vet Med Assoc 2006;228:403–407.

Kouti VI et al: Short-bowel syndrome in dogs and cats. Compend Contin Educ Pract Vet 2006;28:182–195.

Milovancev M et al: Foreign body attachment to polypropylene suture material extruded into the small intestine lumen after enteric closure in three dogs. J Am Vet Med Assoc 2004;225:1713–1715.

Ralphs SC et al: Risk factors for leakage following intestinal anastomosis in dogs and cats: 115 cases (1991–2000). J Am Vet Med Assoc 2003;223:73–77.
Snowdon KA, Smeak DD, Chiang S: Risk factors for dehiscence of stapled functional end-to-end intestinal anastomoses in dogs: 53 cases (2001–2012). Vet Surg 2016;45:91–99.
Sweet DC et al: Preservation versus excision of the ileocolic junction during colectomy for megacolon: a study of 22 cats. J Small Anim Pract 1994;35:358–363.
Weisman DL et al: Comparison of a continuous suture pattern with a simple interrupted for enteric closure in dogs and cats: 83 cases (1991–1997). J Am Vet Med Assoc 1999;214:1507–1510.

Chapter 24
Enterostomy Tube Placement

Tube feeding may be required in animals that are unable or unwilling to eat, or when the oral cavity must be bypassed to allow healing after trauma or surgery. Compared to parenteral nutrition, delivery of nutrients to the gastrointestinal tract is physiologic and cost effective; maintains gastrointestinal mucosal health and immune function; and reduces the risk of catheter-associated infection, vasculitis, metabolic disturbances, bacterial translocation, and sepsis. When oral, esophageal, or gastric feeding is contraindicated, the preferred method for nutritional support is via an enteric feeding tube. Enterostomy tubes can be placed through the nose (nasoenteral) or through a gastrostomy tube (G-J tube). If a laparotomy or endoscopy is to be performed, the end of a naso- or gastro-enteral tube can be guided through the pylorus manually or with an instrument, respectively. These techniques avoid the risk of intestinal incision. Enterostomy tubes inserted through the abdominal wall into the duodenum are usually placed during laparotomy for other issues, but they can be placed through a limited approach in the flank or with laparoscopic assistance through a small ventral midline approach. Contraindications for enteral feeding tubes include intestinal obstruction distal to the tube and adynamic intestinal ileus.

Preoperative management

Preoperative diagnostics and treatment depend on the underlying condition. Clipping and prepping of the abdomen should include the right lateral abdominal wall, which is the most common site for tube egress.

Surgery

Although most reports describe placement of enterostomy tubes through the jejunum, insertion through the descending duodenum is also acceptable and, in fact, may be preferable because the tube is usually fed downstream for 10–25 cm. Tubes for enteral feeding are available commercially; alternatively, red rubber catheters can be used. A 5-French tube is often placed in cats and small dogs; 8-French catheters can be used in medium and large dogs,

Manual of Small Animal Soft Tissue Surgery, Second Edition. Karen Tobias.
© 2017 John Wiley & Sons, Inc. Published 2017 by John Wiley & Sons, Inc.

depending on intestinal diameter. The tip of a closed-ended enterostomy tube can be removed to reduce the chance of food impaction and clogging. Once the surgeon has determined the length of tube to be fed aborally within the intestine, the tube should be marked at that site with a sterile marker. Alternatively, a second tube of similar size and length can be used to estimate the length of tubing within the intestine.

Enterostomy tubes can be placed surgically with a needle- or catheter-assisted technique or an incisional enterostomy with or without a serosal flap. The needle/catheter-assisted technique is primarily used for placement of small (e.g., 5-French) tubes. Once an enterostomy tube is in place, an enteropexy is performed to immobilize the intestine and encourage formation of a fibrous seal around the tube. The intestines can be pexied to the abdominal wall with interrupted mattress sutures or an interlocking box technique, and after the pexy is complete, omentum can be wrapped around the site to help provide a seal. The interlocking box technique is more complicated than interrupted mattress sutures but may permit removal of jejunostomy tubes within 2 to 3 days after placement in some animals. Essentially a 4 bite suture is placed loosely around the tube, alternating from body wall to jejunum, with each bite perpendicular and 90 degrees to the previous one. A second 4 bite suture is similarly placed, alternating from jejunum to body wall and starting at 90 degrees to the first suture. Both sutures are then tightened and tied. When completed, the tube perforation sites through the jejunum and body wall will each be surrounded by four bites of suture.

After enteropexy and laparotomy closure are completed and the tube is secured to the skin, a line should be drawn on the tube at skin level with a permanent marker so that tube position can be monitored after recovery. Unless the incision is large, a purse-string suture around the skin egress site is not necessary and may predispose the animal to cellulitis if there is inflammation or intestinal content leakage around the tube.

Surgical technique: needle- or catheter-assisted enterostomy tube placement

1. Select a large-bore needle or over-the-needle catheter with a lumen slightly larger than the diameter of the feeding tube.
2. After performing a midline celiotomy, choose a site for tube passage along the right ventrolateral body wall, near the proposed enterostomy site, that will allow pexy of the selected intestine segment without tension or kinking.
3. Insert the catheter or needle through the peritoneum and abdominal wall and out the skin. Insert the tube into the tip of the catheter or needle and feed it into the peritoneal cavity. Remove the catheter or needle from the abdominal wall.
4. Identify the normal direction of ingesta flow (oral to aboral) at the proposed enterostomy site. Insert the catheter or needle through the antimesenteric surface of the aboral (downstream) intestinal segment and exit it out of the intestines 2 to 4 cm orally (upstream; fig. 24-1).
   a. If a needle is used, pass the needle through the intestine walls with the bevel up.
   b. If an over-the-needle catheter is used, remove the catheter needle after the catheter has exited fully from the orad site.

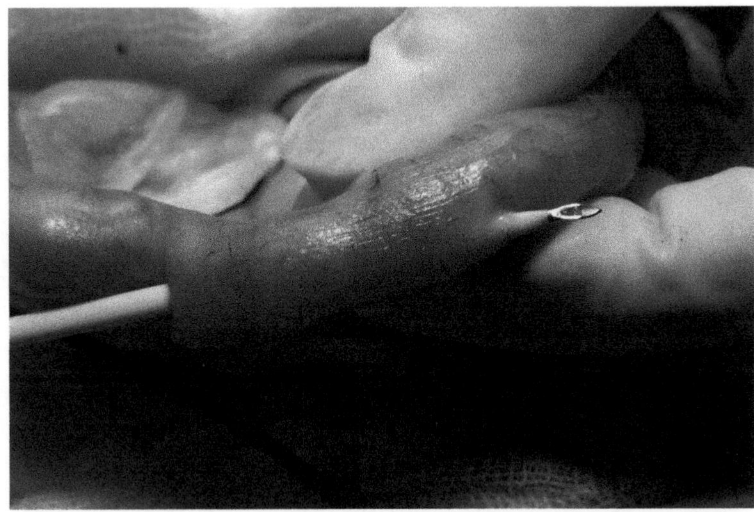

Figure 24-1 Pass the catheter in an aboral direction through the intestinal wall.

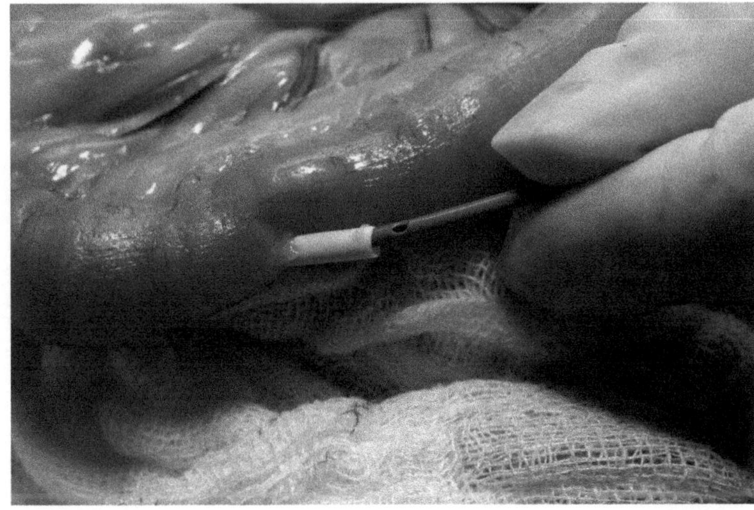

Figure 24-2 Insert the feeding tube into the catheter end. Note that the needle stylet has been removed and the tapered tip of the catheter has been trimmed to make the opening wider.

5. Insert the tip of the feeding tube 1 cm into the open end of the needle or catheter (fig. 24-2). If the tube does not fit into the tapered end of the over-the-needle catheter, cut the catheter end off.
6. Retract the needle/catheter through the orad (upstream) perforation into the intestinal lumen (fig. 24-3).
7. Holding the feeding tube securely, remove needle/catheter from the intestines, leaving the tube tip in the intestinal lumen.
8. Advance the feeding tube 10 to 25 cm aborally in the intestinal lumen (fig. 24-4). If the tube is placed in the descending duodenum, palpate the intestine to verify that the tube has not kinked or bent and that it has been advanced beyond the caudal duodenal flexure, which is located at the attachment of the duodenocolic ligament.
9. Close the aboral enterostomy site with a single interrupted or cruciate suture of 3-0 or 4-0 absorbable monofilament material.

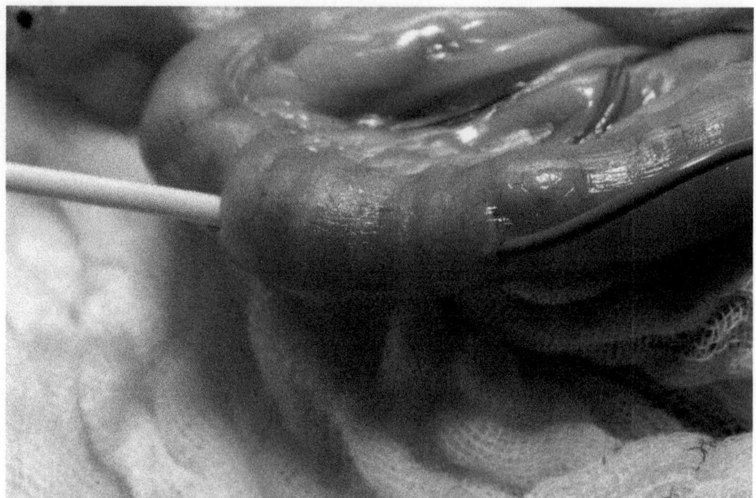

Figure 24-3 Retract the catheter with enclosed feeding tube into the intestinal lumen, then remove the catheter from the intestine.

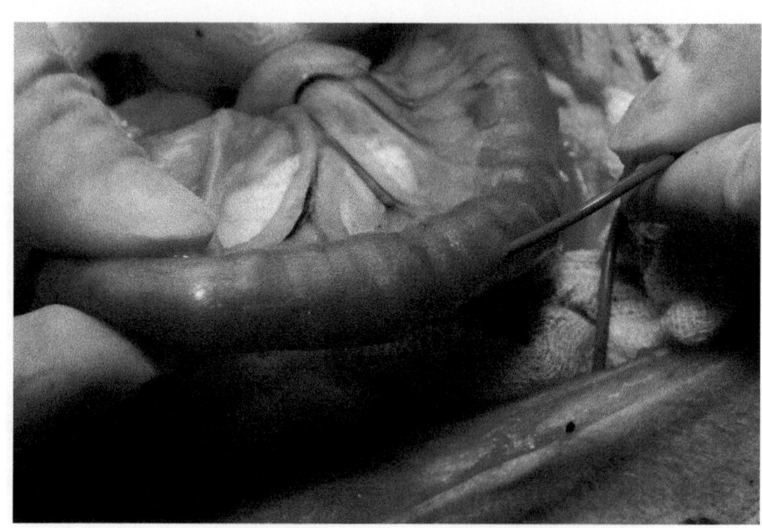

Figure 24-4 Advance the feeding tube 10 to 25 cm aborally in the intestinal lumen.

10. Place a purse-string or mattress suture of 3-0 or 4-0 absorbable monofilament in the intestinal wall around the tube at the oral enterostomy site (fig. 24-5). Tighten the purse string to appose the intestinal wall securely around the tube without blanching the tissues.
11. Using 3-0 absorbable monofilament suture, place four mattress sutures around the enteral stoma to form a box-shaped pexy (fig. 24-6). Place sutures 1 to 2 cm from the stoma and include intestinal submucosa and abdominal wall muscle in each bite. Place the dorsal-most suture first.
12. Tighten the pexy sutures to appose the body wall to the intestines. If desired, wrap omentum around the pexy site and tack it back to itself with an interrupted suture of absorbable material.
13. Secure the tube to the external body wall with a butterfly tape suture or fingertrap pattern (see pp. 497–501). In cats and dogs with mobile skin, include bites of underlying musculature in the fingertrap suture to prevent migration of the tube with skin movement.

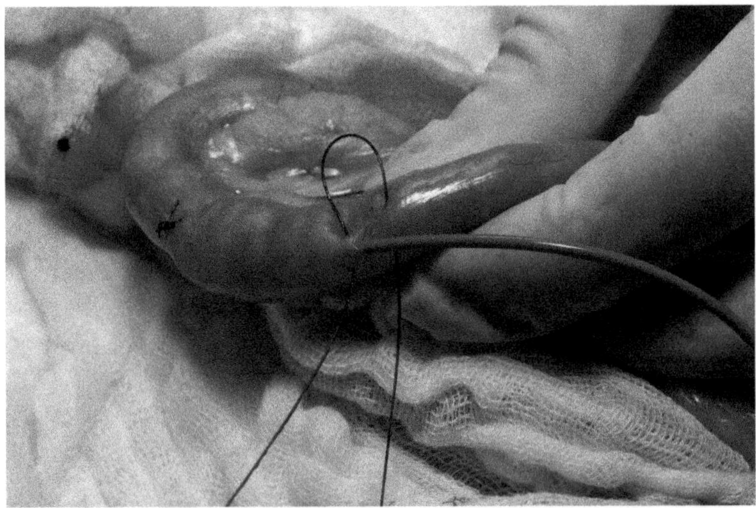

Figure 24-5 Close the distal perforation with a simple interrupted or cruciate suture and place a purse string or mattress suture in the intestinal wall around the tube entry site.

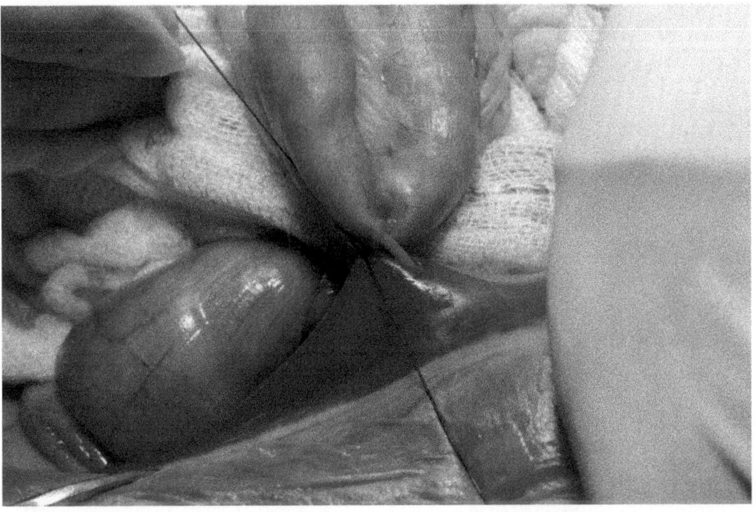

Figure 24-6 Pexy the intestinal wall surrounding the tube to the abdominal wall at the tube exit site.

14. After abdominal closure, measure and record the length of the external tubing or mark the tube at skin level with a permanent marker before bandaging the abdomen.

Surgical technique: enterostomy tube placement using a seromuscular flap technique

1. Insert fine-tipped hemostats through the peritoneum and abdominal wall at the proposed enteropexy site. Incise the skin over the tips of the hemostats to expose the tips, then use the tips to grasp the tube and pull it through the body wall and into the abdominal cavity.
2. At the proposed enterostomy site, make a 1.5- to 2-cm-long incision through the seromuscular layer of the antimesenteric intestinal wall with a no. 11 or no.15 blade to expose the intestinal mucosa (fig. 24-7).
3. With a fine-tipped hemostat or no. 11 blade, perforate the mucosa near the aboral (downstream) end of seromuscular incision (figs. 24-8 and 24-9).

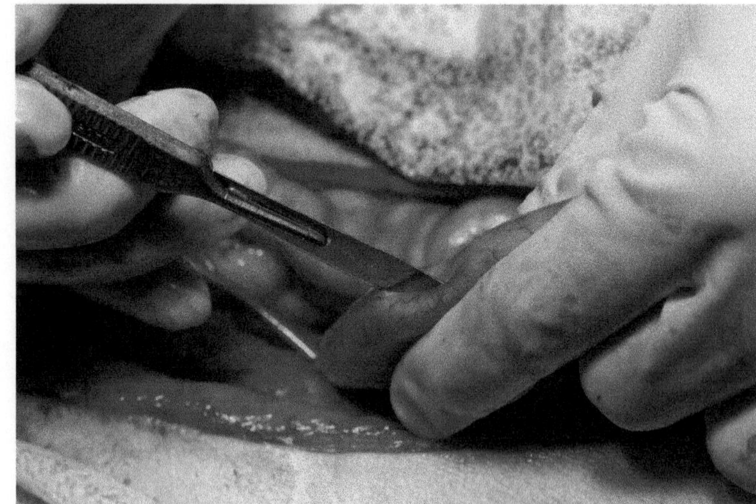

Figure 24-7 Incise through the seromuscular layer to expose the intestinal mucosa.

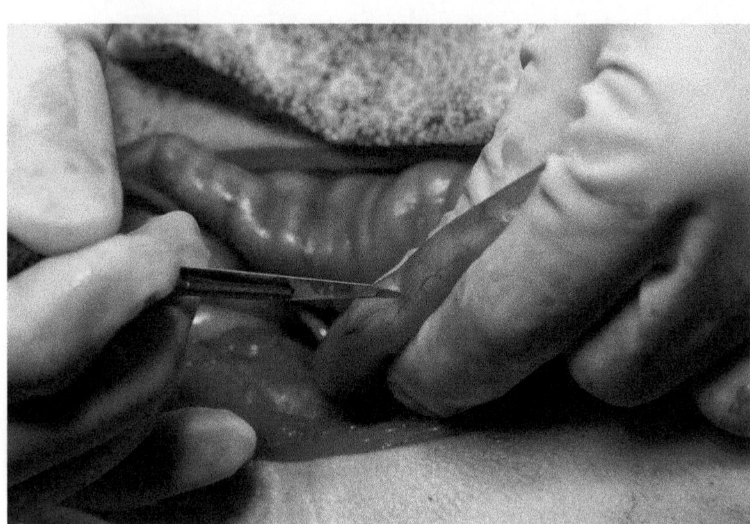

Figure 24-8 Perforate the mucosa at the aboral end of the seromuscular incision with a no. 11 blade.

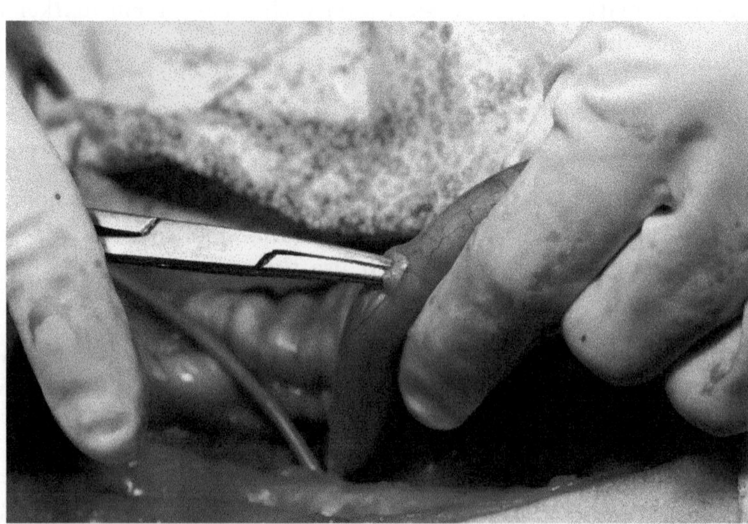

Figure 24-9 Insert fine hemostats through the perforation to verify that the mucosa has been fully penetrated.

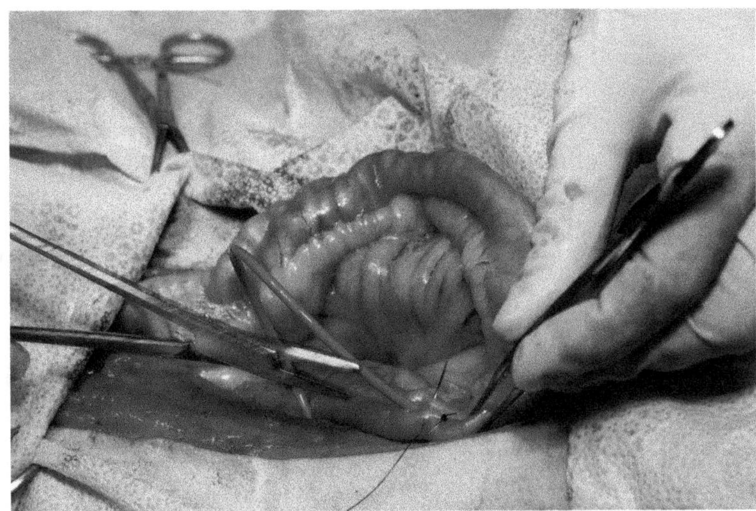

Figure 24-10 Close the seromuscular layer over the tube, and place a purse string or mattress suture in the intestinal wall around the tube exit site.

Insert the feeding tube through the perforation into the intestinal lumen. Advance the tube 10 to 25 cm aborally, as described above.

4. Using 3-0 or 4-0 monofilament suture, close the seromuscular incision over the top of the tube with a simple interrupted pattern (fig. 24-10).
5. Place a purse-string or mattress suture of 3-0 or 4-0 absorbable monofilament in the intestinal wall around the tube (along the orad side of the seromuscular flap). Tighten the purse string to appose the intestinal wall securely around the tube without blanching the tissues.
6. Pexy the tube and secure it to the skin as described above.

Postoperative considerations

Elizabethan collars or side-bar braces are recommended to prevent premature tube dislodgement. Feeding through enterostomy tubes can be started immediately. Initially, liquid diets can be diluted 50% and administered at a slow rate (e.g., 0.5 to 1 mL/kg/hour) with a motorized fluid pump. Concentration and rate are gradually increased over 2 to 3 days as long as feedings are tolerated. Tubes may require flushing with water or saline every 4 to 6 hours to prevent obstruction. Feeding should be calculated to meet resting energy requirements (formula: $70 \times \text{kg BW}^{0.75}$) and maintenance fluid needs. Commercial diets are preferred since they are less likely to clog the tube than homemade, blenderized formulas. Most commercial liquid diets contain 0.9 to 1.0 Kcal/mL.

Minor diarrhea is common with liquid diets. If vomiting, persistent diarrhea, or evidence of nausea (e.g., ptyalism) occurs, rate of administration and concentration of the diet should be decreased and the animal should be examined for ileus. Feeding tubes are usually left in place 6 to 10 days before removal to permit formation of a fibrous seal around the enterostomy site. Tubes can be pulled earlier, however, if an interlocking box technique is used to secure the intestine to the abdominal wall. The tube is removed by cutting the finger trap or butterfly tape suture and pulling gently while kinking off the tube. The skin exit site usually seals by second intention within 24 to 48 hours after the tube is removed.

Complications are seen in 18% to 44% of animals and may include peritonitis; retrograde tube migration; cellulitis at the skin exit site; tube blockage, kinking, or clogging; and inadvertent removal by the patient or caretakers. Vomiting or diarrhea may occur with rapid feeding, ileus, or peritonitis. Cellulitis at the skin site usually resolves with tube removal, unless food or intestinal secretions have pocketed subcutaneously. Animals that have had severe malnutrition, prolonged anorexia, starvation, or diuresis are at risk for refeeding syndrome, which causes a rapid shift of cations into intracellular spaces. Resulting hypophosphatemia, hypokalemia, or hypomagnesemia may cause muscle weakness, intravascular hemolysis, cardiac or respiratory dysfunction, and death. Feeding should be introduced slowly in predisposed patients, and electrolytes should be monitored frequently and supplemented as needed.

Bibliography

Daye RM, Huber ML, Henderson RA: Interlocking box jejunostomy: a new technique for enteral feeding. J Am Anim Hosp Assoc 1999;35:129–134.

Heuter K: Placement of jejunal feeding tubes for post-gastric feeding. Clin Techniques Small Anim Pract 2004;19:32–42.

Orton EC: Enteral hyperalimentation administered via needle catheter–jejunostoma as an adjunct to cranial abdominal surgery in dogs and cats. J Am Vet Med Assoc 1986;188:1406–1411.

Swann HM et al: Complications associated with use of jejunostomy tubes in dogs and cats: 40 cases (1989–1994). J Am Vet Med Assoc 1997;12:1764–1767.

Tsuruta K, Mann FA, Backus RC: Evaluation of jejunostomy tube feeding after abdominal surgery in dogs. J Vet Emerg Crit Care 2016;26:502–508.

Yagil-Kelmer E et al: Postoperative complications associated with jejunostomy tube placement using the interlocking box technique compared with other jejunopexy methods in dogs and cats: 76 cases (1999–2003). J Vet Emerg Crit Care 2006;16: S14–S20.

Chapter 25
Colopexy

Fixation of the colon to the abdominal wall is called colopexy. Indications for this procedure include treatment of recurrent rectal prolapse and reduction of rectal sacculation and deviation associated with perineal hernias. In animals that have complicated perineal hernias, herniorrhaphy can be performed immediately after colopexy or delayed for several weeks to decrease stress on the hernia repair.

Preoperative management

Prolonged fasting and enemas are unnecessary before colopexy. Because the colon may be inadvertently penetrated with suture during the procedure, prophylactic antibiotics are given intravenously at induction and repeated 2 to 6 hours later. Antimicrobials with Gram negative and anaerobic spectrum are commonly used (e.g., cefoxitin). Epidural regional block may reduce postoperative straining, particularly in dogs with rectal disease.

Surgery

Colopexy is usually performed through a caudal midline incision, although a laparoscopic-assisted technique has also been described. To increase the likelihood of permanent adhesion, the peritoneum is incised, scarified, or parted with electrocautery to produce local inflammation. The colonic serosa can be scarified with a blade or gauze sponge, or the serosa and muscularis can be incised, before the colon is sutured to the abdominal wall. There is no difference in outcome when comparing incisional and nonincisional colopexies, and many surgeons therefore prefer the nonincisional technique because it avoids the risk of inadvertent full thickness perforation.

Surgical technique: colopexy

1. Once the caudal abdomen is open, place Balfour retractors, or grasp and elevate the free edge of the left abdominal wall incision with towel clamps, to expose the left lateral peritoneal surface.
2. Scarify the antimesenteric surface of the descending colon at a level 5 to 10 cm cranial to the pubis by scraping it with a scalpel blade or dry gauze sponge (fig. 25-1). Alternatively, incise the colonic serosa (fig. 25-2).

Manual of Small Animal Soft Tissue Surgery, Second Edition. Karen Tobias.
© 2017 John Wiley & Sons, Inc. Published 2017 by John Wiley & Sons, Inc.

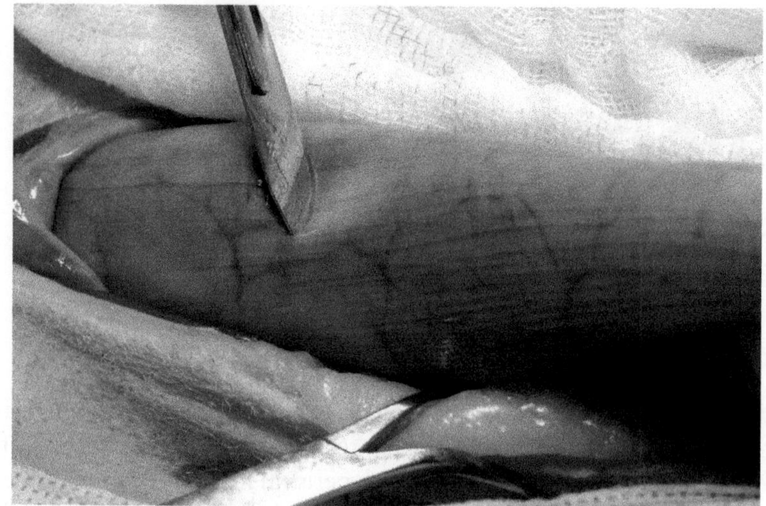

Figure 25-1 Scarify the colonic serosa by scraping it with a scalpel blade.

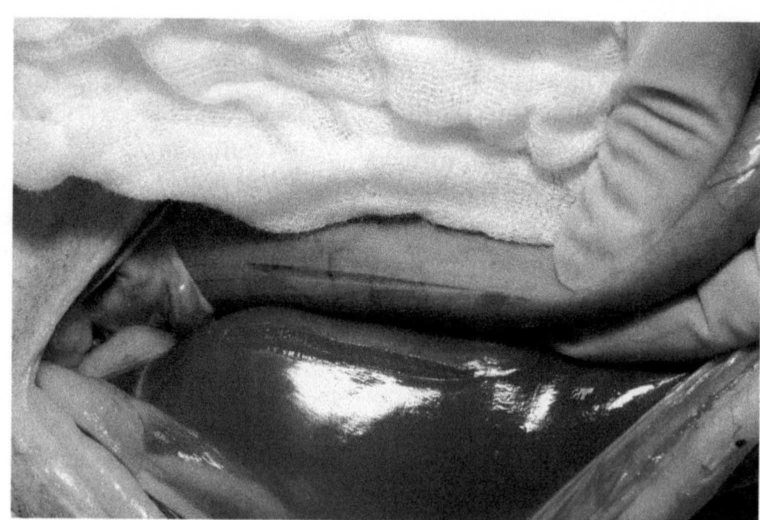

Figure 25-2 Pull the colon cranially to reduce any rectal sacculations or prolapse, then make an incision through the peritoneum of the lateral abdominal wall, adjacent to the site of colonic scarification/incision.

3. Pull the descending colon cranially to remove any rectal sacculation, deviation, or prolapse.
   a. If desired, have a nonsterile assistant perform a digital rectal exam simultaneously to verify that the rectum is straight and any prolapse is reduced.
   b. Check the color of the descending colon and the vessels to make sure tension is not excessive as the colon is pulled cranially. If there is too much tension, the colon will turn white, and its arteries will pulsate strongly.
4. With a scalpel blade or cautery, make a 4- to 6-cm incision in the peritoneum over the left ventrolateral abdominal wall at a level comparable to that of the colonic scarification or incision (fig. 25-2). The incision will usually lie just cranial to the level of the wing of the ileum.

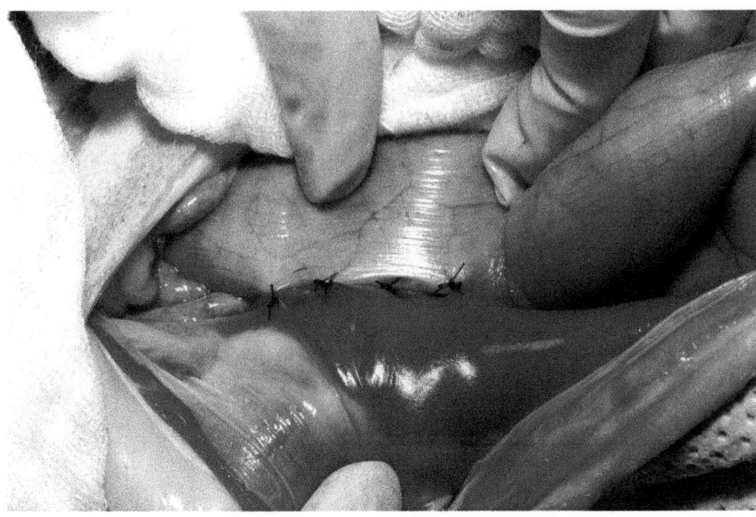

Figure 25-3 Secure the colon to the abdominal wall with interrupted sutures.

5. Place interrupted sutures from the incised body wall to the scarified wall of the descending colon (fig. 25-3).
   a. Use monofilament, slowly absorbable suture material on a taper needle.
   b. In the abdominal wall bites, include transversus abdominis muscle along both sides of the peritoneal incision.
   c. In the colonic bites, include submucosa without penetrating the mucosa. To determine thickness of the seromuscular layer, pinch the colon between thumb and index finger and let the mucosa fall out of the pinch.
   d. Take 1-cm-wide bites of each structure, and tie the sutures gently to appose the tissues without necrosing them.
   e. Place a total of four to eight sutures, spaced 1 to 1.5 cm apart.
6. Close the abdomen routinely.
7. Perform a digital rectal exam to verify that the rectum has been straightened and any prolapsed or redundant folds have been eliminated.

Postoperative considerations

Analgesics are usually administered for 1 to 3 days. Patients may require lactulose or other stool softeners, depending on the underlying condition. The most common complication is recurrence of clinical signs from poor surgical technique, breakdown of the pexy site, or persistence of the underlying condition. Penetration into the colonic lumen during pexy could permit contamination of the abdominal cavity. This is easier to avoid when the serosa is scarified instead of incised. Excessive tension could result in necrosis of the colon wall or breakdown of the pexy site. Patients that develop lethargy, anorexia, fever, or other signs of systemic illness should be evaluated for peritonitis (see Chapter 15).

Bibliography

Brissot HN et al: Use of laparotomy in a staged approach for resolution of bilateral or complicated perineal hernia in 41 dogs. Vet Surg 2004;33:412–421.

Gilley RS et al: Treatment with a combined cystopexy-colopexy for dysuria and rectal prolapse after bilateral perineal herniorrhaphy in a dog. J Am Vet Med Assoc 2003;222:1717–1721.

Mathon DH, Palierne S, Meynaud-Collard P, et al: Laparoscopic-assisted colopexy and sterilization in male dogs: short-term results and physiologic consequences. Vet Surg 2011;40:500–508.

Popovitch CA et al: Colopexy as a treatment for rectal prolapse in dogs and cats: a retrospective study of 14 cases. Vet Surg 1994;23:115–118.

Chapter 26
Rectal Polyp Resection

The most common intestinal masses in dogs are colorectal adenocarcinomas and polyps. Rectal polyps are usually singular and can have a pedunculated or broad base. They are often located within 5 cm of the anus (fig. 26-1) and can be exposed for resection by prolapsing the mass and surrounding rectal mucosa with stay sutures. Although benign in behavior, many polyps in dogs exhibit histologic evidence of malignant transformation. Affected animals may be asymptomatic or develop tenesmus, hematochezia, dyschezia, diarrhea, or intermittent or persistent rectal prolapse. Diagnosis is based on digital palpation or proctoscopy and biopsy. Surgical removal of single masses is recommended. Medical management with piroxicam will reduce clinical signs in dogs with rectal polyps and is an acceptable alternative therapy when multiple polyps are present or owners decline surgery. Inflammatory colorectal polyps, common in miniature dachshunds, may respond to immunosuppression with leflunomide or a combination of cyclosporine and prednisolone.

Preoperative management

If proctoscopy is to be performed before surgery, food is withheld for 24 hours, and multiple enemas are administered. For surgery alone, enemas are not necessary and increase the risk of fecal leakage during the procedure. Epidural administration of analgesics facilitates anal dilation and polyp exposure, and reduces postoperative discomfort. Prophylactic antibiotics are not required if excision is limited to the rectal mucosa and submucosa. If the procedure is performed with the patient in a perineal position, ventilation should be assisted. If solid feces are present, the rectum is digitally evacuated before surgery.

Surgery

Techniques for rectal polyp removal include surgical resection with primary closure of the mucosal defect using suture or staples, or transection of the mass at the level of the mucosa followed by freezing or cauterizing the base with cryosurgery or electrosurgery, respectively. Electrosurgical removal of polyps may result in rectal perforation if the mucosa cannot be separated from the seromuscular layer.

Manual of Small Animal Soft Tissue Surgery, Second Edition. Karen Tobias.
© 2017 John Wiley & Sons, Inc. Published 2017 by John Wiley & Sons, Inc.

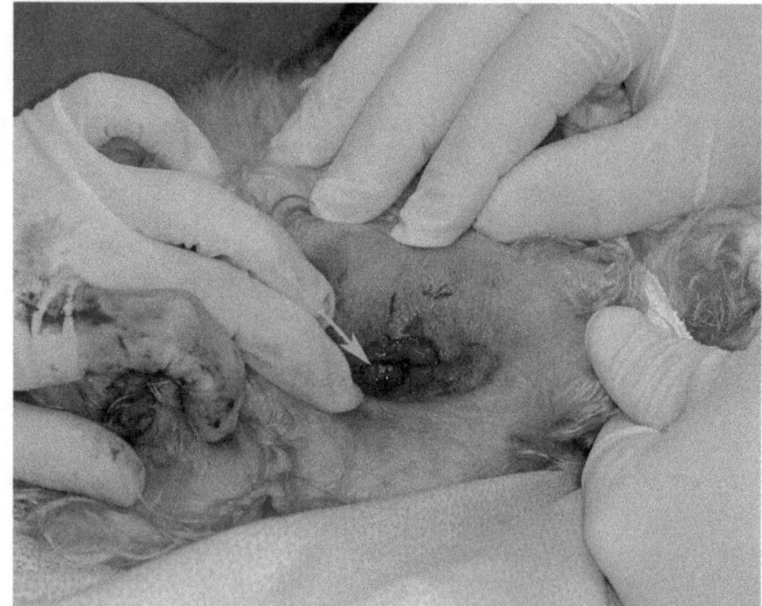

Figure 26-1 This rectal polyp (arrow) is located at the 6 o'clock position in the distal rectum and can be easily exposed by spreading the anus.

Surgical technique: rectal polyp resection

1. If the polyp can be prolapsed digitally, insert stay sutures through the mucosa and submucosa orad (cranial) to the polyp and cranial to the proposed margin of excision. Attach the stay sutures to hemostats.
2. If the polyp cannot be easily prolapsed, grasp the rectal mucosa caudal to the polyp with atraumatic forceps and place stay sutures into the rectal mucosa and submucosa. Retract gently but firmly on the stay sutures to expose more orad mucosa, and place additional stay sutures farther cranially for retraction (fig. 26-2). Continue to place stay sutures cranially for further retraction until the polyp is prolapsed out of the anus.
3. If needed, attach an additional stay suture or atraumatic (e.g., Babcock) forceps to the polyp to assist in retraction.

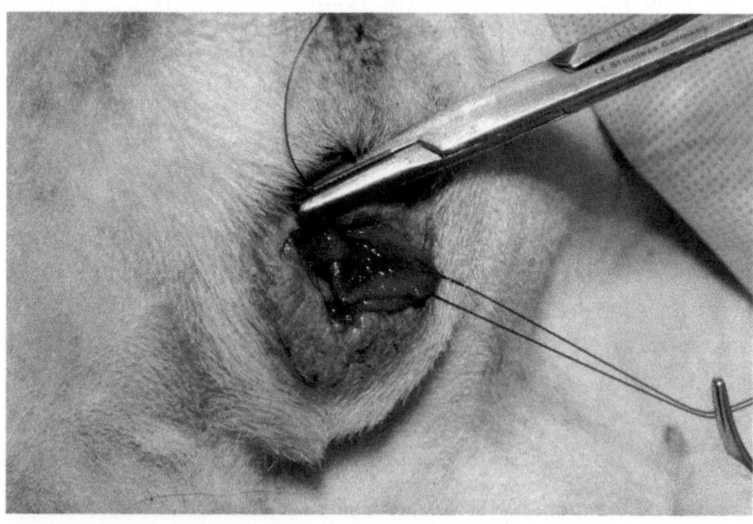

Figure 26-2 Place stay sutures in the mucosa and submucosa cranial to the polyp to keep the mucosa prolapsed.

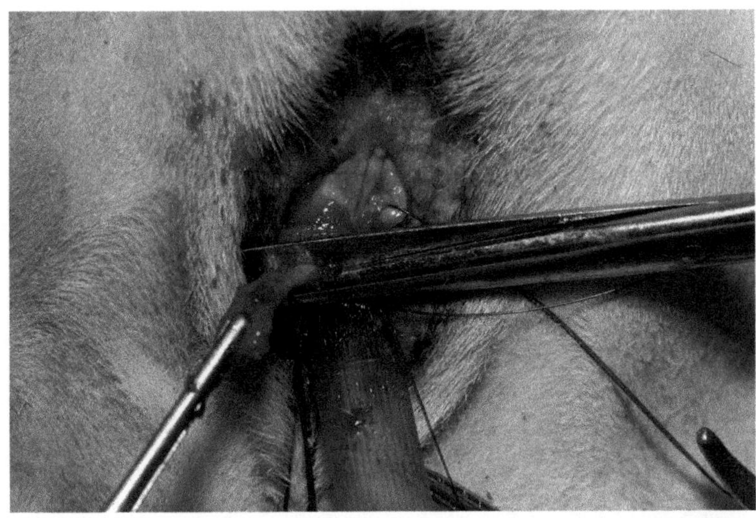

Figure 26-3 Transect half of the mucosal base around the mass. In this dog, a tube was placed in the rectum to help the surgeon identify the rectal lumen.

4. Transect one half of the mucosal base around the mass, including about 1 cm of normal tissue (fig. 26-3). The incision should be caudal to the cranial-most stay sutures.
5. With 3-0 or 4-0 rapidly absorbable monofilament suture on a taper needle, begin to close the mucosal defect with a simple continuous pattern (fig. 26-4). Note that bleeding is expected with mucosal transection but should cease with mucosal apposition.
6. Once the defect is partially closed, resect the remaining mass with its attached mucosa and submucosa and complete the defect closure. Remove the stay sutures.
7. Alternatively, if the mass base is narrow, ligate the base and some healthy mucosa beyond it with rapidly absorbable monofilament suture, and transect the tissue distal to the ligature.

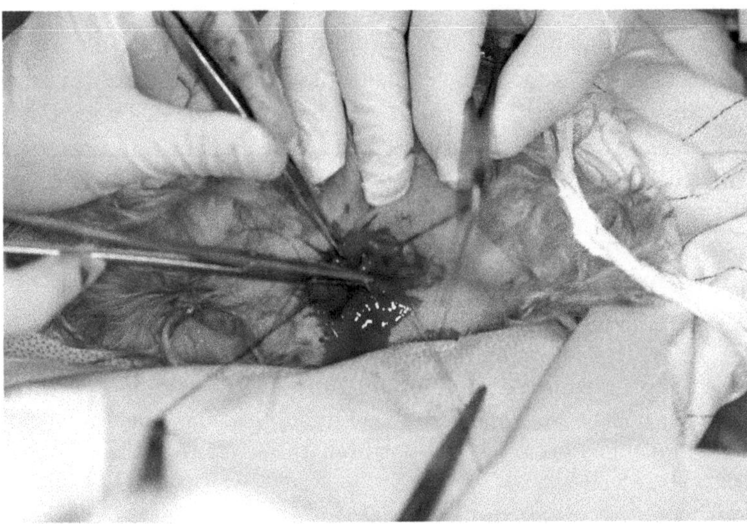

Figure 26-4 Appose the mucosa with a continuous pattern.

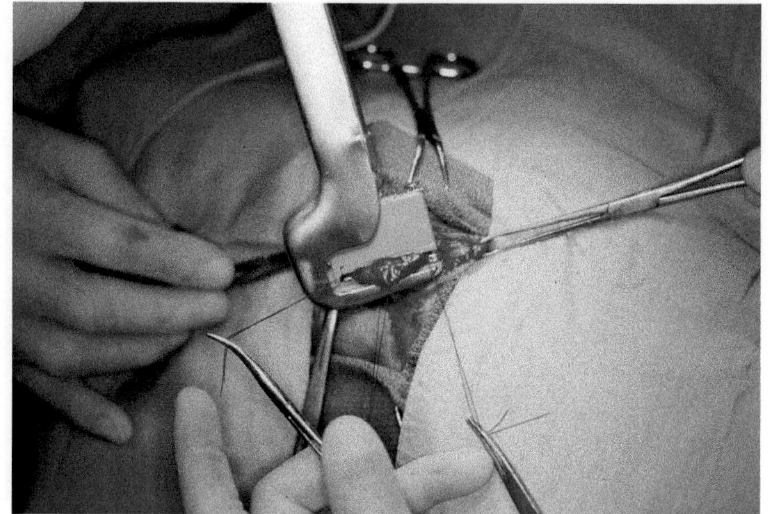

Figure 26-5 Retract the mass from the rectal wall with stay sutures, and place a TA stapler across healthy mucosa below the base of the polyp.

8. Remove large masses rapidly with a thoracoabdominal stapler:
   a. Place stay sutures in the mass to retract it away from surrounding mucosa.
   b. Place a TA30 or TA55 stapler (blue cartridge) across the base of the mass and fire the stapler (fig. 26-5).
   c. Transect the mass distal to the staples before releasing the stapler.
9. Perform a digital rectal examination to verify that the rectal lumen is patent and that there are no palpable mucosal defects.

Postoperative considerations

Before placing the polyp in formalin, the tissue base should be stained so that surgical margins can be evaluated. Rectal temperatures are usually avoided during recovery because of potential damage to the surgery site. Animals with tenesmus may require stool softeners (e.g., lactulose) and analgesics.

Rectal hemorrhage and tenesmus usually resolve within 2 days and 7 days after mass resection, respectively. Persistent straining or significant inflammation may result in rectal prolapse (see Chapter 48). Dogs with large, wide-based, diffuse, or multiple masses or histologic evidence of malignant transformation are more likely to have recurrence after surgical excision.

Bibliography

Danova NA et al: Surgical excision of primary canine rectal tumors by an anal approach in twenty-three dogs. Vet Surg 2006;35:337–340.

Fukushima K, Eguchi N, Ohno K, et al: Efficacy of leflunomide for treatment of refractory inflammatory colorectal polyps in 15 miniature dachshunds. J Vet Med Sci 2016;78:265–269.

Holt PE and Durdey P: Evaluation of transanal endoscopic treatment of benign canine rectal neoplasia. J Small Anim Pract 2007;48:17–25.

Knottenbelt CM et al: Preliminary clinical observations of the use of piroxicam in the management of rectal tubulopapillary polyps. J Small Anim Pract 2000;41:393–397.

Valerius KD et al: Aenomatous polyps and carcinoma in situ of the canine colon and rectum: 334 cases (1982–1994). J Am Anim Hosp Assoc 1997;33:156–160.

Section 4 Surgery of the Reproductive Tract

Chapter 27

Prepubertal Gonadectomy

The most common reason for prepubertal gonadectomy is to reduce the likelihood of reproduction of animals adopted from shelters. Other benefits include decreased anesthetic and materials requirements, simplicity of the procedure, rapid recovery, and reduced complication rate.

In cats, prepubertal gonadectomy has no effect on immune function, bone density, or prevalence of obesity or diabetes mellitus as compared with cats neutered at the traditional time. In male cats, early castration does not significantly decrease urethral diameter or increase the incidence of lower urinary tract disease and obstruction. Benefits to castration before 5.5 months of age include decreases in aggression, sexual behavior, urine spraying, and occurrence of abscesses in male cats. In male and female cats, early gonadectomy reduces the incidence of asthma, gingivitis, and hyperactivity. Potential side effects of prepubertal gonadectomy in cats include increased shyness and immaturity of external genitalia. In male cats castrated at 7 weeks of age, the balanopreputial fold may persist. While this does not affect urination, it may make urethral catheterization more difficult. Physeal closure is delayed in cats castrated at or before 7 months of age; however, this may have no effect on the risk of physeal fracture development.

Prepubertal gonadectomy will reduce the risk of mammary neoplasia by 95% in female dogs spayed before their first heat and by 25% for dogs spayed after their third heat. However, risk of other cancers may increase, depending on the breed. For example, osteosarcoma in Rottweilers gonadectomized at less than 1 year of age is two to four times greater than in intact Rottweilers. Potential side effects of prepubertal gonadectomy in dogs include urogenital abnormalities, delayed physeal closure, and joint incongruity. Compared with dogs gonadectomized at a later age, castration or ovariohysterectomy before 5.5 months of age increases the risk of mild hip dysplasia. Risk of joint disease in golden retrievers spayed or castrated at less than 6 months of age is 20% and 27%, respectively, compared to 5% for those dogs left intact. Prepubertal ovariohysterectomy increases the risk of urinary incontinence, particularly for dogs spayed at 2 months of age. Additionally, dogs spayed at that age may retain infantile vulvas, predisposing them to vaginitis and cystitis. Bitches should therefore be at least 3 months of age before ovariohysterectomy, and those with infantile vulvas or increased risk of incontinence should be spayed after puberty.

Manual of Small Animal Soft Tissue Surgery, Second Edition. Karen Tobias.
© 2017 John Wiley & Sons, Inc. Published 2017 by John Wiley & Sons, Inc.

Preoperative considerations

To reduce the risk of hypoglycemia, pediatric patients are fasted a maximum of 4 to 8 hours, depending on their age, health, and body condition. If needed, fluids with dextrose can be administered during ovariohysterectomy. Cat spays and castrations reportedly can be performed after a subcutaneous injection of a nonsteroidal anti-inflammatory drug and an intramuscular injection of dexmedetomidine/buprenorphine, or medetomidine/buprenorphine/ketamine. To reduce the risk of hypothermia, prep solutions should be heated to body temperature, and the patient should be placed on a forced-air warming blanket or circulating warm water pad during surgery. Anesthesia and surgery time should be kept to a minimum, and the patient should be placed in a warm environment for recovery.

Surgery

The technique for pediatric gonadectomy is similar to that for older animals (see Chapters 28, 29, and 33), with a few exceptions. In puppies undergoing ovariohysterectomy, the abdominal incision is farther caudal than usual. Substantial amounts of serous fluid may be encountered when the abdomen is opened. Tissues in young animals can be friable and therefore must be handled gently. Spay hooks should be used cautiously, if at all. Very tiny pedicles may require only one ligature. In cats, ovarian vessels can be sealed with a pedicle tie, similar to castration, with no increased risk of complications. During abdominal closure, sutures should include the fascia of the external rectus sheath. If this is hard to differentiate from subcutaneous tissues, the subcutaneous fat can be cleared off of the fascia at the linea with Metzenbaum scissors using a push-cut method (pp. 84–85).

Kittens are castrated like adult cats (pp. 231–237), although the spermatic cord cannot be exteriorized as far and must be handled more gently. Prepubertal puppies can be castrated through a prescrotal or scrotal incision. Prescrotal castration can be difficult because the testicles will migrate into the inguinal canals when pushed cranially. If a scrotal approach is used, the scrotum is clipped before the procedure. In very young puppies, the spermatic cord can be tied onto itself, similar to the closed castration technique used for cats. When castrating puppies with this technique, it is important to know that cremaster muscle seems to break closer to the testicle than in a cat, and with an abruptness that could increase the risk for vascular tearing. Many surgeons will therefore leave the muscle intact. The size of the spermatic cord is thicker, especially if the cremaster muscle is not broken, making it more difficult to tie a secure knot in the cord with a pedicle tie. If the cord is too thick to tie on itself, the pedicle should be ligated with suture.

Surgical technique: prepubertal ovariohysterectomy with pedicle ligation for kittens and puppies

1. Make a 2- to 3-cm abdominal approach over the middle third of the distance between umbilicus and pubis (fig. 27-1).
2. Use the handle end of thumb forceps or spay hook to retract the bladder medially and expose the uterus near the colon and dorsal body wall.

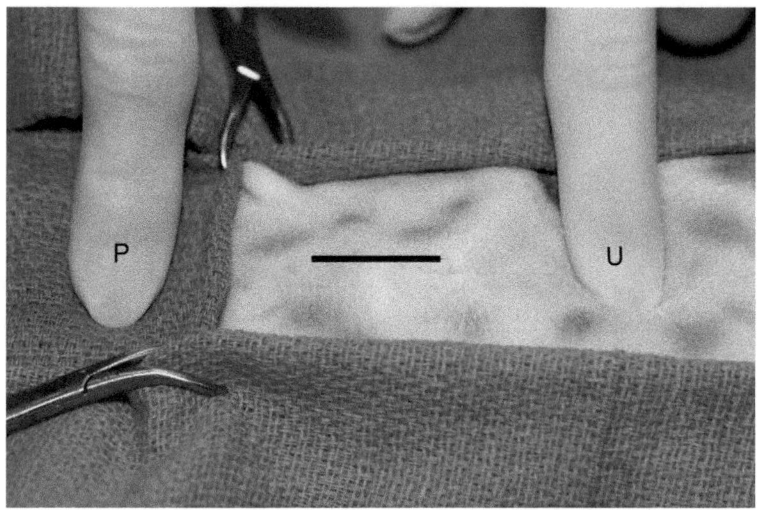

Figure 27-1 For ovariohysterectomy in young animals, make the incision (line) midway between the umbilicus (U) and pubis (P).

3. Place a clamp on the proper ligament and gently retract the ovary out of the abdomen. If necessary, gently stretch the suspensory ligament with an index finger until the ovary is exposed (fig. 27-2).
4. If desired, place two mosquito hemostatic forceps across the ovarian pedicle below the ovary. Use only the tips of the forceps to clamp the pedicle. Transect the pedicle between the clamps and ligate each ovarian pedicle with one or two ligatures of 3-0 or 4-0 absorbable suture or with a hemostatic clip. Alternatively, use a pedicle tie (described below) to occlude the vessels.
5. Ligate the uterine body with one or two encircling sutures (fig. 27-3).
6. Close the abdominal wall musculature with 3-0 or 4-0 monofilament absorbable suture in a simple continuous pattern. Place sutures full thickness or only in the external rectus sheath. If subcutaneous fat is present, appose the subcutis with a simple continuous pattern using 3-0 or 4-0 rapidly absorbable suture. Appose skin with an intradermal pattern, skin sutures, or tissue glue.

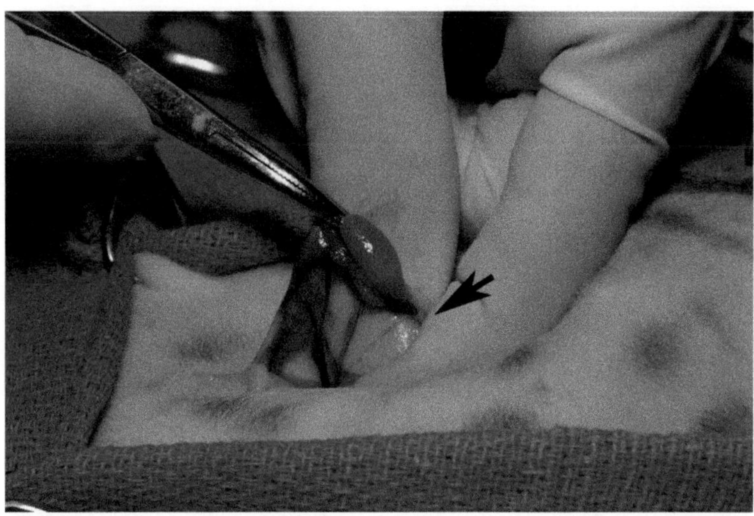

Figure 27-2 Place a clamp on the proper ligament to expose the ovary and pedicle; if necessary, stretch the suspensory ligament (arrow) to improve exposure.

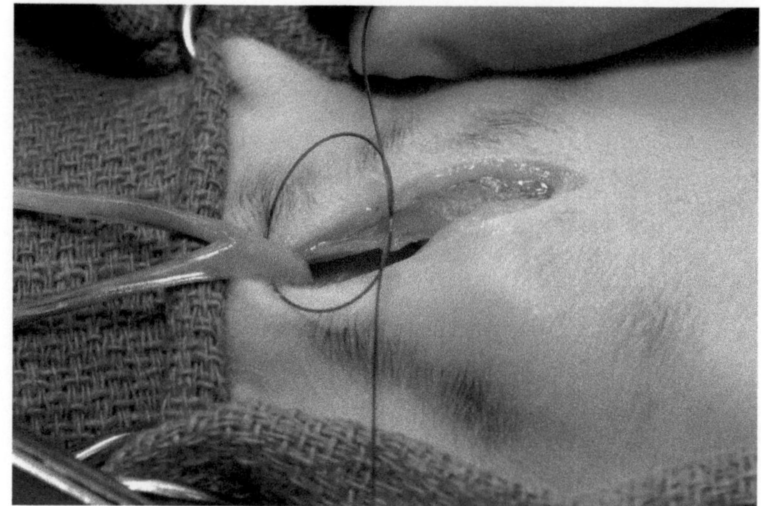

Figure 27-3 Ligate the uterine body near the bifurcation.

Surgical technique: ovarian pedicle tie for cats and kittens

1. Incise the abdomen and locate the ovary as described above.
2. Place a clamp on the proper ligament, if desired, and retract the ovary from the abdomen.
3. With a hemostat, make an opening (fig. 27-4) between the suspensory ligament and ovarian vessels, opening the jaws of the hemostat parallel to the vessels.
4. Using the hemostat, grasp the suspensory ligament distal to the ovary and tear it (fig. 27-5). Alternatively, cut the suspensory ligament with a blade.
5. Tie the pedicle on itself (fig. 27-6).
    a. Place the closed jaws of a curved hemostat adjacent to (parallel with) the pedicle and pointing down toward the abdomen.

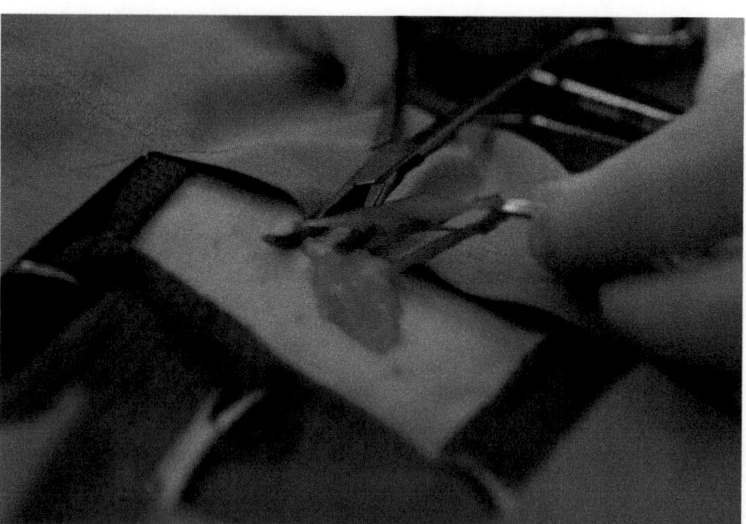

Figure 27-4 Make a window between the suspensory ligament and ovarian vessels by inserting a hemostat at the site and opening the jaws parallel to the vessels.

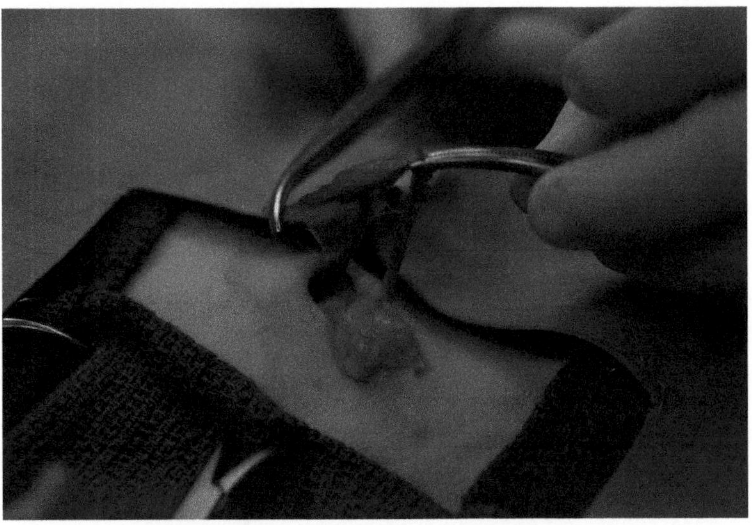

Figure 27-5 Tear or cut the suspensory ligament.

b. Circle the hemostat tips around the pedicle, keeping the tips pointed down toward the abdomen, until the cord is 360° around the hemostat tips.

c. Rotate the hemostat so the tips are pointed up toward the ovary, then open the hemostat jaws and drop the proximal portion of the pedicle into them. Clamp the cord.

d. Transect the pedicle between the hemostat and ovary.

e. Tilt the hemostat tips so they are parallel to the remaining pedicle and pointed toward the abdomen, then push the loop of pedicle off the hemostat tips and over the cord to make a knot.

f. Tighten the knot carefully with thumb and index finger, then release the end of the knotted pedicle from the hemostats.

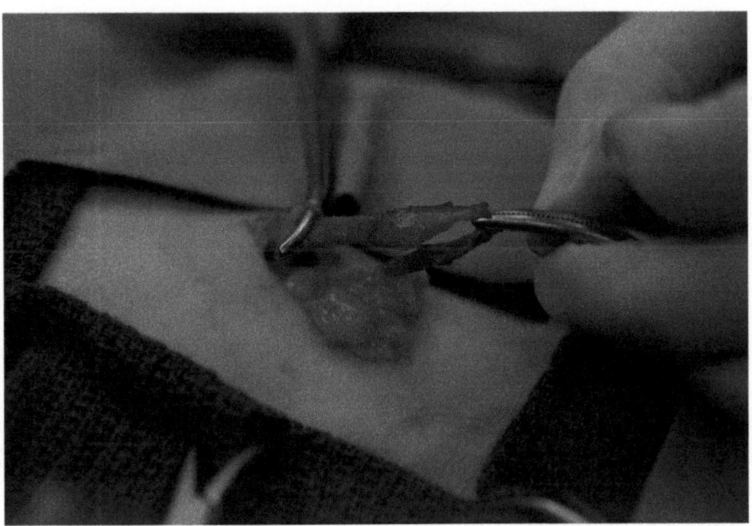

Figure 27-6 Ovarian pedicle tie is similar to a cat castration. In this figure the pedicle is encircling the hemostat and its proximal end has been grasped between the hemostat tips. The pedicle will be cut near the hemostat and distal to the ovary, and the looped portion will be pushed over the pedicle end and off the hemostat tips to make a single tie.

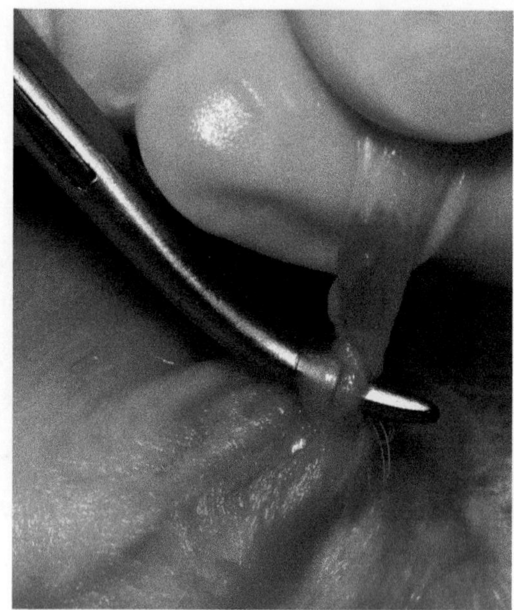

Figure 27-7 Compared with cats, the spermatic cord in this puppy is shorter and wider and therefore may be more difficult to tie securely onto itself.

Surgical technique: closed castration of puppies

1. Clip and prep the scrotal region.
2. Stabilize the base of the testicle between your thumb and index finger. Incise the skin over one testicle near the scrotal midline.
3. Pop the testicle out through the incision.
4. Grasp the testicle with thumb and index finger or hemostat and strip away fascial attachments with a sponge.
5. Ligate the cord with 3-0 absorbable suture or hemostatic clips. Alternatively, tie the cord onto itself (fig. 27-7, similar to a cat castration (p. 233).
6. Push the second testicle over to the initial scrotal incision and incise the overlying subcutaneous tissue and fascia to expose the testicle. Alternatively, make a second scrotal incision to expose the testicle. Exteriorize the testicle and ligate the cord.
7. Leave the skin open, or hold the skin edges apposed and secure them with a drop of tissue glue.

Postoperative considerations

Puppies and kittens usually recover rapidly after prepubertal gonadectomy and often can be released the same day of surgery. To prevent hypoglycemia, they should be fed as soon as they are fully recovered from anesthesia. Postoperative analgesics should be administered for at least 6 hours. Scarring is minimal after prepubertal ovariohysterectomy, and tattooing of females is recommended to prevent future exploratory surgeries.

Mortality rates and surgical complications are similar to those of dogs and cats neutered after 5 months of age. Because they are at an increased risk for infectious diseases, young puppies are more prone to development of parvoviral infections after surgery.

Bibliography

Beauvais W. et al: The effect of neutering on the risk of mammary tumours in dogs – a systematic review. J Small Anim Pract 2012;53:314–322.

Cooley DM et al: Endogenous gonadal hormone exposure and bone sarcoma risk. Cancer Epidem Biomarkers Prev 2002;11:1434–1440.

Hart BL et al: Long-term health effects of neutering dogs: comparison of Labrador retrievers with golden retrievers. PLoS ONE 2014;9 (7): e102241. Doi: 10.1371/journal.pone.0102241

Howe LM: Surgical methods of contraception and sterilization. Theriogenology 2006;66:500–509.

Kustritz MVR: Early spay-neuter: clinical considerations. Clin Tech Small Anim Pract 2002;17:124–128.

Miller KP, Rekers W, Ellis K, et al: Pedicle ties provide a rapid and safe method for feline ovariohysterectomy. J Feline Med Surg 2016;18:160–164.

Porters N, de Rooster H, Moons CPH, et al: Prepubertal gonadectomy in cats: different injectable anaesthetic combinations and comparison with gonadectomy at traditional age. J Feline Med Surg 2015;17:458–467.

Spain CV et al: Long-term risks and benefits of early-age gonadectomy in cats. J Am Vet Med Assoc 2004;224:372–379.

Spain CV et al: Long-term risks and benefits of early-age gonadectomy in dogs. J Am Vet Med Assoc 2004;224:380–387.

Torres de la Riva G et al. Neutering dogs: effects on joint disorders and cancers in golden retrievers. PLOS ONE 2013;8 (2): e55937. doi: 10.1371/journal.pone.0055937

Chapter 28
Feline Castration

Castrated male cats are usually preferred over intact toms as companion animals because they are more affectionate toward people and less aggressive to other animals. Castration also reduces marking behavior and "toileting" problems (urination and defecation outside of the litter box). Because roaming behavior is decreased, neutered male cats live longer and have less exposure to intestinal parasites and other diseases. Castrated cats, however, are prone to weight gain and therefore to diseases associated with obesity. Benefits of castration usually outweigh the risks, however, and complications of the procedure are rare.

Preoperative management

In preparation for surgery, scrotal hair can be removed by gently clipping or "plucking." Peeling the hair down toward the base of the scrotum during plucking is less traumatic than pulling it straight out. Cats can be positioned in lateral or dorsal recumbency with the rear legs and tail pulled cranially. A hemostat can be used to clip tail hair and back hair together to keep the tail retracted. After surgical prep, the scrotal area can be draped with a cloth or paper drape, glove wrapper, or dental dam. Paper drapes will stay in place more readily if the perineal area is soaked with antiseptic spray.

Surgery

Castrations can be performed in an open or closed method, using spermatic cord contents to form hemostatic knots. With open castration, the ductus deferens and vessels are tied to each other with four throws to form two square knots. Failure of this technique occurs when half hitches are thrown, usually because tension is applied unevenly during knot formation. With closed castration, the cord is tied on itself in a single throw. Failure of this technique usually occurs from insufficient tightening of the throw. Suture ligatures or hemoclips can also be used for hemostasis.

Surgical technique: closed castration

1. With thumb and forefinger, compress the base of the scrotum to force the testicle against the skin.

Manual of Small Animal Soft Tissue Surgery, Second Edition. Karen Tobias.
© 2017 John Wiley & Sons, Inc. Published 2017 by John Wiley & Sons, Inc.

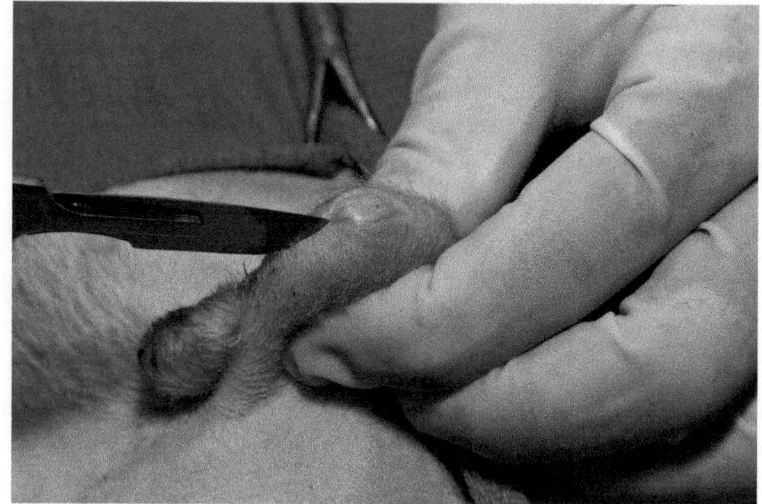

Figure 28-1 Elevate one testicle firmly into the scrotum and incise the skin over it longitudinally.

2. Make a longitudinal incision through skin and subcutis over the testicle (to one side of midline), leaving the tunics intact (fig. 28-1). A small web of subcutaneous fascia may need to be incised further to allow the testicle to pop out of the incision.
3. Grasp the testicle in one hand and pull it away from the cat while using a dry sponge to simultaneously strip away the scrotal attachments (fig. 28-2).
4. Using slow steady traction, pull on the testicle with one hand while pushing against the cat's perineum with a sponge in the other hand. Stretch the cord until the cremaster muscle breaks.
5. Insert a curved hemostatic forceps under, around, and over the cord, initially keeping the tips pointed downward and toward the cat (fig. 28-3A,B).
    a. Palm the hemostats to maneuver them around the cord more easily.
    b. To facilitate knot tying, adjust the position of the cord so that it is wrapped around the hemostats close to the tips and to the cat. Slide the hemostats perpendicular to the cord to reposition (fig. 23-3C).

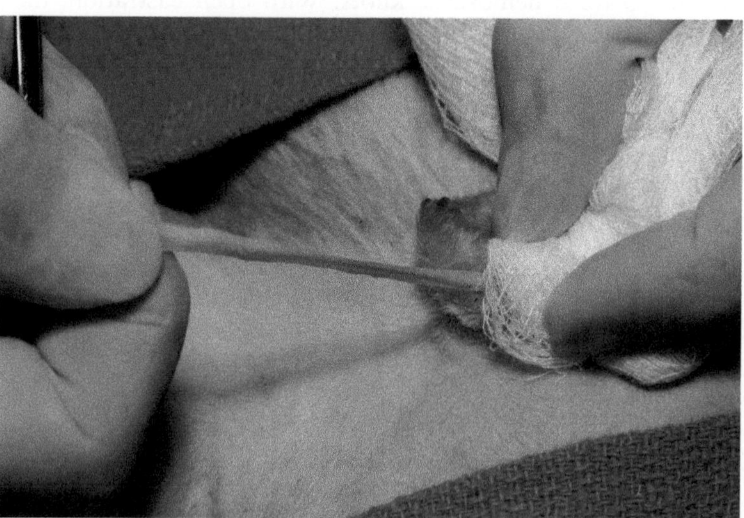

Figure 28-2 Strip away the scrotal attachments, then break the cremaster with slow steady traction.

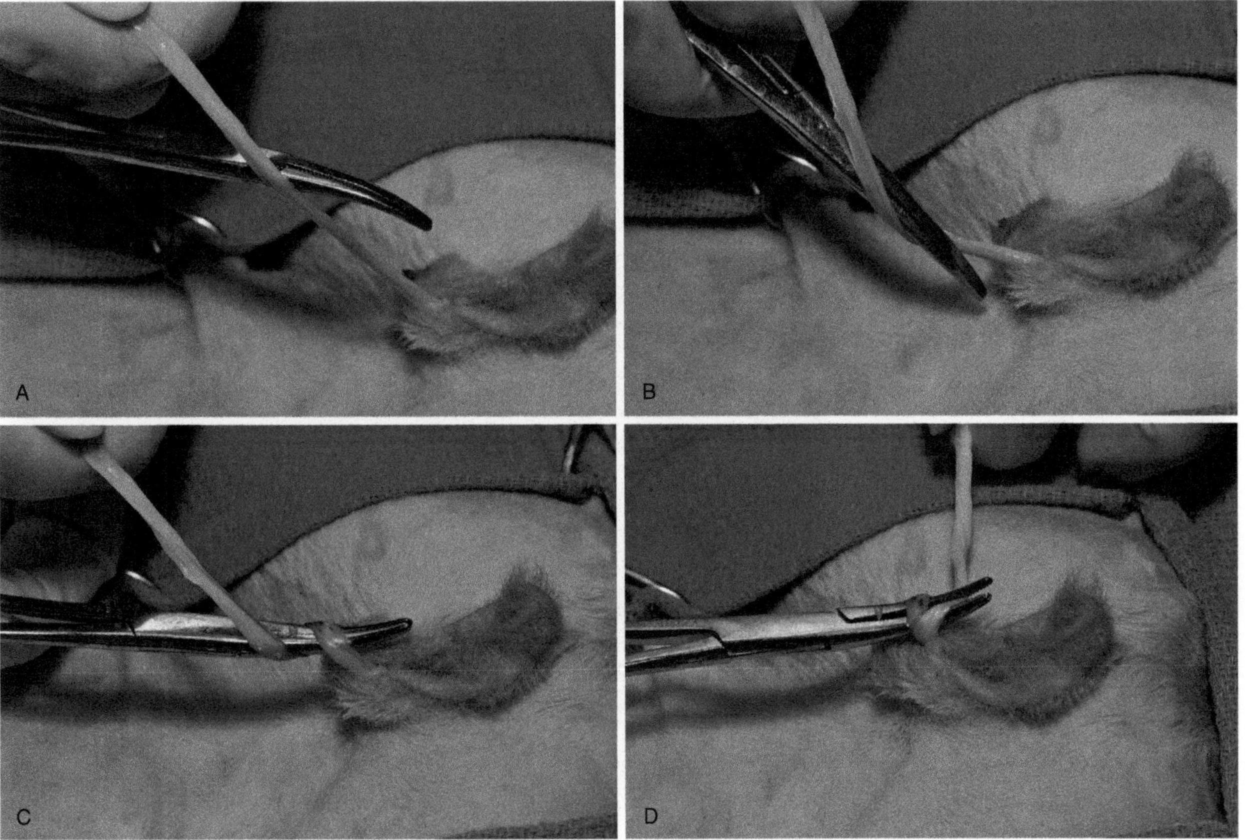

Figure 28-3 Closed castration. Palm the closed hemostat and slide the curved tips under (A), over (B), and around (C) the cord, keeping the tips pointed toward the cat. Slide the hemostat as close to the cat as possible before clamping the cord near the tips of the hemostat (D).

6. Open the jaws of the hemostats and drop the cord between the tips (fig. 28-3D), either from above or from below the jaws.
7. Transect the cord 1 to 2 mm distal to the clamp to remove the testicle and remaining cord (fig. 28-4).

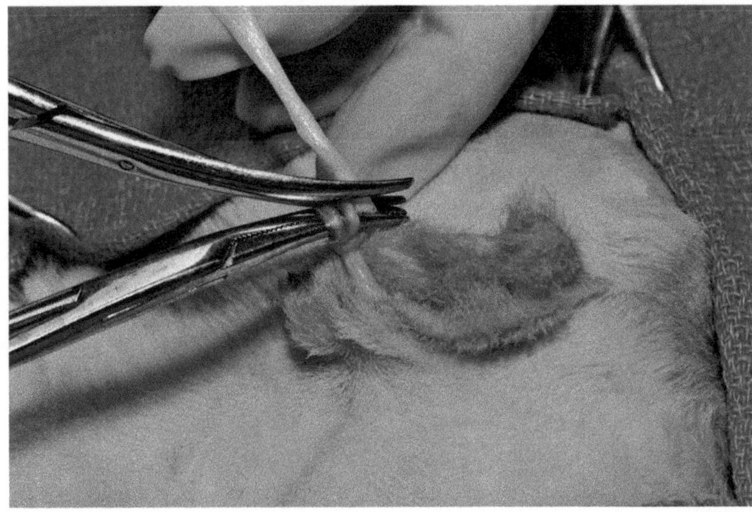

Figure 28-4 Transect the cord close to the hemostat.

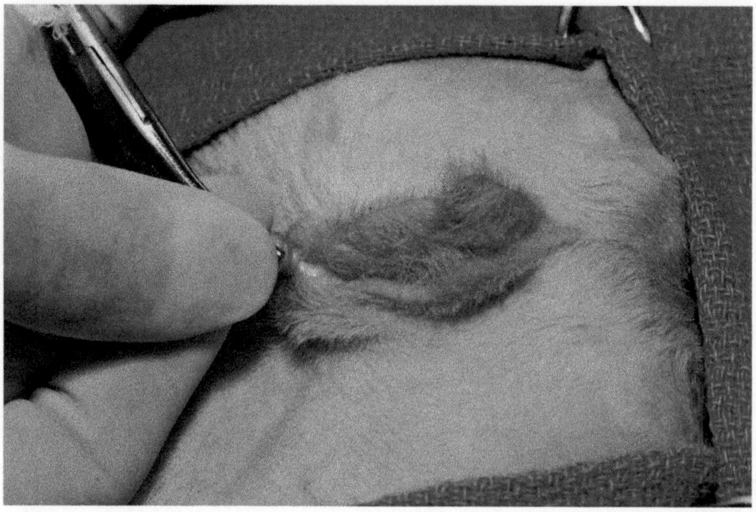

Figure 28-5 Hold the hemostat tips parallel to the remaining cord and slide the encircling portion of the cord off the end of the hemostat with a gauze sponge or fingers.

8. To form a knot, push the encircling portion of the cord over the transected cord end and off of the hemostat with a sponge or fingers (fig. 28-5). Hold the hemostat tips parallel to the cord to make it easier to slide the cord off.
9. Before releasing the hemostat, tighten the throw in the cord: place your thumbnail between the hemostat and throw and slide the throw toward the cat (fig. 28-6).
10. Make a second scrotal incision over the remaining testicle and repeat steps 3–9.
11. Grasp the scrotum between thumb and first two fingers and pull it caudally to help approximate the incision edges. Leave the wounds open.

Surgical technique: open castration

1. While stabilizing the testicle against the scrotum, incise longitudinally through the skin and parietal vaginal tunic (fig. 28-7) to expose the glistening surface (visceral tunic) of the testicle and epididymis.

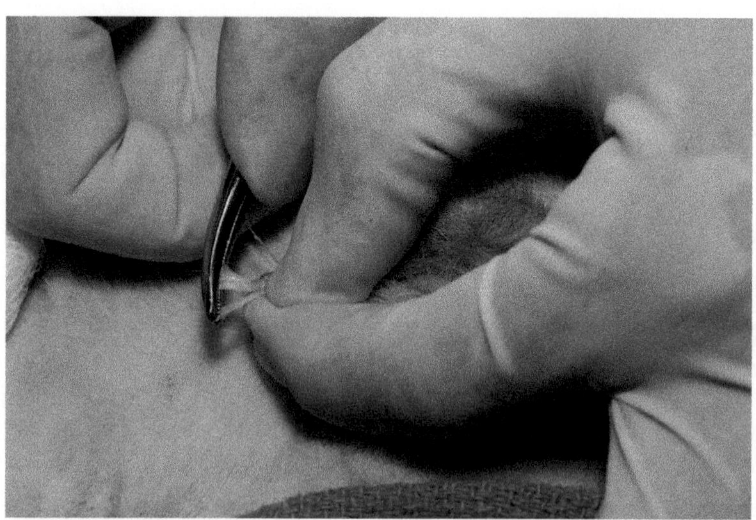

Figure 28-6 With finger and thumb placed between the throw in the cord and the hemostat, slide the throw toward the cat to tighten.

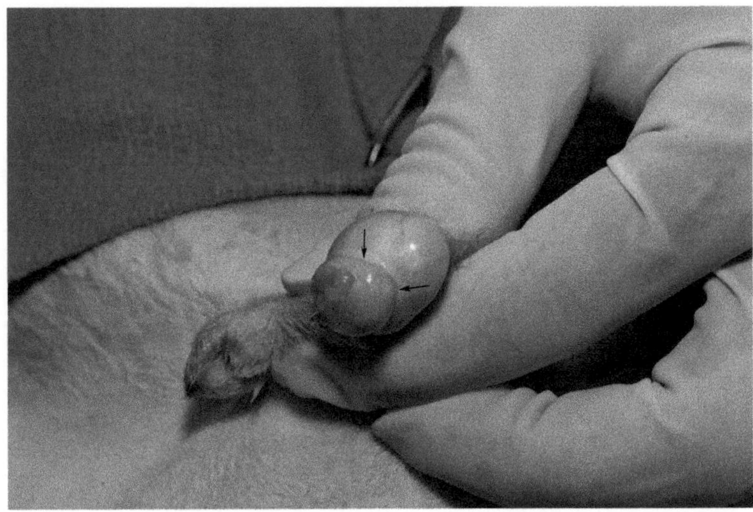

Figure 28-7 Open castration. Incise the parietal tunic (arrows) to expose the visceral tunic.

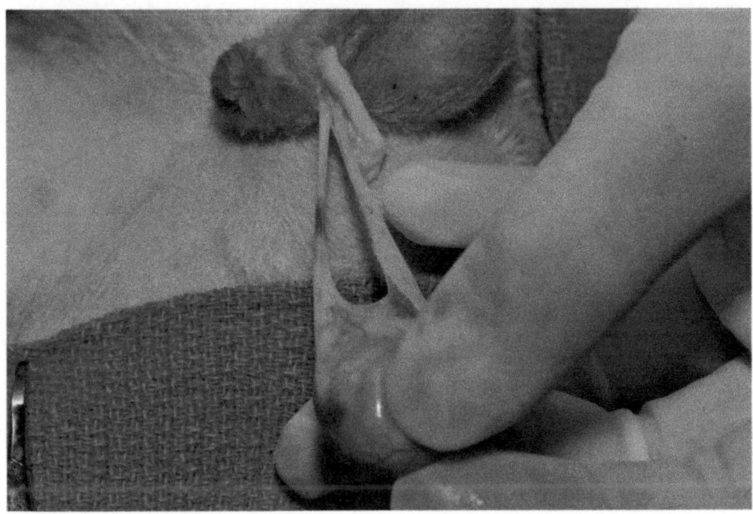

Figure 28-8 The parietal tunic has been separated from the testicle and cord, exposing the vessels and ductus deferens.

2. Extend the parietal tunic incision and pull the testicle out to expose the cord contents.
3. Separate the parietal tunic from the testicle (fig. 28-8). If desired, excise the tunic with scissors.
4. Separate the ductus deferens from the testicular vessels and detach it from the testicle (fig. 28-9).
5. With the ductus deferens and vessels, tie four square throws to make two knots (fig. 28-10). Watch the throws as they lower toward the scrotal incision to confirm that tension is evenly distributed and the throws are square.
6. Transect the cord distal to the knots to remove the testicle. Repeat all steps to remove the second testicle.

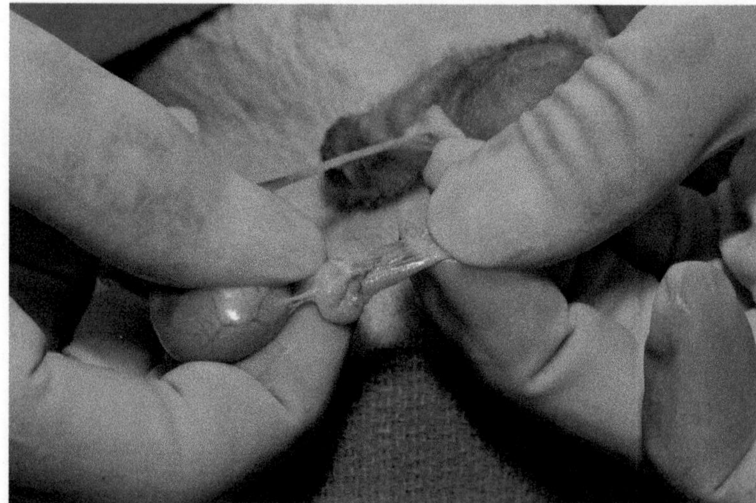

Figure 28-9 Detach the ductus deferens from the testicle.

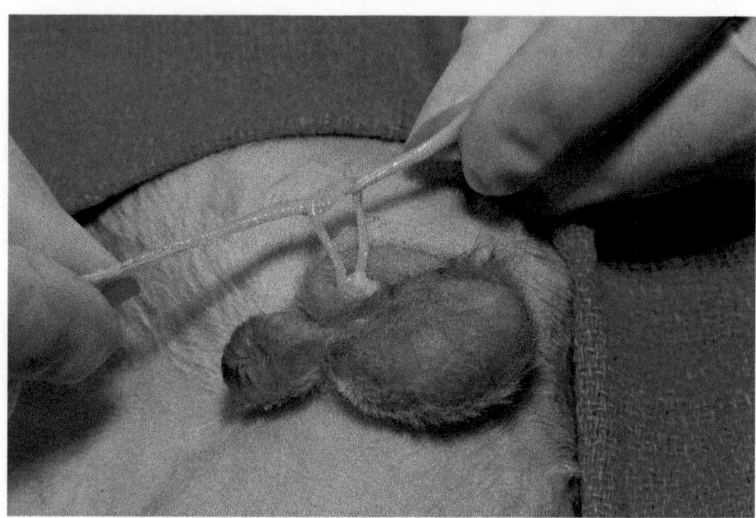

Figure 28-10 Tie four square throws, using the ductus deferens for one side and the vessels for the other.

Postoperative considerations

Because scrotal incisions are left open, paper litter is often recommended for several days after the procedure. Castrated cats have a decreased metabolic rate, and caloric intake should be reduced if unhealthy weight gain is noted.

Postoperative complications are rare (<1%). Scrotal hemorrhage may occur if testicular vessels tear during exposure or the knot fails. If this occurs during surgery, the scrotal incision on the affected side can be extended in an attempt to find the dropped vessel. Occasionally it can be grasped blindly with a hemostat, but often the cord retracts enough to prevent retrieval. If the bleeding vessel cannot be found, pressure should be placed on the inguinal ring (where the vessel exits the inguinal ring) and scrotal regions for 5 to 15 minutes. The cat should be sedated and fitted with an Elizabethan collar upon recovery to reduce the risk of bleeding. Unligated vessels rarely cause significant intra-abdominal bleeding in cats. Serial hematocrits can be monitored if hemorrhage is a concern. If significant anemia develops, the vessel should be located through an abdominal incision and ligated.

Clinical signs of postoperative infection include anorexia and perineal pain. Most cats respond to oral antibiotics and do not need surgical wound drainage.

Bibliography

Neilson J: Thinking outside the box: feline elimination. J Fel Med Surg 2004;6:5–11.

Petit GD: There's more than one way to castrate a cat. Mod Vet Pract 1981;62: 713–716.

Porters N, Polis I, Moons C, et al: Prepubertal gonadectomy in cats: different surgical techniques and comparison with gonadectomy at traditional age. Vet Rec 2014; 175:223 doi: 10.1136/vr.102337; Downloaded 8/10/16

Root MV et al: The effect of prepuberal and postpuberal gonadectomy on radial physeal closure in male and female domestic cats. Vet Radiol Ultrasound 1997; 38:42–47.

Scott KC et al: Body condition of feral cats and the effect of neutering. J Appl Anim Welf Sci 2002;5:203–213.

Spain VC et al: Long-term risks and benefits of early-age gonadectomy in cats. J Am Vet Med Assoc 2004;224:372–379.

Chapter 29
Canine Castration

The most common reasons for canine castration are prevention of certain behaviors (e.g., mounting, roaming, and marking), unwanted breedings, and testicular tumors, which occur in 29% of intact male dogs. Castration is also indicated for removal of infected, torsed, or traumatized testicles and prevention or treatment of perianal adenomas, prostatic cysts, prostatitis, benign prostatic hyperplasia, prostatic abscesses, and sex hormone–associated alopecia. In dogs with uncomplicated benign prostatic hyperplasia, prostate size decreases by 50% within 3 weeks of castration, and clinical signs resolve within 2 to 3 months. Resolution of perianal adenomas is reported in 95% of dogs after castration.

Unfortunately, canine castration has also been associated with negative effects. Risk of prostatic carcinoma, hemangiosarcoma, osteosarcoma, transitional cell carcinoma, and joint disease may increase after gonadectomy, particularly in certain breeds. For example, incidence of joint disease (e.g., cruciate ligament ruptures and hip dysplasia) in golden retrievers castrated at less than 12 months of age is 3 to 5 times that of intact males. Risk of osteosarcoma in Rottweilers castrated at less than 12 months of age is increased as compared with intact Rottweilers. Timing (and necessity) of castration should therefore be made on a case-by-case basis, taking into consideration such things as breed, lifestyle, concurrent diseases, and owner preference.

Preoperative management

Most dogs undergoing castration require minimal preoperative diagnostics. Dogs with testicular neoplasia should be evaluated for metastases and for myelotoxicity, particularly if anemia or feminization is present. Myelotoxicity usually resolves within 2 to 3 weeks after tumor removal but can be fatal, despite appropriate therapy. Testicular torsion most often occurs from torsion of cryptochid neoplastic testicles but can also occur with scrotal testes. Clinical signs include shock and abdominal or scrotal pain; diagnosis is made on ultrasonography and exploratory surgery.

Clipping the surgical field depends on the planned approach. For a prescrotal approach, clipping is often limited to the prescrotal region. Long scrotal hairs are cut short, and the scrotum is sprayed with antiseptic solution during surgical prep. For dogs undergoing scrotal ablation or scrotal castration, the scrotum itself is clipped so that the hairs are very short but the skin has not been traumatized.

Manual of Small Animal Soft Tissue Surgery, Second Edition. Karen Tobias.
© 2017 John Wiley & Sons, Inc. Published 2017 by John Wiley & Sons, Inc.

Intratesticular lidocaine blocks can reduce the anesthetic requirements of dogs undergoing castration. After sterile preparation of the scrotum, 1 mg/kg of 2% lidocaine is slowly injected into the body of each testicle using a one inch 22 gauge needle. The injection is stopped if the testicular pressure seems excessive. Testicular blocks may cause mild hematoma formation or hemorrhage within the tunica or testes.

Surgery

Whether the procedure is performed through a scrotal or prescrotal incision depends on surgeon preference, age of the dog (castration of young puppies is more easily performed through a scrotal incision; see page 228), and need for concurrent scrotal resection (e.g., for neoplasia or scrotal dermatitis). In studies comparing scrotal and prescrotal approaches, complication rates for each are very low; surprisingly, a scrotal approach can be faster and lead to less self-trauma than a prescrotal approach.

For a right-handed surgeon, prescrotal castration of an adult dog is more easily performed from the dog's left side; the left hand pushes the testicle forward while the right hand makes the incision. Scrotal castration can be performed from either side of the table.

Testicles are removed using a closed or open technique, the former of which leaves parietal tunic intact. Closed castration can be used in any size dog, as long as the spermatic cord is stretched and stripped to a narrow diameter (less than 1 cm). Small cords are double-ligated with encircling sutures of 2-0 or 3-0 absorbable monofilament material; cords larger than 5 mm in diameter are ligated with at least one transfixing/encircling suture. Cords can be clamped during ligation; however, large cords are easier to transfix if they are not clamped.

Surgical technique: closed castration through a prescrotal approach

1. After pushing the testicle cranially to protect the urethra, make an incision through the prescrotal skin and subcutaneous tissues over the testicle (fig. 29-1). A small conglomeration of fat is usually present on the surface of the parietal tunic, which indicates the incision depth is appropriate for a closed castration.

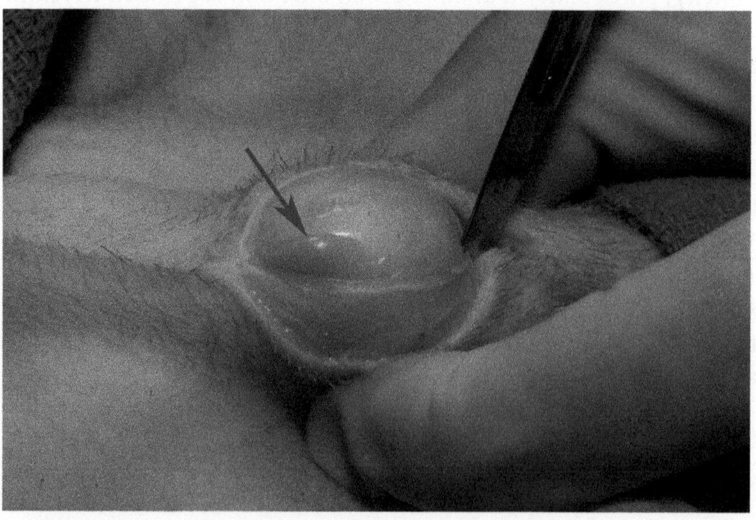

Figure 29-1 Prescrotal closed castration. Push the testicle cranially and incise the overlying prescrotal skin and subcutis to the level of the parietal tunic. A small conglomeration of fat (arrow) is usually visible on the parietal tunic.

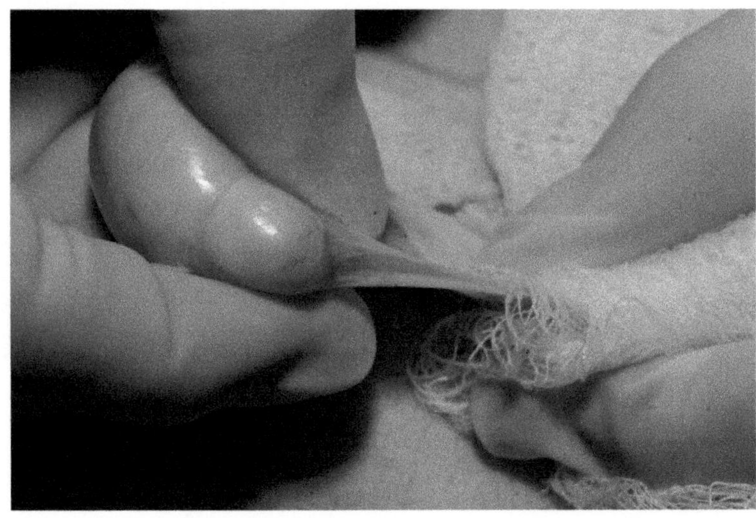

Figure 29-2 Break down the scrotal ligament to detach the testicle from the scrotum.

2. Using both hands, tilt the cranial pole of the testicle up to the incision and squeeze below the testicle to force it out of the incision.
3. Grab the testicle with one hand and use a sponge in the other hand to break down the scrotal ligament (fig. 29-2), which attaches the scrotum to the caudal pole of the testicle. If the ligament will not tear, transect it with scissors. During ligament stripping, the scrotum may invert itself and appear as a white "mass" within the surgery site.
4. Identify the white line (fig. 29-3) that indicates the junction between the spermatic cord and surrounding soft tissues.
5. Lift the testicle straight up with one hand while stripping downward at the base of the cord with the other hand, using a dry sponge (fig. 29-4). This will separate the spermatic cord from surrounding tissues and stretch it out to less than 1 cm in diameter. Wipe the cord upward toward the testicle to remove any remaining fat.

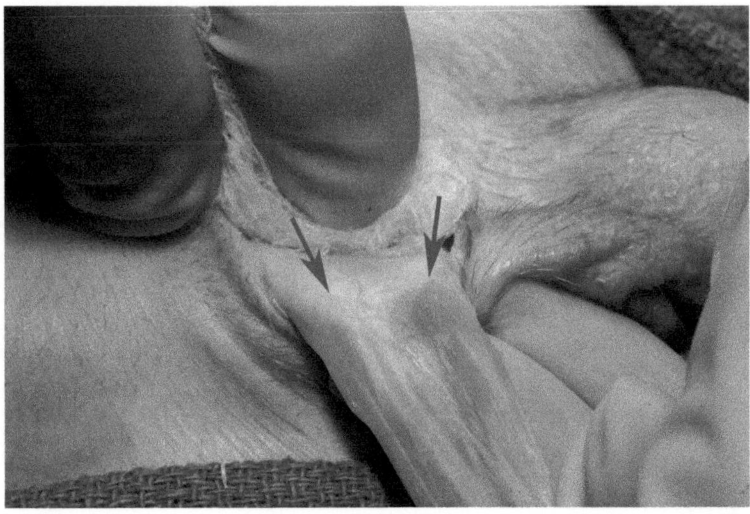

Figure 29-3 Identify the junction between the spermatic cord and surrounding soft tissues (arrows).

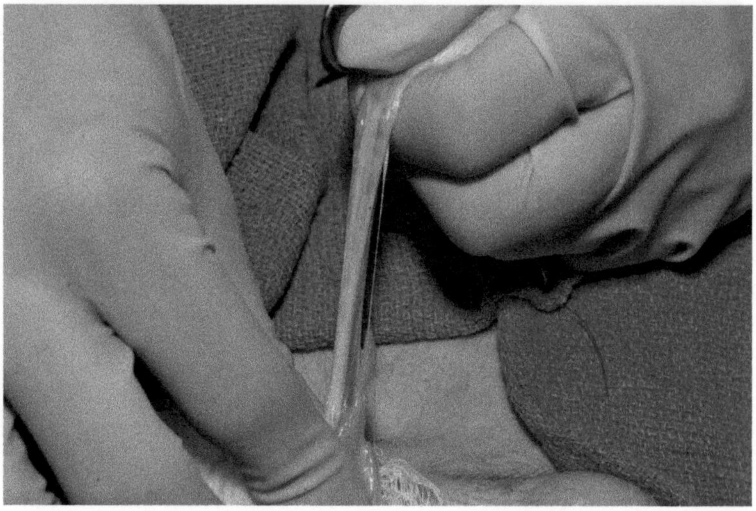

Figure 29-4 Lift the testicle upwards while stripping the base of the cord with a sponge. The cord will elongate as it separates from the soft tissues at the junction noted in figure 29-3.

6. Place the first ligature. For transfixing/encircling ligatures, fan out the cord over one index finger to separate the structures and pass the needle between the cremaster muscle and the vessels (fig. 29-5). Tie two simple throws on the vessel side, then encircle the entire cord and tie four more throws (fig. 29-6). If the cord is large, use a surgeon's throw for the first throw of the encircling ligature.
7. Place an encircling ligature or a second transfixing/encircling ligature above or below the first ligature, spacing ligatures at least 0.5 cm apart.
8. Clamp the cord several centimeters below the testicle, then grasp the cord above the ligatures with thumb forceps and transect the cord between the thumb forceps and clamp.
9. Lower the cord toward the dog and release it, inspecting the end for hemorrhage.
10. Push the second testicle up to the incision site and incise through the overlying fascia (the scrotal septum). Proceed with the second testicle as outlined above.

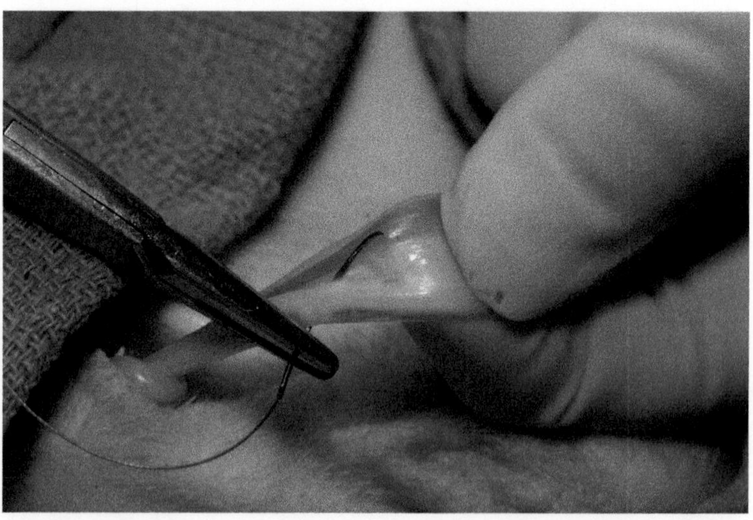

Figure 29-5 Flatten the cord between thumb and index finger to separate the cremaster muscle from the vessels, and pass a suture through the cord and around the vessels.

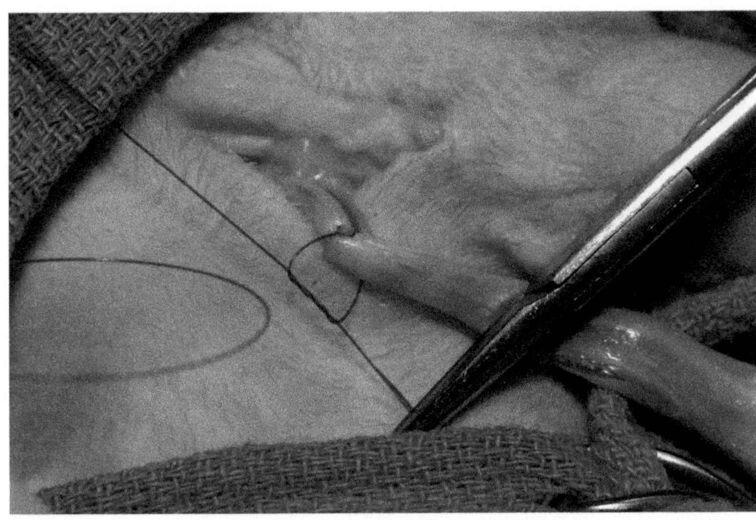

Figure 29-6 Ligate the vessels first with two throws, then pass the end of the suture around the entire cord and tie four throws.

11. Close the incision with an intradermal or subcutaneous-to-intradermal pattern (pp. 5–7).
    a. To identify the subcutaneous layer, retract the skin laterally with thumb forceps to visualize two ring-like openings laterally and the septal remnant on midline above the urethra.
    b. Take bites of the subcutaneous tissue (those ring-like edges, usually 5–7 mm below the incision edge) and, if desired, include the superficial edge of the septal remnant on midline. Avoid the urethra in the middle.

Surgical technique: open castration

1. Advance the testicle and incise the skin as described above.
2. Incise through the parietal tunic to expose the testicle and epididymis (fig. 29-7).

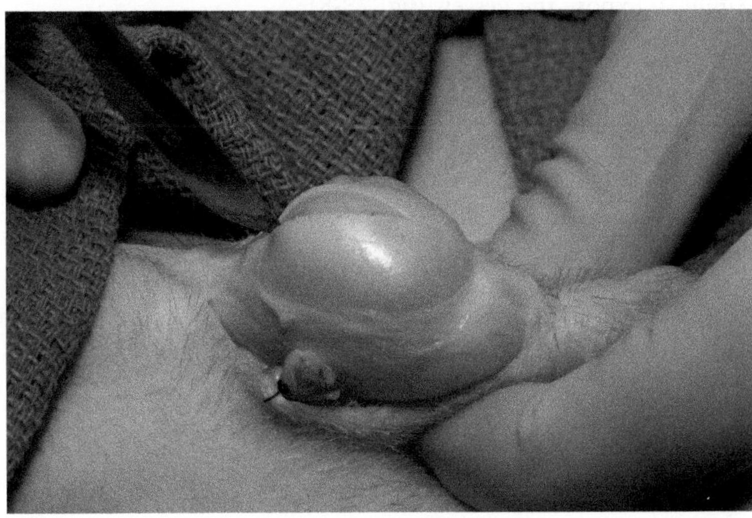

Figure 29-7 Open castration. Incise through the parietal tunic.

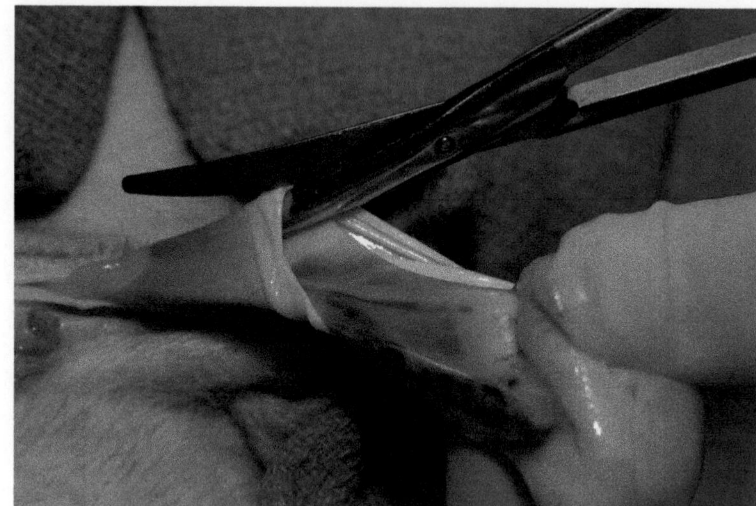

Figure 29-8 Extend the parietal tunic incision with scissors to expose the vessels.

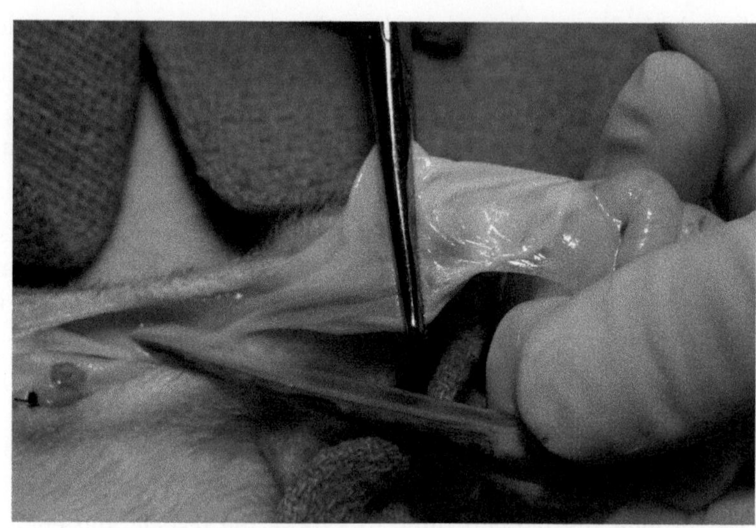

Figure 29-9 Separate the vessels from the cremaster muscle. If necessary, ligate the cremaster muscle and parietal tunic en masse before transecting the tissues.

3. Pop the testicle out of the tunic incision and, with scissors, extend the tunic opening to expose the vessels (fig. 29-8).
4. Ligate the parietal tunic and cremaster muscle en masse, using transfixing-encircling ligatures if the tunic is more than 1 cm wide, and transect and remove the tissues (fig. 29-9).
5. Double ligate and transect the vessels (fig. 29-10).

Surgical technique: scrotal castration of adult dogs

1. Elevate the testicle caudoventrally so that the scrotal skin is taut over the testicle.
2. Make a longitudinal incision, parallel to and to one side of the median raphe, over one-third to one-half the length of the testicle.
3. Proceed with a closed or open castration as described above.

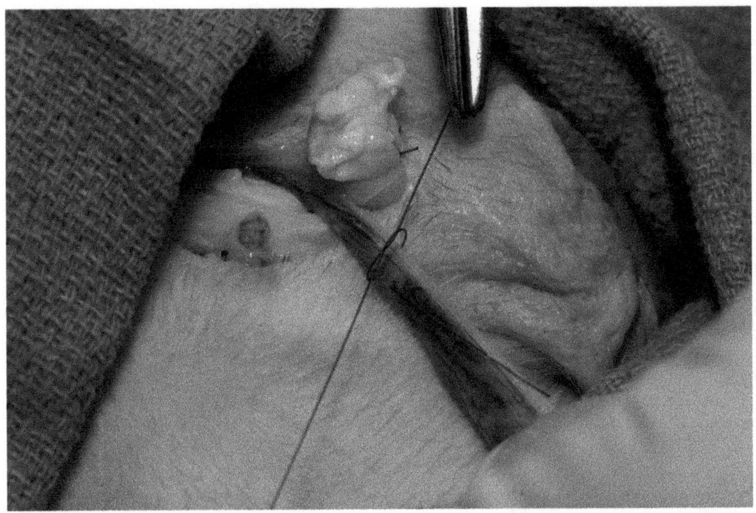

Figure 29-10 Double ligate the vessels. In this dog, the ductus deferens was included in the ligatures.

4. Once the first testicle has been removed, position the second testicle under the skin incision and incise through the scrotal septum and spermatic fascia.
5. Exteriorize the second testicle and proceed with a closed or open castration.
6. Once both testicles have been removed, gently compress the incision edges together manually (puppies), or place one buried interrupted subcutaneous suture, using fine absorbable monofilament. Do not handle the scrotal skin with thumb forceps.

Surgical technique: scrotal ablation with castration

1. Incise the skin around the base of the scrotum (fig. 29-11). Ligate or cauterize the vascular supply, which occurs primarily along the lateral aspects of the scrotum.

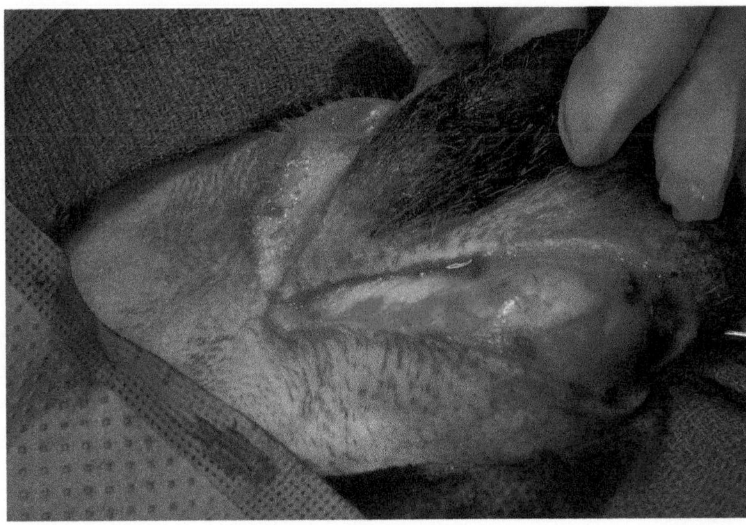

Figure 29-11 Scrotal ablation. Incise the skin around the base of the scrotum.

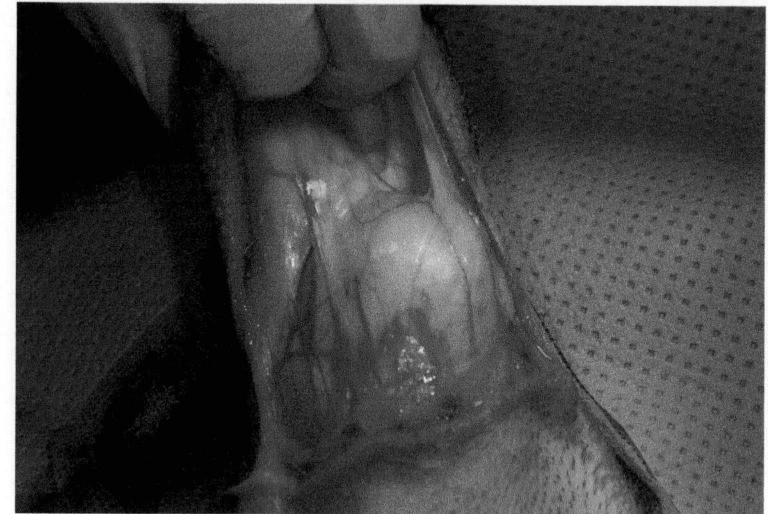

Figure 29-12 In intact dogs, transect the subcutaneous tissues and scrotal ligaments to expose the testicles.

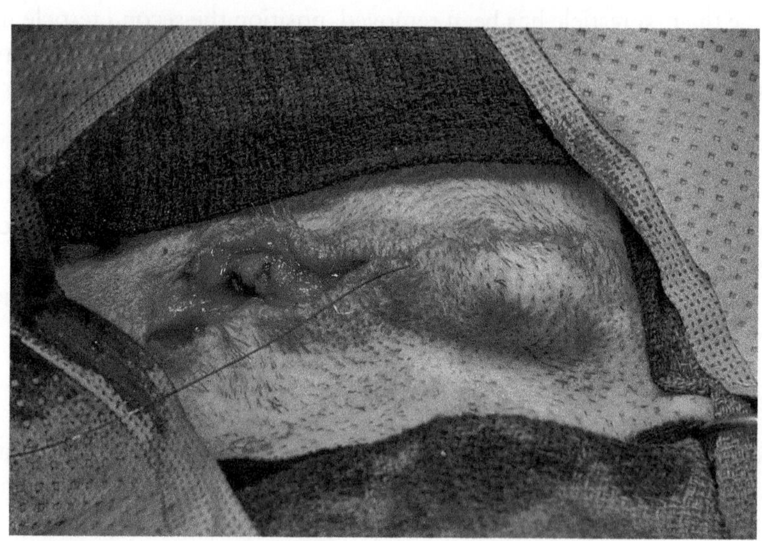

Figure 29-13 After apposing the subcutaneous tissues, close the skin with an intradermal pattern.

2. Using Metzenbaum scissors, transect the subcutaneous tissues and scrotal septum. If the dog is intact, strip the resected scrotum from the testicles (fig. 29-12) and then castrate as described above.
3. Appose the subcutaneous tissues with 3-0 rapidly absorbable synthetic monofilament suture, and close the skin with an intradermal or cutaneous pattern (fig. 29-13).

Postoperative considerations

Complications of castration include self-trauma, swelling, bruising, scrotal hematoma, dehiscence, and infection. Swelling is common, particularly after an open castration, and may be limited by exercise restriction, cold packs, and use of Elizabethan collars postoperatively. Hemorrhage most often occurs from bleeding subcutaneous and septal vessels and is managed with sedation and pressure. Severe scrotal hemorrhage, swelling, or infection may require scrotal ablation. Rarely, a poorly ligated vascular pedicle retracts into the abdomen and bleeds. Bleeding patients are monitored with serial hematocrits; laparotomy and abdominal exploration should be performed if life-threatening hemorrhage occurs. Testicular vessels can retract to the level of the kidney, so a long celiotomy incision may be required. In dogs with myelotoxicity from testicular neoplasia, hemograms are rechecked weekly to verify improvement. Digital rectal examination is repeated 2 weeks after surgery in dogs with prostatic disease; in dogs with benign prostatic hyperplasia, the prostate should be palpably smaller within 10 days after castration.

Delayed postoperative bleeding is noted in 30% of retired racing greyhounds after elective gonadectomy. The risk of bleeding can be reduced by administering epsilon aminocaproic acid (500 mg PO q8h for 5 days), beginning the treatment once the dogs are awake from surgery.

Bibliography

Bryan JN et al: A population study of neutering status as a risk factor for canine prostate cancer. Prostate 2007;67:1174–1181.

Cooley DM et al: Endogenous gonadal hormone exposure and bone sarcoma risk. Cancer Epidem Biomark Prevent 2002;11:1434–1440.

Digangi BA, Johnson M, Isaza N: Scrotal approach to canine orchiectomy (Procedures Pro). Clinician's Brief 2016;14:87–93.

Hart BL, Hart LA, Thigpen AP et al: Long-term health effects of neutering dogs: comparison of Labrador Retrievers with Golden Retrievers. PLoS ONE 2014; (7):e102241. doi: 10.1371/journal.pone.0102241

Kustritz MVR: Determining the optimal age for gonadectomy of dogs and cats. J Am Vet Med Assoc 2007;231:1665–1675.

Marin LM, Iazbik MD, Alsdivar-Lopez S, et al: Epsilon aminocaproic acid for the prevention of delayed postoperative bleeding in retired racing greyhounds undergoing gonadectomy. Vet Surg 2012;41:594–603.

McMillan MW, Seymour CJ, Brearley JC. Effect of intratesticular lidocaine on isoflurane requirements in dogs undergoing routine castration. J Small Anim Pract 2012;53:393–397.

Wilson GP and Hayes HM: Castration for treatment of perianal gland neoplasms in dogs. J Am Vet Med Assoc 1979;174:1301–1303.

Woodruff K, Bushby PA, Rigdon-Brestle K, et al: Scrotal castration versus prescrotal castration in dogs. Vet Med 2015;110:131–135.

and pressure. Severe scrotal hemorrhage, swelling, or infection may require scrotal ablation. Rarely, a poorly ligated vascular pedicle retracts into the abdomen and bleeds. Bleeding patients are monitored with serial hematocrits. A laparotomy and abdominal exploration should be performed if life-threatening hemorrhage occurs. Testicular vessels can retract to the level of the kidney, so a long celiotomy incision may be required. In dogs with myelotoxicity from testicular neoplasia, hemograms are rechecked weekly to verify improvement. Digital rectal examination is repeated 2 weeks after surgery in dogs with prostatic diseases; in dogs with benign prostatic hyperplasia, the prostate should be palpably smaller within 10 days after castration.

Delayed postoperative bleeding is noted in 30% of retired racing greyhounds after elective gonadectomy. The risk of bleeding can be reduced by administering epsilon aminocaproic acid (500 mg PO q8h for 5 days), beginning the treatment once the dogs are awake from surgery.

Bibliography

Bryan JN et al. A population study of neutering status as a risk factor for canine prostate cancer. Prostate 2007;67(11):1174–1181.

Cooley DM et al. Endogenous gonadal hormone exposure and bone sarcoma risk. Cancer Epidemiol Biomarkers Prev 2002;11:1434–1440.

D[illegible] EA, [illegible] N. Scrotal approach [illegible] orchiectomy [illegible]. Top Companion Anim Med 2016 [illegible].

Hart BL, Hart LA, Thigpen AP et al. Long-term health effects of neutering dogs: comparison of Labrador Retrievers with Golden Retrievers. PLoS One 2014;9(7):e102241. doi:10.1371/journal.pone.0102241.

Kustritz MVR. Determining the optimal age for gonadectomy of dogs and cats. J Am Vet Med Assoc 2007;231:1665–1675.

[illegible] LM, [illegible]. [illegible] dogs: [illegible] effects on joint disorders and cancers in golden retrievers [illegible]. PLoS One 2013 [illegible].

N[illegible] W, [illegible] C. [illegible] effect of [illegible] in dogs [illegible] volume reduction. [illegible]

[illegible] and [illegible] LM. [illegible] treatment of [illegible] dogs. J Am Vet Med Assoc [illegible].

[illegible] in dogs. [illegible] Vet Med 20[illegible];1[illegible]:1[illegible]–13[illegible].

Chapter 30
Cryptorchid Castration

Testicles normally descend from the caudal pole of the kidneys, through the inguinal canal, and into the scrotum by 40 days after birth. Retention of testicles in the inguinal region or abdominal cavity is termed cryptorchidism. Cryptorchidism is most commonly unilateral. Retained testicles are usually found in the inguinal region, and, in dogs, the right testicle is most likely to be affected. Removal of the retained testicle is recommended because of continued hormone production, increased risk for neoplasia and torsion, and trait heritability. Cryptorchid testicles are nine times more likely to be neoplastic than scrotal testes. In dogs with retained testicles, Sertoli cell tumors develop at a younger age and are more likely to induce clinical signs of hyperandrogenism than dogs with scrotal testicles.

Cryptorchidism is most often an incidental finding on physical examination; however, animals with torsion of cryptorchid testicles can present with clinical signs of an acute abdomen. Dogs with Sertoli cell tumors may have mammary gland development, alopecia, prostatitis, and bone marrow hypoplasia. Diagnosis of cryptorchidism is usually made by scrotal palpation. Additionally, cats with retained testicles will continue to display penile barbs. When the animal's history is unknown, ultrasonography can be performed. Ultrasound is highly sensitive for detecting retained testicles, particularly when they are neoplastic or located inguinally. Cryptorchidism can also be diagnosed by measuring increased blood testosterone concentrations after stimulation with gonadotropin-releasing hormone or human chorionic gonadotropin. Laparoscopic exploration for retained abdominal testicles permits concurrent removal.

Preoperative management

Young patients undergoing cryptorchid castration are usually healthy and require minimal preoperative diagnostics. Animals with neoplasia or testicular torsion should undergo a complete blood count, serum biochemistry, and urinalysis, and in some cases abdominal imaging. Metastases are reported in 10% to 20% of dogs with Sertoli cell tumors; in patients with suspected neoplasia, abdominal ultrasound should be performed to evaluate regional lymph nodes, kidney, liver, and spleen, which are the most common sites for metastases. Sertoli and interstitial cell tumors may cause aplastic anemia. Bone marrow samples are evaluated if nonregenerative anemia is detected on complete blood count.

Manual of Small Animal Soft Tissue Surgery, Second Edition. Karen Tobias.
© 2017 John Wiley & Sons, Inc. Published 2017 by John Wiley & Sons, Inc.

The bladder should be manually expressed or drained by catheter before surgery. Because cryptorchidectomy may require an abdominal incision, the abdomen and inguinum should be clipped and prepped. The prepuce should be flushed with an antiseptic solution before the final skin prep is completed.

Surgery

Some retained testicles can be forced back to the prescrotal region and removed through a routine castration approach. Testicles retained in the inguinal region are easiest to remove through an incision directly over the testicle or superficial inguinal ring. The superficial inguinal ring is a slit in the external abdominal oblique aponeurosis (see fig. 11-1, p. 98). If not obscured by fat, it can be palpated caudolateral to the last nipple, about 1 cm craniomedial to the femoral ring and pectineus. Occasionally, inguinal cryptorchid testicles are accidentally pushed into the inguinal canal during palpation and must be removed through an abdominal incision. If an inguinal retained testicle cannot be found during surgery, simultaneous abdominal and inguinal approaches may be necessary.

In animals with unilateral abdominal cryptorchidism, the affected side can be determined by pushing the normal testicle cranially toward its inguinal ring. In dogs, unilateral abdominal testicles that are small can be removed through a paramedian abdominal wall incision. In dogs with bilateral abdominal cryptorchidism or unilateral testicular torsion or neoplasia, retained testicles are removed through a midline celiotomy. The approach is similar to an ovariohysterectomy, but the incision may need to be extended caudal to the prepuce, if the testicles are resting near the inguinal rings, or cranial to the umbilicus if they are resting near the kidneys. In cats, abdominal testicles are removed through a caudal midline celiotomy. Cryptorchid abdominal testicles are located by following the ductus deferens or testicular vessels to the testicle. The ductus deferens are located dorsal to the bladder at the prostate, while the testicular vessels are followed caudally from the kidney region. Alternatively, the testicle can be located by finding the inguinal extension of the gubernacular remnant (the ligament of the tail of the epididymis), which exits the superficial inguinal ring; retracting it to identify the vaginal process at the level of the superficial inguinal ring; and opening the vaginal process to identify the ductus deferens or tail of the epididymis. Either of these two structures can be retracted carefully to pull small testicles out of the inguinal canal. In some adult dogs, however, the superficial ring must be enlarged to allow the testicle to exit the abdominal wall.

In animals with unilateral cryptorchidism and large inguinal fat pads, locating an atrophied cryptorchid testicle may be difficult. If the testicle location is uncertain, the initial skin incision should be made paramedian in the dog and on the caudal midline in the cat. The skin is retracted, and the superficial inguinal ring is examined. If the testicle is not found, the incision is extended into the abdomen.

Surgical technique: inguinal cryptorchidectomy

1. Incise the skin over the palpable inguinal testicle or over the inguinal ring.
2. With Metzenbaum scissors, spread the subcutaneous tissues longitudinally to expose the retained testicle (fig. 30-1).
3. Break down the fascial attachments to the base of the testicle with a dry sponge (fig. 30-2) or Metzenbaum scissors, and retract the testicle from the incision.

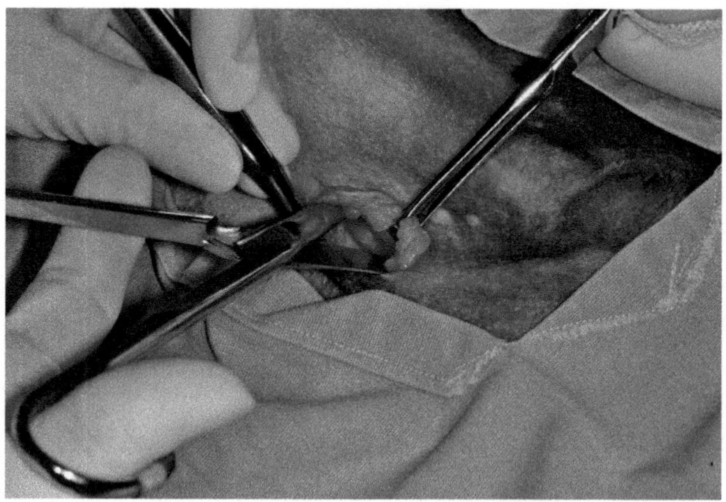

Figure 30-1 Make an incision over the palpable inguinal testicle or inguinal ring, and spread the subcutaneous tissues longitudinally to expose the testicle.

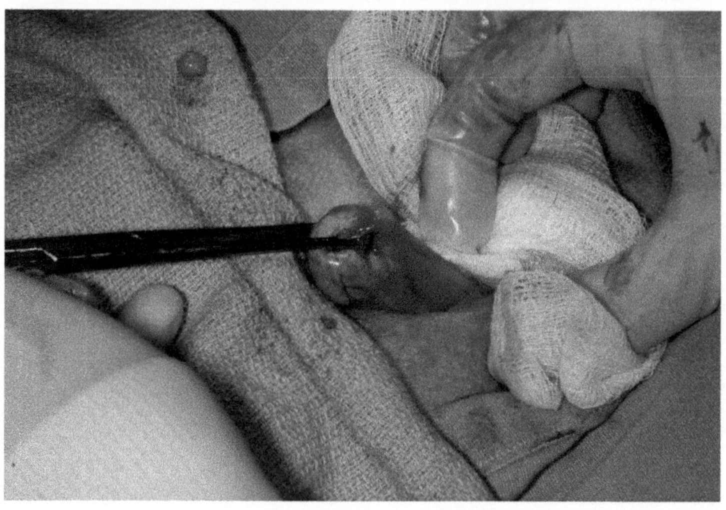

Figure 30-2 Break down the fascial attachments to retract the testicle from the incision before ligating the cord.

4. Double ligate and transect the spermatic cord (see p. 242).
5. Close the subcutaneous tissues with 3-0 absorbable suture in an interrupted pattern. In fat animals, place two layers of subcutaneous sutures to close the dead space.
6. Appose the skin routinely.

Surgical technique: paramedian abdominal cryptorchidectomy in male dogs

1. Make a 3- to 5-cm longitudinal incision in the skin several centimeters lateral to the prepuce and last nipple, ending over the inguinal ring.
2. Spread the subcutaneous tissues longitudinally with Metzenbaum scissors to expose the external rectus sheath. If desired, retract the subcutis with Gelpi retractors.
3. Incise the rectus sheath with a blade. Separate and spread the underlying muscle fibers longitudinally with scissors or index fingers to expose the peritoneum (fig. 30-3).

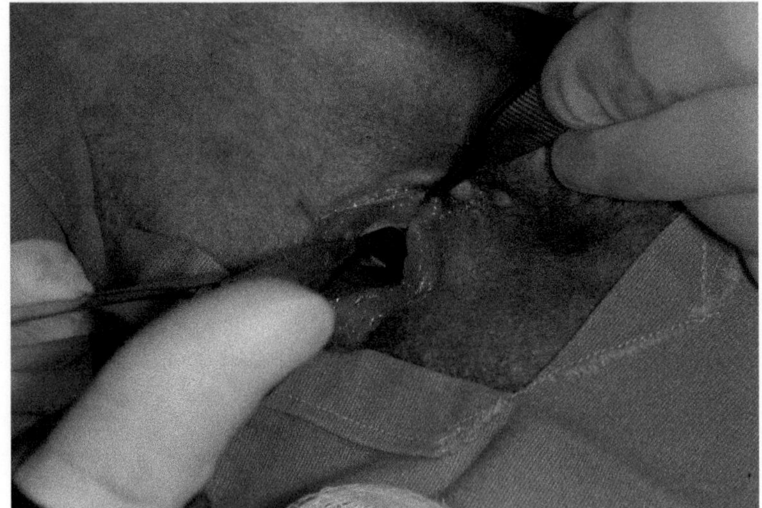

Figure 30-3 Paramedian abdominal approach. Incise the external rectus sheath, then separate the muscle fibers by spreading the scissor blades longitudinally.

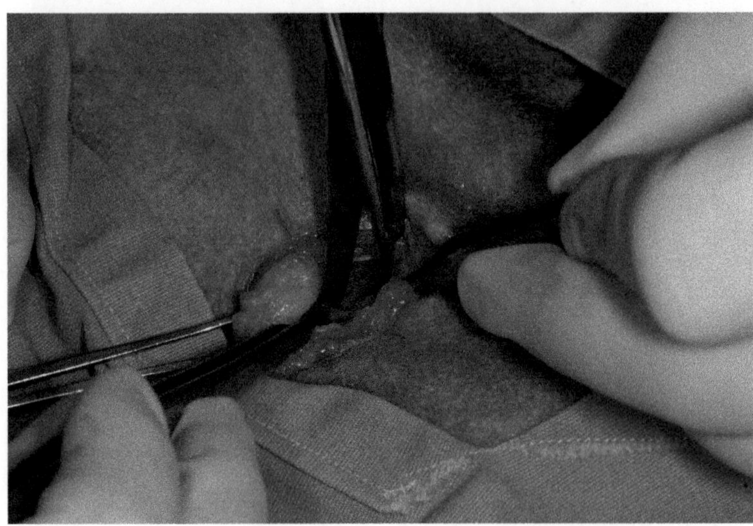

Figure 30-4 Incise the underlying peritoneum and spread it to expose the ductus deferens, testicular vessels, or testicle.

4. Pick up the peritoneum carefully with thumb forceps and perforate it with a blade or scissors (fig. 30-4). The bladder may be directly under the site and can be accidentally incised.
5. Spread or retract the body wall to expose the ductus deferens. If the ductus deferens is not visible, push the abdominal viscera medially with the blunt wide end of a spay hook or scalpel handle. The ductus deferens and testicular vessels are usually found in the dorsolateral portion of the caudal abdomen.
6. Grasp the ductus deferens and retract it out of the incision to expose the testicle (fig. 30-5). If the testicle is not visible, follow the ductus deferens caudally to determine whether the testicle has entered the inguinal canal. Extend the skin and subcutaneous incisions over the superficial inguinal ring to increase exposure.
7. Break down any residual ligamentous tissue (fig. 30-6), then ligate and transect the testicular vessels and ductus deferens en masse (fig. 30-7).

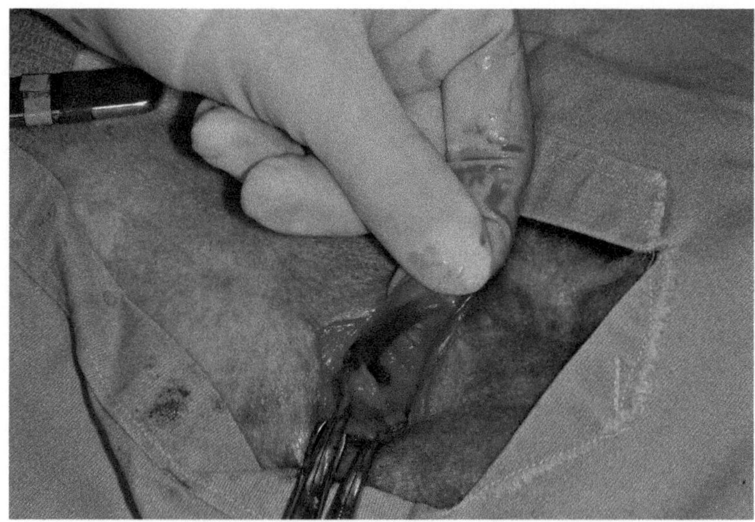

Figure 30-5 Gently retract ductus deferens and testicular vessels from the abdomen to expose the testicle.

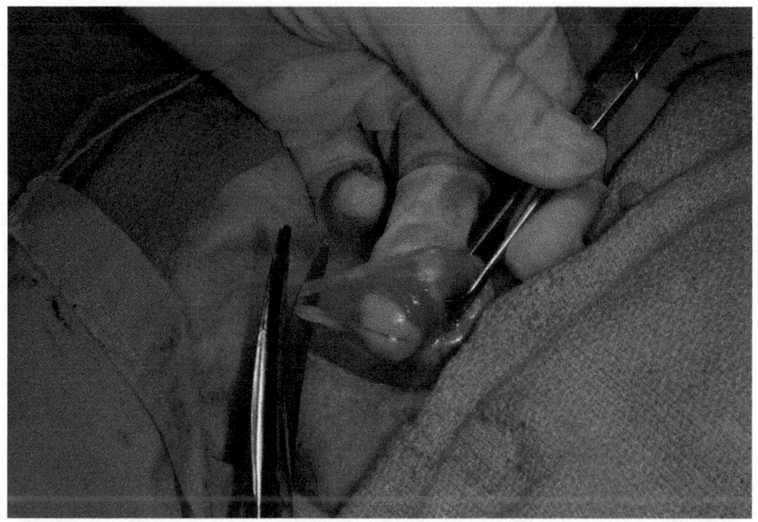

Figure 30-6 Transect or tear the ligamentous tissue attached to the caudal pole of the testicle.

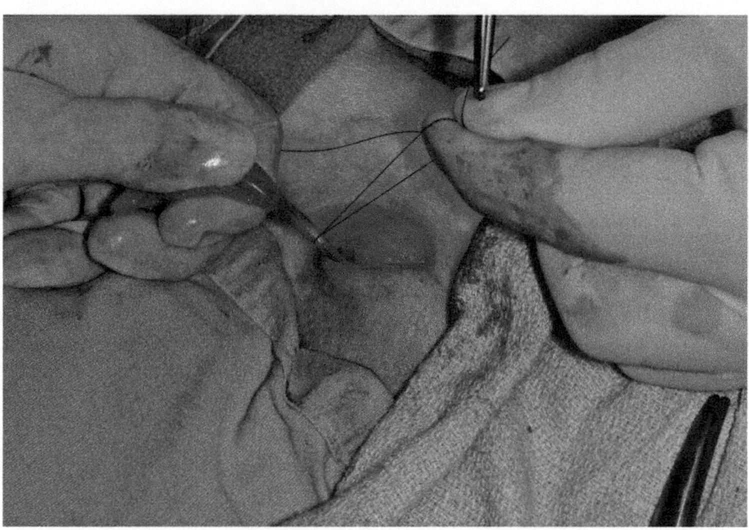

Figure 30-7 Ligate and transect the vessels and ductus deferens and remove the testicle.

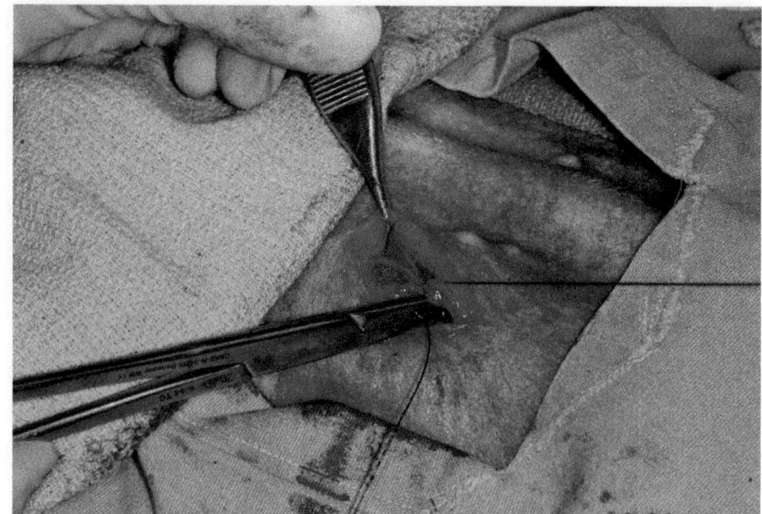

Figure 30-8 Appose the external rectus fascia before closing subcutis and skin.

8. Close the external rectus sheath with 2-0 or 3-0 absorbable suture in a simple continuous or interrupted pattern (fig. 30-8). Close subcutis and skin routinely; if there is dead space, tack down the subcutis to the rectus fascia before closing skin.

Postoperative considerations

After surgery, the testicles are submitted for histologic evaluation when neoplasia is suspected, and analgesics are administered for 1 to 3 days. Swelling commonly occurs at the surgical sites, particularly in active dogs that have undergone paramedian incisions. Intraoperative closure of dead space will limit seroma formation.

Serious complications after cryptorchidectomy are rare. Iatrogenic damage to the urethra has occurred when spay hooks were used to blindly locate the testicle. The prostate has also been mistakenly identified as a retained testicle and removed, resulting in inadvertent urethral transection. In animals with hyperandrogenism, clinical signs usually resolve after castration. Bone marrow hypoplasia is irreversible and fatal in some patients.

Bibliography

Birchard SJ and Nappier M: Cryptorchidism. Compend Contin Educ 2008;30: 325–336.

Hecht S et al: Ultrasound diagnosis: intra-abdominal torsion of a non-neoplastic testicle in a cryptorchid dog. Vet Radiol Ultrasound 2004;45:58–61.

Schulz KS et al: Inadvertent prostatectomy as a complication of cryptorchidectomy in four dogs. J Am Anim Hosp Assoc 1996;32:211–214.

Steckel RR: Use of an inguinal approach adapted from equine surgery for cryptorchidectomy in dogs and cats: 26 cases (1999–2010). J Am Vet Med Assoc 2011;239: 1098–1103.

Yates D et al: Incidence of cryptorchidism in dogs and cats. Vet Rec 2003;152: 502–504.

Chapter 31
Prostatic Biopsy

Prostatic disease is common in intact male dogs over 10 years of age. Some dogs are asymptomatic as long as the prostate remains relatively small. As the prostate enlarges, it may compress the colon or urethra, resulting in tenesmus or stranguria. Animals with severe prostatic enlargement may develop rear limb edema from compression of nearby lymphatics or veins. Dogs with inflammation, infection, or neoplasia may develop hematuria, pain, or signs of systemic illness.

Preoperative management

Initial evaluation of animals with prostatic disease usually includes a complete blood count, biochemistry panel, urine analysis and culture, and digital rectal examination. On rectal exam, prostates with benign hyperplasia are firm, symmetrical, and nonpainful. Dogs with acute bacterial prostatitis have enlarged, firm, painful prostates. With chronic infection, however, the prostate may become small, hard, and nonpainful. Prostatic abscesses and cysts are often enlarged and asymmetric, and may feel firm or fluctuant. Dogs with prostatic abscesses are usually painful on digital rectal palpation.

Ultrasound is helpful for examining prostate size and character. It is frequently used to facilitate collection of percutaneous aspirates and needle (e.g., Tru-cut) biopsies. Unfortunately, aspirates and needle biopsies provide insufficient samples in 50% and 75% of dogs, respectively. Incisional biopsy may be recommended to definitively diagnose prostatic disease, particularly in dogs undergoing laparotomy for other reasons.

Before surgery, dogs with systemic illness should be stabilized. The abdomen should be clipped and prepped from the xiphoid to the cranial scrotum. Intact dogs should also be prepped for castration, including gentle clipping and aseptic preparation of the scrotum. The prepuce should be flushed with an antiseptic solution before the final scrub.

Surgery

The prostate is approached through a caudal ventral midline incision (p. 83). The skin incision starts on midline and then extends along the peripreputial region. Ipsilateral branches of the external pudendal vessels to the prepuce will need to be ligated during subcutaneous dissection. After subcutaneous dissection, the penile body is retracted and the abdominal wall is incised on the

Manual of Small Animal Soft Tissue Surgery, Second Edition. Karen Tobias.
© 2017 John Wiley & Sons, Inc. Published 2017 by John Wiley & Sons, Inc.

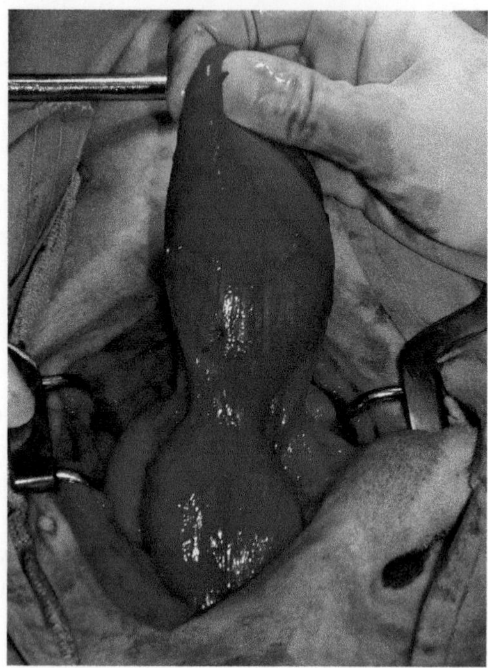

Figure 31-1 Retract the bladder cranially to expose the prostate. In this dog, the prepuce is clamped over to the side to improve exposure and reduce contamination.

midline; the linea is usually not visible near the pubis. The prostate is exposed by retracting the bladder cranially (fig. 31-1) and should be isolated with moistened laparotomy pads. To improve exposure, stay sutures can be placed in the bladder or prostate and retracted cranially. Alternatively, a Penrose drain can be placed around the prostate and urethra and retracted cranially. Excessive retraction may damage innervation to the bladder, however.

The urethra is catheterized so that it can be identified before biopsy. The hypogastric and pelvic nerves are closely associated with the larger vascular branches dorsal and dorsolateral to the prostate gland. If possible, prostate manipulation and biopsy should be limited to the gland's ventral half to avoid urinary incontinence. In dogs with generalized disease, biopsies are taken from the ventrolateral surface of the gland to avoid damaging the urethra, which passes through the gland on the midline just dorsal to its center (fig. 31-2). The subcapsular vessels and parenchyma can bleed vigorously when incised.

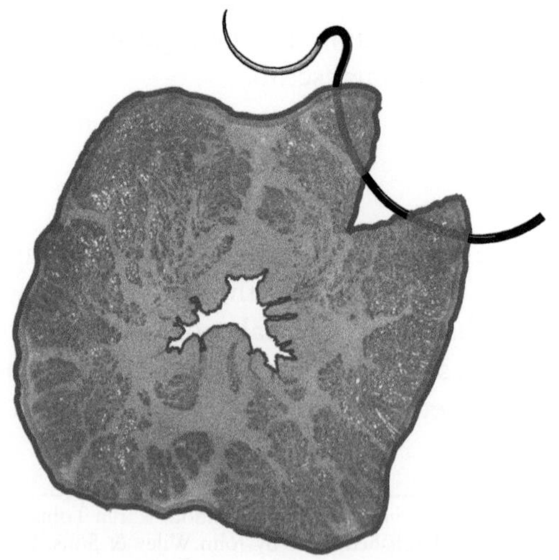

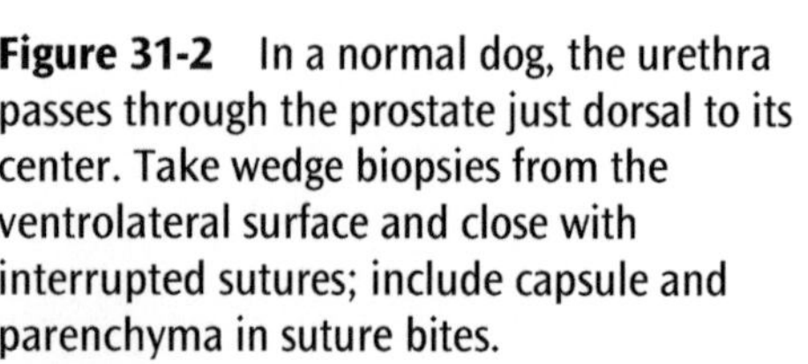

Figure 31-2 In a normal dog, the urethra passes through the prostate just dorsal to its center. Take wedge biopsies from the ventrolateral surface and close with interrupted sutures; include capsule and parenchyma in suture bites.

Bleeding usually slows when the incised edges are apposed; however, use of bipolar cautery may be necessary in some dogs.

Because testosterone exacerbates many prostatic conditions, intact males are usually castrated at the time of biopsy. Castration is performed after the abdominal incision is closed.

Surgical technique: prostatic biopsy

1. Elevate any periprostatic fat away from the biopsy site with Metzenbaum scissors.
   a. Grasp the fat with thumb forceps and insert the scissor tips at the base of the fat near its prostatic attachments.
   b. Spread the scissor tips gently to expose the underlying prostatic capsule.
   c. If desired, sharply transect avascular tissue attachments on the ventrolateral surface of the prostate. Do not transect any dorsal attachments.
2. With a no. 11 or no. 15 blade, make an elliptical incision in the prostate (fig. 31-3). The incision should include capsule and parenchyma.
   a. For focal disease, choose a site farthest from the urethra and nerves.
   b. For diffuse disease, incise the ventrolateral surface of the prostate.
   c. Make the incision 1 to 1.5 cm long and 0.5 to 1 cm deep, depending on the prostate size.
   d. Angle the blade inward as you incise to remove a wedge of tissue.
3. Remove the tissue gently by elevating it with the scalpel blade or by grasping the capsule with the thumb forceps.
4. Place digital pressure to encourage hemostasis.
5. Close the biopsy site with one or two cruciate or mattress sutures of 3-0 absorbable monofilament.
   a. If the capsule is thin, include a superficial bite of the parenchyma on each side of the incision.
   b. Tie the initial throw as a surgeon's throw to appose the tissues firmly; do not overtighten, or the capsule will tear.
   c. Tie three more throws and cut the suture ends short.

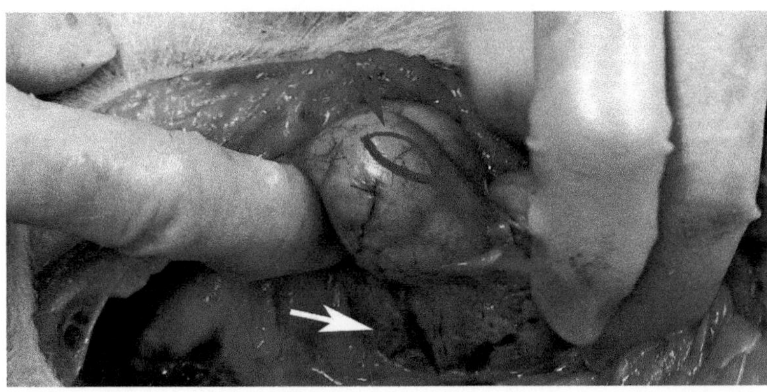

Figure 31-3 For generalized disease, take an elliptical wedge of the ventrolateral prostatic parenchyma and capsule (blue arrow). Note the neurovascular pedicle (white arrow) dorsal to the prostate.

6. If hemorrhage continues, place additional sutures or tack omentum over the site with interrupted sutures of absorbable material.

Postoperative considerations

Prostatic biopsy samples should be submitted for culture and histologic evaluation. If purulent material or a cavitary lesion is detected during biopsy, omentalization (see Chapter 32) may be required. Complications such as postoperative hemorrhage and urethral fistula are rare. If hemorrhage is a concern, packed cell volume is monitored after surgery. If significant anemia develops, the animal should be evaluated for coagulopathies and transfused. Most hemorrhage will respond to nonsurgical management. If the urethra is accidentally incised during prostatic biopsy, primary closure can be attempted; alternatively, the prostatic parenchyma can be apposed over the defect. A transurethral catheter is left in place for 5 to 7 days until damaged urethral mucosa has healed.

Bibliography

Barsanti JA et al: Evaluation of diagnostic techniques for canine prostatic diseases. J Am Vet Med Assoc 1980;177:160–163.

Freitag T et al: Surgical management of common canine prostatic conditions. Compend Contin Educ Pract Vet 2007;29:656–672.

Powe JR et al: Evaluation of the cytologic diagnosis of canine prostatic disorders. Vet Clin Path 2004;33:150–154.

Chapter 32
Prostatic Omentalization

Fluid-filled pockets associated with the prostate can take several forms. Parenchymal "retention" cysts result from an obstruction of prostatic ducts, creating a coalescing, fluid-filled cavity within the prostatic parenchyma that occasionally connects with the urethra. Paraprostatic cysts are thought to be vestigial Müllerian ducts (uterus masculinus). These cysts attach to the prostate but do not communicate with the urethra. Hematogenous spread of bacteria or infection of a prostatic cyst may result in prostatic abscess (fig. 32-1).

Prostatic cysts and abscesses most commonly occur in older, intact, medium-to-large breed dogs. Clinical signs may include stranguria, hematuria, dysuria, tenesmus, and urinary incontinence. Dogs with abscesses will also have signs of systemic illness, such as lethargy, fever, abdominal pain, and anorexia and may have hind limb stiffness and edema. If the abscess ruptures, peritonitis, shock, and death may occur.

Diagnosis of prostatic cysts and abscesses is initially based on results of rectal examination and ultrasound. On digital rectal exam, the prostate is asymmetrically enlarged and can be painful, particularly if an abscess is present. On ultrasound, cysts are usually anechoic cavitary lesions with regular, well-defined margins, while abscesses may be hypoechoic with irregular margins. A retrograde contrast urethrogram may be needed to differentiate the bladder from cystic structures on radiographs.

Dogs with small cysts and abscesses and mild clinical signs may respond to treatment with castration, percutaneous ultrasound-guided drainage under anesthesia, and long-term antibiotics (at least 6 weeks) if there is infection. Multiple drainage procedures are required in 65% of dogs; 90% to 100% will have complete resolution after one to four treatments. Dogs with moderate or severe clinical signs, peritonitis, or large cysts and abscesses require surgical treatment. Omentalization of the prostate is effective for resolving prostatic cysts or abscesses with minimal complications. The omentum provides a source of blood supply to deliver antibiotics, white blood cells, and angiogenic factors and serves as a physiologic drain. Because abscesses are suctioned and flushed during the procedure, omentalization does not increase the risk of sepsis or peritonitis.

Manual of Small Animal Soft Tissue Surgery, Second Edition. Karen Tobias.
© 2017 John Wiley & Sons, Inc. Published 2017 by John Wiley & Sons, Inc.

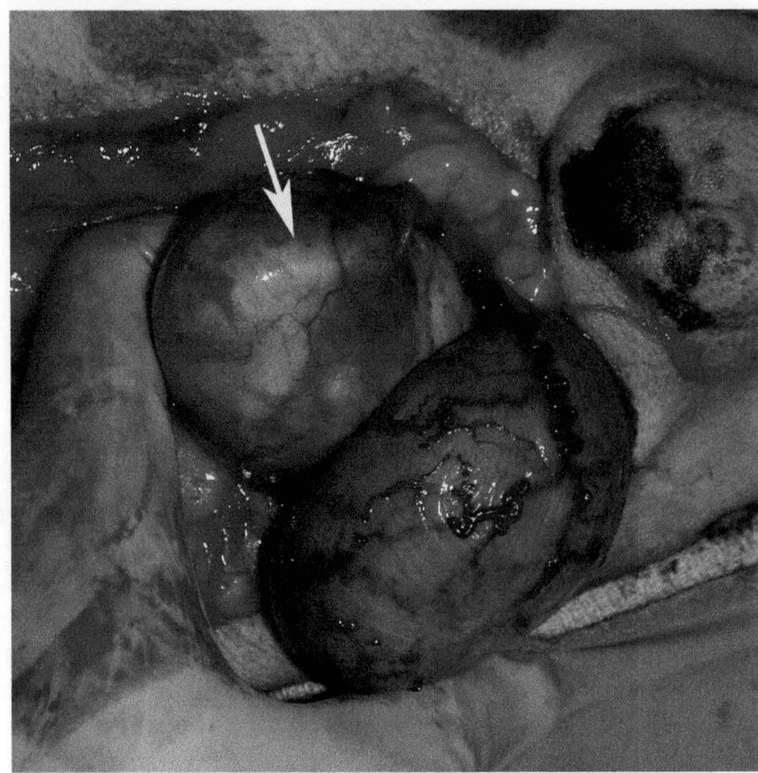

Figure 32-1 Prostatic abscess (arrow) adjacent to the bladder.

Preoperative management

Dogs with abscesses are more likely to have hypoglycemia, azotemia, leukocytosis, pyuria, and bacteriuria. These patients should receive fluid and antibiotic therapy before surgery. A urine culture should be obtained by urethral catheterization. To reduce the risk of rupture, large prostatic cysts and abscesses are usually not cultured until surgery. The most common bacterium cultured from prostatic abscesses is *Escherichia coli*; infections with *Staphylococcus*, *Streptococcus*, *Klebsiella*, *Proteus*, *Pseudomonas*, *Mycoplasma*, and *Brucella* species have also been reported. Initial antibiotic selection should be based on effectiveness against these organisms until urine and tissue culture results are available. The abdomen should be clipped from umbilicus to pubis, including the prescrotal region in intact males. The prepuce should be flushed with an antiseptic solution.

Surgery

If an abscess is suspected, sterile instruments should be set aside for abdominal closure. The prepuce is usually included within the surgical field to permit intraoperative urethral catheterization. The prostate is approached by a ventral midline caudal celiotomy (p. 83) and isolated with moistened laparotomy pads. If needed, a urine sample is obtained by cystocentesis once the bladder is exposed. The cyst or abscess wall should be opened ventrally or ventrolaterally to avoid damage to urethral and bladder innervation. After the cavity is drained, samples are obtained for biopsy and culture, and the cavity is omentalized. In most dogs, omentum easily reaches the cyst cavity; occasionally, however, the omental pedicle must be lengthened by incising its dorsal attachments with electrocautery or with ligation and transection of its vascular attachments. If peritonitis is present, continuous suction drainage may be required (pp. 125–127). The dog should be castrated at the end of the procedure if it is intact.

Surgical technique: prostatic omentalization

1. To expose the prostate, place stay sutures in the bladder or fibrous capsule of the cyst and pull them cranially.
2. To facilitate urethral identification, place a urinary catheter.
3. Perforate the ventrolateral portion of the cyst or abscess wall (away from the urethra) with Metzenbaum scissors, a blade, or hemostats. Remove the contents with suction (fig. 32-2).
4. Digitally break down any septa within the cavity, and suction and flush the cavity with sterile saline.
5. If a urethral fistula is identified, close it with 4-0 or 5-0 monofilament absorbable suture.
6. Using scissors, excise a portion of the incised edge of the cyst wall for culture and histologic evaluation. For large cysts, resect half of the cyst wall.
7. Insert the free edge of the omentum into the evacuated cavity, packing it in to fill the entire space.
    a. If the cavity is large, pass a Carmalt forceps through one wall of the prostate and out the incision. Grasp the omentum with the tips of the forceps and pull it through the cavity and out the opposite wall (fig. 32-3).

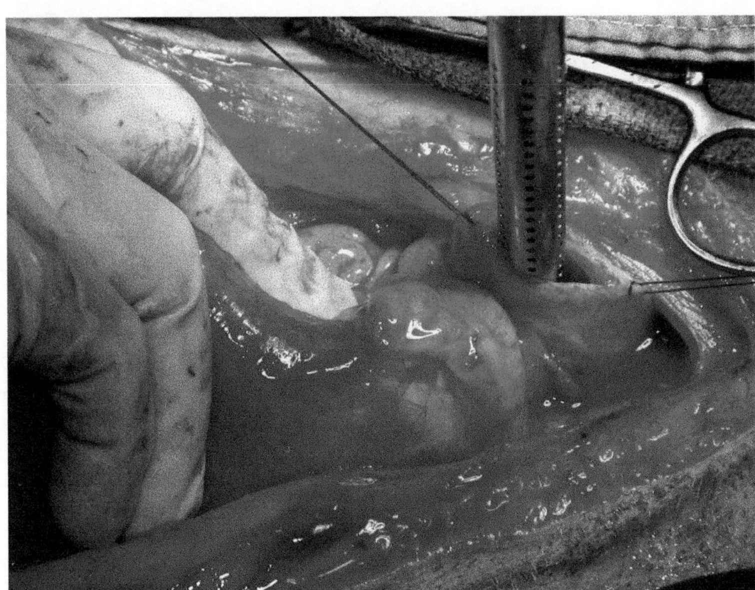

Figure 32-2 After passing a urinary catheter, incise through the cyst wall and suction out the contents. Place stay sutures in the cyst wall to facilitate manipulation.

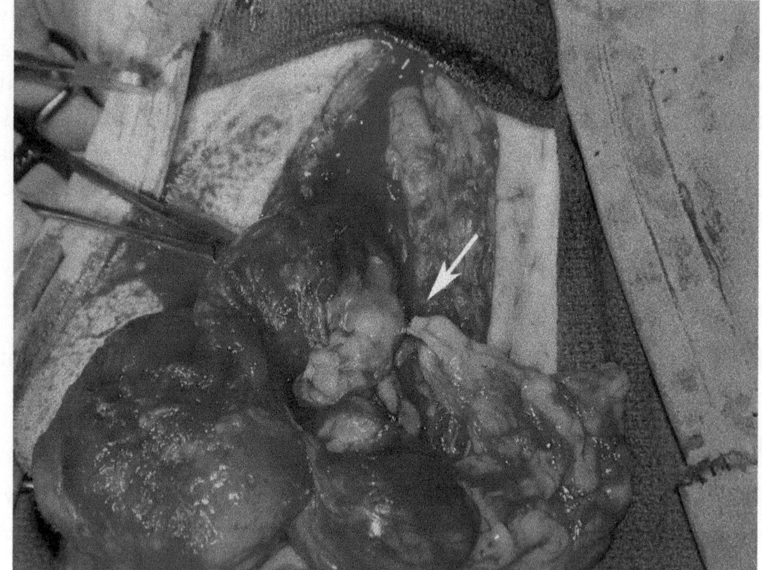

Figure 32-3 Pass a Carmalt forceps through the cyst or abscess wall and grasp the omentum with the tips of the forceps (arrow) to pull it through the cavity and out the opposite wall.

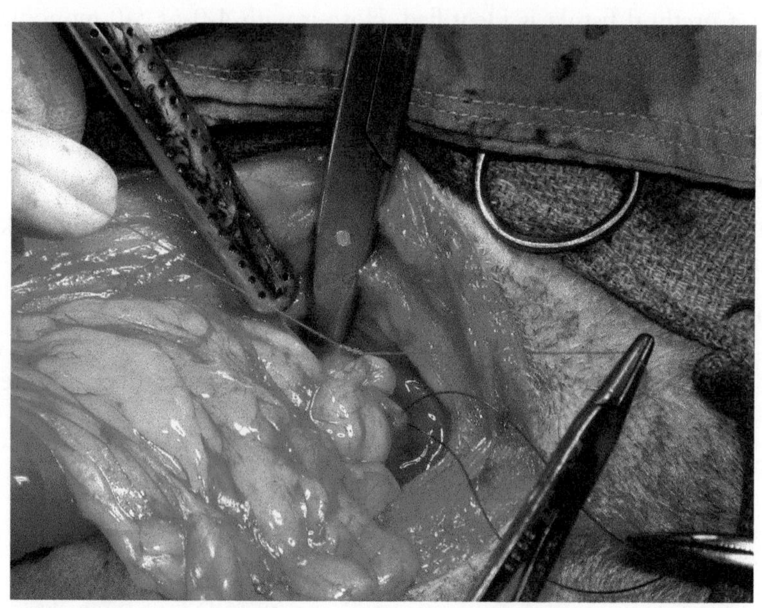

Figure 32-4 Tack the omentum to the exterior surface of the prostate with simple interrupted sutures.

   b. Alternatively, if the cavity is bilateral, insert omentum in both sides of the cavity, taking care not to constrict or compress the urethra.

8. Tack the omentum to the prostate near the incision edges or forceps perforation site with two to four simple interrupted absorbable monofilament sutures (figs. 32-4 and 32-5).
9. Change gloves and instruments, if an abscess was present, and then flush and suction out the abdomen and close routinely.
10. Castrate the dog.

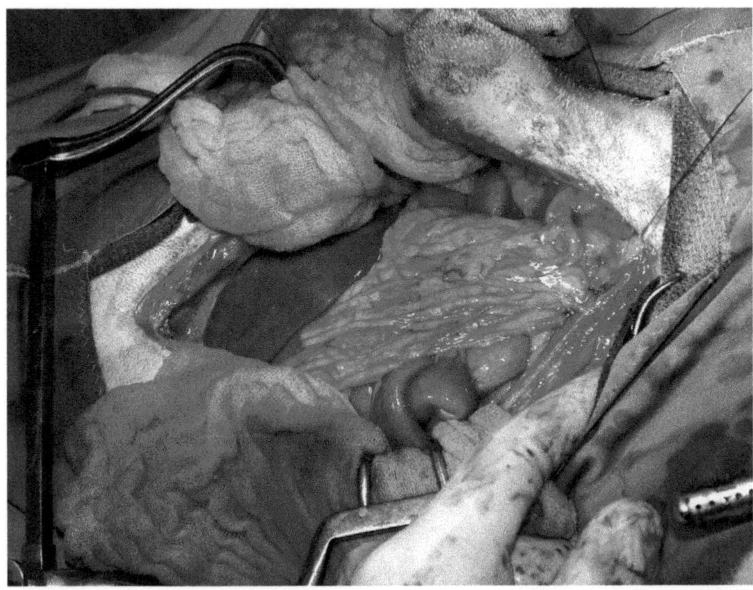

Figure 32-5 Final appearance.

Postoperative considerations

Antibiotics are continued for at least 1 week in dogs with omentalized abscesses. Urine cultures should be re-evaluated after antibiotic treatment is completed. Acute postoperative complications include vomiting or urine retention in 7% of dogs. Death may occur in dogs with sepsis or peritonitis. Transient urinary incontinence is reported in up to 20% of dogs after prostatic omentalization. Incontinence may be secondary to neurologic damage from excessive dissection or traction during surgery. Affected dogs should be evaluated for cystitis and urethral obstruction from continued prostatic enlargement. Incontinence is responsive to phenylpropanolamine and usually resolves in 8 weeks. Metastasis along the omental pedicle has been reported in a dog with prostatic carcinoma and a previous omentalization.

Bibliography

Bokemeyer J, Peppler C, Thiel C, et al: Prostatic cavitary lesions containing urine in dogs. J Small Anim Pract 2011;52:132–138.

Boland LE et al: Ultrasound-guided percutaneous drainage as the primary treatment for prostatic abscesses and cysts in dogs. J Am Anim Hosp Assoc 2003;39:151–159.

Bray JP et al: Partial resection and omentalization: a new technique for management of prostatic retention cysts in dogs. Vet Surg 1997;26:202–209.

Freitag T et al: Surgical management of common canine prostatic conditions. Compendium Contin Educ 2007;29:656–673.

Jacobs TM, Hoppe BR, Poehlmann CE, et al: Metastasis of a prostatic carcinoma along an omental graft in a dog. Case Rep Vet Med 2013;2013(0):141094. 1–5.

Polisca A, Troisi A, Fontaine E, et al: A retrospective study of canine prostatic diseases from 2002 to 2009 at the Alfort Veterinary College in France. Theriogenol 2016;85: 835–840.

White RAS et al: Intracapsular prostatic omentalization: a new technique for management of prostatic abscesses in dogs. Vet Surg 1995;24:390–395.

Chapter 33
Ovariohysterectomy and Ovariectomy

Elective ovariohysterectomy ("spay") is commonly performed to prevent estrous cycles and unwanted pregnancy. Additional benefits include prevention of pyometra and ovarian or uterine neoplasia. Spaying dogs and cats before their first estrus dramatically decreases their lifetime risk of mammary neoplasia, while spaying cats after 2 years of age or dogs after 2.5–4 years of age has minimal effect on mammary tumor development.

Ovariohysterectomy is performed therapeutically in animals with pyometra, dystocia, uterine or ovarian cancer, and vaginal hyperplasia or prolapse. In dogs with congenital clotting disorders, ovariohysterectomy prevents life-threatening hemorrhage that can occur during estrus. Ovariohysterectomy or ovariectomy also eliminates hormonal changes that can interfere with medical therapy for diabetes mellitus or epilepsy.

Adverse effects of ovary removal include obesity and a greater potential for urinary incontinence, particularly in those dogs spayed at a very young age. Ovariohysterectomy has also been associated with an increased risk for development of transitional cell carcinoma, osteosarcoma, mast cell tumor, lymphoma, hemangiosarcoma, and joint disease in some dog breeds. For example, golden retrievers spayed before 6 months of age have a 20% risk of risk of joint diseases (e.g., cranial cruciate ligament rupture), compared with a 5% risk in intact dogs. Whether these conditions result directly from hormonal deficiencies or as a consequence of obesity or selection bias is unknown; however, the fact that they occur at higher rates illustrates the importance of considering breed and other issues in determining when and if a dog should be gonadectomized.

Ovariectomy without hysterectomy is becoming more common, particularly with laparoscopic spays. Ovariectomy alone does not increase the risk of pyometra, since development of endometritis, pyometra, or stump pyometra requires endogenous or exogenous progestogens. Ovariectomy may be less traumatic than ovariohysterectomy because the incision size is smaller and tissues are handled less. The only increased risk compared with ovariohysterectomy is for uterine tumor development. Incidence of uterine tumors in dogs is low (0.03%), and 90% of the tumors are benign leiomyomas.

Manual of Small Animal Soft Tissue Surgery, Second Edition. Karen Tobias.
© 2017 John Wiley & Sons, Inc. Published 2017 by John Wiley & Sons, Inc.

Preoperative management

In young healthy animals, packed cell volume and total protein should be assessed. Blood glucose should be measured in toy breeds and any animal predisposed to hypoglycemia. Other diagnostics are based on breed predisposition for various conditions and on the animal's age and health status.

In dogs with clotting disorders, such as von Willebrand disease, preoperative transfusion with fresh frozen plasma or cryoprecipitate may be necessary. Intramuscular injections should be avoided in these patients. Owners of greyhounds should be warned about the risk of delayed postoperative bleeding.

Before surgery, the bladder is manually expressed in nonpregnant animals to make locating the uterus easier. The abdomen is clipped and prepped from xiphoid to the pubis and the surgery site should be draped widely to permit extension of the incision cranially or caudally, respectively, if an ovarian pedicle is dropped or the uterus cannot be found. In dogs with clotting disorders, skin penetration with towel clamps should be avoided.

Surgery

Ovariectomy and ovariohysterectomy are usually performed during anestrus, since reproductive and mammary tissues are more vascular under the influence of estrogen. Additionally, the uterus is more friable during estrus and may tear when crushed by clamps.

In patients with clotting disorders, the abdomen should be entered directly on midline (through the linea). Subcutaneous hemostasis must be meticulous to reduce the risk of postoperative hemorrhage. Suspensory and broad ligaments should be ligated in these patients, and the abdomen should be bandaged with a pressure wrap after surgery.

During elective ovariohysterectomy, the uterus can be located and retrieved with an index finger or spay hook. Spay hooks should be inserted and retracted cautiously to prevent inadvertent damage to the spleen or mesenteric vessels. Spay hooks should not be used in animals with pyometra, bleeding disorders, or a gravid or fragile uterus. If the uterus or ovaries cannot be found easily, the incision should be extended and the areas dorsal to the bladder and caudal to the kidneys examined.

Breaking the suspensory ligaments is often the most frightening part of ovariohysterectomy. The suspensory ligament extends from the cranial pole of the ovary to the caudal pole of the kidney or the body wall dorsolateral to the kidney. The ovarian vessels extend from dorsal midline laterally toward the ovary. If the suspensory ligament is broken at its cranial-most extent, the ovarian vessels are less likely to be damaged (fig. 33-1). If the ovary is pulled too vigorously when the suspensory ligament is broken, the vessels could be torn. The final goal is to be able to elevate the ovary from the abdomen enough to visualize the pedicle; in some animals, particularly cats or animals that are pregnant or in estrus, stretching the suspensory ligament may be sufficient to accomplish this goal.

A three-clamp technique is commonly used on adult canine ovarian pedicles. If possible, all clamps are placed on the vascular pedicle between the ovary and aorta. The pedicle will be transected between the two clamps closest to the ovary. If the pedicle is short, two clamps are placed across the pedicle below the

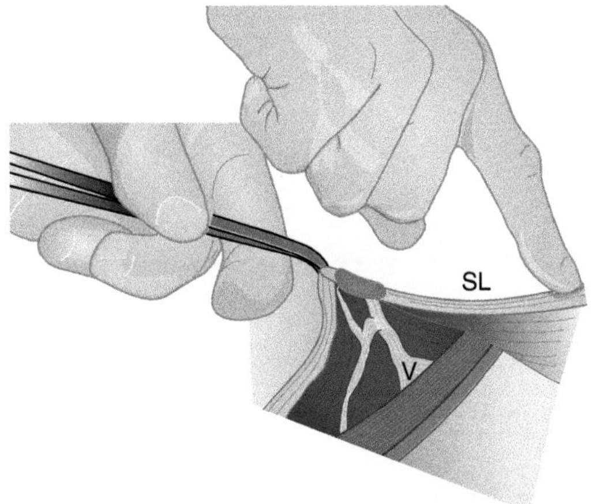

Figure 33-1 Hand position for breaking the suspensory ligament (SL). The clamp is on the proper ligament. Vessels (V) will be caudal and medial to the ligament.

ovary, and a third clamp is placed across the uterine horn and uterine artery and vein. In this case, the ovarian pedicle will be transected between the ovary and the middle clamp. When closed, larger clamps may have a gap between their jaws near the hinge. Pedicles should therefore be clamped within the tips of the hemostatic forceps. Small pedicles can be transected before ligation. Large pedicles should be ligated first to reduce the risk of tearing during pedicle manipulation. Ovarian pedicles should be ligated with absorbable material; ligature size depends on the size of the pedicle and ranges from 3-0 to 0. Ligatures should be placed as far as possible from the clamps so that they will tighten properly. Ligatures can be secured with hand or instrument ties; instrument ties will use less suture material, while hand ties provide the surgeon with more tactile information about the throw. If the pedicle is wide or the surgeon tends to lift up when tying, the first throw of a simple encircling ligature should be a surgeon's throw to provide more knot security when the ligature is under tension.

Alternatives for pedicle ligation include Miller's, modified Miller's, constrictor, strangle, and single double knots, and transfixing-encircling ligatures; experimentally, these sutures provide more knot security than simple or surgeon's throws. With the modified Miller's knot, the suture is wrapped 720° around the pedicle and over the surgeon's finger, with the strands parallel to one another (fig. 33-2A). With a strangle knot, the strands cross one another (fig. 33-2B). With either knot, the wrapped suture is secured between thumb and index finger, and the needle holder is passed under the wrapped suture to grasp the free end and pull it back through (fig. 33-2C). Because the free end has passed under two sutures, the throw remains secure after tightening, even when under tension (fig. 33-2D). Three additional throws are added to make 2 full knots.

The contralateral uterine horn should be located by following the first uterine horn to the uterine bifurcation. If the second horn is retrieved without exposure of the bifurcation, it may end up on the opposite side of the colon or urethra, inadvertently encircling and compressing the organ.

After the ovarian pedicles are ligated, the broad ligament is torn to allow uterine exteriorization. The broad ligament is usually ligated in animals with

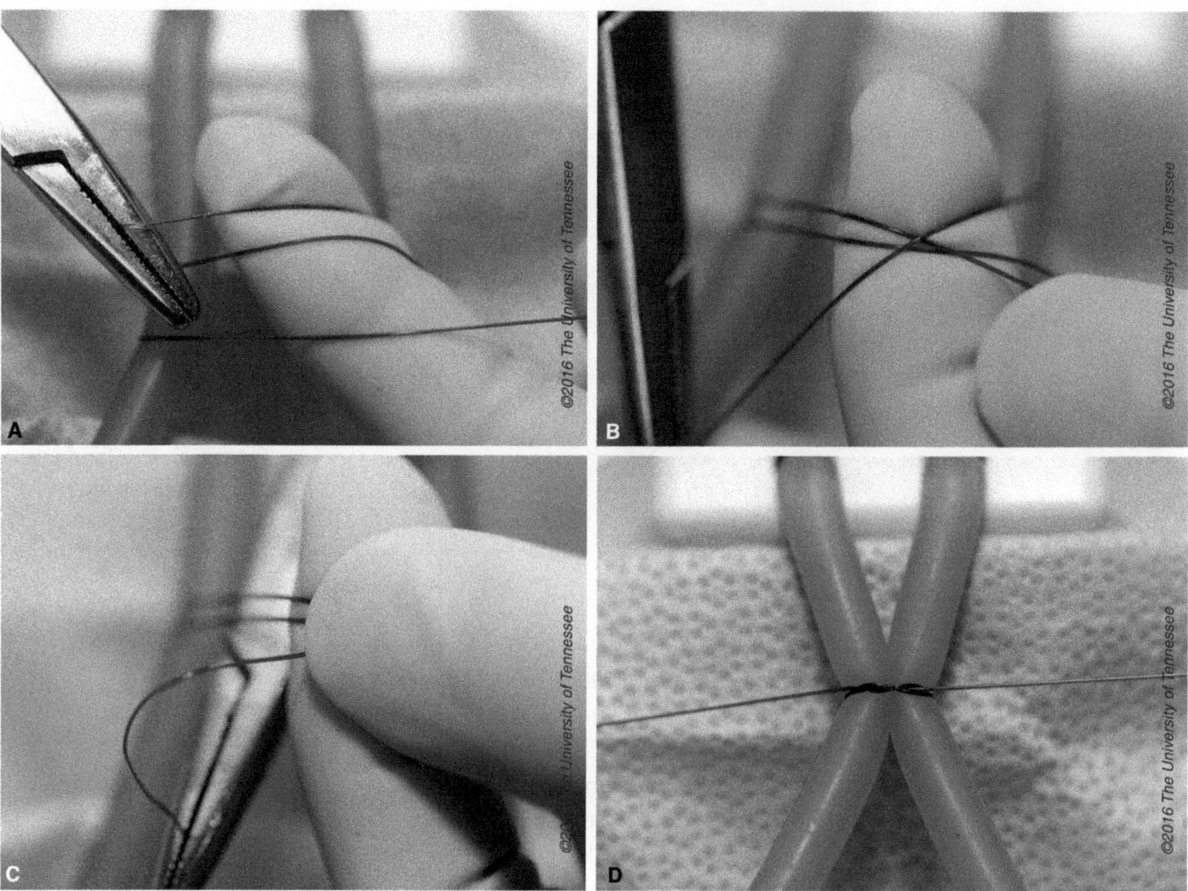

Figure 33-2 A. For a Miller's knot, wrap the suture 720° around the pedicle and your finger to make 2 complete loops. B. For a strangle knot, cross the suture as you make 2 loops around your finger and the pedicle. C. Pass the needle holder between the pedicle and your finger, and pull the free end of the suture back through both loops. D. Pull evenly to tighten the throw. © 2016 The University of Tennessee.

coagulopathies. Once the round ligament of the uterus has been transected, the uterine body can be retracted from the abdomen. If the uterine body is difficult to expose, the horns should be retracted cranially before they are elevated from the abdomen. If the uterine body still cannot be seen, the incision should be extended caudally. Some veterinarians use a three-clamp technique on the uterine body before ligation. If the uterus is small, however, clamping is unnecessary, and if the animal is in heat, the uterus may tear off at the bottom clamp. Technique for uterine ligation depends on the size of the uterus. A small uterus can be ligated with two encircling sutures, while a large uterus is often ligated with two transfixing-encircling sutures. Monofilament synthetic absorbable material is commonly used for ligation. Suture size depends on uterine diameter; most commonly, 3-0 or 2-0 material is used.

Transfixing-encircling sutures are placed on thick, wide uterine bodies and ovarian pedicles. The needle is passed forward (tip first) or backward (suture end first) through the center of the tissue, and two simple throws are tied to crush the encircled tissue. The suture is then passed around all the tissue and tied again with four throws, using a surgeon's throw and 3 simple throws. Transfixing-encircling ligatures are less likely to pull free from the tissues.

Potential complications during suture placement include tearing of the tissue or inadvertent vessel penetration. Usually, the bleeding from the latter stops once the ligature is tied.

Significant intraoperative hemorrhage may occur if the ovarian or uterine vessels are dropped, torn, or inadequately ligated. Bleeding should be controlled temporarily with pressure in the general region of the pedicle until the vessel can be found. The uterine stump is exposed by extending the abdominal incision caudally and retracting the bladder caudoventrally from the abdomen. The ovarian pedicles are exposed by extending the incision cranially and retracting the viscera with the intestinal mesentery. To find the left ovarian pedicle, the intestines are retracted to the right behind the mesocolon; to find the right ovarian pedicle, the intestines are retracted to the left behind the mesoduodenum. Balfour retractors will improve exposure. The ovarian pedicles often retract over the ureter just caudal to the kidney. To avoid damaging the ureter, the dropped vessel should be picked up with thumb forceps before it is clamped.

Canine Ovariohysterectomy

In adult dogs, the ovaries can be difficult to reach and retract. Therefore, the abdominal incision should start at the umbilicus and extend over the cranial third of the distance between the umbilicus and pubis. In puppies, the incision is made over the middle third of this distance since the ovaries are farther caudal (see p. 202). Subcutaneous fat attaches externally to the midline in dogs, making the linea difficult to find. Fat attachments should be transected at their base (only along midline) with a push-cut technique (pp. 84–85). Once the abdomen is open, the uterine horn can be found with a finger or spay hook. If a spay hook is used to find the uterine horn, it should be inserted into the caudal end of the abdominal incision in adult dogs to avoid inadvertently hooking the ovary or spleen. Small- or medium-sized pedicles are usually ligated with two encircling sutures. Large pedicles may require an additional transfixing-encircling suture. After the ovaries and uterus are removed, the abdomen should be examined for excessive hemorrhage. Some blood will normally pool on top of the intestines or in the paraspinal regions because of subcutaneous bleeding, especially if dogs are in heat, lactating, or pregnant during ovariohysterectomy.

Surgical technique: canine ovariohysterectomy

1. Make a midline abdominal incision (see Chapter 9).
2. Locate the left uterine horn with a spay hook.
    a. Hold the instrument so that the hook is pointing cranially or caudally.
    b. Insert the spay hook into the caudal end of the incision and press it against the left ventrolateral peritoneal surface (fig. 33-3).
    c. Angle the hook 30 to 40 degrees caudally.
    d. Slide the instrument laterally and dorsally along the left body wall until you feel resistance near the midline from the colon or spine.
    e. Turn the hook toward midline and straighten the handle so that it is perpendicular to the ventral abdominal wall.
    f. Slowly lift the hook straight up and extract it from the abdomen. Stop if there is any resistance during elevation (the spleen, ovary, or colon may be hooked).

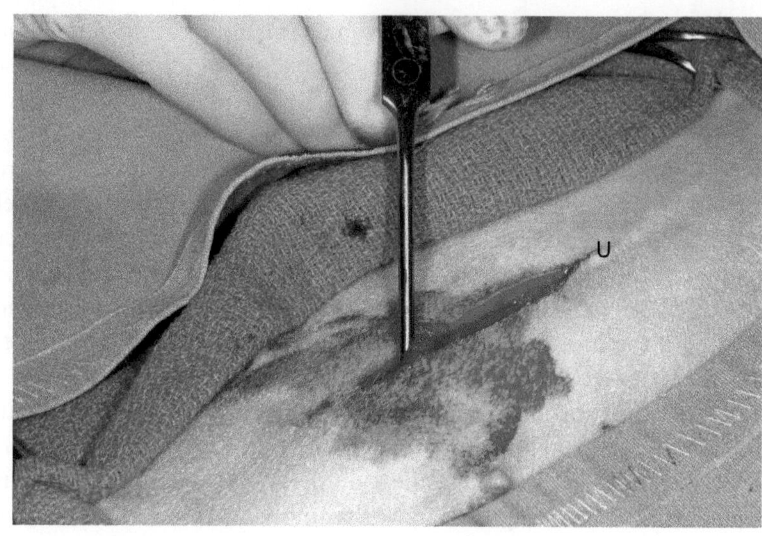

Figure 33-3 In the dog, insert the spay hook into the caudal end of the incision, with the hook tip pointing cranially. Angle the hook caudally and laterally and sweep it down the lateral body wall and across the dorsum of the dog. U = umbilicus.

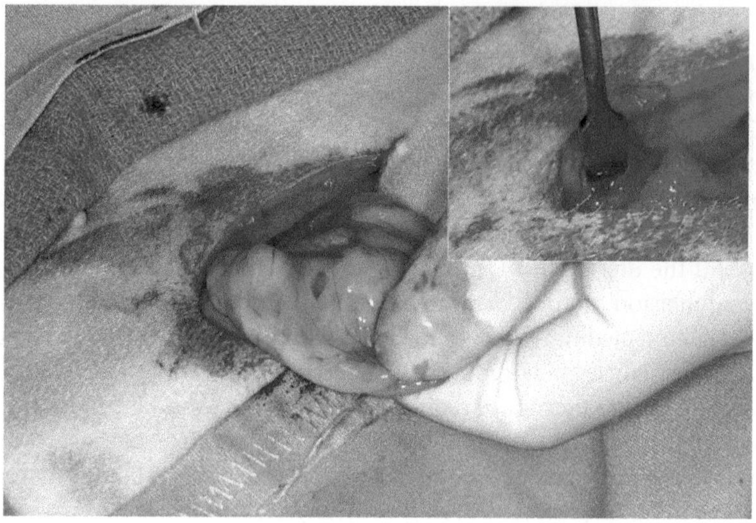

Figure 33-4 Sweep the hook across midline, then turn the tip toward midline and pull upward to expose the broad ligament (inset). Grasp the broad ligament and follow its medial surface dorsally to find the uterine body.

   g. Gently remove any omentum caught on the hook.

   h. Examine the remaining tissue on the hook (fig. 33-4). If it is fatty, it may be broad ligament. In that case, follow the medial surface of the tissue toward midline to find the attached uterine horn.

3. Retract the uterine horn to expose the proper ligament. The proper ligament is a small white band that extends from the ovary to the uterine horn.

4. Using tips of a hemostatic forceps, place a clamp on the proper ligament (see fig. 33-1).

5. Retract the proper ligament clamp caudally and upward to expose the ovary. If the ovary cannot be visualized or the pedicle is short, break the suspensory ligament.

   a. Retract the proper ligament clamp caudally.

   b. Insert an index finger into the abdominal incision and palpate the suspensory ligament as far cranially as possible (fig. 33-5).

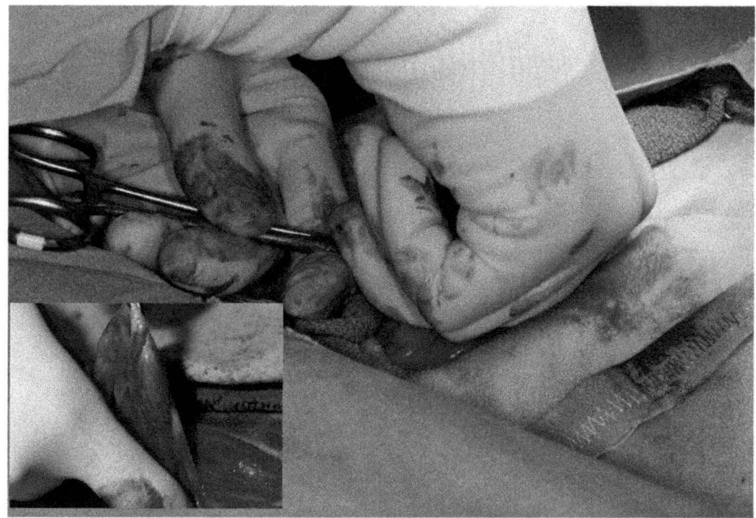

Figure 33-5 Grasp the proper ligament with a hemostat and retract it caudally as you stretch or break the most cranial extent of the suspensory ligament with your index finger. Press caudally and medially to stretch the ligament (inset).

   c. Strum the cranial extent of the ligament dorsally and toward midline while gently pulling the clamp caudally (see fig. 33-1).

   d. Alternatively, grasp the cranial end of the suspensory ligament between thumb and index finger. Rotate the index finger around your thumb toward midline. This will twist the ligament inward, stretching it where it crosses your index finger.

   e. If the suspensory ligament cannot be broken easily or the pedicle is fragile, extend the abdominal incision cranially so you can see the ligament and cut it with scissors.

6. Once the ovary is elevated out of the incision, make a window in the broad ligament caudal to the vessels.

   a. Perforate the broad ligament caudal to the pedicle with closed Kelly or Carmalt forceps.

      i. Many pedicles have multiple tortuous vessels. Make sure that the perforation is caudal to all the ovarian vessels.

      ii. Make the perforation dorsal to (below) the anastomosing branches of the ovarian and uterine vessels so these are included in the pedicle ligatures.

      iii. In many dogs, there is a translucent area caudolateral to the ovarian vessels that is an excellent site for broad ligament perforation.

   b. Open the forceps parallel to the ovarian vessels to reduce the chance of tearing a vessel (fig. 33-6).

7. Triple clamp the pedicle as far below the ovary as possible.

   a. Grasp a Kelly or Carmalt forceps with the tips facing upward and toward you. Clamp the pedicle with the tips of the forceps.

   b. Place the second clamp below the first one. To keep the ovary from slipping back into the abdomen, place the second clamp so that the

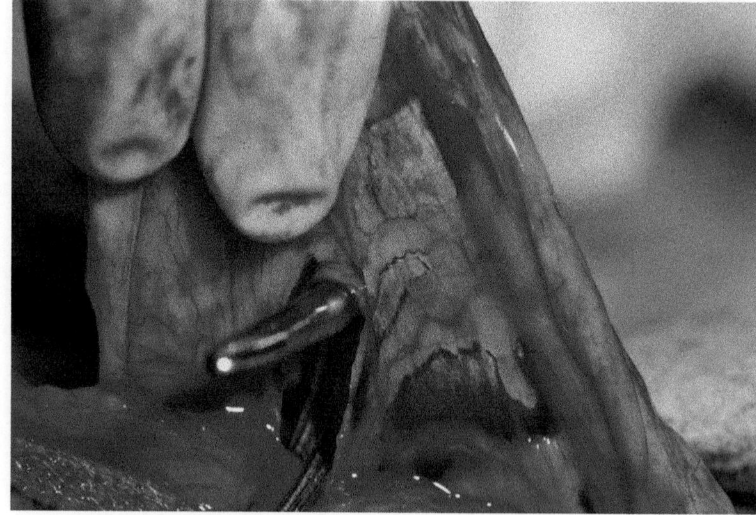

Figure 33-6 Open the forceps parallel to the ovarian vessels to make a window in the broad ligament.

tips are facing upward and away from you (so that the clamps will be pointed in opposite directions). This will keep the pedicle out of the abdomen while you place your first ligature.

i. To place the lowest clamp without an assistant, grasp the first clamp in your palm with your ring and pinky fingers under the clamp (fig. 33-7).

ii. Lift up on the clamp with your ring and pinky fingers. At the same time, push down on the body wall with your thumb and index or middle finger. This will expose more pedicle.

iii. Place the second clamp below and opposite to the first (this holds the pedicle out of the abdomen). Make sure skin and subcutis have not been included in the clamp.

c. Place a third clamp on the pedicle or across the uterine horn and associated vessels.

8. Ligate the pedicle (fig. 33-8).

a. Place an encircling ligature as far below the bottom clamp as possible. If desired, release the bottom clamp while tightening the first throw of the suture. This can be difficult to do without an assistant.

i. To place a modified Miller's knot, loop the suture around the pedicle and your finger twice. Pass the needle holder between the pedicle and the looped suture; grasp the free end of the suture and pull it under the crossing sutures and out the opposite side (see fig. 33-2). Tighten the suture to make an initial throw, then add 3 additional throws.

ii. To place a single-double ligature, pass the suture around the pedicle and tie one or two simple throws, then pass the suture ends around to the opposite side and tie one surgeon's throw and three simple throws.

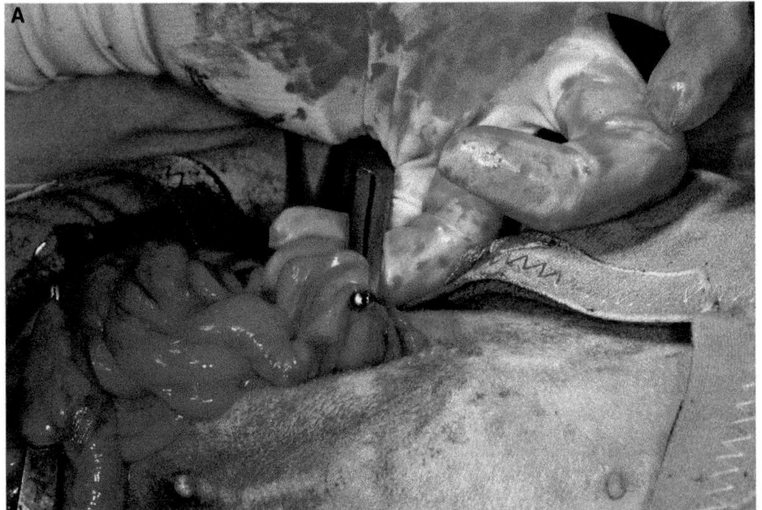

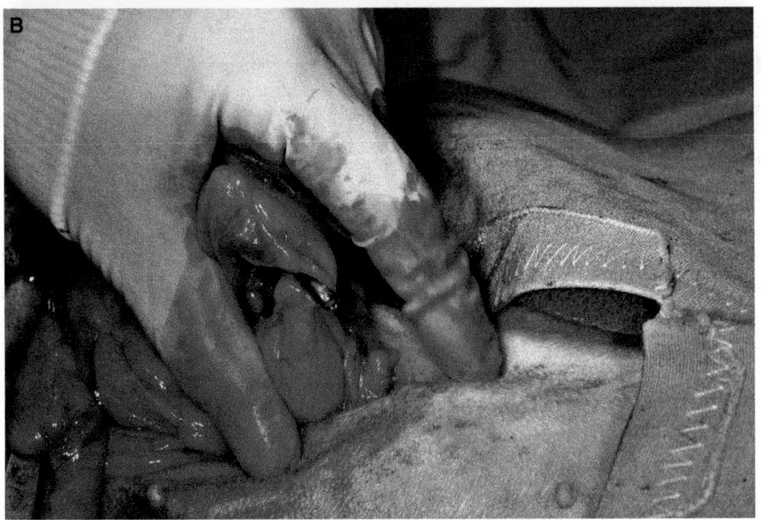

Figure 33-7 To expose more of the pedicle, elevate the clamp with ring and pinky fingers (A) while pushing the body wall away with thumb and index finger (B). This will allow you to place a second clamp below the first.

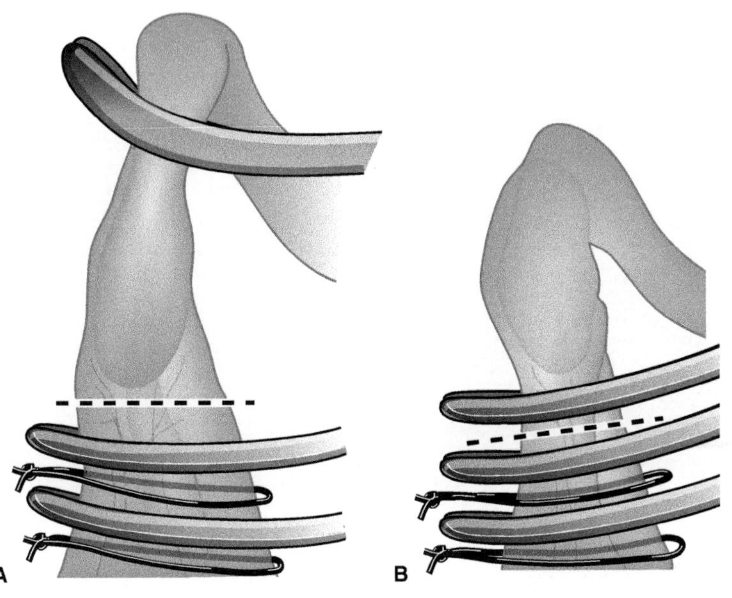

Figure 33-8 Triple clamp the pedicle; if the pedicle is short (left illustration), place two clamps on the pedicle below the ovary and one above. Ligate below and between the bottom two clamps, and cut above the second clamp.

b. Place a second ligature at the site crushed by the bottom clamp.
   i. If the pedicle is large, place a transfixing-encircling ligature (described above under Surgery).
   ii. If the pedicle is small, use an encircling ligature.

9. Transect the pedicle.
   a. Transect the pedicle between the two remaining clamps so that one clamp remains on the pedicle and one clamp prevents bleeding from the ovary and uterine horn.
   b. Use scissors when cutting the pedicle so that a small amount of tissue remains above the clamp. This will make the pedicle easier to grasp distal to the ligature.
   c. Make sure all ovarian tissue is removed.
10. Grasp an edge of the remaining pedicle adjacent to the clamp with thumb forceps. Do not lift up on the forceps or the tissue will tear.
11. Release the clamp and check the pedicle stump for bleeding. Return the pedicle to the abdomen.
12. Follow the uterine horn to the contralateral horn and ovary (fig. 33-9).
    a. If the bifurcation is not visible, grasp the uterine body without including the broad ligament in your fingers. Gently and firmly pull the horn cranially and upward and then caudally to expose the bifurcation.
    b. Alternatively, extend the incision caudally if the bifurcation cannot be visualized.
13. Break the suspensory ligament and ligate the second ovarian pedicle as described above.
14. Gently pull the uterine body out of the abdomen so that the bifurcation is exposed. Spread the broad ligament to identify the uterine artery and vein near the uterine body.

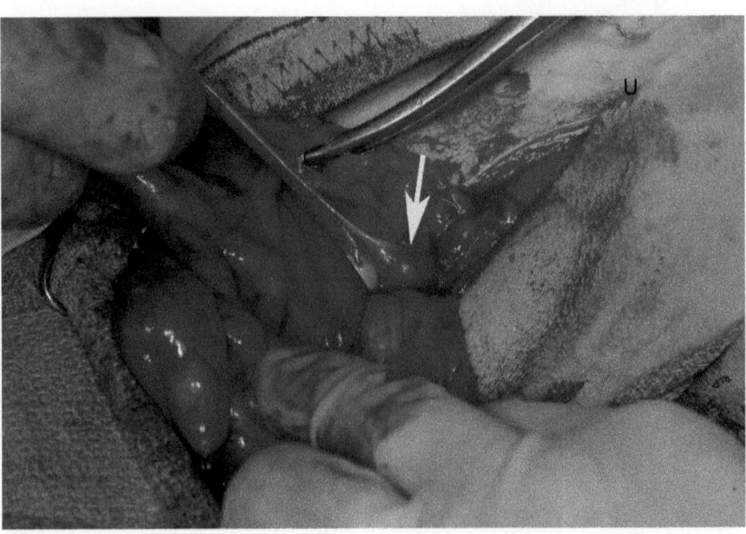

Figure 33-9 Pull the uterine horn forward (cranially), up, and back (caudally) to expose the bifurcation and second uterine horn (arrow). U = umbilicus.

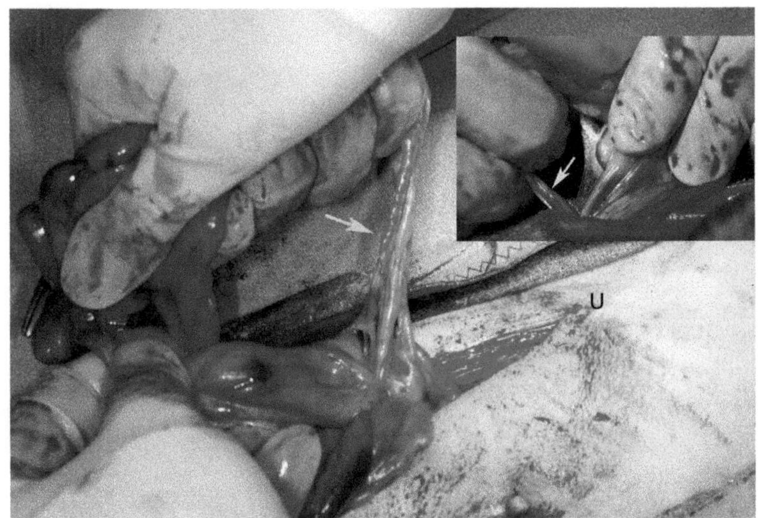

Figure 33-10 While protecting the uterine vessels and uterus with one hand, grasp the round ligament (arrow) and associated broad ligament with the other hand and pull it from the caudal abdomen. In small animals, grasp the round ligament with thumb and index finger (inset). U = umbilicus.

15. Tear the broad and round ligaments (fig. 33-10).
    a. Position your left hand with the pinky down and thumb up (like gripping a steering wheel).
    b. Wrap that hand around one broad ligament and the uterine body.
    c. With your right hand, spread out the remaining broad ligament so that you can see the uterine artery and vein and the round ligament of the uterus.
    d. While holding the uterus and opposite broad ligament in your left fist, protect the uterine vessels in the remaining broad ligament between your left thumb and middle finger (fig. 33-10 inset). Make sure the vessels are protected as low as possible along the uterine body.
    e. With a hemostat or your right thumb and forefingers, make a large opening in the remaining broad ligament lateral and parallel to the vessels and medial to the round ligament of the uterus.
    f. Grasp the remaining broad ligament with associated round ligament in your right fist. Make sure your right fist is positioned with the pinky down and thumb up.
    g. Twisting at the wrist, rotate your right hand inward toward the uterine body (pronate) to stretch and tear the broad and round ligaments out of the abdomen.
        i. The ligaments should tear beyond your right pinky and near the inguinal ring.
        ii. You may need to move your right fist lower on the ligaments to regrasp them as they stretch.
    h. Repeat on the opposite side, switching hand positions.
16. Ligate the uterine body above the cervix and below the bifurcation (fig. 33-11). Include the uterine arteries in the ligatures.
    a. Ligate a small uterine body with two encircling sutures.

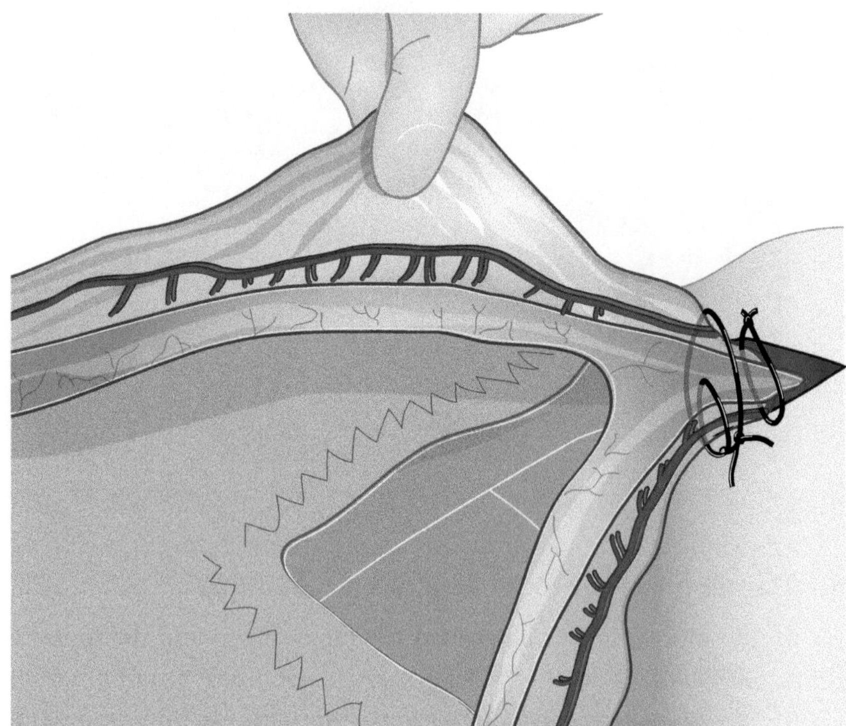

Figure 33-11 Ligate the uterus and uterine arteries and veins en masse with encircling and transfixing-encircling sutures.

b. Ligate a large uterine body with one encircling suture closer to the cervix and one or two transfixing-encircling sutures farther from the cervix. To place a transfixing-encircling suture on the uterus:
   i. Pass the needle through the lateral one-third of the uterine body.
   ii. Ligate the encircled tissue and uterine vessels with two simple throws.
   iii. Pass the suture around the remaining uterine body and vessels.
   iv. Ligate the entire uterine body and uterine vessels with two knots, starting with a surgeon's throw.

17. Clamp and transect the uterine body.
    a. Clamp the uterine body between the bifurcation and the ligatures.
    b. With thumb forceps, gently grasp the middle of the uterine body between the ligatures and the clamp.
    c. With Mayo scissors, transect the uterine body between the clamp and thumb forceps.
    d. Examine the uterine stump for hemorrhage and return it to the abdomen.

18. Check for bleeding before routinely closing the abdomen.
    a. Compress the abdomen from side to side to see if blood wells up.
    b. Some surgeons "sweep the gutters" with a gauze sponge: this should be performed with caution because ligatures are occasionally "wiped off" with this technique.

Feline Ovariohysterectomy

Cats can be spayed through a ventral midline or lateral flank approach. Surgical duration and complication rates are similar with flank and ventral midline approaches, except that cats that have undergone flank spays are more likely to develop postoperative wound drainage. Some veterinarians prefer flank ovariohysterectomy in lactating cats because the mammary glands can be difficult to separate on the abdominal midline. Because milk is sterile, subcutaneous leakage from mammary glands usually does not cause serious postoperative problems. Flank ovariohysterectomy is recommended in cats with mammary fibroadenomatous hyperplasia.

In cats, the ovaries are relatively easy to retract from the abdomen, but the uterine body is harder to expose. Therefore, the abdomen should be incised in the middle third of the distance between the umbilicus and pubis. The external rectus midline is easy to see once the subcutaneous fat has been incised; however, the linea can be very narrow. Falciform fat attaches internally along the abdominal midline, which can interfere with visualization and spay hook insertion. The uterus can be located with a spay hook or index finger. In the cat, the omentum is easier to hook than the broad ligament, so finding the uterus with a spay hook can be frustrating. The cervix is not visible in cats, and the ureters may be located in the broad ligament near the cervical region. To avoid damaging the ureters, the uterine body is ligated just below the bifurcation.

Surgical technique: feline ovariohysterectomy

1. Make a midline abdominal incision.
2. Locate the left uterine horn with a spay hook.
    a. Insert the spay hook into the abdomen at the cranial end of the incision.
    b. Hook the left uterine horn as described for the dog.
3. Clamp the proper ligament with the tips of a mosquito hemostatic forceps.
4. Retract caudally on the proper ligament clamp to expose the ovary.
5. If the ovary cannot be elevated from the abdomen, stretch the suspensory ligament.
    a. Retract the proper ligament clamp caudally to tense the ligament.
    b. Stretch the suspensory ligament. It is usually unnecessary to break it.
        i. Insert your index finger into the abdomen and press the cranial end of the suspensory ligament dorsally or medially (see fig. 33-1).
        ii. Alternatively, stretch the suspensory ligament with external compression (fig. 33-12). Place an index finger on the external surface of the body wall over the ligament. Press down on the

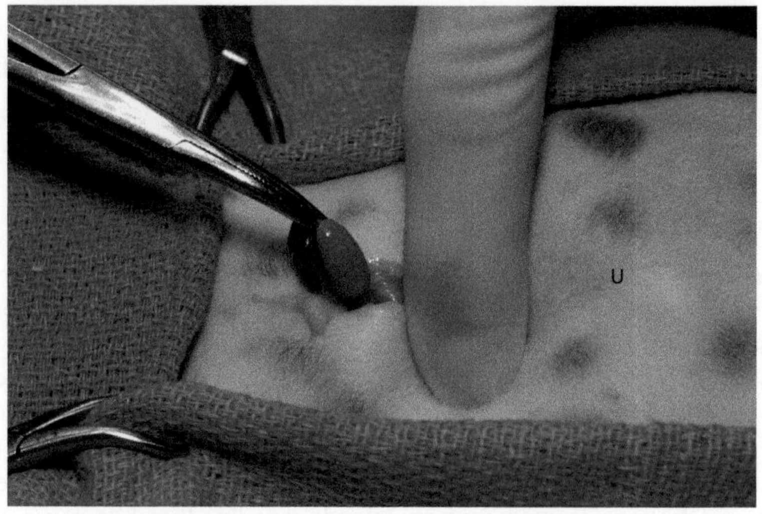

Figure 33-12 In cats, break or stretch the suspensory ligament by pulling caudally on the proper ligament clamp while pressing down on the abdominal wall over the palpable, taut suspensory ligament. U = umbilicus.

skin and abdominal wall over the suspensory ligament as you gently retract on the proper ligament clamp.

6. Ligate the ovarian pedicle with suture or a pedicle tie.
   a. Triple clamp large pedicles as in the dog. Ligate with encircling ligatures, placing one ligature below the bottom clamp and one ligature in the crush of the bottom clamp. Transect before or after ligation.
   b. Double clamp and transect small pedicles before ligating. Place one or two encircling ligatures below the bottom clamp.
   c. Use a pedicle tie on juvenile or small pedicles (see fig. 27-6 and pp. 226-227).
7. Transect the pedicle and check for bleeding, then follow the uterine body to the other ovary and repeat the process.
8. Use a hemostat to make openings in the broad ligament between the round ligaments and uterine vessels. Tear the round ligament of the uterus (fig. 33-13) using your thumb and index finger.

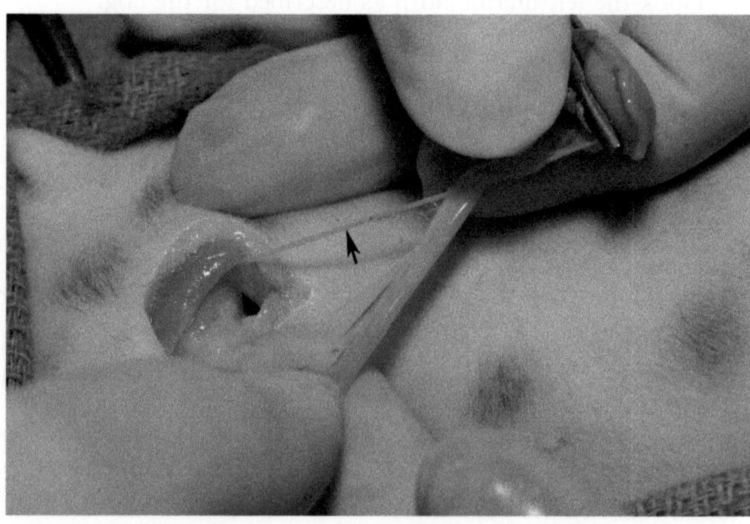

Figure 33-13 Round ligament of the uterus (arrow) in a cat.

9. Ligate the uterine body with two encircling ligatures or one encircling and one transfixing-encircling ligature 0.5 to 1 cm below the uterine bifurcation. Transect the uterus and check for bleeding.
10. Close the abdomen routinely.

Surgical technique: canine or feline ovariectomy

1. Make a midline or flank incision into the abdomen.
2. Locate the ovary and place a clamp on the proper ligament.
3. With a hemostat, fenestrate the mesovarium caudal to the ovarian vessels to make 1.5 to 2 cm window.
4. Pass a suture through the fenestration and around the ovarian vessels, and ligate the vessels, leaving sufficient space between the ovary and the ligature. Ligate the pedicle with one or two sutures.
5. Pass another suture through the fenestration and around the uterine horn 1–3 cm caudal to the proper ligament and ligate the uterine horn.
6. Remove the ovary.
   a. Sever the ovarian pedicle between the ovary and pedicle ligation, and sever the uterine horn between the ovary and uterine ligation, then remove the ovary.
   b. Alternatively, place 2 clamps between the pedicle ligature and ovary and 2 more between the uterine ligature and ovary, and sever the tissues between the clamps. Release the pedicle clamps and check for bleeding.

Postoperative considerations

Complications of ovariohysterectomy include abdominal hemorrhage, seroma formation, incisional infection, skin dehiscence, incisional hernia, urinary incontinence, and vaginal bleeding. More unusual complications include suture granulomas, ureterovaginal fistula formation, tetanus, colonic or urethral obstruction, and ureteral obstruction from ligation or adhesions. If a ureter is accidentally ligated during surgery, the ligature should be removed immediately. Once fibrosis occurs, ureteral resection and transplantation (ureteroneocystostomy) will be required. Permanent damage occurs with total ureteral occlusion of 4 or more weeks; affected animals will require ureteronephrectomy (Chapter 39).

Swelling is common after ovariohysterectomy, particularly in active animals. Some cats will develop a ridge of thick tissue along the incision line that can look like a hernia. The swelling is firm, nonpainful, and not reducible, however, and will resolve with time.

Ligated ovarian pedicles may bleed postoperatively because of poor technique. Ligature knots may be loose from half hitching, which is usually caused by upward tension on the suture during knot tying. Ligatures will not tighten properly if placed too close to a clamp, which prevents full compression of the tissue. If the subcutis is accidentally included in an ovarian pedicle ligature, the pedicle may be torn or the ligature pulled off as the rectus sheath is being apposed, or the rectus sheath will be missed during abdominal wall closure, increasing the risk of abdominal hernia formation. Abdominal bleeding can be slowed with sedation and a compressive abdominal bandage. If postoperative hemorrhage is a concern, temperature, pulse, mucous membrane color, capillary refill time, and packed cell volume should be monitored. The abdomen can also be examined with ultrasound to determine whether significant hemorrhage has occurred and surgical ligation is needed.

Postoperative vaginal bleeding may occur with uterine stump infections or poor ligation technique. Large vessels within the uterine wall may be penetrated inadvertently during transfixing suture placement. Bleeding may also occur if uterine ligatures are too loose or erode through the tissues. If vaginal hemorrhage develops immediately after surgery, the patient is sedated and monitored for anemia. Animals with significant or persistent hemorrhage should be evaluated for coagulopathies and infection. Rarely, animals may require ligation, transection, and culture of the uterine stump.

Delayed postoperative bleeding is noted in 30% of retired racing greyhounds 36 to 72 hours after elective surgery. The risk of bleeding can be reduced by administering epsilon-aminocaproic acid (500 mg PO q8h for 5 days), with the first dose given once the dog is able to eat and drink after surgery.

Clinical signs of estrus may develop if ovarian remnants are left in the abdomen ("ovarian remnant syndrome"). Most commonly, an entire ovary remains; however, pieces of ovarian tissue can also revascularize (fig. 33-14). Diagnosis of ovarian remnant syndrome in dogs is made by measuring baseline progesterone concentrations. In cats, progesterone concentrations are measured 7 days after administration of human chorionic gonadotropin. Affected animals should be explored while in estrus to facilitate visualization of the ovarian remnant or associated vessels.

Granulomas may develop when nonabsorbable sutures, especially braided reactive material or nylon bands, are used to ligate ovarian pedicles. Clinical signs include abdominal pain or sinus tracts that drain out the flanks or sublumbar region. Granulomas are usually removed through an abdominal approach.

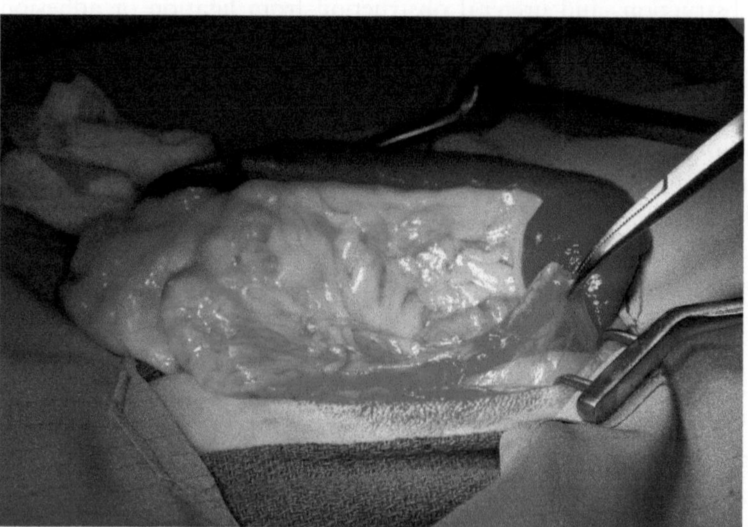

Figure 33-14 Ovarian remnant in a cat displaying signs of estrus.

Bibliography

Burrow R et al: Complications observed during and after ovariohysterectomy of 142 bitches at a veterinary teaching hospital. Vet Rec 2005;157:829–833.

Coe RJ et al: Feline ovariohysterectomy: comparison of flank and midline surgical approaches. Vet Rec 2006;159:303–313.

Ehrhardt EE: Performing an ovariectomy in dogs and cats. Vet Med 2012; V 107: 273-L 278.

Goethem BV et al: Making a rational choice between ovariectomy and ovariohysterectomy in the dog: a discussion of the benefits of either technique. Vet Surg 2006;35:136–143.

Hart BL, Hart LA, Thigpen AP, et al: Long-term health effects of enutering dogs: comparison of Labrador retrievers with golden retrievers. PLoS ONE 9 (7): e102241. Doc10.1371/journal.pone.0102241. Downloaded 8/10/16.

Hazenfield KM, Smeak DD: In vitro holding security of six friction knots used as a first throw in the creation of va vascular ligation. J am Vet Med Assoc 2014; V 245: 571-L 577.

Kustritz MR: Determining the optimal age for gonadectomy of dogs and cats. J Am Vet Med Assoc 2007;231:1665–1667.

Leitch BJ, Bray JP, Kim MJG, et al: Pedicle ligation in ovariohysterectomy: an in vitro study of ligation techniques. J Small Anim Pract 2012;53:592–598.

Marin LM, Iazbik MD, Alsdivar-Lopez S, et al: Epsilon aminocaproic acid for the prevention of delayed postoperative bleeding in retired racing greyhounds undergoing gonadectomy. Vet Surg 2012;41:594–603.

Salomon JF et al: Experimental study of urodynamic changes after ovariectomy in 10 dogs. Vet Rec 2006;159:807–811.

Smith AN: The role of neutering in cancer development. Vet Clin Small Anim 2014;44:965–975.

Chapter 34
Cesarean Section

The primary indication for cesarean section is treatment or prevention of dystocia. Dystocia may result from maternal factors, such as uterine inertia or pelvic canal narrowing, or fetal factors, such as malformed or malpositioned fetuses. For Boston terriers and English and French bulldogs, with their large heads and small pelvic canals, the rate of cesarean section is over 80%. Other breeds with high cesarean rates include Scottish terrier, Chihuahua, miniature and Staffordshire bull terriers, mastiff, German wirehaired pointer, Clumber spaniel, Pekingese, and Dandie Dinmont terrier. These high rates may indicate a preference by breeders or an actual increased risk of dystocia; in the case of the latter, veterinarians must be prepared to intervene surgically.

Preoperative management

Elective cesarean section should be performed as close to full term as possible. Gestation period is usually 63 days but can vary from 57 to 72 days. A reliable indicator of impending labor in dogs is a decrease in core body temperature to less than 100°F, which occurs within 24 hours of parturition. Serum progesterone concentrations also decrease to <2 ng/mL within 24 hours of parturition. In-house commercial assays for progesterone, however, are not highly accurate.

Before surgery, abdominal radiography or ultrasonography can be performed to determine the number of fetuses. On ultrasound, fetal heart rate less than 150 beats per minute indicates fetal distress. The animal is examined by digital rectal or vaginal palpation for the presence of a fetus in the pelvic canal. Blood work is evaluated for hypocalcemia, hypoglycemia, and toxemia. Pregnant animals normally have a packed cell volume of 30% to 35%, lower than normal because of increased maternal blood volume. A normal packed cell volume may indicate dehydration.

An intravenous catheter is placed, and intravenous fluid administration is initiated before anesthetic induction. Injectible antibiotics, such as first-generation cephalosporins, are given to animals that are toxic, septic, or carrying dead fetuses. Antibiotic therapy may also be initiated during surgery if there is a break in aseptic technique.

Anesthesia time should be kept to a minimum to improve neonatal survival. Before induction, the patient should be clipped and prepped. The surgery suite should be set up with appropriate equipment, and additional personnel should

Manual of Small Animal Soft Tissue Surgery, Second Edition. Karen Tobias.
© 2017 John Wiley & Sons, Inc. Published 2017 by John Wiley & Sons, Inc.

be available to resuscitate the neonates. If possible, the surgeon should be scrubbed and gowned by the time the animal is induced.

Animals can be premedicated with reversible agents such as opioids and midazolam. Drugs that pass rapidly through the placenta, such as phenothiazines, barbiturates, and ketamine, are usually avoided. Anticholinergic use depends on maternal and fetal status. Unlike glycopyrrolate, atropine crosses the placental barrier and will increase fetal heart rate. Oxygen is administered by mask before and during induction to reduce maternal and fetal hypoxia. The animal is induced in the surgery suite with propofol and then intubated and maintained on oxygen. If possible, anesthetic gas (e.g., isoflurane) is withheld until the neonates are delivered. Anesthesia can be maintained with an additional dose of propofol, or with a minimal amount of isoflurane. A midline lidocaine block (maximum, 10 mg/kg SQ) may reduce intraoperative anesthetic requirements. A final prep is performed before the patient is draped in. The surgery table can be tilted to elevate the head slightly, reducing pressure on the maternal diaphragm.

Surgery

Cesarean section is performed through a midline celiotomy. The incision should be long enough to expose the entire uterine body; the linea must be opened carefully to avoid damaging the gravid uterus. If a routine cesarean section is performed, the uterus is elevated gently from the abdomen and isolated with moistened laparotomy pads before it is incised.

In animals with dystocia that are undergoing concurrent ovariohysterectomy, a rapid en bloc uterine resection can be performed. After the uterus and ovaries are exteriorized, the broad ligament is broken down. The ovarian pedicles and uterine body are double or triple clamped, making sure that neonates are cranial to the transuterine clamps. The ovarian pedicles and uterus are transected within 30 to 60 seconds of clamping. The uterus is immediately handed to a team of assistants who immediately open it and remove the neonates. The remaining surgery on the dam is completed as for an ovariohysterectomy (see Chapter 33). Neonatal survival rates after en bloc resection are similar to those following cesarean section.

After extraction, the neonates are cleaned, dried, and briskly rubbed to stimulate respiration. If necessary, amniotic fluid can be suctioned from the nares and nasopharynx. If spontaneous respiration does not occur, oxygen delivery by mask or intubation should be initiated. Opioids transmitted from the dam's bloodstream to the neonate can be reversed by placing a drop of naloxone under the tongue; a second dose may be required after recovery. Doxapram does not improve oxygenation in neonates that are already breathing but can be tried (one drop under the tongue) as a last resort in those that have not responded to vigorous rubbing and oxygen supplementation. The umbilical cord should be ligated several centimeters distal to the body wall, transected, and disinfected. If the cord is of sufficient length, the enclosed umbilical vein can be used for intravenous injections. The neonate should be checked for congenital abnormalities before being placed in a 90°F incubator or warmed container.

Surgical technique: cesarean section

1. Perform a long midline celiotomy. Gently retract the uterus from the abdomen and isolate it with moistened laparotomy pads.

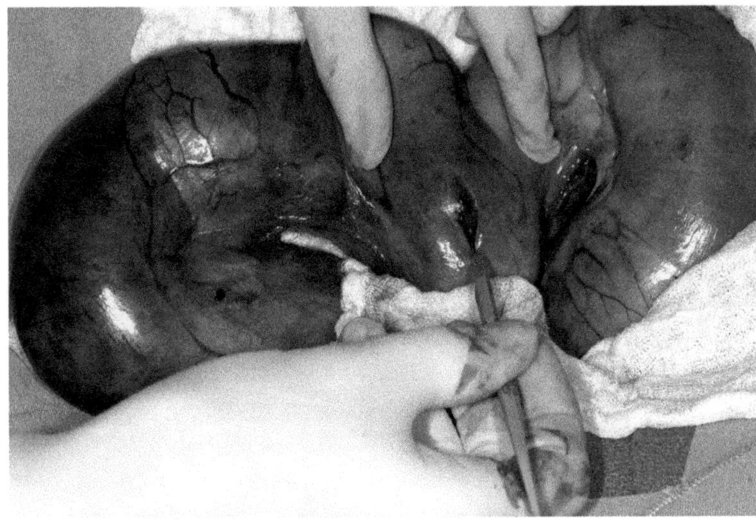

Figure 34-1 Incise the uterine wall carefully to avoid damaging the fetus.

2. Tent the uterine body with thumb forceps or tense between thumb and finger and gently make a midline partial incision through the uterine wall (fig. 34-1).
3. With Metzenbaum scissors, carefully extend the incision so that the fetus can be removed easily.
4. Extract the fetus through the incision (fig. 34-2). Break the amniotic membrane surrounding its muzzle with fingers or scissors.
5. Clamp the umbilical cord at least 3 cm distal to the neonate's abdominal wall (fig. 34-3) and transect it distal to the clamp. Aseptically pass the neonate to an assistant.
6. With gentle traction, remove the placenta (fig. 34-4) from the uterus if possible. If the placenta does not separate quickly and easily from the uterine wall, leave it in place and extract the next fetus.

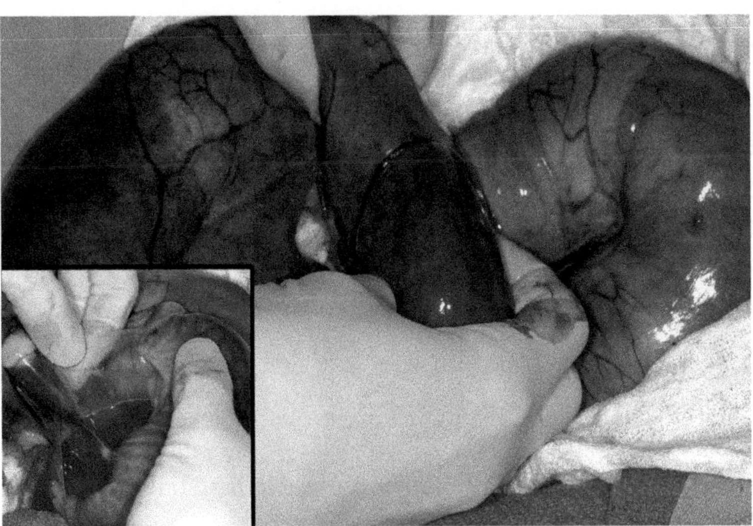

Figure 34-2 Extract the fetus through the midbody uterine incision and break the membranes around the neonate's muzzle (inset).

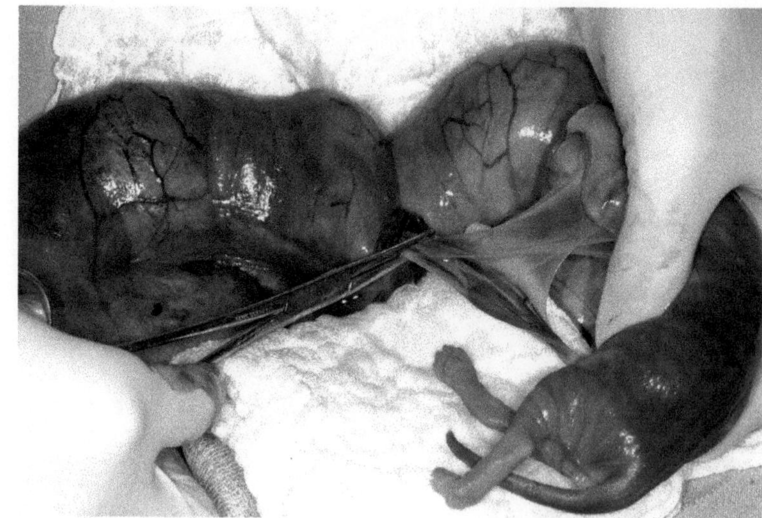

Figure 34-3 Clamp the umbilical cord at least 3 cm distal to the neonate's abdominal wall.

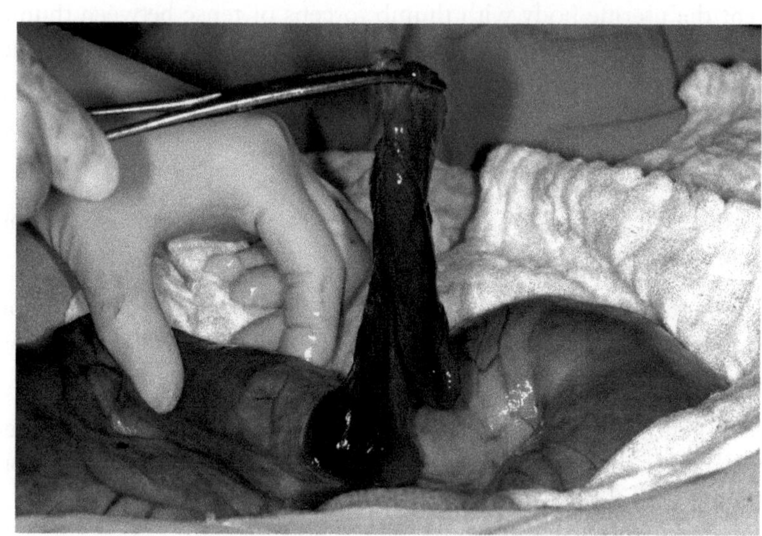

Figure 34-4 Remove the placenta from the uterus by gentle traction after delivery of each neonate.

7. Milk each subsequent fetus down the uterine horn, and manually extract it through the uterine incision (fig. 34-5).
8. Palpate the uterus to verify that all fetuses have been removed.
9. Close the uterine incision with 3-0 or 4-0 rapidly absorbable, synthetic monofilament suture in a one- or two-layer continuous appositional or inverting pattern (fig. 34-6). Sutures do not need to penetrate the mucosa.
10. After the uterus is closed, lavage and suction the abdomen to remove contaminants.
11. Appose the abdominal musculature with monofilament absorbable suture in a continuous pattern.
12. Close the skin with 3-0 rapidly absorbable material in an intradermal pattern.

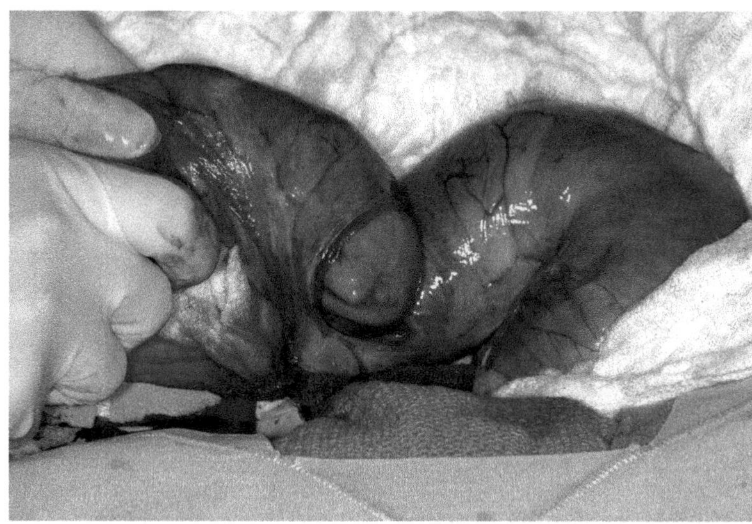

Figure 34-5 Milk each subsequent fetus down the uterine horn, and manually extract it from the uterine incision.

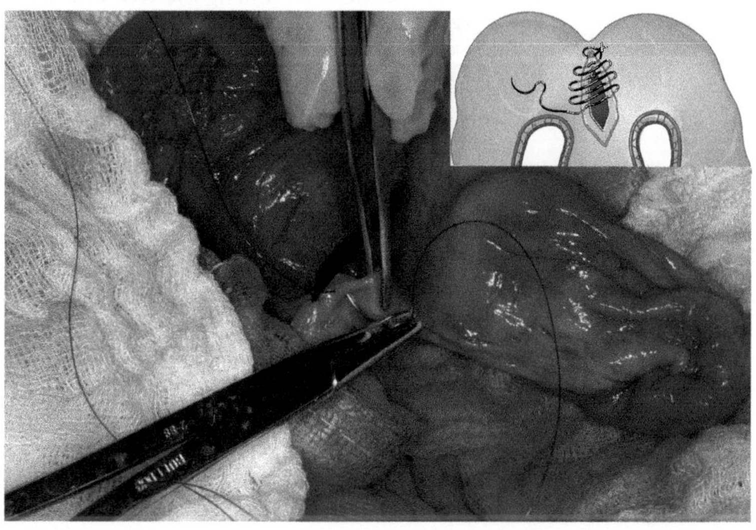

Figure 34-6 Close the uterine wall in a continuous pattern with partial thickness bites (inset).

Postoperative considerations

The abdominal skin should be cleaned to remove antiseptics and debris before neonates are placed with the dam. Neonates should be allowed to nurse as soon as possible to ensure colostrum intake. Mothers are monitored postoperatively for hypothermia, hypotension, hypocalcemia, neonatal rejection, and agalactia and are released from the hospital as soon as they are sufficiently awake. Ovariohysterectomy does not affect mothering ability or milk production.

Maternal complications may include hemorrhage, peritonitis, endometritis, mastitis, or wound infections. An odorless vaginal discharge should be expected for several weeks. Hemorrhage is more likely to occur with forcible separation of the placenta from the endometrium and may respond to oxytocin administration. Maternal mortality rates after cesarean section are 1%. Neonatal mortality rates range from 5% to 20%. Mortality rates are higher after prolonged dystocia or in puppies from brachycephalic dams or large litters. Neonatal mortality is increased when ketamine, barbiturates, xylazine, or methoxyflurane are used for anesthesia.

Bibliography

Evans KM, Adams VJ: Proportion of litters of purebred dogs born by caesarean section. J Small Anim Pract 2010;81:113–118.

Gendler A et al: Canine dystocia: medical and surgical management. Compend Contin Educ Pract Vet 2007;29:551–562.

Moon-Massat PF and Erb HN: Perioperative factors associated with puppy vigor after delivery by cesarean section. J Am Anim Hosp Assoc 2002;38:90–96.

Robbins MA and Mullin HS: En bloc ovariohysterectomy as a treatment for dystocia in dogs and cats. Vet Surg 1994;23:48.

Ryan SD and Wagner AE: Cesarean section in dogs: anesthetic management. Compend Contin Educ Pract Vet 2006;28:44–54.

Ryan SD and Wagner AE: Cesarean section in dogs: physiology and perioperative considerations. Compend Contin Educ Pract Vet 2006;28:34–42.

Smith FO: Challenges in small animal parturition: timing elective and emergency cesarean sections. Theriogenol 2007;68:348–353.

Chapter 35 Pyometra

Pyometra is the accumulation of purulent material within the uterus. This condition is reported in up to 25% of intact bitches by the age of 10 but occurs in less than 0.2% of female cats. In dogs pyometra occurs most commonly 1 to 3 months after the last estrus. Under the influence of progesterone, endometrial gland secretions increase and myometrial contractions decrease, resulting in fluid accumulation within the uterus. Subsequent bacterial contamination can lead to severe infection. Feline pyometra is more likely to occur after sterile matings, since cats are induced ovulators. Stump pyometra in spayed animals occurs only in those animals with residual ovarian tissue or that have received exogenous progestational compounds.

Animals with open pyometras may have vaginal discharge and mild, nonspecific clinical signs. Closed pyometra, however, can lead to sepsis, peritonitis, and death and is therefore considered a surgical emergency.

Preoperative management

Diagnosis of pyometra can often be based on history and clinical signs. In dogs uterine enlargement may be palpable and is often evident on abdominal radiographs; however, ultrasound is the most accurate preoperative test. Ultrasonographic findings that are characteristic for pyometra include uterine wall thickening and intraluminal fluid accumulation. Stump pyometra appears as a fluid-filled mass between the bladder or urethra and colon. In animals with open pyometra, large numbers of degenerate neutrophils and intracellular and extracellular bacteria are found on vaginal cytology.

Animals with closed pyometra should be evaluated for anemia, dehydration, azotemia, hypoglycemia, and electrolyte imbalances. Coagulation panels, platelet count, and blood pressure measurements should be assessed in patients with shock, sepsis, or suspected toxemia. Bacterial cystitis is found in at least 25% of dogs with pyometra; cystocentesis for urine culture is usually performed intraoperatively, when the bladder can be directly visualized, so that the uterus is not perforated inadvertently.

Before anesthesia, animals should receive fluids to correct dehydration and electrolyte and glucose abnormalities. Intravenous broad spectrum antibiotics, such as first-generation cephalosporins or ampicillin/sulbactam, should also be administered. The most common bacterial species is *Escherichia coli*, which has a specific affinity for progesterone-sensitized endometrium. Hetastarch,

Manual of Small Animal Soft Tissue Surgery, Second Edition. Karen Tobias.
© 2017 John Wiley & Sons, Inc. Published 2017 by John Wiley & Sons, Inc.

fresh frozen plasma, dopamine, and central venous pressure measurements may be required in septic or toxic animals (see pp. 122–124 for more information). In preparation for surgery, the abdomen should be clipped from xiphoid to pubis to permit sufficient exposure of the enlarged uterus.

Surgery

During linea incision, the abdomen is entered cautiously to prevent damage to the uterus. The affected uterus, which is usually large and friable, must be handled gently to prevent rupture. Risk of contamination can be reduced by isolating the exposed uterus with laparotomy pads. Pyometra removal is similar to routine ovariohysterectomy, except that the suspensory ligaments are often stretched out from increased uterine weight and do not need to be broken down. Although ovarian vessels are larger in dogs with pyometra, total ovarian pedicle diameter is often smaller than expected because of stretching and lack of fat.

After the uterus is removed, the uterine stump is cultured and then cleaned of any remaining discharge. Oversewing the uterine stump is not necessary and may increase the risk of granuloma or abscess formation. Laparotomy pads are discarded and gloves and instruments are changed before abdominal closure. A cystocentesis can be performed for urine culture. If contamination has occurred, the abdomen should be lavaged with several liters of sterile saline and cultured. Peritonitis may require treatment with abdominal drain placement (see pp. 125–127).

If stump pyometra is present, the abdomen is explored for ovarian remnants near the caudal poles of the kidneys. Ovarian remnants are easier to find when an animal is in estrus, which increases the vascularity to the remnant, or in diestrus, when the corpora lutea are evident. Ovarian remnants are located by retracting the intestines behind the mesoduodenum or mesocolon so that the dorsal abdominal walls, omentum, and regions around the caudal poles of the kidneys can be examined. If ovarian tissue cannot be identified, any thick tissue around the previously ligated pedicle sites is carefully resected and submitted for histologic examination. The ureters should be identified first, since they are often located directly dorsal to these sites. The uterine stump is dissected free from surrounding tissues and ligated, transected, and removed. Nonresectable stumps can be opened and omentalized, similar to prostatic abscesses (see Chapter 33).

Surgical technique: ovariohysterectomy for pyometra

1. Make a midline abdominal incision from pubis to midway between the umbilicus and xiphoid.

2. Gently exteriorize the uterus (fig. 35-1) and isolate it with moistened laparotomy pads.

3. If the ovaries are not readily accessible, place a clamp on the proper ligament to retract the ovary from the abdomen (fig. 35-2). Triple clamp, ligate, and transect ovarian pedicles as usual (see Chapter 33).

4. Tear the broad ligaments, as described for routine ovariohysterectomy (see fig. 33-10).

5. Triple clamp the uterine body above the cervix and transect it between the top two clamps before ligation. Remove the uterus from the surgical area.

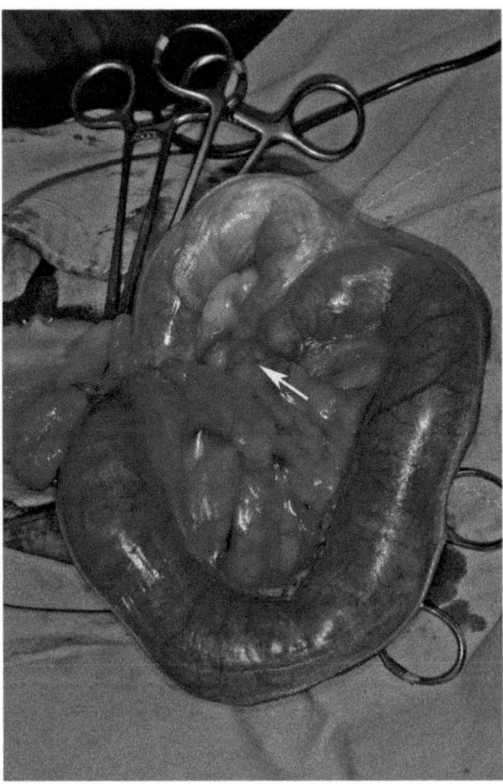

Figure 35-1 Exteriorize the entire uterus, including the cervix (arrow) through a large ventral midline abdominal incision.

6. Alternatively, ligate the uterus before transection.
   a. Place a clamp across the uterine body.
   b. With 0, 2-0, or 3-0 monofilament absorbable suture (depending on uterine size), place an encircling ligature at least 2 cm below the clamp and tie two knots, starting with a surgeon's throw or modified Miller's knot (see Fig 33-2). If the ligature is near the clamp, loosen ("flash") the clamp as the first throw is tightened.

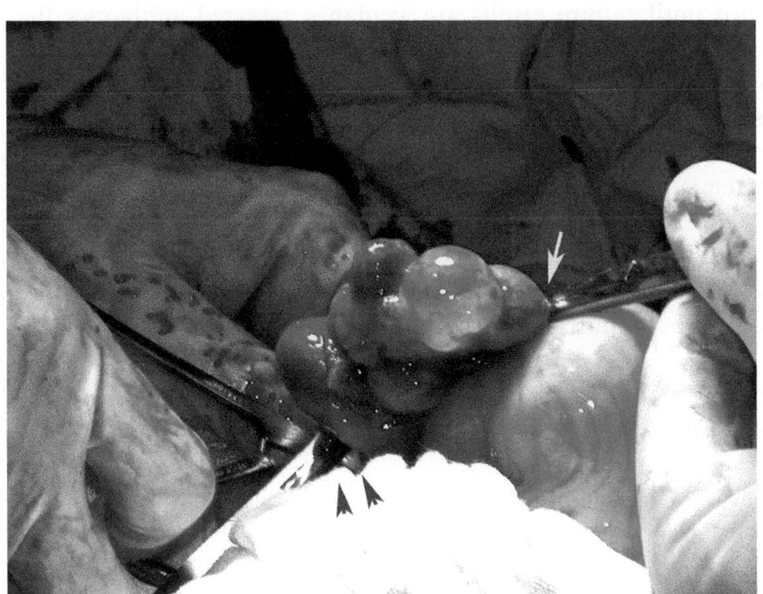

Figure 35-2 Place a clamp on the proper ligament (white arrow) to retract the ovary from the abdomen, then triple clamp (blue arrowheads) the ovarian pedicle.

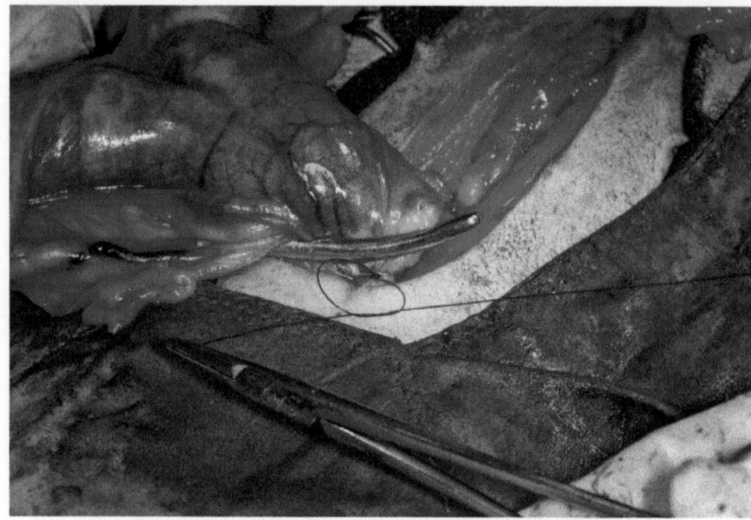

Figure 35-3 Ligate the uterus with encircling and encircling-transfixing sutures.

   c. Place one or two transfixing-encircling ligatures above the first ligature (see fig. 33-11), and below the clamp, using 0, 2-0, or 3-0 absorbable monofilament suture (fig. 35-3).

7. Wipe the stump clean of any discharge. If desired, suture the omentum to the stump with interrupted sutures of absorbable monofilament. Change gloves and instruments.
8. If contamination has occurred, lavage and suction the abdomen before closure.

Postoperative considerations

After surgery, supportive care is continued as needed. White blood cell count will often increase dramatically one day after surgery (e.g., a mature neutrophilia >50,000 cells/μL) but should improve after 2 to 3 days, once concentrations of chemotactic factors decrease. Empirical antibiotic treatment is continued until culture results are available; targeted antibiotics (based on sensitivity results) are continued for a minimum of 1 week when urinary or peritoneal infection is present. Urine should be cultured 1 week after antibiotics are discontinued to verify resolution of bacterial cystitis.

Complications after surgery are usually related to preoperative sepsis, endotoxemia, or peritonitis. Neurologic abnormalities, osteomyelitis, and splenic infarction from sepsis and vascular thrombosis have been reported 5 to 6 days after pyometra surgery. Postoperative mortality in bitches with pyometra is 3% to 8% but is increased to 57% in dogs with ruptured pyometra. In cats postoperative mortality is 5 to 6%.

Bibliography

Campbell BG: Omentalization of a nonresectable uterine stump abscess in a dog. J Am Vet Med Assoc 2004;224:1799–1803.

Dennis J, Hamm BL: Surgical and medical treatment of pyometra. Vet Med 2012;107:228.

Gibson A, Dean R, Yates D, et al: A retrospective study of pyometra at five RSPCA hospitals in the UK: 1728 cases from 2006 to 2011. Vet Rec 2013;173:396 doi: 10.1136/vr.101514; downloaded 8/11/16

Hagman R, Holst BS, Moller L, et al: Incidence of pyometra in Swedish insured cats. Theriogenol 2014;82:114–120.

Hamm BL, Dennis J: Canine pyometra: Early recognition and diagnosis. Vet Med 2012;107:226–228.

Kenney KJ, Matthiesen DT, et al: Pyometra in cats: 183 cases (1979–1984). J Am Vet Med Assoc 1987;191:1130–1132.

Chapter 36
Episiotomy

Episiotomy may be performed to facilitate vaginal mass or prolapse resection, laceration repair, urethral catheterization, or correction of vaginal strictures or congenital malformations. Episiotomy may be also necessary to assist in vaginal delivery of neonates.

Preoperative management

Intravenous broad spectrum antibiotics (e.g., first-generation cephalosporins) are administered prophylactically at induction and again in 2 to 6 hours. A caudal epidural block provides excellent intraoperative and early postoperative analgesia. If a rapid episiotomy is required (e.g., to remove a neonate), the vulva skin and muscle can be blocked on midline with 0.2 mL/kg of bupivicaine or lidocaine.

The perineal region is clipped around the vulva and anus. The vestibule and vagina are flushed with a dilute chlorhexidine or iodinated antiseptic solution during the surgical prep. The animal is placed in a perineal position with a purse-string suture in the anus (pp. 382–383), which is covered during draping.

Surgery

Episiotomy incisions usually extend from the dorsal commissure of the vulva to the vagina, which starts at the level of the urethral tubercle. Before incising the tissues, the vestibule should be palpated digitally or with a hemostat to identify its dorsal boundary. This will help prevent accidental damage to the anus. The skin incision can be made with a blade, followed by transection of underlying muscle and mucosa with scissors. Alternatively, one blade of a straight Mayo scissors can be inserted into the vulva until the tips reach the dorsal recess, and then all tissue layers are cut simultaneously. Hemorrhage can be controlled with electrocautery or pressure. In large dogs, Doyen clamps can be placed abaxial to the cut edges of the labia to reduce bleeding. Some surgeons crush all the tissues on midline with a Doyen or straight hemostatic forceps before incising; because the area is so vascular, subsequent necrosis from tissue crushing is uncommon.

Vaginal masses or prolapsed tissue are usually removed with a cut and sew technique, similar to rectal polyp removal (p. 217). The base of the tissue is partially transected, and the cut mucosal edges are reapposed before the remaining tissue is amputated and sutured. A urinary catheter should be placed before mass removal is attempted.

Manual of Small Animal Soft Tissue Surgery, Second Edition. Karen Tobias.
© 2017 John Wiley & Sons, Inc. Published 2017 by John Wiley & Sons, Inc.

Surgical technique: episiotomy

1. Incise the skin on midline with a blade (fig. 36-1). Cut the remaining subcutis, muscle, and mucosa on midline with Mayo scissors (fig. 36-2).
2. For a rapid episiotomy, insert one blade of a straight Mayo scissors (fig. 36-3) carefully into the vestibule without damaging any contents (e.g., masses or fetuses) and transect all layers simultaneously.
3. To improve exposure, place stay sutures in the cut edges and retract them laterally (fig. 36-4) or use a Gelpi retractor.
4. Identify the urethral opening and catheterize the urethra if tissue is to be resected.
5. If a mass resection is performed, appose mucosal margins with 3-0 or 4-0 rapidly absorbable monofilament suture.
6. Reappose the vestibular mucosa in a simple continuous pattern with 3-0 or 4-0 rapidly absorbable suture (fig. 36-5). Start the suture at the dorsal vulvar commissure to reappose the margins.

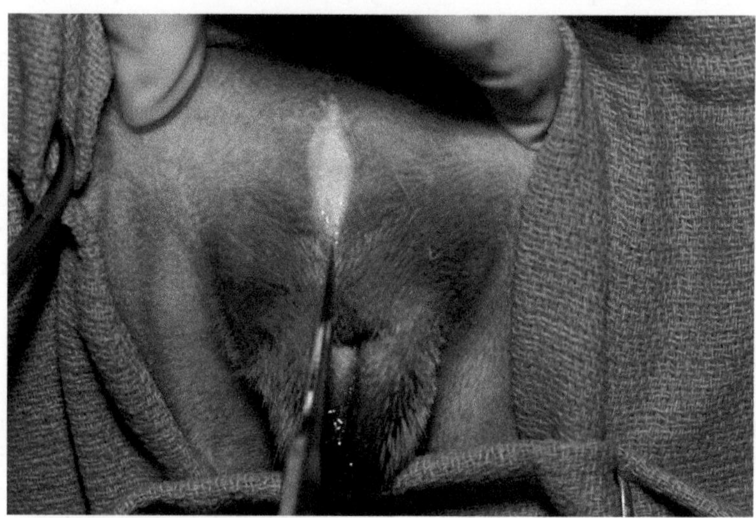

Figure 36-1 For an elective episiotomy, incise the skin on midline with a blade.

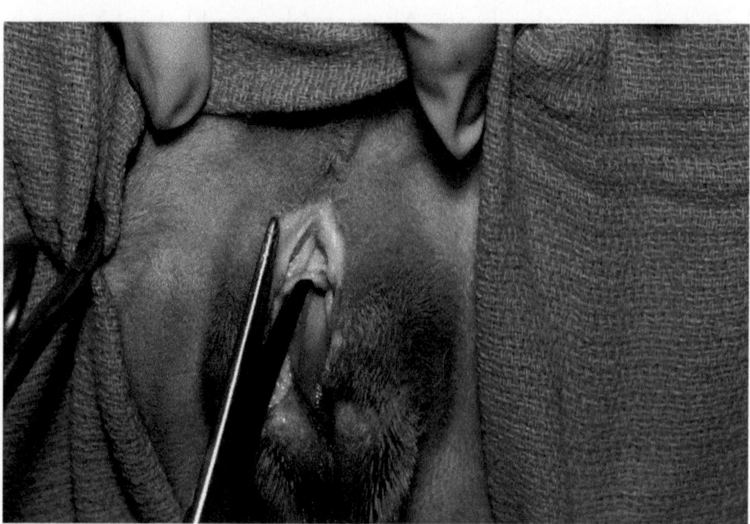

Figure 36-2 Transect the remaining layers with scissors.

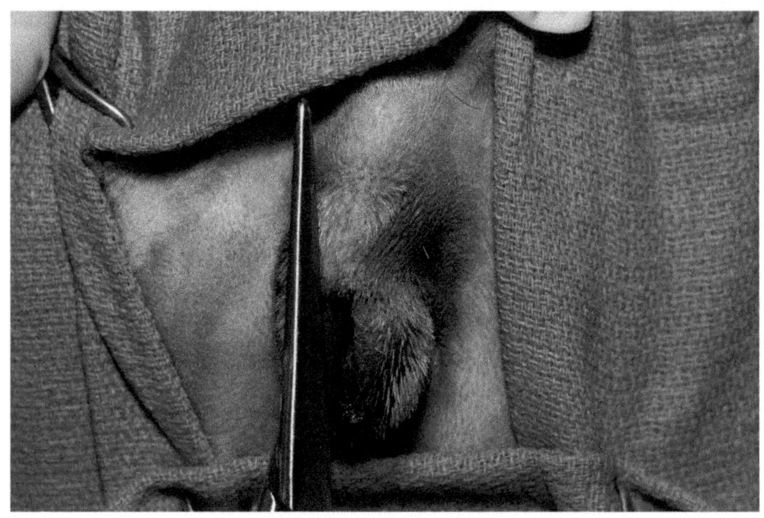

Figure 36-3 For emergency episiotomy, insert a straight Mayo scissors blade carefully into the vestibule and transect all tissue layers simultaneously

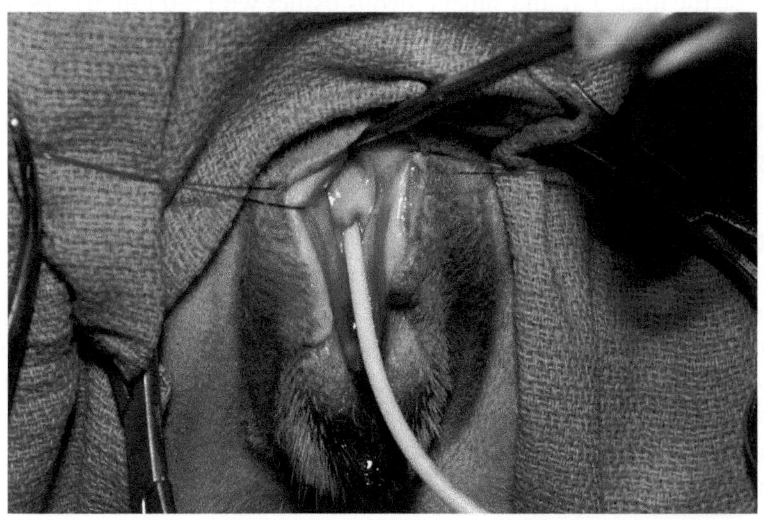

Figure 36-4 Retract the vestibular wall with stay sutures and place a urinary catheter before performing any tissue resection.

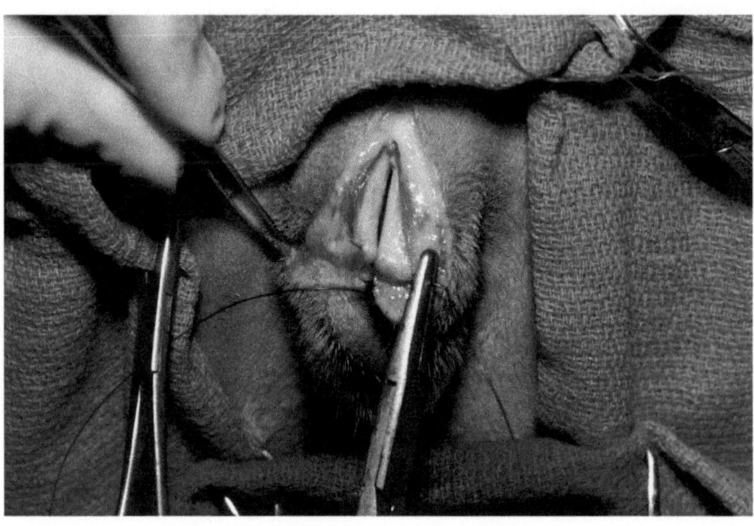

Figure 36-5 Reappose the vestibular mucosa in a continuous pattern, starting ventrally to reappose the dorsal vulvar commissure.

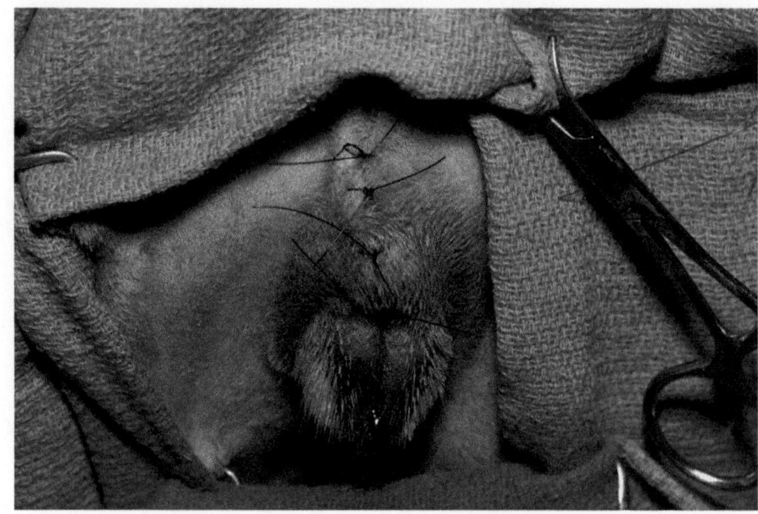

Figure 36-6 Final appearance after skin closure.

7. Close the muscular and subcutaneous tissues with 3-0 rapidly absorbable suture in a simple continuous or simple interrupted pattern.
8. Appose skin edges with interrupted nylon sutures, starting at the ventral extent of the incision to realign the vulvar edges (fig. 36-6). Alternatively, appose the skin with an intradermal pattern.

Postoperative considerations

After surgery, animals should wear an Elizabethan collar for 7 to 10 days to prevent self-trauma. The most common complications are swelling and discomfort. Other complications are rare and most likely associated with the underlying condition. Most vaginal tumors are benign tumors of fibrous tissue or smooth muscle origin; recurrence of these is unlikely with appropriate excision.

Bibliography

Cain JL. An overview of canine reproduction services. Vet Clin N Am Small Anim Pract 2001;31:209–218.

Kydd DM and Burnie AG. Vaginal neoplasia in the bitch: a review of forty clinical cases. J Small Anim Pract 1986;27:255–263.

Mathews KG. Surgery of the canine vagina and vulva. Vet Clin N Am Small Anim 2001;31:271–290.

Nelissen P and White RAS. Subtotal vaginectomy for management of extensive vaginal disease in 11 dogs. Vet Surg 2012;41:495–500.

Chapter 37
Episioplasty

Resection of the perivulvar folds is known as vulvoplasty or episioplasty. Indications for episioplasty include perivulvar dermatitis, vaginitis, cystitis, or incontinence. In dogs that are obese or have small, cranially positioned ("recessed") vulvas (fig. 37-1), surrounding folds of skin and fat can trap material around and within the vulva. Local friction and accumulated moisture predispose affected animals to vaginitis, dermatitis, ulcerations, and thickening of the skin, which exacerbates the problem. Skin folds overlying the vulva may also trap urine within the vagina, resulting in ascending cystitis and apparent urinary incontinence. Affected animals are often obese medium- or large-breed dogs. Clinical signs may include excessive grooming, frequent scooting, malodor, dermatitis, positional urine leakage, or vaginal discharge.

Preoperative management

Before surgery, urine and vaginal cultures are obtained by cystocentesis and sterile swab, respectively. Skin scrapes and cytology should be performed to determine if the animal has parasites or a local or generalized yeast or bacterial infection. Coagulase-positive Staphylococci are the most common bacteria present in skin fold dermatitis. If the dermatitis is severe, the animal should be treated with systemic and topical antimicrobials and anti-inflammatories. In these patients, surgery should be delayed until the skin is improved. Culture and sensitivity are important, as dogs with chronic or nonresponsive dermatitis may have developed a resistant infection.

If antibiotics have not been administered before the procedure, they should be given intravenously immediately after anesthetic induction and again 2 to 6 hours later. Antibiotics are usually continued for at least 7 days after surgery in dogs with infections. If possible, a caudal epidural nerve block is performed to provide additional analgesia during and immediately after surgery. A purse-string suture is placed in the anus to limit contamination. The perivulvar and perianal region is clipped and prepped, including the base of the tail. The animal is placed in a perineal position with the legs hanging over the padded edge of the surgery table, and the tail is pulled forward.

Manual of Small Animal Soft Tissue Surgery, Second Edition. Karen Tobias.
© 2017 John Wiley & Sons, Inc. Published 2017 by John Wiley & Sons, Inc.

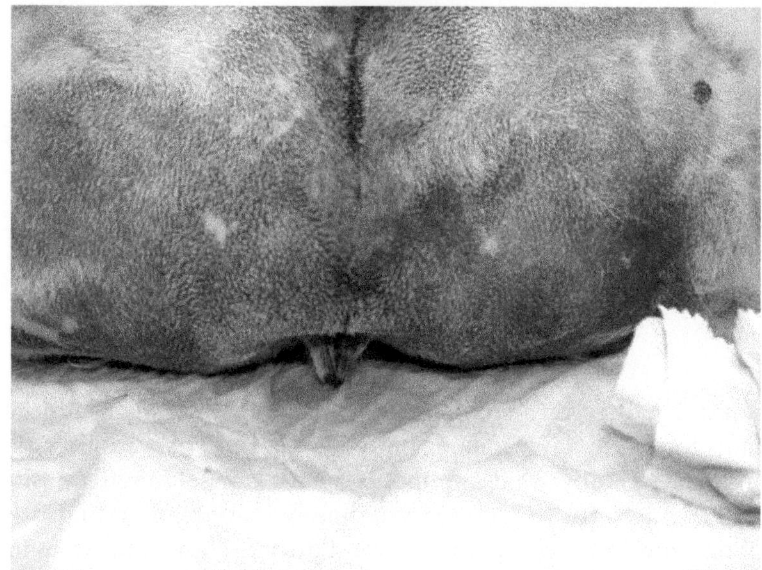

Figure 37-1 Obstruction of the vestibular opening in a dog with obesity and an underdeveloped ("infantile") vulva. This dog was presented for urinary incontinence and recurrent cystitis.

Surgery

The amount of skin to be removed can be estimated by grasping the redundant folds of skin dorsal and lateral to the vulva with fingertips (fig. 37-2). The amount of skin grasped should be gradually increased until the vulva is repositioned caudally and slightly dorsally. The proposed skin incision sites can be outlined with a sterile marker or crushed with Allis tissue forceps (fig. 37-3). After incision, the incised skin is freed from its subcutaneous attachments with a combination of blunt and sharp dissection. On the dorsal midline, dissection must proceed cautiously, since the vestibular wall is more superficial at this location. The surgeon can insert a sterile probe through the vulvar opening into the vestibule to confirm its location. Lateral to the

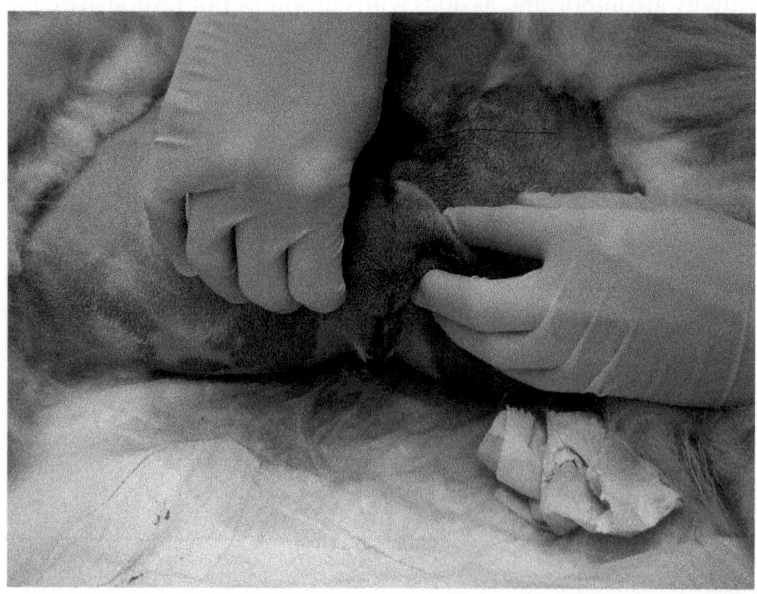

Figure 37-2 Grasp the redundant folds at their base to determine the amount of resection needed.

vestibule, fat can be resected or left in place. Subcutaneous closure is optional but is recommended in animals with excessive or traumatic perivulvar fat resection or incision-line tension. The skin is apposed with interrupted sutures of 3-0 nonabsorbable, monofilament material. If the sutures are under tension, the tail can be released to provide more laxity during closure.

Surgical technique: episioplasty

1. Grasp the folds of skin with the fingers of your nondominant hand until the vulva is exposed and no longer recessed (fig. 37-2).
2. Place the jaws of an Allis tissue forceps around the grasped fold. Close the forceps to crush the flap at its base (fig. 37-3). Repeat the process at five or six sites around the vulva. This will produce two rows of crush marks: an outer, more dorsal row and an inner, ventral row. The resulting crush marks will serve as landmarks for the two skin incisions. Alternatively, use a sterile marker to outline skin to be resected.
3. Make a horseshoe-shaped skin incision along the outer row of marks dorsal and dorsolateral to the vulva (fig. 37-4).

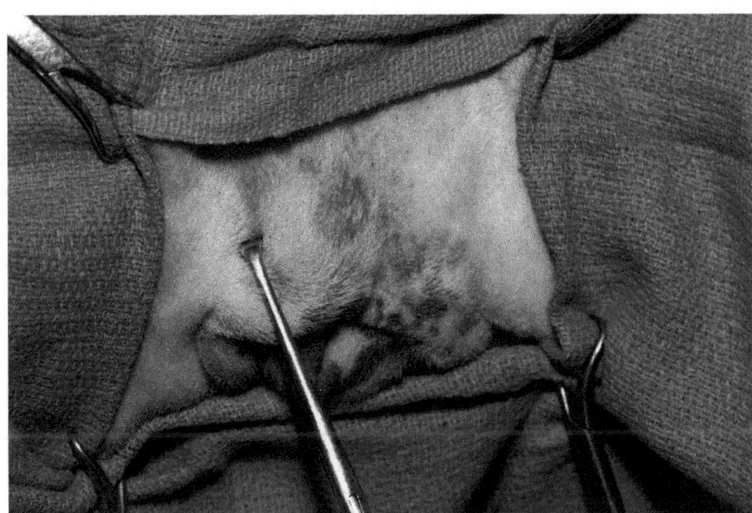

Figure 37-3 Compress the fold at its base with Allis tissue forceps; repeat at several sites. Use the resultant crush marks as landmarks for tissue incision.

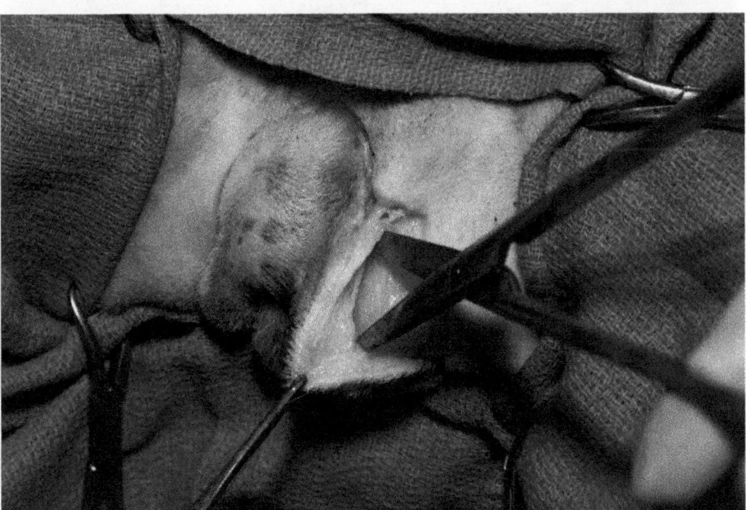

Figure 37-4 Incise the dorsal skin in a horseshoe shape, and elevate the skin from the underlying tissues with sharp and blunt dissection.

4. Continue the skin incision along the outer row of marks lateral to the vulva.
    a. The incision should extend to the level of the ventral vulvar commissure on either side of the vulva.
    b. The skin incision will be close to the vulva ventrolaterally and far from the vulva dorsally and dorsolaterally.
5. Before making the second skin incision, check the position of the inner row of crush marks to make sure that the amount of skin to be removed is appropriate.
    a. Grasp the ventral edge of the incised skin.
    b. Pull the associated flap of skin dorsally until the vulva is repositioned to the desired location.
    c. Compare the location of the inner row of crush marks to the dorsal edge of the skin incision.
        i. Because the dorsal skin edge will retract, the inner row of crush marks will likely be 0.5 to 1cm below the dorsal skin edge when the vulva is properly repositioned.
        ii. If the amount of skin to be removed seems excessive, redraw the ventral incision line. The final closure should not be under excessive tension.
6. Make the ventral, inner incision in a gentler arc (fig. 37-5). The resected area will be crescent-shaped and should extend to a level parallel with the ventral vulvar commissure.
7. With Metzenbaum scissors, dissect and transect the subcutaneous tissue to remove the skin. Avoid damaging the vestibule on the midline (fig. 37-6).
8. If desired, remove any excess subcutaneous fat laterally with sharp transection.

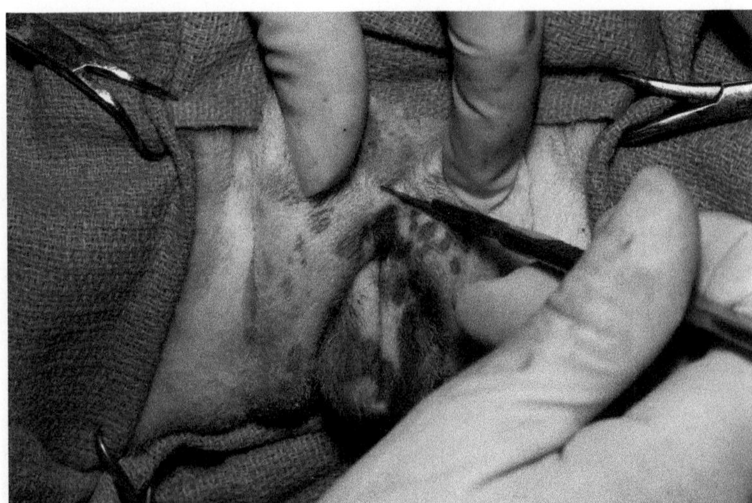

Figure 37-5 Pull the flap dorsally to check the final position of the vulva; then make the ventral, inner incision.

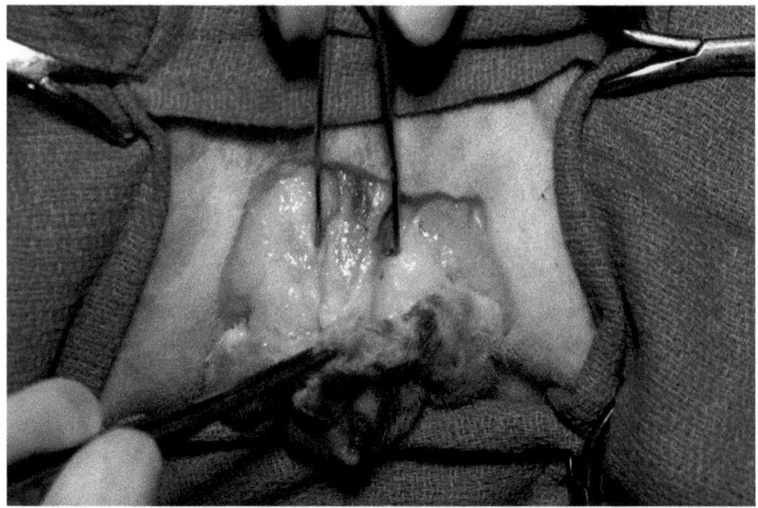

Figure 37-6 Appearance after skin resection. Note that the vestibule and overlying retractor clitoridis muscles (between thumb forceps jaws) are very superficial on the dorsal midline.

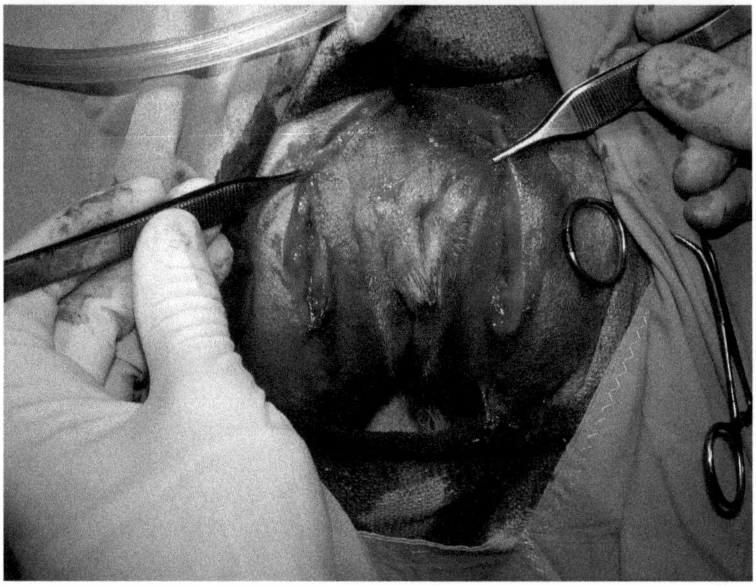

Figure 37-7 Place the first three skin sutures at the 10, 12, and 2 o'clock positions (thumb forceps). Note that the skin resection extends to the level of the ventral vulvar commissure.

9. Place three interrupted skin sutures around the dorsal third of the incision to evaluate the final vulvar position (fig. 37-7).
   a. Place the first skin suture on dorsal midline (the 12 o'clock position).
   b. Grasp the ventral edge of the skin incision at the 10 o'clock position. Pull the skin dorsally and laterally. Adjust the skin position so that the vulva remains exposed but does not gape open. Place a skin suture to keep the vulva in the appropriate position.
   c. Repeat the process at the 2 o'clock position.
   d. If the vulvar position needs to be readjusted, remove and replace the dorsolateral sutures as needed. If the vulva is still recessed, remove all the skin sutures and resect more skin.
10. If desired, appose the subcutaneous tissues in the remaining gaps with interrupted absorbable sutures, burying the knots.
11. Complete the skin closure with simple interrupted sutures (fig. 37-8). Remove the anal purse-string suture.

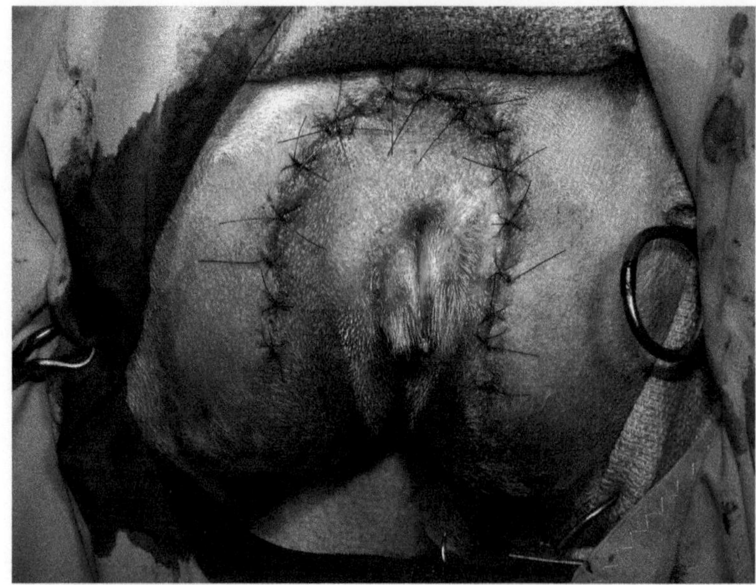

Figure 37-8 Final appearance. The vulva will relax to a more ventral position once the tail is released.

Postoperative considerations

To prevent self-trauma, the animal should wear an Elizabethan collar until the skin is healed. Residual yeast pyoderma should be treated with antifungal shampoos and topical medications. Weight reduction should be instituted in obese animals.

Potential complications may include swelling, bruising, dehiscence, and recurrence of clinical signs. Dehiscence usually occurs from self-trauma. Animals with perineal sutures tend to rub the surgical site on furniture and carpets; affected animals may require sedatives or antihistamines to reduce this behavior and decrease pruritus. Additionally, owners can use boy's briefs, boxer shorts, or a child's onesie (one piece body suit) with the "fly" facing upward or a hole cut in the cloth to provide a gap for the tail to exit. The clothing is removed or, in the case of the onesie, unsnapped when the dog is taken out to urinate and defecate.

Clinical signs may reoccur with insufficient skin removal or progressive obesity. When the procedure is performed appropriately, however, almost all dogs with vaginitis and recurrent urinary tract infections from a recessed vulva have resolution of signs. Urine pooling resolves when urine retention is secondary to vulvar obstruction by perivulvar folds. Urine pooling may persist if vaginal stricture or vestibulovaginal stenosis is present.

Bibliography

Crawford JT and Adams WM: Influence of vestibulovaginal stenosis, pelvic bladder, and recessed vulva on response to treatment for clinical signs of lower urinary tract disease in dogs: 38 cases (1990–1999). J Am Vet Med Assoc 2002;221:995–999.

Hammel SP and Bjorling DE: Results of vulvoplasty for treatment of recessed vulva in dogs. J An Anim Hosp Assoc 2002;38:79–83.

Lightner BA et al: Episoplasty for the treatment of perivulvar dermatitis or recurrent urinary tract infections in dogs with excessive perivulvar skin folds: 31 cases (1983–2000). J Am Vet Med Assoc 2001;219:1577–1581.

Section 5 Surgery of the Urinary Tract

Chapter 38
Renal Biopsy

Renal biopsies are most useful for determining the underlying etiology of renal dysfunction in animals with acute renal failure of unknown cause or with persistent, marked proteinuria (UPC ≥ 3.5) of glomerular origin. In patients with chronic renal failure or end-stage kidney disease, biopsy is unlikely to change the treatment and may further reduce renal function. Renal biopsies are also contraindicated in animals with moderate to severe thrombocytopenia or coagulopathies, uncontrolled systemic hypertension, severe azotemia, severe hydronephrosis, large renal cysts, perirenal abscesses, or extensive pyelonephritis.

Needle (e.g., Tru-cut) biopsy of the kidneys can be performed under ultrasound guidance or through a lateral, keyhole approach. A surgical approach provides higher-quality samples and has fewer complications. Surgery is particularly recommended for dogs less than 5 kg or animals that require other procedures. In healthy animals, serial needle biopsies have minimal effect on renal function and structure, except when major blood vessels are damaged during the procedure. The effect of biopsy on renal function in dogs and cats with kidney disease, however, has not been evaluated.

Preoperative management

Before renal biopsy, a complete blood count, platelet count, biochemistry panel, urinalysis, and coagulation panel should be evaluated and any serious metabolic abnormalities corrected. Animals with glomerular disease may have significant protein loss that requires treatment with hetastarch or other colloids. Arterial blood pressure and retinal examination should be performed to detect systemic hypertension. Renal size and architecture should be evaluated with ultrasound to detect conditions for which renal biopsy is contraindicated.

Animals should be clipped and prepped from midthorax to the caudal abdomen. Suction and hemostatic gel should be available in case bleeding is excessive.

Surgery

Surgical renal biopsies are performed through a midline abdominal incision. The abdomen is incised from the xiphoid to a point midway between the umbilicus and pubis, and the abdominal wall is retracted with Balfour

Manual of Small Animal Soft Tissue Surgery, Second Edition. Karen Tobias.
© 2017 John Wiley & Sons, Inc. Published 2017 by John Wiley & Sons, Inc.

retractors. To expose the kidneys, the intestines are tucked behind the mesoduodenum or mesocolon, which is retracted away from the kidney. If a needle biopsy is performed, the kidney can usually be stabilized in its normal location. For a wedge biopsy, the kidney is elevated from the paralumbar fossa.

Compared with needle (e.g., Tru-cut) biopsy, a wedge biopsy provides superior-quality samples. To control hemorrhage during wedge biopsy, the renal artery or arteries should be occluded: the left kidney may have more than one artery. Once arterial blood flow is occluded, the kidney should soften in 30 to 60 seconds. The renal parenchyma will still ooze dark blood when cut; if the renal artery is not occluded, however, hemorrhage will be bright red, pulsatile, and copious. After the tissue wedge is removed, the renal capsule must be apposed while the artery is still occluded. Because renal capsule is thin, superficial parenchyma is usually included in the suture bites. The needle and attached suture must be passed gently through the tissues, following the curve of the needle. If the needle is lifted during passage or the suture is tied too tightly, the parenchyma will tear. Renal artery occlusion should be limited to 20 minutes.

In most animals, a needle sample provides sufficient tissue to obtain an accurate diagnosis of the underlying condition. For needle biopsies, 14- to 18-gauge spring-loaded instruments have been recommended. The 14-gauge needle provides larger numbers of glomeruli and less crushing artifact. Needle samples are usually obtained in the cortex across the renal pole or along the length of the convex surface of the kidney. The semi-automated instruments often have a slotted needle surrounded by a cutting sheath. The needle is passed into the tissues, and the spring is released so the sheath slides over the needle, trapping a piece of tissue in the needle slot. To avoid crushing artifact, samples can be dislodged from the biopsy instrument into a container by directing a fine stream of sterile saline onto the open guide with a syringe and needle.

Because sample size is small, at least two samples should be obtained when needle biopsy is performed. In animals with glomerular disease, one sample should be placed in formalin for light microscopy. The second sample should be divided into two pieces containing glomeruli; one piece should be placed in a fixative suitable for electron microscopy, and the second should be frozen for immunofluourescent microscopy. Small samples should be enclosed in fine mesh cassettes before they are placed in formalin so that they can be located easily. Wedge biopsies are also divided into 1 large and 2 small pieces, with the largest portion going in formalin, a small portion placed in chilled 3% glutaraldehyde for electron microscopy, and another small portion snap frozen in Michel's transport medium for immunofluorescence. Kits with media and directions are available from some pathology centers.

Surgical technique: needle biopsy with a semi-automatic core biopsy instrument

1. Spring-load the instrument's sheath.
2. Grasp the kidney with your left hand and elevate it so that the convex surface is facing upwards.
3. With your right hand, position the instrument so that the slotted needle and sheath will remain in the outer third of the renal cortex after firing.
    a. At the cranial or caudal pole of the kidney, position the needle perpendicular to the long axis of the kidney (fig. 38-1).

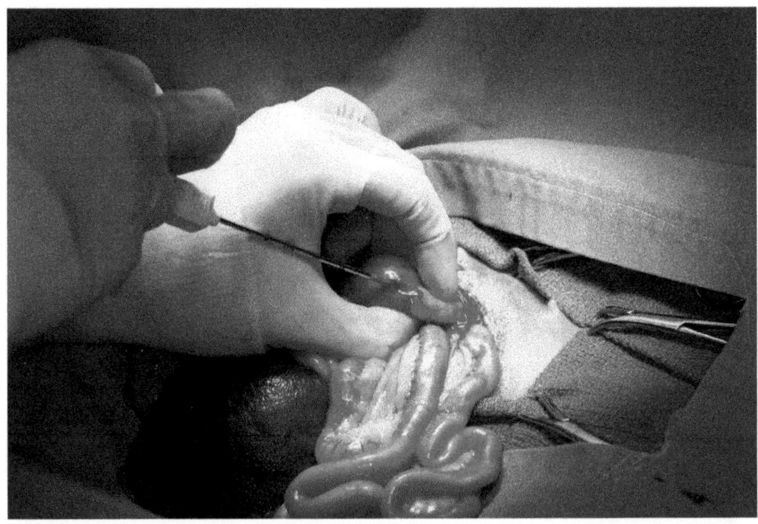

Figure 38-1 Stabilize the kidney and position the needle across the caudal pole.

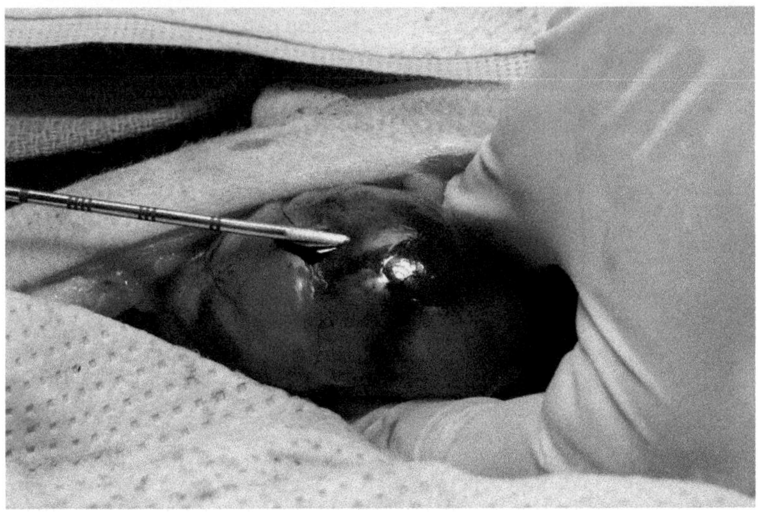

Figure 38-2 Biopsy of the convex surface. Position the device so that the needle is parallel to the outer surface of the kidney and remains in the cortex after firing.

b. Along the convex surface of the kidney, position the needle parallel to the long axis of the kidney (fig. 38-2).

4. Insert the tip of the slotted biopsy needle through the renal capsule to the level of the sheath.
5. Brace the instrument so the sheath does not move. With your right thumb, press on the needle button to advance the needle fully into the renal cortex. Keep the kidney and instrument stable during needle advancement.
6. Trigger the firing mechanism to advance the sheath over the needle and sever the parenchyma.
7. Retract the entire instrument with the enclosed sample (figs. 38-3 and 38-4). Use digital pressure for 2 to 5 minutes to decrease hemorrhage from the biopsy site.
8. If bleeding persists, place an interrupted or cruciate suture of 3-0 or 4-0 absorbable monofilament to appose the capsule and peritoneum over the site.

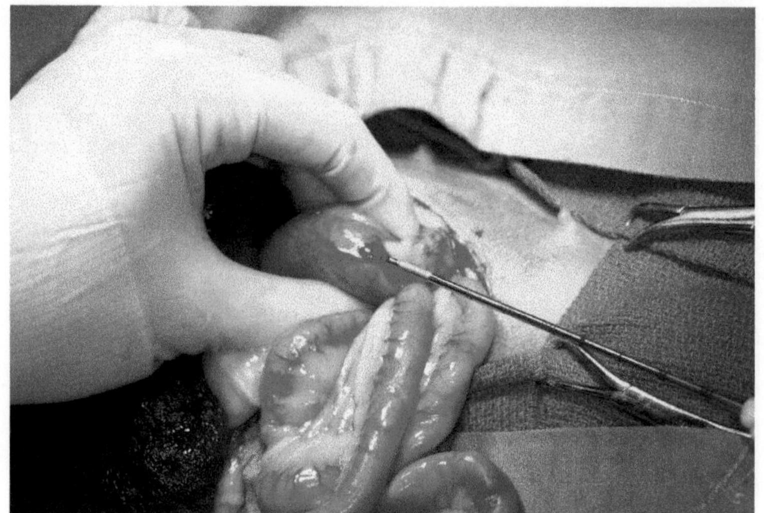

Figure 38-3 As the instrument is removed, the site will bleed. Hemorrhage can usually be controlled with digital pressure.

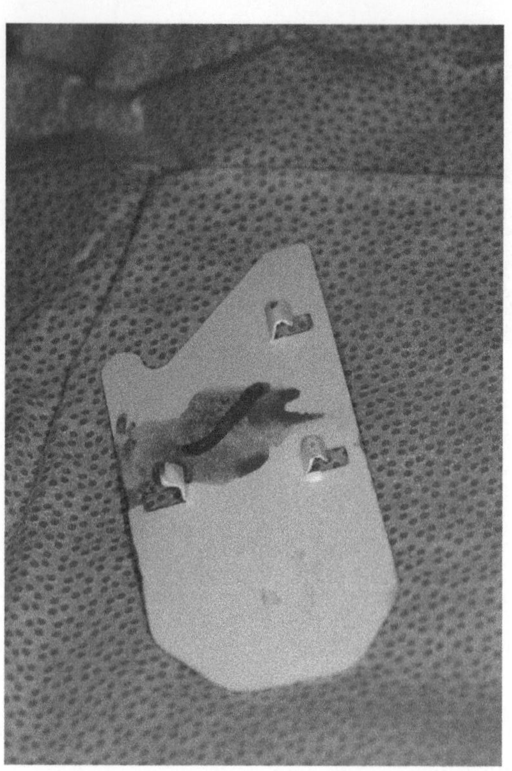

Figure 38-4 Tissue sample from a biopsy needle.

Surgical technique: wedge biopsy

1. Free the kidney from its peritoneal attachments by incising the peritoneum caudal to the kidney with scissors and then digitally tearing the remaining attachments (see figs. 39-1 and 39-2, pp. 316 and 317).
2. Reflect the kidney ventromedially to expose the renal vessels.
3. Occlude the renal artery.
   a. Have an assistant elevate the kidney and occlude the renal artery with thumb and index finger. The assistant should occlude the vessels where the pulse is palpable.

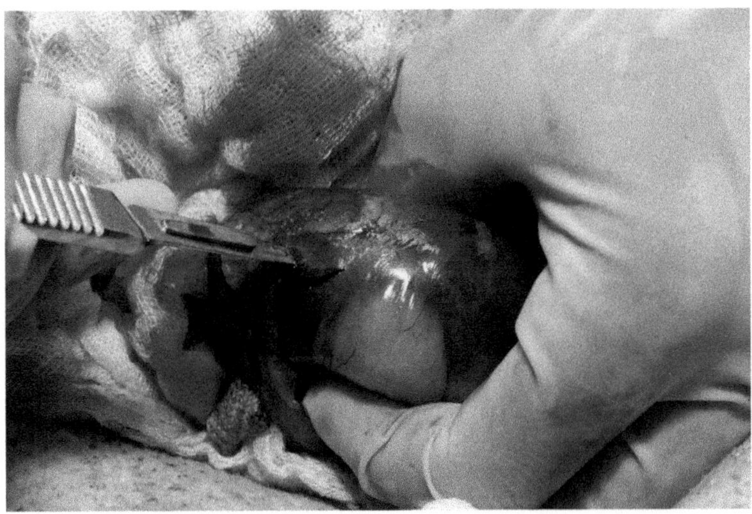

Figure 38-5 Once the renal artery is occluded, make a semicircular cut in the cortex, angling inward.

b. If no assistant is available, reflect the kidney ventromedially and place a vascular clamp or tourniquet around the arteries. Keep the kidney elevated and in view with a laparotomy sponge. The kidney will get darker and softer if the arteries are properly occluded.

4. Once the kidney has become soft, remove a wedge of tissue with a no. 11 or 15 blade.

   a. Make a crescent-shaped incision, about 5 mm long, angling inward into the outer third of the kidney (fig. 38-5). The incision should be 2 to 5 mm deep, depending on the thickness of the cortex.

   b. Make a straight incision to connect the ends of the first incision, angling the blade inward to sever parenchymal attachments at the base of the sample (fig. 38-6).

   c. Remove the specimen by gently elevating it with the blade or grasping the edge of the renal capsule with forceps. Do not handle renal parenchyma with thumb forceps.

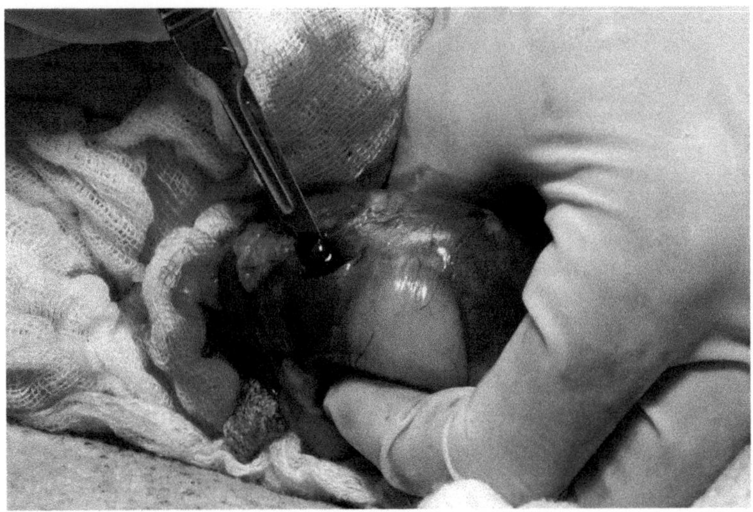

Figure 38-6 Connect the ends of the semicircular cut with a straight incision, angled inward, to sever parenchymal attachments.

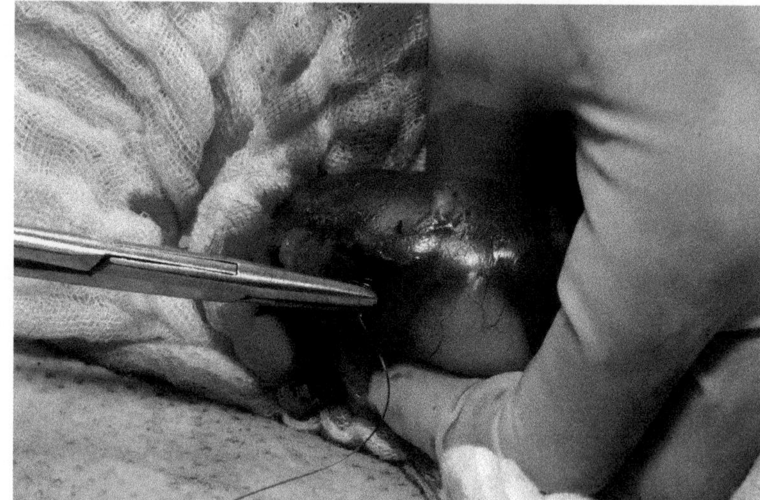

Figure 38-7 Close the biopsy site. Include capsule and parenchyma in the suture bite.

5. Close the renal capsule with an interrupted cruciate suture of 3-0 or 4-0 monofilament absorbable material on a taper needle (fig. 38-7). Use a surgeon's throw and a second throw to gently appose the parenchyma (fig. 38-8) without cutting into the tissues.
   a. Pass the needle through the capsule and parenchyma on either side of the incision, following the curve of the needle during placement and advancement.
   b. When the needle tip protrudes out the capsule on the opposite side, release the needle. Regrab the needle end and ease it through the tissues until more of the needle tip is exposed.
   c. Release the needle again and rotate the needle holder so that your palm is facing downward. Grab the needle near its tip and gently withdraw the needle from the tissues with a rotating (supinating) motion, following the curve of the needle.

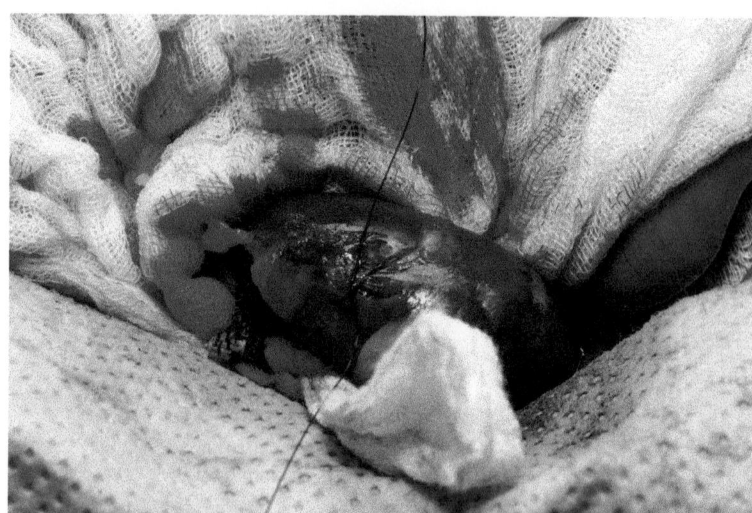

Figure 38-8 Appose the parenchyma with a surgeon's throw. Do not overtighten the suture.

6. If the capsule tears during placement, verify that the renal artery is occluded and place a second suture, including a superficial bite of parenchyma.
7. If bleeding persists, apply direct digital pressure for 5 to 10 minutes or tack omentum or peritoneum over the area with interrupted sutures.

Postoperative considerations

After renal biopsy, patients should be diuresed for several hours to decrease the risk of blood clot obstruction of the renal pelvis or urethra. The hematocrit should be monitored for significant anemia that may require transfusion. Activity should be restricted for 72 hours. Microscopic hematuria is seen in the majority of patients within 48 hours of biopsy. Gross hematuria is uncommon and usually resolves within 24 hours.

Complications are reported in 13% to 19% of patients. Severe perirenal hemorrhage occurs in 3% to 17% of dogs and cats and is usually a result of poor technique. Other complications include damage to renal blood vessels, arteriovenous fistula formation, permanent decrease in renal function, and death. Rarely, the renal pelvis or ureter can be obstructed by blood clots, resulting in hydronephrosis. Complications are more likely to occur in animals with thrombocytopenia, prolonged clotting times, or serum creatinine >5 mg/dL. Complications are also more common in patients more than 4 years of age or weighing less than 5 kg.

Bibliography

Groman RP et al: Effects of serial ultrasound-guided renal biopsies on kidneys of healthy adolescent dogs. Vet Radiol Ultrasound 2004;45:62–69.

Jeraj K et al: Evaluation of renal biopsy in 197 dogs and cats. J Am Vet Med Assoc 1982;181:367–369.

Lees GE et al: Renal biopsy and pathologic evaluation of glomerular disease. Topics in Compan An Med 2011;26:143–153.

Vaden SL et al: Renal biopsy: a retrospective study of methods and complications in 283 dogs and 65 cats. J Vet Int Med 2005;19:794–801.

Chapter 39
Nephrectomy

Indications for nephrectomy include severe renal trauma, large renal abscesses, end-stage hydronephrosis, primary renal tumors, and adrenal tumors that invade the kidney or its vasculature. Nephrectomy is not recommended in animals with unilateral renal calculi unless removal of the nonfunctional kidney will prevent further deterioration of the animal. Nephrectomy may be contraindicated in animals with azotemia, since total renal function is already reduced at least 75%. Animals with large or vascular renal tumors should be referred, preferably to a practice with advanced imaging (e.g., CT) and vessel-sealing devices, since affected kidneys may be revascularized by numerous peritoneal and retroperitoneal vessels.

Preoperative management

If the indication for surgery is not life threatening, animals should be evaluated thoroughly and stabilized before considering nephrectomy. Potential systemic disturbances include anemia, azotemia, electrolyte and acid-base abnormalities, coagulopathies, hypoalbuminemia, hypoproteinemia, and urinary tract infection. Thoracic radiographs and abdominal ultrasound should be performed in animals with primary renal tumors, which frequently metastasize to the lungs and can occur bilaterally. Ultrasound will also provide information about structure of the contralateral kidney and facilitate procurement of samples for cytology or histology. Excretory urography may provide information about function of the unaffected kidney; however, it is not as sensitive as renal scintigraphy and may cause acute renal failure. If excretory urography is performed, the animal should be kept well perfused during and after the procedure.

To prevent overhydration, a jugular catheter should be placed to measure central venous pressures during fluid administration before and during surgery. Urine output should be monitored by placement of an indwelling urinary catheter with attached collection system. Preoperative administration of an anticholinergic agent may help to prevent the transient decrease in cardiac output and peripheral resistance that can occur during nephrectomy. Because the ureter is ligated and transected at the level of the bladder, a wide prep and long incision are required for nephrectomy.

Manual of Small Animal Soft Tissue Surgery, Second Edition. Karen Tobias.
© 2017 John Wiley & Sons, Inc. Published 2017 by John Wiley & Sons, Inc.

Surgery

The left and right kidneys can be exposed by retracting the abdominal viscera away from the kidney with the mesocolon or mesoduodenum, respectively. Presence of a contralateral kidney should be confirmed first before removing the affected kidney. During nephrectomy, kidneys should be checked carefully for multiple or branched renal vessels. Multiple renal arteries occur most commonly on the left side in dogs. In some animals, the kidneys are so atrophied that the vessels will not be visible. If gonads are to be left in the patient, the left renal vein will need to be ligated proximal (abaxial) to its junction with the ovarian or testicular vein. Before performing a nephrectomy, the contralateral ureter should be identified to prevent accidental damage.

Surgical technique: nephrectomy

1. Grasp avascular peritoneum near the caudal pole of the kidney and incise it sharply with Metzenbaum scissors (fig. 39-1).
2. Transect or digitally break down the remaining avascular peritoneal attachments. Transect peritoneal vessels <1 mm in diameter with electrocautery or a radiosurgical scalpel; ligate or seal larger vessels (fig. 39-2) with ligatures, hemoclips, or a vessel-sealing device.
3. Reflect the kidney ventromedially to expose the artery and vein (fig. 39-3). If necessary, gently dissect away the perirenal fat from the hilus with a gauze sponge or curved hemostats, keeping parallel to the long axis of the vessels, to improve visualization.
4. Triple ligate the artery and vein separately with absorbable suture, leaving enough space to allow vessel transection. Alternatively, clamp each vessel before double-ligating the axial portions of the vessels, then transect between the clamp and ligatures.
   a. If ovaries or testicles are to be left in the animal, identify any gonadal tributaries and ligate the renal vessels lateral (abaxial) to their junctions with these vessels.
5. Follow the ureter to the bladder, freeing it with blunt dissection from its peritoneal attachments (fig. 39-4), then clamp and ligate it close to the bladder before transecting.

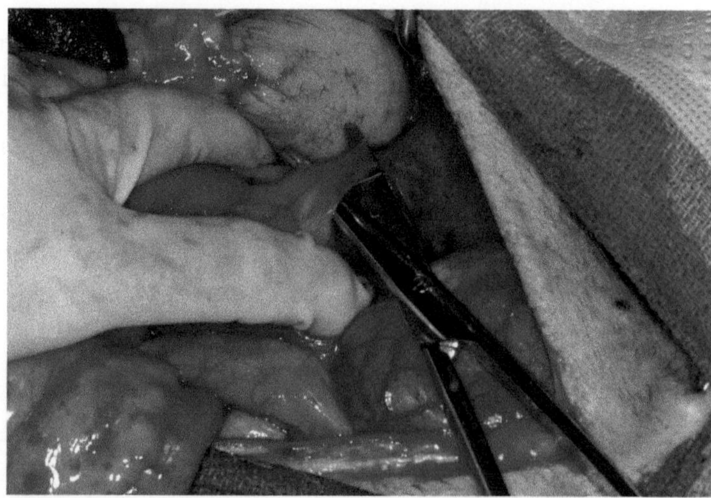

Figure 39-1 Elevate and transect the peritoneum near the caudal pole of the kidney.

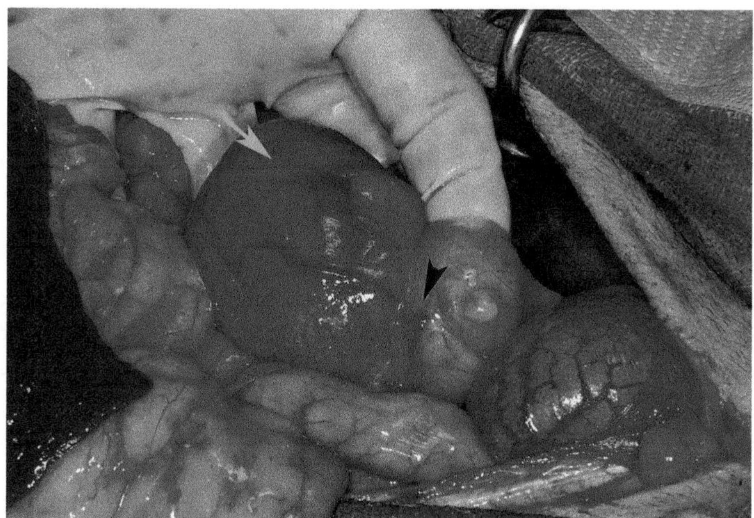

Figure 39-2 Large peritoneal vessels (black arrowhead) to the kidney (green arrow) may need to be ligated or cauterized during peritoneal transection.

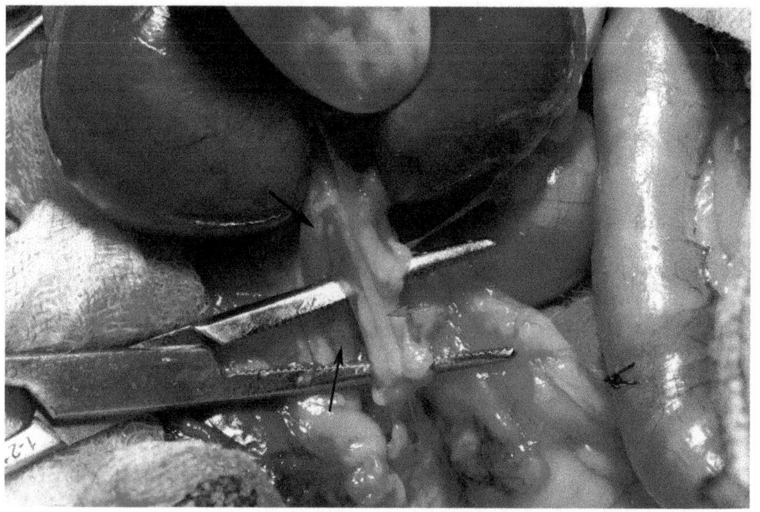

Figure 39-3 Reflect the kidney ventromedially and isolate the renal artery (green arrow) and vein (black arrows). Triple ligate each vessel before transecting.

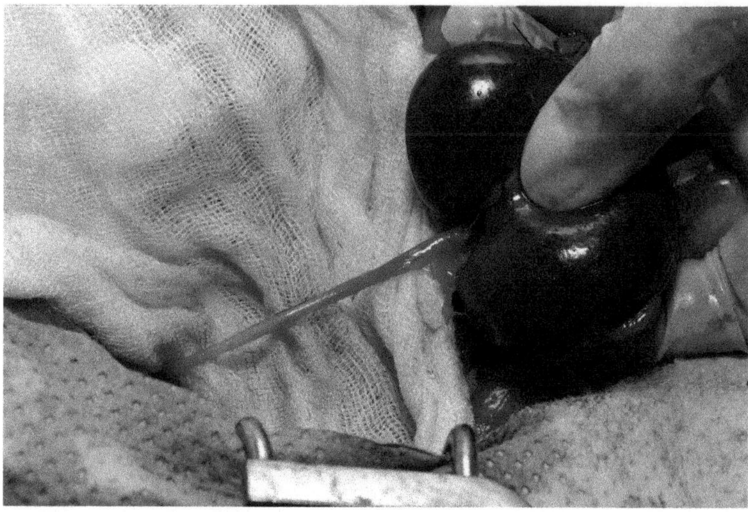

Figure 39-4 Free the ureter from its peritoneal attachments and ligate it close to the bladder.

Postoperative considerations

After surgery, hematocrit, central venous pressure, peripheral blood pressure, electrolytes, creatinine, BUN, and urine output are monitored, and intravenous fluids are continued for at least 24 hours. Postoperative complications are uncommon; the greatest concern is reduced urine production because of persistent renal dysfunction. Overhydration can be a more serious problem, however, if the remaining kidney is unhealthy.

In healthy uninephrectomized animals, the remaining kidney may increase in size because of compensatory hypertrophy. Reduction of protein and salt intake are not obligatory after nephrectomy; in fact, a higher-protein diet can increase glomerular filtration rate and renal plasma flow. In cats with renal dysfunction, decreased dietary sodium chloride may result in hypokalemic nephropathy.

Survival after unilateral nephrectomy depends on the underlying condition; in dogs with renal carcinoma, approximately 8% die or are euthanized in the perioperative period. Median survival for dogs with unilateral renal neoplasia is 16 months and is correlated with the tumor type, grade, and presence of metastatic disease. Dogs with low-grade renal carcinoma mitotic index <10) have a median survival time of 3.2 years. Dogs with renal hemangiosarcoma and hemoperitoneum have a median survival of 2 months. In dogs with renal neoplasia, death or euthanasia is usually a result of metastatic disease.

Bibliography

Bryan JN et al: Primary renal neoplasia of dogs. J Vet Int Med 2006;20:1155–1160.

Buranakarl C et al: Effects of dietary sodium chloride intake on renal function and blood pressure in cats with normal and reduced renal function. Am J Vet Res 2004;65(5):620–627.

Edmonson EF et al: Prognostic significance of histologic features in canine renal cell carcinomas: 70 nephrectomies. Vet Path 2015;52:260–268.

Gookin JL et al: Unilateral nephrectomy in dogs with renal disease: 30 cases (1985–1994). J Am Vet Med Assoc 1996;28(12):2020–2026.

McCarthy RA et al: Effects of dietary protein on glomerular mesangial area and basement membrane thickness in aged uninephrectomized dogs. Can J Vet Res 2001;65:125–130.

Urie BK et al: Evaluation of clinical status, renal function, and hematopoietic variables after unilateral nephrectomy in canine kidney donors. J Am Vet Med Assoc 2007;230:1653–1656.

Chapter 40
Cystotomy

Cystotomies are most frequently performed to remove cystic calculi. Other indications include mass biopsy, foreign-body removal, ureteral catheterization, ureteral reimplantation, and correction of intramural ectopic ureters. Cystotomy can be converted to cystectomy (bladder wall resection) if a cystic mass or urachal diverticulum is detected. Even if 75% of the bladder is removed, the bladder will usually regain its original size within a few months.

Preoperative management

Patient workup depends on the underlying disease process. Most animals undergo a complete blood count, biochemistry panel, urinalysis, urine culture, and radiographic studies. Ultrasound and cystoscopy are also useful for determining the extent of disease. Some patients may require stabilization and urinary tract catheterization before anesthesia, particularly if severe azotemia, dehydration, acidosis, or hyperkalemia is present. In animals with radiopaque cystic calculi, abdominal radiographs should be reviewed to estimate the number and size of stones.

Once the animal is anesthetized, epidural analgesia can be administered to reduce postoperative discomfort during urination. Intravenous antibiotic treatment (e.g., ampicillin or a first-generation cephalosporin) can be initiated before surgery because it does not affect results of bladder tissue cultures taken during surgery. In preparation for surgery, the abdomen is clipped and prepped from xiphoid to pubis. In male dogs, the prepuce is clipped and flushed with antiseptic solution, since it will be included within the sterile surgical site. In females, the perivulvar region should be clipped and cleaned and, preferably, included in the sterile surgical field in the event that any urinary catheter passed antegrade during surgery inadvertently exits the urethra. If a mass is present, clean instruments and gloves should be available for closure, since transitional cell carcinoma can spread to the abdominal wall.

Surgery

Cystotomy is usually performed through a caudal midline abdominal incision. In male dogs, the skin incision may extend lateral to the prepuce to expose the caudal linea. Once the abdomen has been explored, the ureters are identified, and the bladder is palpated for masses. If the bladder is full, it can be emptied

Manual of Small Animal Soft Tissue Surgery, Second Edition. Karen Tobias.
© 2017 John Wiley & Sons, Inc. Published 2017 by John Wiley & Sons, Inc.

with a needle and syringe, or with suction through an initial stab wound. Before the bladder is incised, it should be surrounded with moistened laparotomy pads to reduce peritoneal contamination. A stay suture can be placed at its apex to facilitate retraction.

Cystotomy incisions are usually made in the ventrum or apex of the bladder to avoid damage to the ureteral openings. Ventral cystotomy provides better exposure to the cystic trigone. Extra stay sutures can be placed along the edges of the cystotomy incision to improve visualization of the bladder interior. Bladder mucosa should be handled gently, since trauma from suction tips, sponges, thumb forceps, and calculus retrieval spoons will rapidly cause swelling and will obscure the ureteral openings. A piece of the bladder wall along the margin of the cystotomy can be harvested with scissors for histology and culture. Bladder mucosa or a urolith is preferred over a urine sample for culture, since false negative preoperative urine cultures can occur in dogs with urolithiasis. In male dogs with cystic calculi, the urethra should be catheterized retrograde and flushed multiple times to verify all stones have been removed. In female dogs and cats, a urethral catheter can be passed antegrade through the cystotomy to verify patency. If the catheter exits out the vulva into a nonsterile field during antegrade passage, it should be discarded because of contamination. The proximal urethra can also be evaluated for residual calculi by inserting a sterile scope through the cystotomy.

If intraoperative placement of a urinary catheter is desired in females, the vulva and perineum should be surgically prepped and included in the sterile field. A red rubber catheter can be passed through the cystotomy and urethra and out the vulva. The tip of the red rubber catheter is attached to the end of a Foley catheter with suture, and the red rubber catheter is pulled back into the bladder. Once the tip of the Foley is visible, the suture is cut, and the Foley balloon is inflated. The cystotomy can then be closed.

Cystotomy closure depends on incision location and bladder wall thickness. Continuous appositional patterns are preferred for closure of thick bladders and for incisions near the ureteral openings or trigone. Thin bladders can be closed with a single-layer appositional or double-layer appositional or inverting pattern. Strength of closure is the same for appositional and inverting patterns and for single-and double-layer closures. The bladder regains 100% of its original strength 2 to 3 weeks after cystotomy; therefore, a 3-0 or 4-0 monofilament absorbable suture material that maintains effective wound support for 3 weeks is sufficient for closure. Penetration of absorbable suture material into the bladder lumen may cause calculus formation. If bladder wall integrity or vascularity is questionable, the omentum can be tacked over the entire bladder with interrupted absorbable sutures after cystotomy closure.

Surgical technique: cystotomy

1. Isolate the bladder with laparotomy pads.
2. Place a full-thickness monofilament stay suture in the bladder apex for retraction (fig. 40-1). If desired, add a second stay suture beyond the caudal extent of the proposed incision.
3. While gently lifting up on the stay suture(s), make a stab incision into the bladder in an avascular region (fig. 40-2). Remove any intraluminal urine with a Poole suction tip.
4. Extend the bladder incision with scissors (fig. 40-3). For ventral cystotomies, extend the incision along the long axis of the bladder.

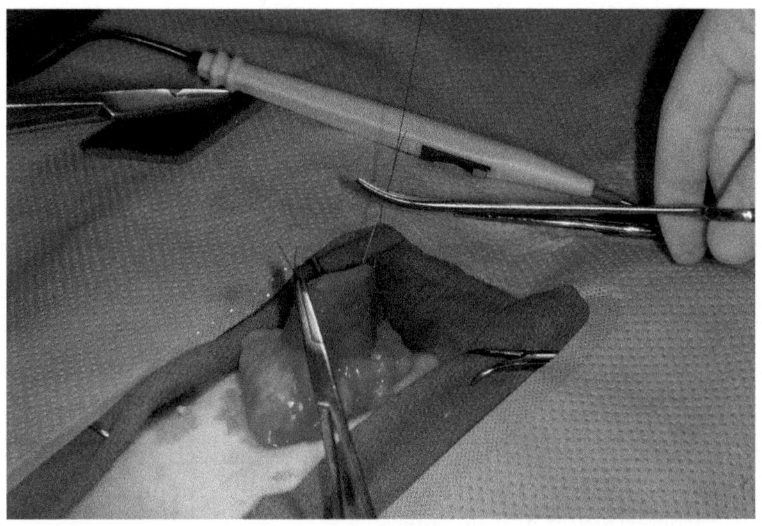

Figure 40-1 Place full-thickness stay sutures in the bladder to facilitate retraction.

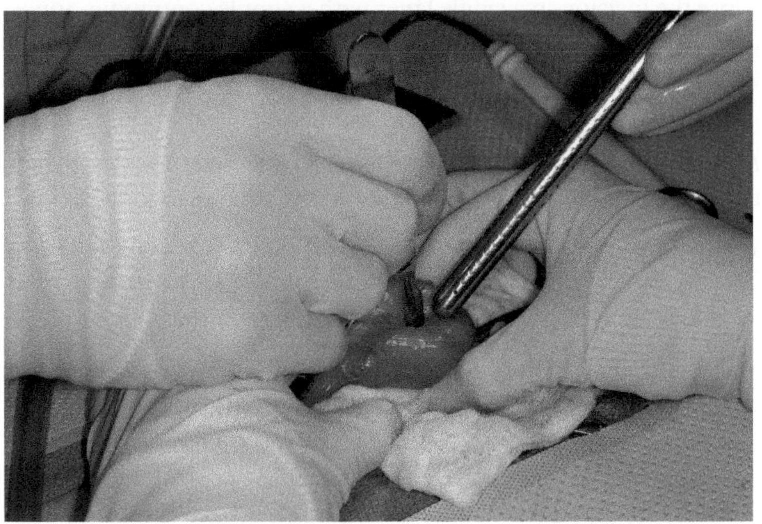

Figure 40-2 Make a stab incision into the bladder lumen and remove urine with suction.

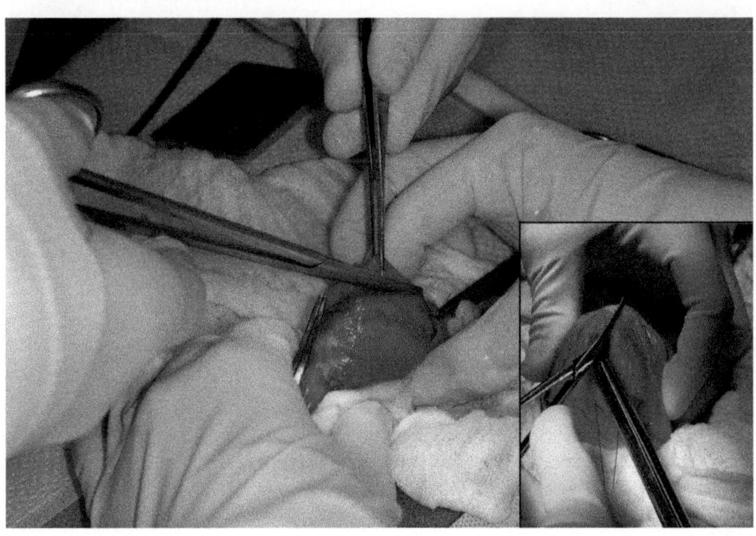

Figure 40-3 Extend the bladder incision with Mayo or Metzenbaum scissors.

5. If the inside of the bladder needs to be explored, place additional stay sutures lateral to the incision site, and retract these to hold open the incision.
6. If calculi are present, remove them gently with a bladder spoon.
   a. After scooping out stones, flush and suction out the bladder.
   b. Verify that the urethra is patent by placing a red rubber catheter retrograde (males) or antegrade (females) through the urethra. Flush through the catheter as you withdraw it.
   c. Repeat flushing and scooping until you get three consecutive negative scoops.
   d. If desired, explore the interior of the bladder and trigone with a gloved finger to verify there are no calculi remaining after urethral catheterization and flushing.
7. Remove a section of bladder mucosa along the incision line for culture.
8. Close the incision in a single layer with a simple continuous appositional pattern (fig. 40-4). Use 3-0 or 4-0 rapidly absorbable monofilament suture on a taper needle, and include submucosa in each suture bite. Be careful not to damage the bladder wall with thumb forceps.
9. Alternatively, if the bladder wall is thin or of questionable health, close the incision with a rapid two-layer inverting pattern.
   a. Just beyond the end of the incision, take a bite perpendicular to the incision line (fig. 40-5) and tie two knots. Leave the suture end of the knot long and tag it with a hemostat.
   b. Perform a Cushing pattern by taking bites parallel to the incision line (fig. 40-6). Contralateral bites should overlap slightly, and the suture should be tightened after each bite to invert the bladder wall.

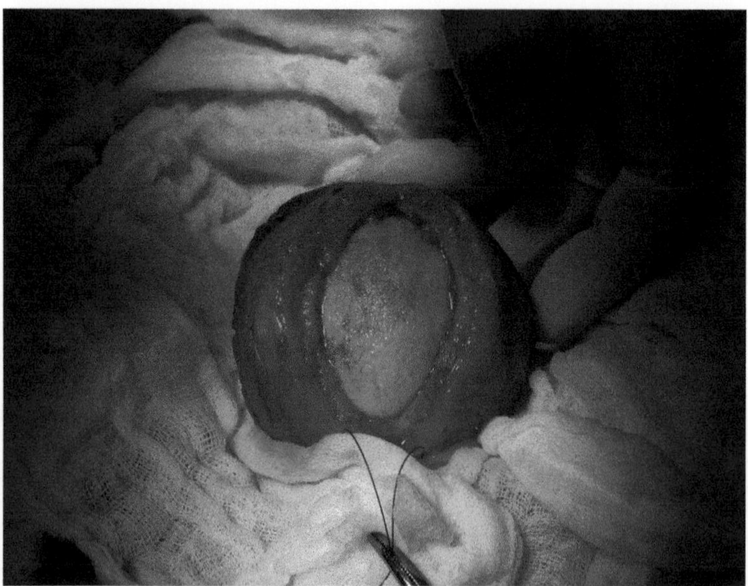

Figure 40-4 Thickened bladder containing a single, large calculus. Closure should be performed with a simple continuous pattern.

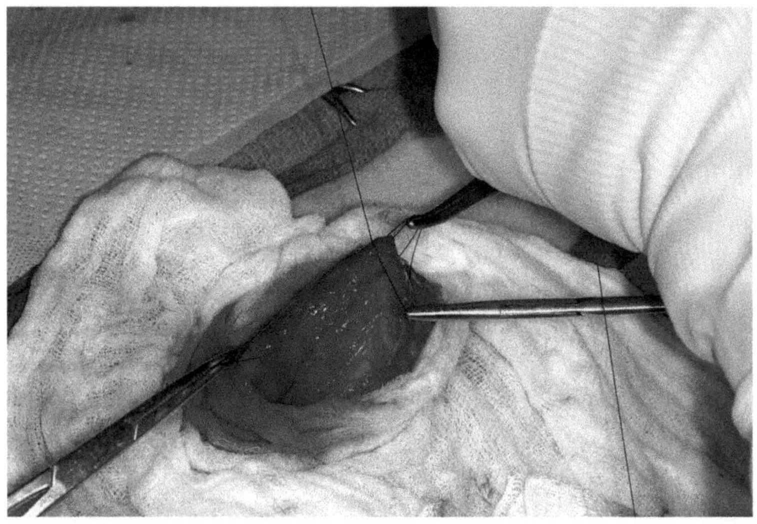

Figure 40-5 Closure of a thin bladder. Take the first suture bite perpendicular to the incision line and tie two knots. Tag the suture end with a hemostat.

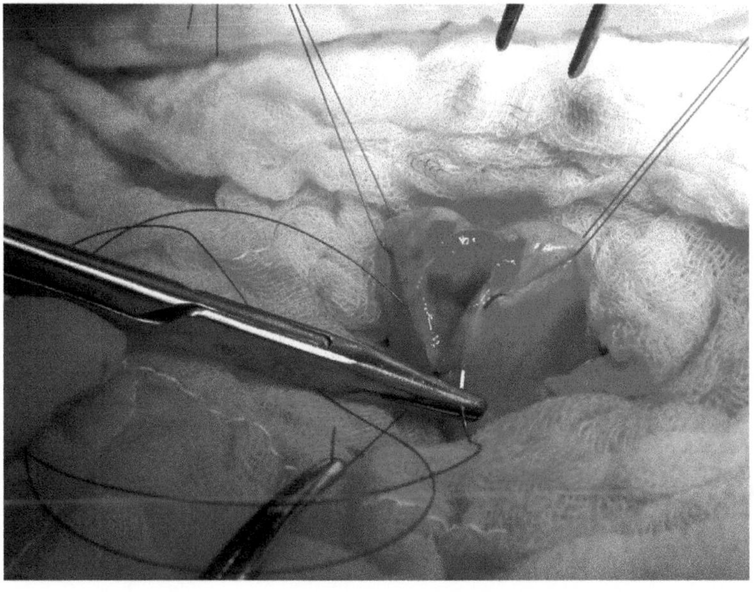

Figure 40-6 Cushing pattern. Take suture bites parallel to the incision line, angling slightly outward. Bites should overlap slightly with those on the contralateral side.

c. Take the final bite beyond the end of the incision line. Do not tie a knot.

d. Immediately begin a Lembert pattern (fig. 40-7), suturing back over the Cushing pattern. Take bites perpendicular to the incision line. To avoid using thumb forceps, keep tension on the suture material as you take tissue bites (fig. 40-8). Because the bladder wall is already inverted, the Lembert pattern is placed just like a simple continuous pattern.

e. After finishing the second layer, tie off to the tagged suture end.

10. If infection or neoplasia is present, change gloves and instruments before closing the abdomen.

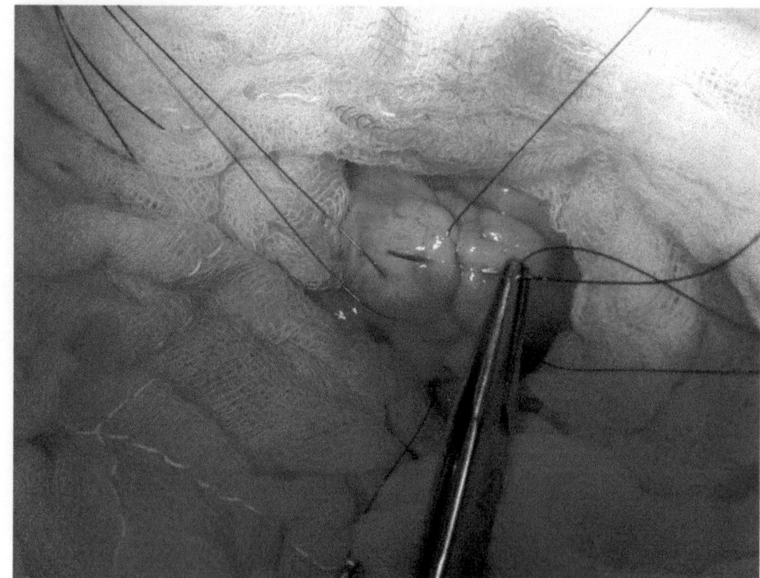

Figure 40-7 Lembert oversew. The pattern looks similar to a simple continuous pattern.

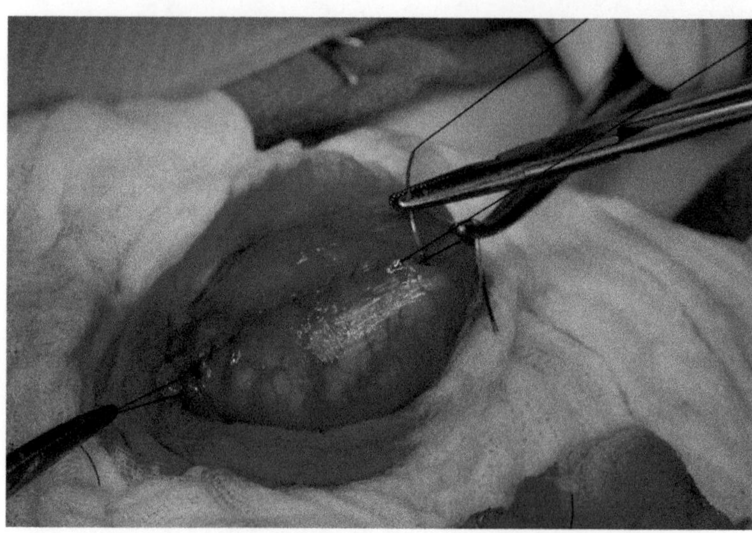

Figure 40-8 Take the last suture bite beyond the incision line and tie the suture back to the original suture end that was secured in a hemostat. Note that thumb forceps are not being used; instead, tension is kept on the bladder by retracting the sutures.

Postoperative considerations

In animals with radiopaque cystic calculi, the abdomen can be radiographed after surgery to verify that all the stones have been removed. Additionally, the proximal urethra can be examined with a sterile arthroscope or cystoscope before cystotomy closure. Residual cystic calculi are noted in 14% to 20% of animals after open cystotomy and 5% or fewer of animals that undergo scope examination before closure.

Intravenous fluids are continued for at least 12 hours, since blood clots from incisional bleeding can cause urinary tract obstruction. If the bladder is poorly vascularized, atonic, or undersized, a transurethral Foley catheter should be left in place for at least 2 to 3 days to keep the bladder decompressed. Urine should be cultured after the catheter is removed and also 1 week after any antibiotic therapy has been discontinued.

Mild hematuria and pollakiuria usually persist for several days after surgery. Serious complications after cystotomy are unusual. Urethral obstruction may occur secondary to persistent or recurrent calculi, blood clots, or mass regrowth. If the bladder wall is unhealthy, animals with urethral obstruction may develop uroabdomen from tears that develop along the suture line.

Bibliography

Appel SL et al: Evaluation of risk factors associated with suture-nidus cystoliths in dogs and cats: 176 cases (1999–2006). J Am Vet Med Assoc 2008;233:1889–1895.

Appel S, Ottos SJ, Weese JS: Cystotomy practices and complications among general small animal practitioners in Ontario, Canada. Can Vet J 2012;53:303–310.

Arulpragasam SP, Case JB, Ellison GW: Evaluation of costs and time required for laparoscopic-assisted versus open cystotomy for urinary cystolith removal in dogs: 43 cases (2009–2012). J Am Vet Med Assoc 2013;243:703–708.

Buote NJ, Kovak-McClaran JR, Loar AS, et al: The effect of preoperative antimicrobial administration on culture results in dogs undergoing cystotomy. J Am Vet Med Assoc 2012;241:1185–1189.

Gatoria IS et al: Comparison of three techniques for the diagnosis of urinary tract infections in dogs with urolithiasis. J Small Anim Pract 2006;47:727–732.

Grant DC, Harper TA, Were SR: Frequency of incomplete urolith removal, complications, and diagnostic imaging following cystotomy for removal of uroliths from the lower urinary tract in dogs: 128 cases (1994–2006). J Am Vet Med Assoc 2010; 236:763–766.

Radasch RM et al: Cystotomy closure. A comparison of the strength of appositional and inverting suture patterns. Vet Surg 1990;19:283–288.

Chapter 41
Cystostomy Tube Placement

Urine diversion may be required to optimize healing after urethral injury or repair, to stabilize a patient before surgical removal of a urethral obstruction, or to decompress distended bladders in animals with neurologic dysfunction, detrusor muscle atony, or nonresectable urethral or trigonal neoplasia. Most frequently, diversion is accomplished with a transurethral catheter; however, urethral catheterization may not be possible in some patients with complete obstruction. In animals with urethral tears, leakage of urine around the catheter could delay healing and increase inflammation, which may predispose animals to stricture. A cystostomy tube provides complete urine diversion and can be used for temporary or long-term bladder decompression.

Foley and mushroom-tip catheters can be used as temporary cystostomy tubes; however, because of their length, they are more likely to be damaged or removed prematurely. Additionally, the balloon in a Foley catheter may gradually deflate over time, increasing the chance of inadvertent removal. When chronic urinary diversion is required, a low-profile cystostomy tube is preferable. Low-profile cystostomy tubes are an adaptation of low-profile gastrostomy ports. They usually protrude a maximum of 1 to 3 cm from the body wall and thus are more difficult to accidently dislodge. The external end has a hinged cap or "antireflux" valve designed to prevent leakage and reduce contamination. Owners drain the bladder with an extension tube tipped with a special adaptor.

Low-profile tubes can be used for the initial cystostomy tube placement or as a replacement for a preexisting Foley or mushroom-tipped catheter 2 to 3 weeks after surgery. Before replacement, the original cystostomy tube is retracted so that the balloon or mushroom tip comes in contact with the bladder wall, and the tube is marked at the level of the skin. The tube is then removed from the bladder with firm traction, and the distance between the marked line and mushroom or balloon is measured to determine the appropriate low-profile tube length. The low-profile tube is straightened with a stylet (see fig. 19-1, p. 156) and inserted immediately through the fistula (figs. 19-2 and 41-1) and then secured to the skin (fig. 19-11, p. 162). Bandaging over low-profile tubes is usually not required.

Manual of Small Animal Soft Tissue Surgery, Second Edition. Karen Tobias.
© 2017 John Wiley & Sons, Inc. Published 2017 by John Wiley & Sons, Inc.

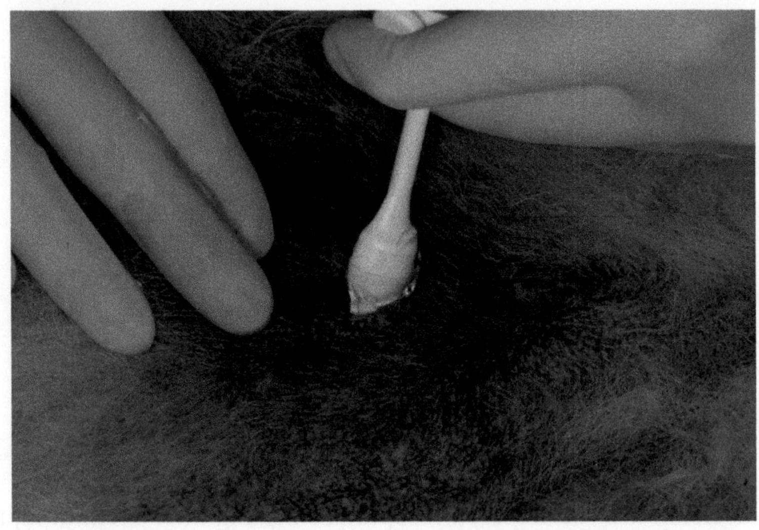

Figure 41-1 Placement of a low-profile cystostomy tube through a pre-existing cystostomy tube wound. Straighten the mushroom tip with a stylet and insert the tube through the stoma. Lubrication with sterile, water-soluble gel may facilitate passage.

Preoperative management

Animals with complete obstruction may have uremia, hyperphosphatemia, acidosis, hyperkalemia, and bradycardia. If possible, patients should be stabilized before anesthesia. For a ventral midline approach, the abdomen is clipped and prepped from xiphoid to pubis. In male dogs, the prepuce should be flushed with antiseptic solution before final prep, or it can be towel-clamped to the side away from the proposed incision site so that it is not included in the surgery field.

Surgery

In animals undergoing concurrent procedures, the bladder is approached through a midline incision and the cystostomy tube is placed through a separate paramedian incision, as described below. An alternative for dogs not undergoing laparotomy (e.g., those requiring only emergency decompression) is a paramedian grid approach. With this approach, the animal is positioned in lateral recumbancy, and a 2–3 cm vertical-oblique skin incision is made in the caudolateral abdomen over the distended bladder. In male dogs, the incision is dorsal to the caudal half of the prepuce and cranial to the flank fold. The external abdominal fascia is incised, and the peritoneal cavity is accessed by spreading the fibers in a grid approach, similar to that described for cryptorchidectomy (see Chapter 30). A purse-string suture is placed in the bladder, and a Foley tube is inserted through a stab incision 2–3 cm cranial to the wound and through the purse string suture via a stab incision in the bladder wall. After the Foley balloon is inflated and the purse-string suture is tightened, the abdominal incision is closed in 3 layers.

Cystostomy tube diameter is based on bladder size; 6 or 8 French tubes are used in animals with undersized bladders while 24 French tubes have been placed in very large dogs. Placement of mushroom-tipped or Foley catheter cystostomy tubes is similar to gastrostomy tube placement (see Chapter 19). If a Foley catheter is used, the balloon integrity should be tested before placement. Low-profile cystostomy tubes are more awkward to place than Foley or mushroom-tipped catheters because of their short length. To facilitate placement, the bladder can be partially pexied to the abdominal wall before inserting the low-profile tube into the bladder. The length of the low profile cystostomy tube is based on body wall and bladder thickness, which can be measured preoperatively with ultrasound or intraoperatively after abdominal incision.

Surgical technique: cystostomy tube placement through a ventral midline approach

1. Expose the bladder through a caudal ventral midline celiotomy and isolate it with moistened laparotomy pads. If needed, place a stay suture in the apex of the bladder to keep it retracted out of the abdomen.
2. In the ventral or ventrolateral midbody of the bladder, place a 1.5- to 2-cm-diameter purse-string suture, using 3-0 rapidly absorbable monofilament suture. Take four to five bites, and engage the bladder submucosa in each bite (fig. 41-2).
3. Using a Carmalt or Kelly hemostatic forceps, perforate the peritoneum and abdominal wall (from inside to outside) 4 to 6 cm lateral to the midline abdominal incision and at a point level with the bladder purse string in a transverse plane. Incise the skin over the forceps (see fig. 19-3, p. 157) and push the forceps through the body wall.
4. Grasp the tube tip within the jaws of the forceps and pull it into the abdomen (see fig. 19-4, p. 158).
5. Make a stab incision through the bladder wall in the center of the purse string, taking care not to cut the suture.
6. Insert the catheter into the bladder. Inflate the Foley catheter balloon with saline, then tighten and tie the purse string suture.
7. Place four to six interrupted sutures of 2-0 or 3-0 absorbable monofilament material between the bladder and body wall around the tube. Pexy sutures should include bladder submucosa and abdominal wall muscle.

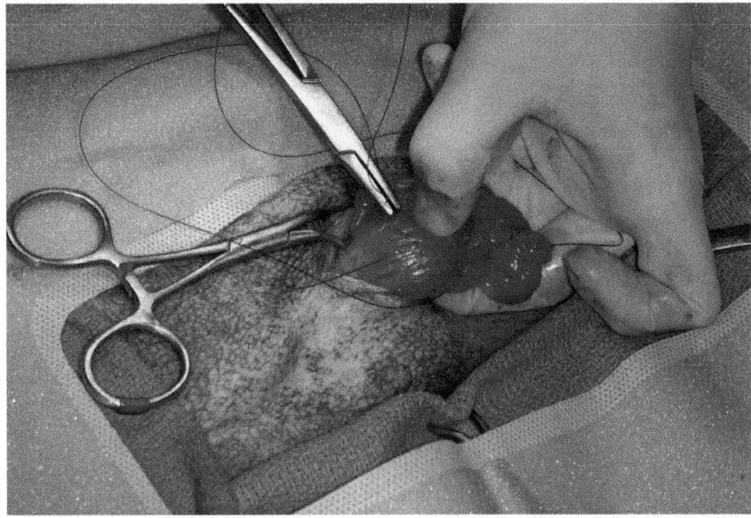

Figure 41-2 Place a purse-string suture in the ventral wall of the bladder.

8. If desired, wrap omentum around the pexy site and tack it in place with interrupted absorbable sutures. Close the abdomen routinely.

9. Place a nylon purse-string suture around the skin exit wound. Secure the tube to the skin with a finger-trap suture pattern (pp. 497–501).

Surgical technique: low-profile cystostomy tube

1. Expose the bladder and place a purse-string suture as described above (see fig. 41-2).

2. At the proposed pexy site, pass closed hemostatic forceps outward through the abdominal wall lateral to the incision, and incise the skin over the tips to expose the forceps.

3. Using the accompanying stylet, straighten out the cystostomy tube before grasping it in the jaws of the forceps and feeding it into the abdomen (fig. 41-3).

4. Place two or three pexy sutures between the bladder and body wall, dorsal and dorsolateral to the tube and purse string (fig. 41-4).

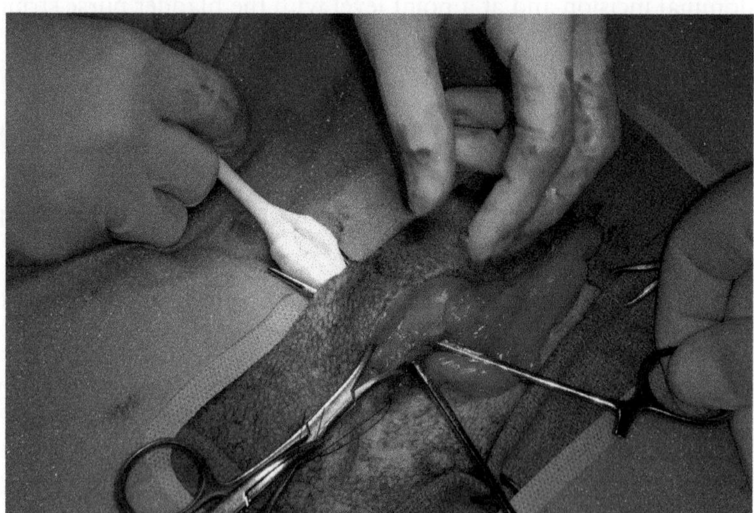

Figure 41-3 Straighten the low-profile tube with a stylet and insert it through the abdominal wall. Passage is facilitated with Kelly forceps.

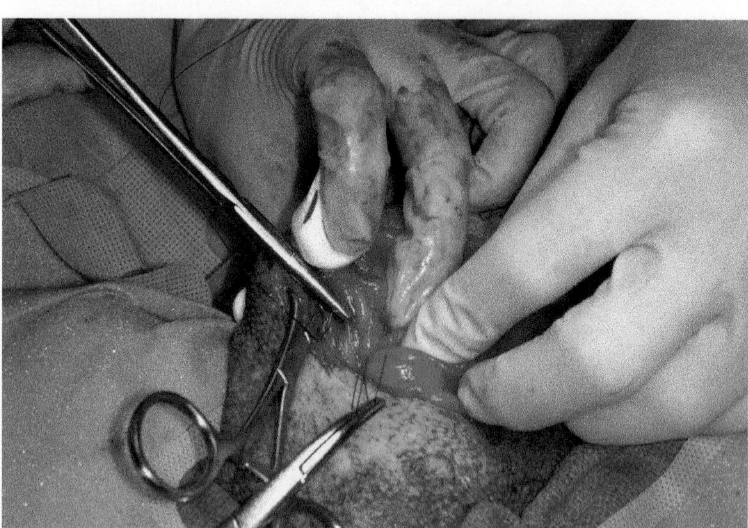

Figure 41-4 Place pexy sutures between the bladder and abdominal walls dorsal to the tube.

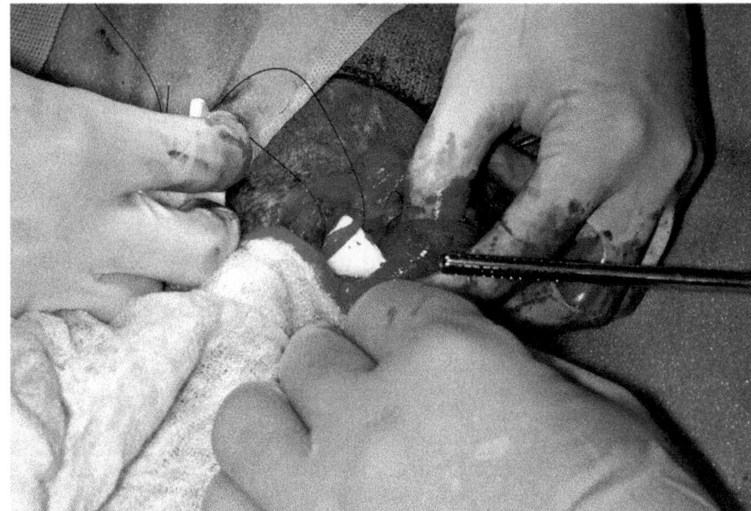

Figure 41-5 Straighten the tube with a stylet and insert it through a stab incision within the purse-string suture.

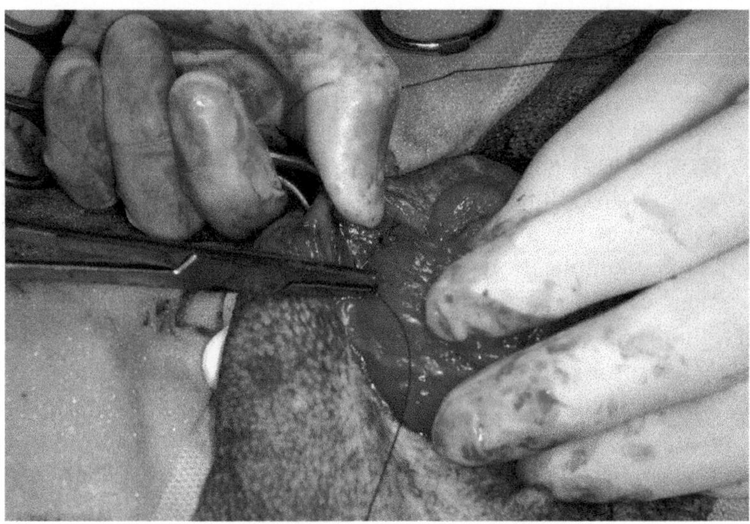

Figure 41-6 Tighten and tie the purse string and pexy the bladder to the abdominal wall ventral to the tube.

5. Make a stab incision through the bladder wall within the purse string, and insert the low-profile tube into the bladder while straightening its tip with the stylet (fig. 41-5).
6. Tighten and tie the purse string, then add additional pexy sutures ventrolaterally and ventrally (fig. 41-6).
7. Close the abdomen routinely. If desired, secure the flange of the tube to the skin with simple interrupted sutures (see fig. 19-11, p. 162).

Postoperative considerations

To reduce the risk of obstruction from blood clots, intravenous fluids can be administered for 12 to 24 hours after cystostomy tube placement. Elizabethan collars, sidebars, or a lycra bodysuit (e.g., K9 Top Coat) will reduce the risk of self-trauma. Exit sites of long tubes are covered with bandage material, while low-profile tubes are usually left uncovered. Tube exit sites may require occasional cleaning with antiseptic solutions. Antibiotics are used only in animals with clinical signs of urinary tract infection.

To prevent urine leakage around the tube, tubes should be hooked to a collection system or drained every 3 to 4 hours for 3 to 5 days after surgery until a good seal has formed between the bladder and body wall. Catheters left in long term are usually drained 4 times a day. Antiseptic technique (e.g., cleansing the catheter insertion site and use of gloves) is recommended when draining the tube.

Tubes can be removed as early as 5 days after placement; however, any urine leakage around the tube will reduce fibrous tissue formation. Without a good fibrous seal around the tube, urine may leak into the abdomen or subcutaneous tissues once the tube has been removed. Tubes should therefore be left in longer in animals with immunosuppression, poor tissue healing, or urine leakage around the tube. If diversion is performed to enhance urethral healing, a contrast cystourethrogram can be performed through the cystostomy tube to evaluate urethral integrity. To remove a Foley catheter, deflate the balloon and pull. To remove a low-profile or mushroom-tip tube, insert a blunt obturator into the tube to extend and narrow the tip before pulling the tube out. If the tube gets stuck at skin level, cut the skin purse string. After the tube is pulled, the stoma is covered with a bandage for 1 to 3 days until it has sealed.

The most common complication in animals with a cystostomy tube is urinary tract infection. Urine should be cultured after tube removal and, in animals with long-term diversion, when clinical signs of urinary tract infection are present. Culture of the urine is more accurate than culture of the tube tip at removal. Other complications of tube cystostomy include inadvertent removal; displacement of the tube from the bladder, resulting in uroabdomen; peristomal celluliltis; tube breakage; and fistula formation. If peristomal dermatitis develops, skin sutures securing the flange can be removed to facilitate cleaning. Pre-existing trigonal tumors may gradually obstruct the ureteral openings; therefore, affected animals should be examined intermittently with ultrasound or contrast radiographs. Transitional cell carcinoma can also spread to the abdominal wall and omentum around the cystostomy tube.

Bibliography

Anderson RB et al: Prognostic factors for successful outcome following urethral rupture in dogs and cats. J Am Anim Hosp Assoc 2006;42:136–146.

Beck AL et al: Outcome of and complications associated with tube cystostomy in dogs and cats: 76 cases (1995–2006). J Am Vet Med Assoc 2007;230:1184–1189.

Bray JP, Doyle RS, Burton CA: Minimally invasive inguinal approach for tube cystostomy. Vet Surg 2009;38:411–416.

Cooley AJ et al: The effects of indwelling transurethral catheterization and tube cystostomy on urethral anastomoses in dogs. J Am Anim Hosp Assoc 1999;35:341–347.

Hayashi K and Hardie RJ: Use of cystostomy tubes in small animals. Compend Contin Educ Pract Vet 2003;25:928–935.

Stiffler KS et al: Clinical use of low-profile cystostomy tubes in four dogs and a cat. J Am Vet Med Assoc 2003;223:325–329.

Chapter 42
Urethrotomy

In dogs, the penile urethra is located in a U-shaped groove in the ventral surface of the os penis. The caudal entrance to this groove is narrow at its base and is a common site for obstruction by urethral calculi. Most urethral calculi can be retropulsed into the bladder with urethral catheterization and flushing, particularly if a dog is under general anesthesia. Rarely, large stones become acutely lodged within the urethra at the base of the os penis and cannot be shifted with a catheter. These stones can be approached by prescrotal urethrotomy. Prescrotal urethrotomy can also be used for passage of a urinary catheter when scrotal urethrostomy has to be delayed. Prescrotal urethrotomy for urolith retrieval is often unsuccessful in dogs with chronic urethral calculi because trapped stones become embedded in the wall of the urethra at the level of the os penis. In those patients, a scrotal urethrostomy (Chapter 43) is often recommended.

Rarely, permanent prescrotal urethrostomy is performed in dogs with recurrent obstructions when owners refuse castration. Though natural breeding is not possible, semen can be collected for artificial insemination; however, some dogs may be uncomfortable during erection after this surgery. Dogs with permanent prescrotal urethrostomy have a greater risk of urine scald and dermatitis compared to scrotal urethrostomy.

Other urethral approaches in male dogs include urethrotomy of the glans penis or the perineal urethra. Both approaches have been used for removal of stones trapped at that level, and perineal urethrotomy has also been used for removal of kinked urinary catheters and for passage of rigid endoscopes to facilitate scope-assisted techniques such as laser lithotripsy and correction of intramural ectopic ureters.

Preoperative management

Before prescrotal urethrotomy in obstructed dogs, metabolic status, including electrolytes and renal function, should be evaluated. When possible, dogs should be stabilized before anesthesia. Dogs with complete obstruction may require cystocentesis to relieve excessive distension; the bladder should be drained completely (using a needle attached to an extension set, 3-way stopcock, and syringe) to prevent leakage of urine into the abdomen through the needle puncture site. General anesthesia is preferred for urethrotomy; however, it can be performed under sedation and a local or epidural nerve block in

Manual of Small Animal Soft Tissue Surgery, Second Edition. Karen Tobias.
© 2017 John Wiley & Sons, Inc. Published 2017 by John Wiley & Sons, Inc.

severely ill dogs. For prescrotal urethrotomy with cystotomy, the caudal abdomen and prepuce are clipped for sterile surgery, and the prepuce is flushed with antiseptic solution before the final prep. Preparation for a scrotal urethrostomy is also recommended in the event that the calculus cannot be removed; alternatively, a catheter can be placed through the prescrotal incision into the bladder so that the dog can be stabilized for surgery at a later date. Several sizes of red rubber catheters should be available during surgery to facilitate shifting the stone.

Surgery

The incision is centered over the site of the obstruction. Since the urethra cannot be catheterized in obstructed dogs, it is identified visually and by palpating the calculus. Because of its vascular wall, the urethra will often have a bluish tint on visual inspection. Hemorrhage is expected during urethrotomy and immediately after surgery. Urethral incisions that are left open to heal by second intention will bleed for 3 to 14 days; therefore, suture closure is recommended. If the obstructing calculus cannot be removed through a prescrotal urethrotomy, a scrotal urethrostomy is performed.

Surgical technique: prescrotal urethrotomy

1. Make a 2- to 3-cm skin incision centered over the caudal aspect of the os penis, staying superficial to the penile body. Dissect through the subcutaneous tissues with Metzenbaum scissors (fig. 42-1).
2. Expose the retractor penis muscle (fig. 42-2); elevate it and retract it laterally (fig. 42-3).
3. Stabilize the penile body between thumb and forefinger, and incise the urethra on midline over the calculus with a no. 11 or no. 15 blade (fig. 42-4).
4. Extend the urethrotomy with tenotomy scissors or blade as needed to remove the calculus. Control hemorrhage with digital pressure.

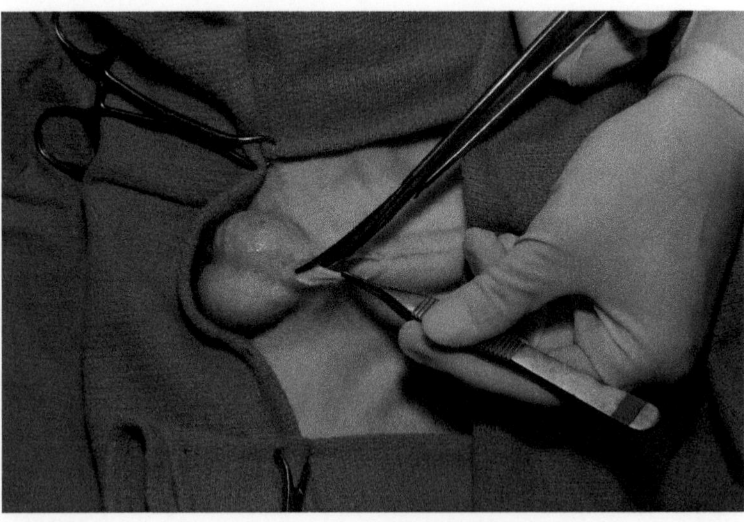

Figure 42-1 Incise the skin over the calculus and transect the subcutaneous tissues with Metzenbaum scissors.

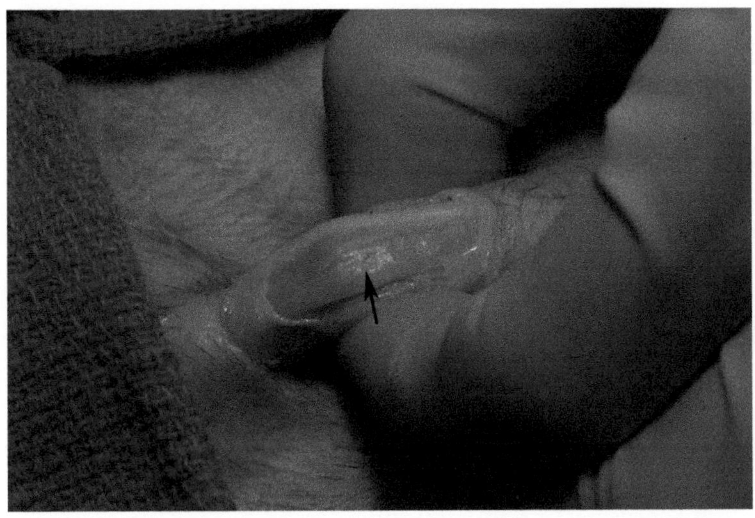

Figure 42-2 Retractor penis muscle (arrow).

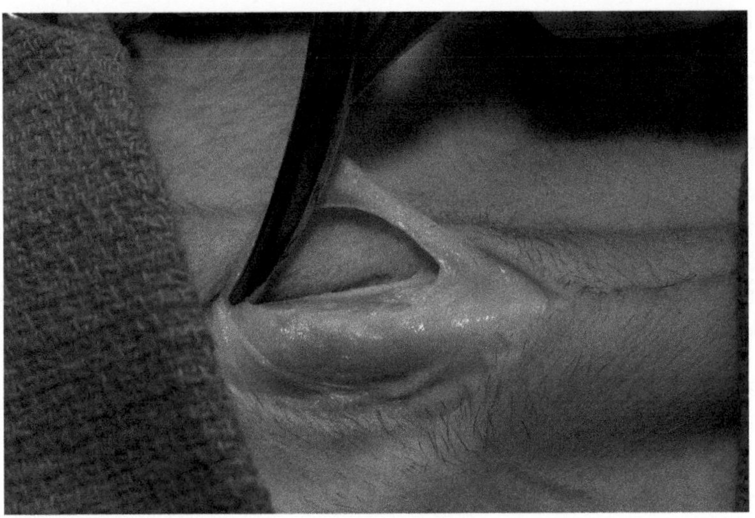

Figure 42-3 Elevate and retract the retractor penis muscle.

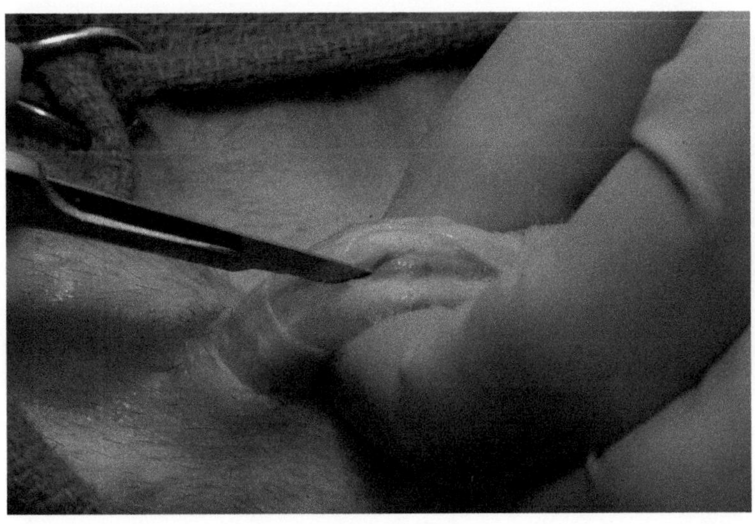

Figure 42-4 Incise the urethra over the calculus.

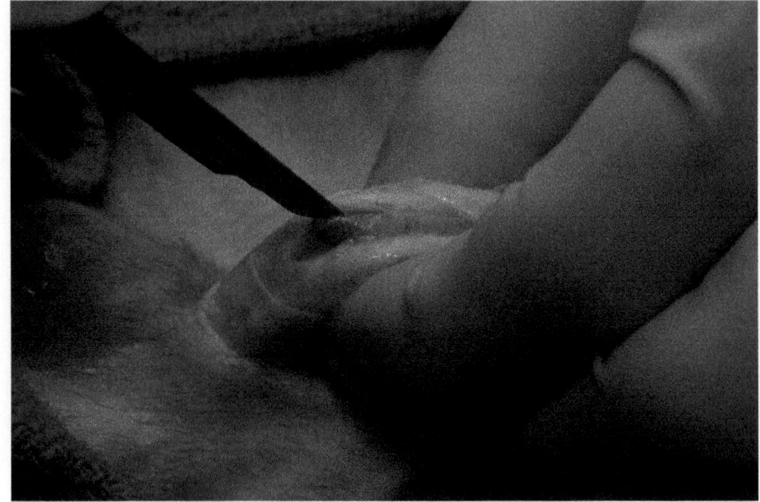

Figure 42-5 Expose and remove the calculus and catheterize the urethra to verify patency.

5. Advance the urethral catheter through the os penis to push any remaining calculi out of the urethrotomy site (fig. 42-5). Flushing with a mixture of sterile water, soluble lubricant, and saline may also help shift the calculus.
6. If the calculus will not move, extend the urethrotomy cranially and attempt to grasp the calculus with Debakey or alligator forceps.
7. Once the calculus is removed, advance the transurethral catheter into the bladder to verify that the urethra is patent, then close the site. Appose the incised urethral edges with 5-0 rapidly absorbable monofilament suture on a taper needle in a simple continuous appositional pattern (fig. 42-6), taking bites 2 mm apart and 2 mm wide.
8. Remove the urethral catheter and close subcutis and skin routinely, or leave them open to permit drainage.

Surgical technique: urethrotomy of the glans penis

1. With the dog in dorsal recumbency, prepare the caudal abdomen, prepuce, and preputial cavity for aseptic surgery.

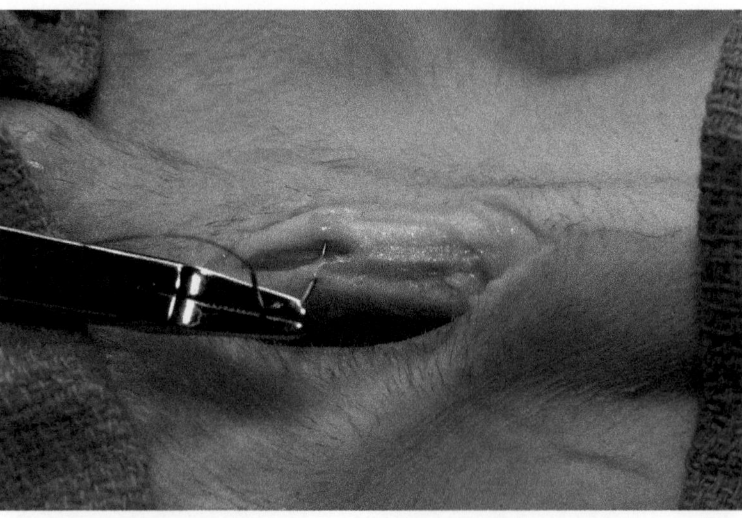

Figure 42-6 Appose the urethral mucosa in a continuous pattern.

2. Exteriorize the penis and catheterize the urethra to the level of the obstruction with a sterile polypropylene catheter.
3. Tie a sterile length of gauze around the base of the penis caudal to the bulbus glandis; pull it caudally to retract the prepuce.
4. Make a longitudinal incision through the ventral midline of the glans penis into the urethra at the level of the obstruction. Extend the incision to 2–2.5 cm. with Metzenbaum scissors to allow removal of the calculus with tissue forceps.
5. Flush and catheterize the urethra to verify that the obstruction is removed.
6. Remove the gauze tie, and reduce the penis back into the prepuce. The wound is allowed to heal by second intention.

Surgical technique: perineal urethrotomy

1. Prep the perineum, prepuce, and caudal abdomen. Place a purse-string suture in the anus and position the dog in sternal recumbency in a perineal position (see fig. 47-2) or on its back with the hind limbs pulled forward (similar to a perineal urethrostomy in a cat).
2. Make an incision along midline, halfway between the anus and scrotum. If the dog is on its back, the level of the incision can be guided by advancement of a urinary catheter to the level of the obstruction.
3. Retract the retractor penis muscle laterally, and separate the paired bulbospongiosus muscles to expose the urethra.
4. Incise the urethral wall over the calculus or obstruction.
5. Once the obstruction is removed, advance the urinary catheter and flush the urethra.
6. Appose the urethral mucosa with 4-0 or 5-0 rapidly absorbable monofilament suture in a simple continuous or simple interrupted pattern. Close subcutaneous tissue and skin routinely.

Postoperative considerations

After the surgery, radiographs are often taken to verify that all stones have been removed. Elizabethan collars or other restraints are placed on the dog to prevent self-trauma. Minimal hemorrhage is reported after urethrotomy of the glans penis, even without suture closure. Hemorrhage usually resolves within 24 hours after prescrotal urethrotomy if the urethra has been closed primarily. Some dogs may require acepromazine and strict exercise restriction, particularly if they are excitable, to stop bleeding. The urethra is usually leakproof within 2 days after primary closure. If evidence of urine leakage is noted (e.g., red and yellow bruising radiating away from the surgery site, fig. 42-7), a urinary catheter should be placed for 2 to 3 days to divert urine and facilitate healing.

Complications of prescrotal urethrotomy are rare with primary closure when tissue handling is gentle and urethral apposition is meticulous and tension free. When urethrotomy sites are allowed to heal by secondary intention, urine leakage from the stoma may continue for up to 2 weeks, and hemorrhage is

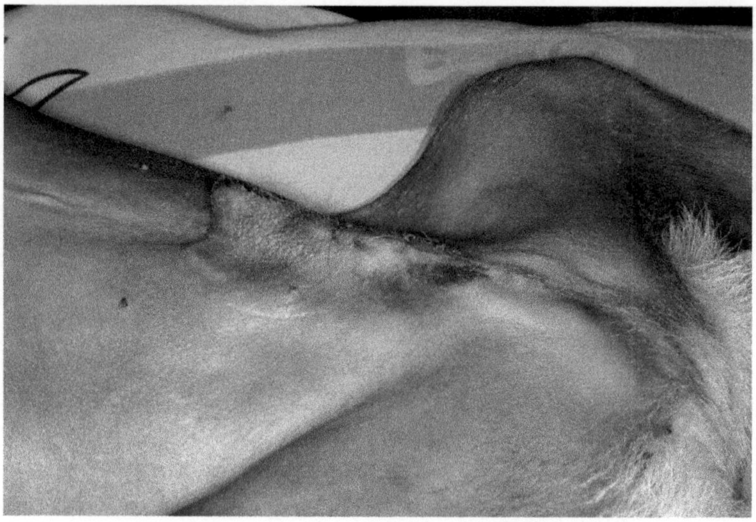

Figure 42-7 Postoperative urine leakage. In this dog, the urethral mucosa was closed with interrupted sutures instead of a continuous pattern. Urine leakage resolved within 3 days after indwelling catheter placement.

much more persistent and severe. More fibrosis is also expected, although stricture is not common.

Bibliography

Basdani E, Papazoglou LG, Kazakos GM, et al: Spontaneous urethral catheter kinking or knotting in male dogs: four cases. J Am Anim Hosp Assoc 2011;47:351–355.

Cinti F, Pisani G, Carusi U, et al: Urethrotomy of the glans penis in three male dogs with urolithiasis. J Small Anim Prac 2015;56:671–674.

Lipscomb V: Surgery of the lower urinary tract in dogs: 2. Urethral surgery. In Pract 2004;26:13–19.

Reimer SB, Kyles AE, Schulz KS, et al: Unusual urethral calculi in two male dogs. J Am Anim Hosp Assoc 2004;40:157–161.

Smeak DD: Urethrotomy and urethrostomy in the dog. Clin Tech Small Anim Pract 2000;15:25–34.

Waldron DR et al: The canine urethra. A comparison of first and second intention healing. Vet Surg 1985;14:213–217.

Weber WJ et al: Comparison of the healing of prescrotal urethrotomy incisions in the dog: sutured versus nonsutured. Am J Vet Res 1985;46:1309–1325.

Weisse C: Percutaneous perineal approach to the canine urethra. In Weisse C, Berent A (ed.): Veterinary Image-Guided Interventions. John Wiley & Sons, Ames IA, 2015: 415–418.

Chapter 43
Scrotal Urethrostomy

Scrotal urethrostomy is most commonly performed in dogs with recurrent cystic and urethral calculi. Other indications include penile neoplasia, necrosis, trauma, or urethral stricture. In dogs, the scrotal urethra is wide, distensible, and superficial, which makes it the preferred site for permanent urethrostomy. Compared with prescrotal or perineal urethrostomy, scrotal urethrostomy also reduces the risk of urine scald.

Preoperative management

Before surgery, dogs should be evaluated for cystic and urethral calculi, cystitis, and metabolic abnormalities such as uremia and hyperkalemia. Intravenous fluids are administered to correct hydration, electrolyte, and acid-base imbalances. If the dog is obstructed, urethral catheterization should be attempted and any urethral calculi retropulsed into the bladder. Calculi can then be removed by cystotomy (Chapter 40). If the obstruction cannot be relieved, intermittent cystocentesis may be required until the animal is stable. If intermittent cystocentesis is performed, the bladder should be completely drained each time so urine does not leak from the puncture wound. This is best accomplished with a needle attached to an extension set, 3-way stopcock, and syringe.

Ultrasound or abdominal and perineal radiographs are recommended to determine the number and location of stones. If ultrasound is not available, contrast cystourethrogram may be required for dogs with radiolucent (e.g., urate) calculi.

In preparation for surgery, the scrotum and caudal abdomen are shaved and prepped. The prepuce is flushed with antiseptic solution before scrubbing the area. For dogs undergoing concurrent cystotomy, the entire abdomen is included in the prep. Epidurals provide excellent intraoperative and post-operative analgesia. Dogs should be monitored after surgery to make sure they urinate after epidural regional block.

Surgery

In unobstructed dogs, the urethra is catheterized during surgery to facilitate urethral identification and dissection. Intact dogs are castrated after the scrotum has been incised. Urethrostomy is performed over the caudoventral

Manual of Small Animal Soft Tissue Surgery, Second Edition. Karen Tobias.
© 2017 John Wiley & Sons, Inc. Published 2017 by John Wiley & Sons, Inc.

curve of the penile body where the urethra is most superficial. Corpus spongiosum surrounds the urethra at this site, and bleeding is expected until the urethrocutaneous anastomosis is complete. Apposition of urethral mucosa and skin is usually performed with a simple continuous pattern using 4-0 rapidly absorbable monofilament suture. Postoperative hemorrhage can be prolonged and significant when an interrupted pattern is used. Some clinicians include bites of tunica albuguinea in the urethrocutaneous closure to improve the holding power of the suture and decrease hemorrhage from the cut edge of the corpus spongiosum. Because the direction of the needle must be altered to remain parallel with each tissue as it is included, the bites of each tissue should be taken separately, especially at the beginning of the pattern, to prevent damage to the urethral mucosa. Because the mucosa can be hard to identify, magnification is recommended. If the surgeon has normal eyesight, a simple pair of reading glasses may be sufficient to improve visibility.

In dogs with cystic calculi and urethral obstruction, scrotal urethrostomy is performed simultaneously with cystotomy. This allows retrograde and antegrade catheterization and flushing of the urethra before cystotomy closure. Calculi that are lodged within the urethra distal to the urethrostomy site do not need to be removed.

Surgical technique: scrotal urethrostomy

1. Make an incision through the scrotal skin.
    a. If the scrotum is not evident, make the incision over the caudoventral curve of the penile body.
    b. If the scrotum is pendulous, make an elliptical incision around redundant scrotal tissue. Leave enough skin so that there will be no tension on the urethrostomy closure.
    c. If the dog is intact, perform a scrotal ablation (see figs. 29-11 and 29-12, pp. 245–246) and closed castration to expose the urethra.
2. With Metzenbaum scissors, dissect away the subcutis to expose the retractor penis muscle ventral to the penile body. Resect the retractor penis muscle or elevate it and retract it laterally (fig. 43-1).
3. Identify the urethra, which often looks like a prominent vein on the ventral midline of the penile body (fig. 43-2).
4. Make a small midline incision in the urethra over the caudoventral curve of the penile body with a no. 11 or no. 15 blade. Use digital pressure to slow hemorrhage.
5. With tenotomy scissors, extend the midline urethral incision to 2 to 3 cm in length, centering it over the curve of the penile body.
6. Identify the cut edge of mucosa, which usually retracts away from the edge of the penile body (fig. 43-3).
7. Suture the skin and mucosa together with a simple continuous pattern, using 4-0 rapidly absorbable monofilament suture on a taper or tapercut needle.
    a. At one end of the incision, take a bite of urethral mucosa (less than one-fourth the diameter of the urethra, if possible) and then the skin, and tie two knots.

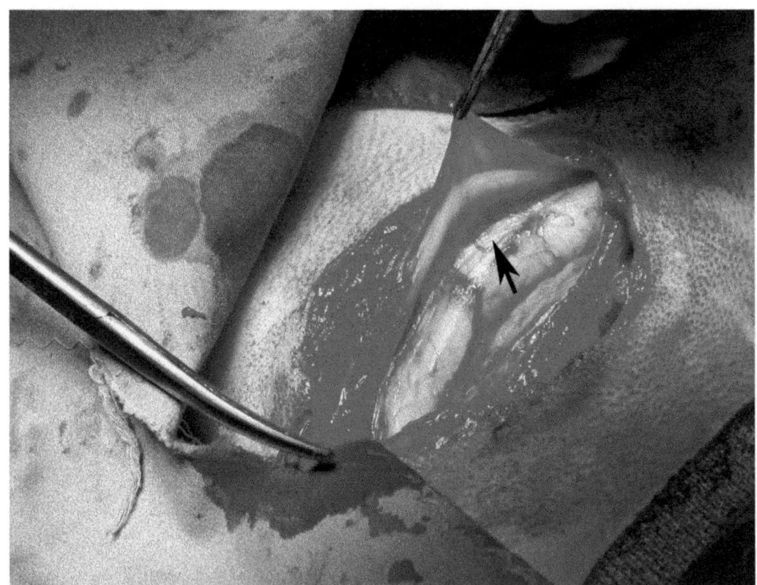

Figure 43-1 Dissect subcutaneous fat away from the penile body and elevate and retract or resect the retractor penis muscle. The urethra (arrow) is pale blue.

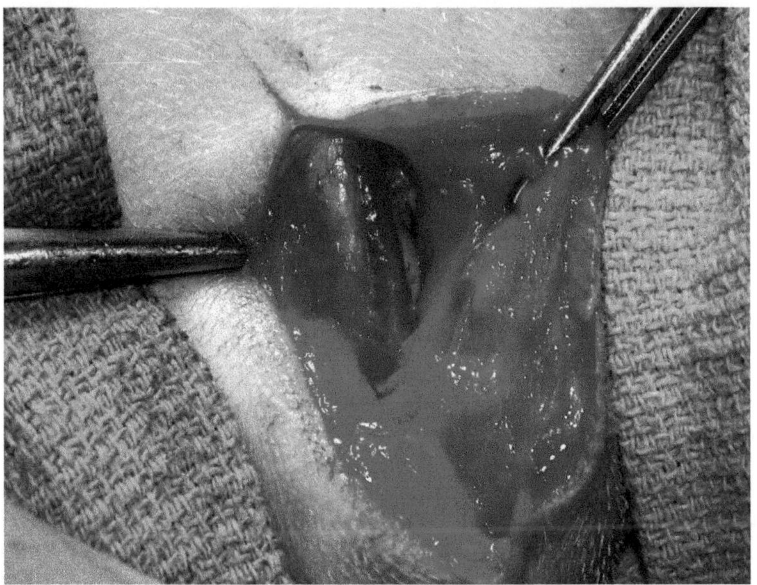

Figure 43-2 In this dog, the urethra is rotated to one side and looks like a large vein.

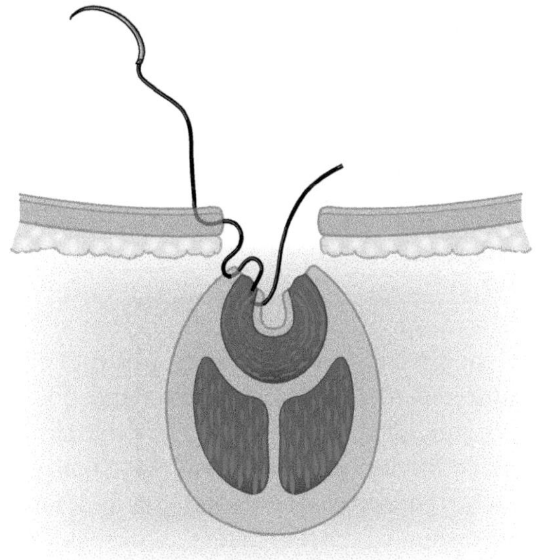

Figure 43-3 Take a bite of mucosa, then a bite of tunica albuguinea, and finally a bite of skin. Courtesy of Samantha Elmurst.

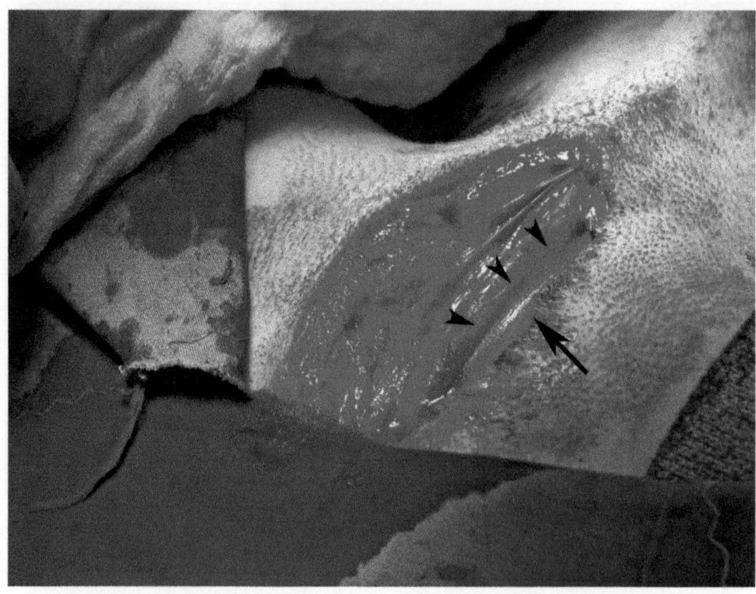

Figure 43-4 The urethral mucosa along one side has been sutured to the skin with a simple continuous pattern (arrow). The cut edge of the mucosa (arrowheads) usually retracts away from the edge of the penile body.

b. Appose skin and mucosa along one side with a continuous pattern. If desired, include tunica albuginea in each bite (fig. 43-3).

    i. Take bites 2 to 3 mm apart.

    ii. Take bites of skin, tunica albuginea, and mucosa separately (pull the needle through each tissue before taking the next bite) to avoid tearing mucosa.

    iii. Include at least 2 mm of each tissue in the bite. If the skin is thick, take a partial thickness bite.

    iv. Avoid handling mucosa with thumb forceps.

c. Complete the closure on the first side (fig. 43-4), then tie off and cut the suture. Repeat the process on the opposite side.

8. Insert a hemostat or catheter into the urethral opening at the caudal end of the incision and place an interrupted suture to appose the skin and ventral urethral mucosa at the "crotch" of the incision. Close the cranial end similarly (fig. 43-5) to reduce the risk of subcutaneous urine leakage and hemorrhage at the incision ends.
9. Close the remaining subcutis and skin as needed.
10. Pass a urinary catheter through the stoma into the bladder to verify that the urethra is unobstructed.

Postoperative considerations

Dogs that have undergone simultaneous cystotomy should receive intravenous fluids for 12 to 24 hours to prevent urinary obstruction by blood clots. Sedatives are administered to reduce excitement and postoperative hemorrhage. If urine scald occurs, clean and dry the peristomal skin and coat the skin with a thin layer of petroleum jelly or liquid bandage. Dogs should wear Elizabethan collars and be exercise-restricted for at least 7 days after the surgery to reduce self-trauma and hemorrhage. Absorbable stomal sutures are

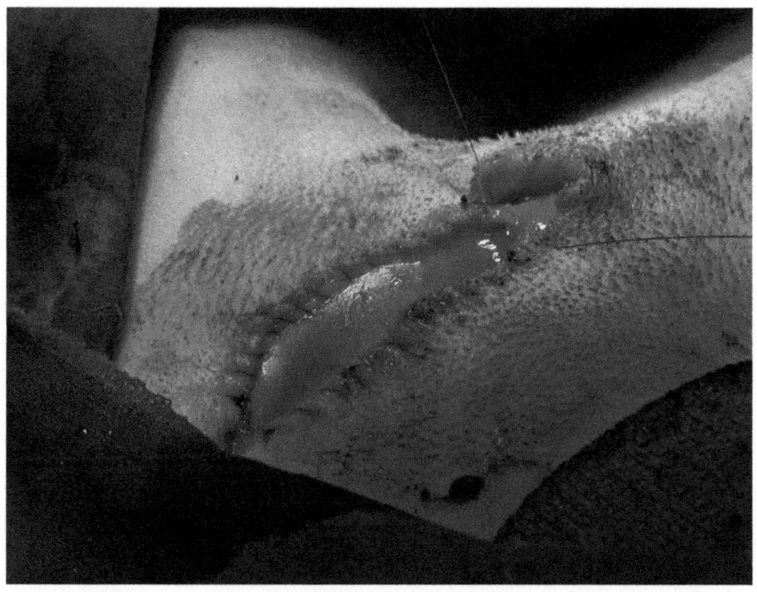

Figure 43-5 At each end of the stoma, suture the ventral urethral mucosa to the skin with an interrupted suture. Before placing the suture, insert hemostat tips or a catheter into the urethra to limit the bite to the ventral aspect of the urethra.

left in place and usually fall out, or are removed by self-grooming, within 3 weeks after surgery.

Complications of scrotal urethrostomy include hemorrhage, stricture, urine scald, incisional infection, dehiscence, and obstruction or cystitis from recurrence of cystic calculi. Hemorrhage is uncommon when continuous suture patterns are used, unless the mucosa was inadvertently excluded from the urethrostomy closure, and anecdotally when tunica albuginea is included in the closure. Animals with persistent hemorrhage should be sedated for 1 to 2 weeks. If hemorrhage is severe, a urinary catheter is placed so that a pressure wrap can be positioned over the site. Urine scald may occur if the urethrostomy site is cranial to the scrotum or too high on the perineum. Stricture is rare as long as the original stoma is sufficient in size and the mucosa has been accurately apposed to the skin.

Bibliography

Bilbrey SA et al: Scrotal urethrostomy: a retrospective review of 38 dogs (1973 through 1988). J Am Anim Hosp Assoc 1991;27:561–564.

Burrow RD, Gregory SP, Giejda AA, et al: Penile amputation and scrotal urethrostomy in 18 dogs. Vet Rec 2011;169:657.

Newton J and Smeak D: Simple continuous closure of canine scrotal urethrostomy: results in 20 cases. J Am Anim Hosp Assoc 1996;32:531–534.

Smeak DD: Urethrotomy and urethrostomy in the dog. Clin Tech Small Anim Pract 2000;5:25–34.

Chapter 44
Perineal Urethrostomy in Cats

Permanent enlargement of the urethral opening may be recommended in male cats with recurrent urinary-tract obstruction from calculi or mucoid plugs. Perineal urethrostomy is also indicated for irresolvable obstruction, strictures, irreparable distal urethral injuries, or neoplasia. Because perineal urethrostomy (PU) increases the risk for bacterial cystitis in cats with underlying urinary tract disease, conservative management of cats with obstructive urolithiasis should be attempted before considering surgery.

Preoperative management

Cats with urethral obstruction may present with dysuria, stranguria, abdominal pain, and lethargy. With complete obstruction, they develop uremia, acidosis, hyperphosphatemia, hyperkalemia, ionized hypocalcemia, and bradycardia and eventually die. Initial management should focus on relieving the obstruction and providing intravenous fluids to correct electrolyte abnormalities and dehydration. Cats may require general anesthesia (e.g., opioids and gas anesthetic) to unplug the penile urethra. If the obstruction cannot be relieved by catheterization, the bladder should be completely emptied by cystocentesis. Cystocentesis must be performed carefully, since overdistended bladders can rupture, and can be facilitated by use of a needle attached to an extension set, 3-way stopcock, and syringe and with ultrasound guidance. Besides routine blood work and urinalysis, survey and contrast radiographic studies of the bladder and urethra are recommended to rule out conditions that can be treated by other means or that require concurrent cystotomy. Permanent urethral stenosis can be difficult to rule out on contrast cystourethrography, since the urethra may swell or spasm after traumatic catheterization.

In preparation for surgery, the caudal abdomen, perineum, and base of the tail are clipped, and a purse-string suture is placed in the anus. If possible, an epidural is performed to provide postoperative analgesia. Traditionally cats have been placed in a perineal position, with the tail pulled forward and the legs either hanging over the table edge or placed in a crouched position under the cat. If the cat is positioned with legs hanging over the table, the table edge

Manual of Small Animal Soft Tissue Surgery, Second Edition. Karen Tobias.
© 2017 John Wiley & Sons, Inc. Published 2017 by John Wiley & Sons, Inc.

should be padded and the cat's chest elevated (e.g., using a rolled towel placed under the axilla) to reduce pressure on the diaphragm.

Cats that require concurrent cystotomy, perineal urethrostomy revision, correction of a urethral stricture, or antegrade catheterization can be positioned in dorsal recumbency with the rear legs pulled forward, tail resting on the table, and perineum facing upwards. For veterinarians accustomed to performing perineal urethrostomy with the cat in a perineal position, the dorsal position is confusing at first. Understanding orientation is easier when veterinarians consider that positioning in dorsal recumbency places the external genitalia in an orientation similar to a canine scrotal urethrostomy. The cats in this chapter's photo series are all in dorsal recumbency.

Surgery

If the cat is intact, castration can be performed routinely through individual apical scrotal incisions or after the initial periscrotal incision has been made. The penile body, which is attached to the pelvis by the ventral penile ligament and ischiourethralis and ischiocavernosus muscles, must be completely mobilized to prevent postoperative stricture. Dorsal and lateral dissection cranial to these muscles should be avoided to reduce the risk of fecal or urinary incontinence secondary to pelvic nerve damage.

The urethra should be opened to the level of the bulbourethral glands. These glands may be difficult to visualize during dissection in a castrated cat, however, so the ostium diameter should be tested with a closed hemostat or a 5 or 8 French red rubber catheter, as described below. Urethrocutaneous apposition is performed with synthetic, rapidly absorbable 4-0 or 5-0 monofilament suture. Fine-tipped needle holders, thumb forceps, and iris scissors are used when manipulating and dissecting urethral tissues. The urethral mucosa, which must be included in each suture bite, often retracts away from the cut edge of the penile body. Reading glasses provide excellent magnification for improving visibility of the urethral mucosa.

If a cystotomy is performed simultaneously, the bladder and urethra can be flushed, in turn, with a catheter advanced retrograde through the urethrostomy and antegrade through the cystotomy. In overweight cats, elliptical pieces of skin and underlying subcutaneous fat can be resected lateral to the finished urethrostomy to evert the stomal edges.

Surgical technique: perineal urethrostomy

1. Make an elliptical incision along the base of the scrotum and prepuce, leaving enough skin for a tension-free closure. Retract the scrotum and prepuce away from the blade as each side is incised (fig. 44-1).
2. After incising through the subcutis, use a gauze sponge to strip any remaining fatty attachments to the penile body (fig. 44-2) in a motion similar to that used for castration. The retractor penis muscle is sometimes removed during this part of the dissection. Alternatively, use scissors to dissect away subcutis.
3. Palpate between the penile body and pelvis to identify the ventral penile ligament. Transect the ligament with Metzenbaum scissors (fig. 44-3), gradually rotating the scissors so they are parallel with the penile body

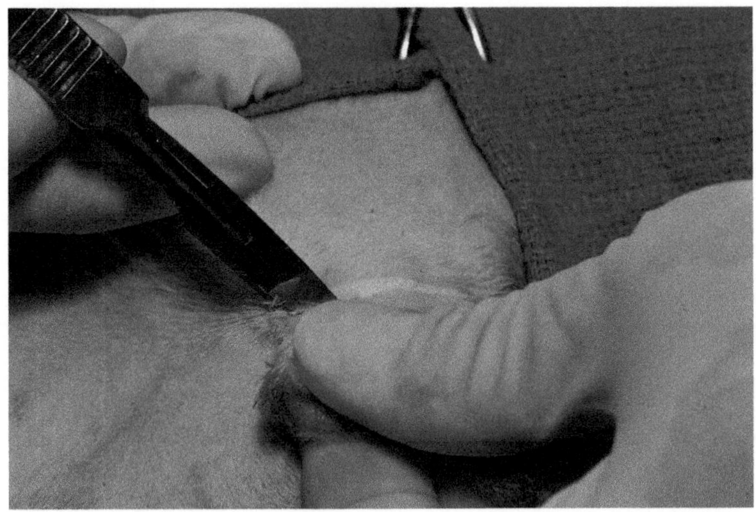

Figure 44-1 Make an incision along the base of the scrotum and prepuce. In this photo series, the cat is in dorsal recumbency with its tail and anus to the right.

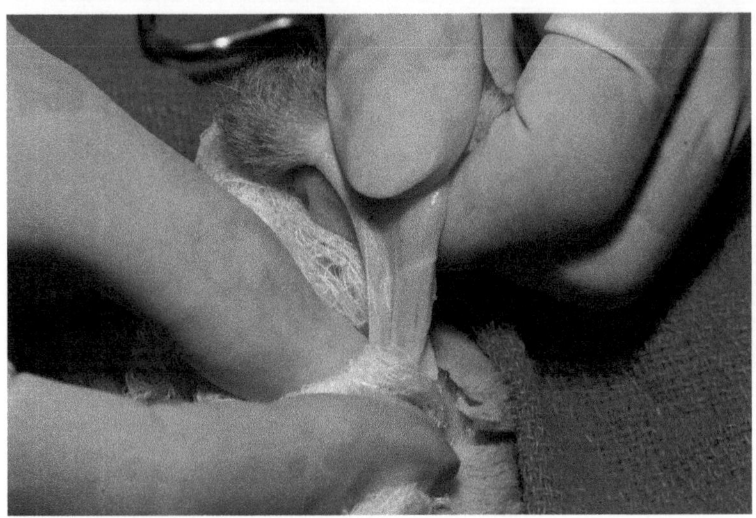

Figure 44-2 Remove any subcutaneous attachments with Metzenbaum scissors or a gauze sponge.

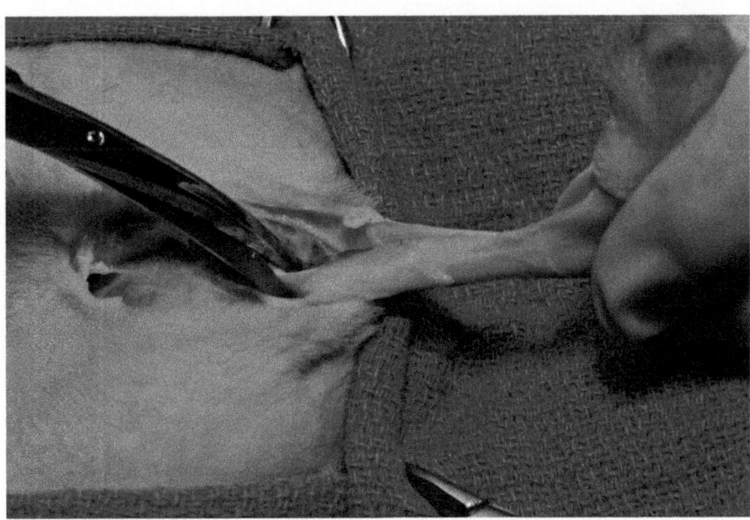

Figure 44-3 Transect the ventral penile ligament.

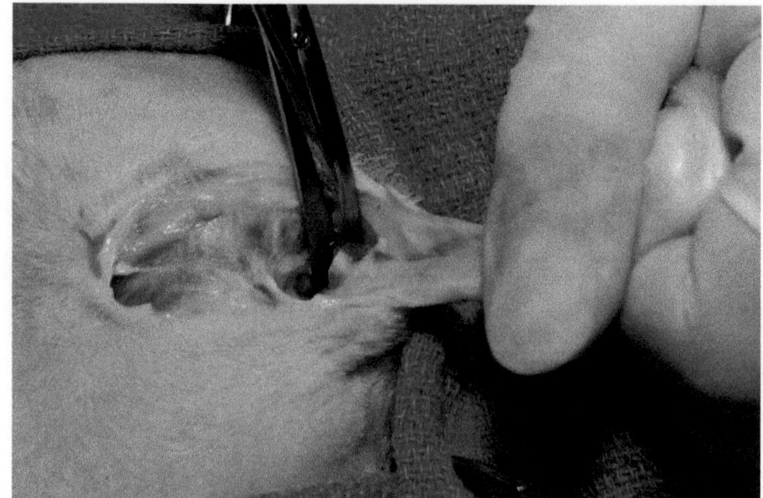

Figure 44-4 Transect the ischiocavernosus and ischiourethralis muscles at their ischial attachments.

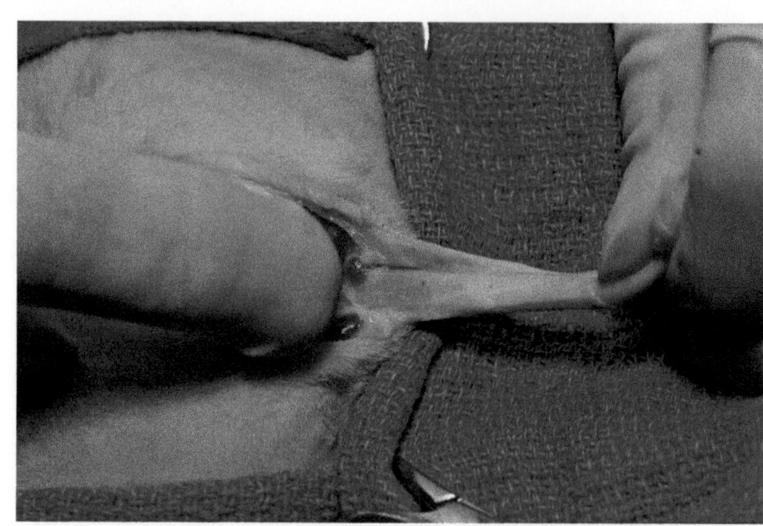

Figure 44-5 Palpate between the penile body and ischium to verify that all attachments have been transected.

with the tips pointed cranially. Gently disrupt any ligamentous remnants with digital pressure.

4. Retract the penile body laterally to identify the ischiocavernosus and ischiourethralis muscles. Place a scissor blade on either side of the muscle group and cut the muscle origins immediately adjacent to the ischium (fig. 44-4). Alternatively, elevate them off the ischium with a periosteal elevate. Repeat on the opposite side.
5. Palpate ventral to the penile body to verify that the penis is freely moveable from the caudal half of the pelvic floor (fig. 44-5).
6. Flip the penile body so it is resting on the ventrum of the animal and facing cranially.
   a. Note that the cat's penile body is now in a position similar to that of a dog undergoing scrotal urethrostomy.
   b. The normally dorsal portion of the cat's penile body will now be facing upward away from the abdomen.

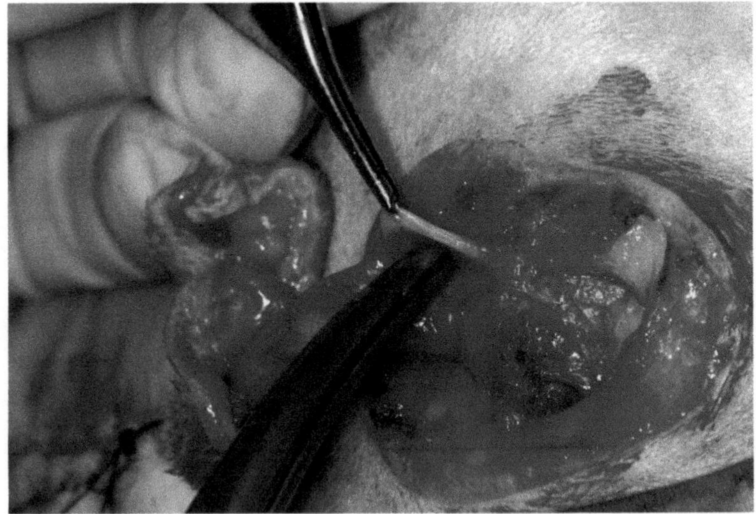

Figure 44-6 Remove the retractor penis muscle if still present.

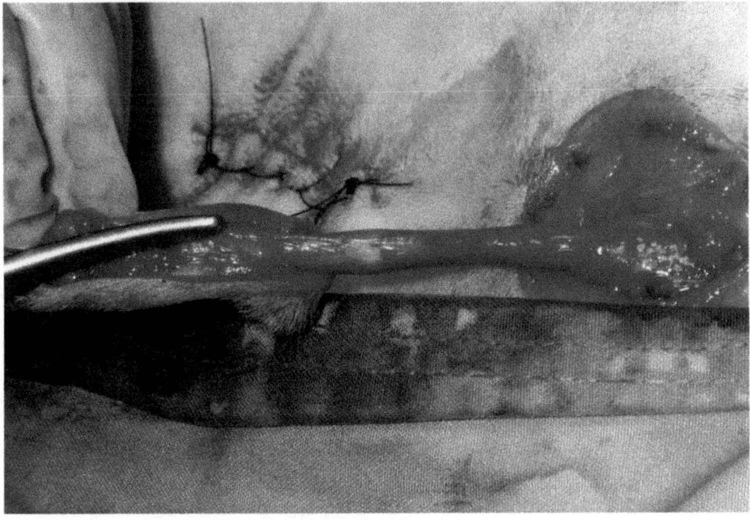

Figure 44-7 Incise the prepuce to expose the penile tip.

7. If it is still present, elevate and resect the retractor penis muscle from the dorsal penile body (fig. 44-6).
8. Incise the dorsal prepuce (the side facing toward the surgeon and the anus) to expose the penile tip (fig. 44-7).
9. Insert one blade of the tenotomy scissors into the tip of the urethra and cut the urethra along the dorsal surface of the penile body (fig. 44-8) to the level of the bulbourethral glands.
    a. Note: with the cat in dorsal recumbency, the cat's "dorsal" penile body surface is on the side facing upward (toward the surgeon) or, with the penis pulled upward, the side closest to the anus.
    b. A distinct crunch can often be felt at the level of the bulbourethral glands when cutting with scissors.
10. Test the diameter of the urethra (fig. 44-9). The opening should be large enough to accommodate a 5 French red rubber catheter or the closed tips of a Halsted mosquito hemostats. If a fine-tipped hemostat is used, you

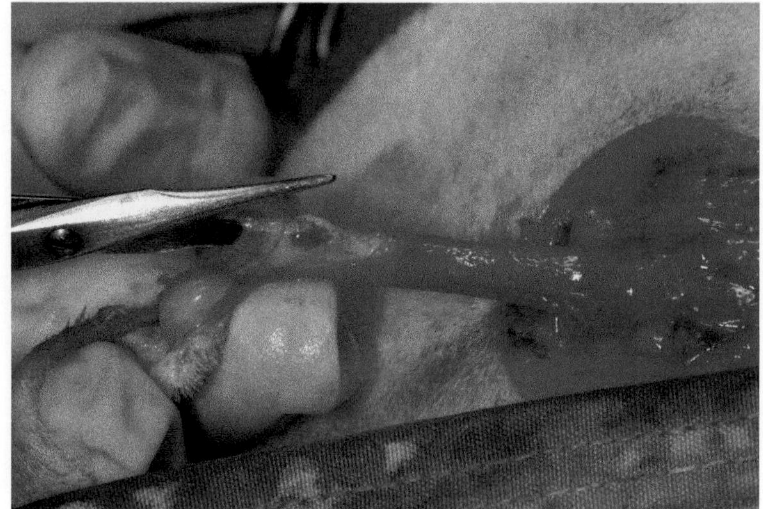

Figure 44-8 Cut open the urethra with fine scissors to the level of the bulbourethral glands.

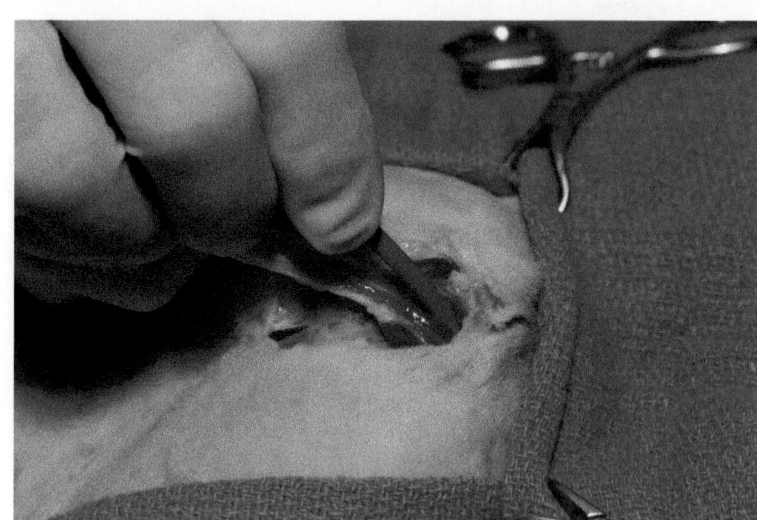

Figure 44-9 Test the diameter of the urethra with a 5 French red rubber catheter or hemostat tips.

should be able to insert the tips to the level of the box locks so that the jaws are no longer visible. Extend the urethral incision proximally (toward the anus) as needed to enlarge the opening.

11. Preplace the first two sutures from the urethral mucosa to the skin at the 10 and 2 o'clock positions (fig. 44-10A), securing each in hemostats.
    a. Identify the mucosa, which commonly retracts from the cut edge of the penile body (fig. 44-11).
    b. Take bites of mucosa that are less than one-third of the urethral diameter.
    c. To reduce the risk of mucosal tearing, take the mucosal and skin bites separately, pulling the needle through the tissue between each bite.
12. Place the dorsal most (12 o'clock) suture (fig. 44-12).
    a. Take a bite of skin 2 mm dorsal/caudal to the 10 or 2 o'clock preplaced suture (see Figure 44-10A), and pull the needle through. Note: Taking this skin bite laterally, versus dorsally, decreases

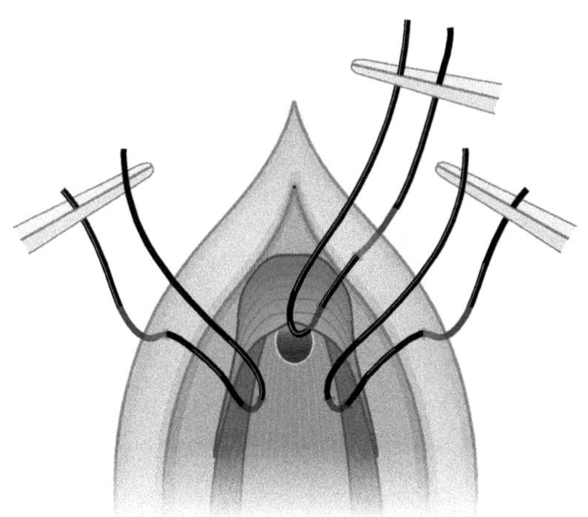

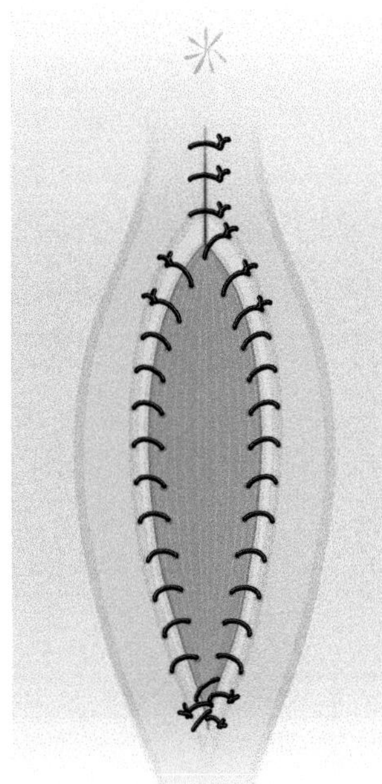

Figure 44-10 A. The first 3 sutures are preplaced between skin and urethral mucosa at 10 o'clock, 2 o'clock, and 12 o'clock. Note that the skin bite in the 12 o'clock suture is laterally placed. **B.** Once the first 3 sutures are tied, the remaining urethrostomy is formed with a simple continuous pattern down each side of the site. Gaps in skin dorsal to the urethrostomy are closed with interrupted sutures.

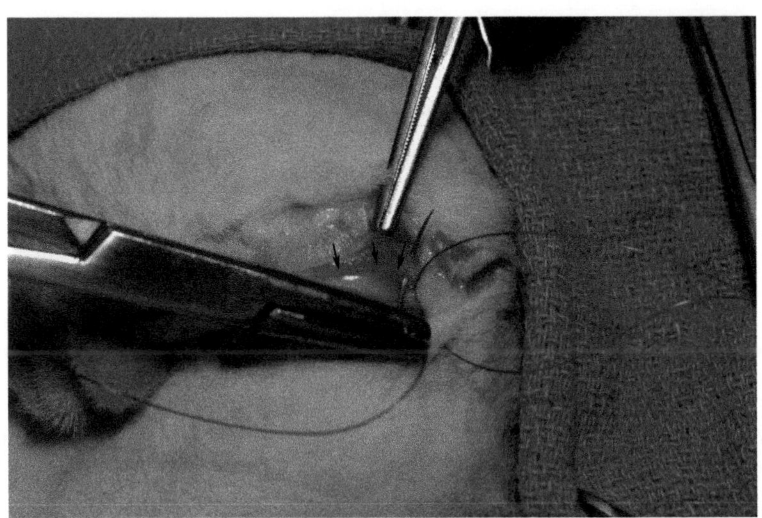

Figure 44-11 Note how the mucosal edge (arrows) retracts from the cut edge of the penile body (held with a hemostat in this cadaver photo).

tension on the urethrostomy and leaves a greater distance between the urethrostomy and the anus as compared with taking the skin bite at the dorsal "crotch" of the skin incision.

b. Insert the closed jaws of a straight Halsted mosquito hemostat into the urethra.

c. Open the jaws of the hemostat slightly and pass the needle through the dorsal urethral mucosa (fig. 44-12), exiting the urethral lumen between the hemostat jaws. This improves visualization of the dorsal urethral wall and prevents accidental inclusion of urethral mucosa from the opposite side.

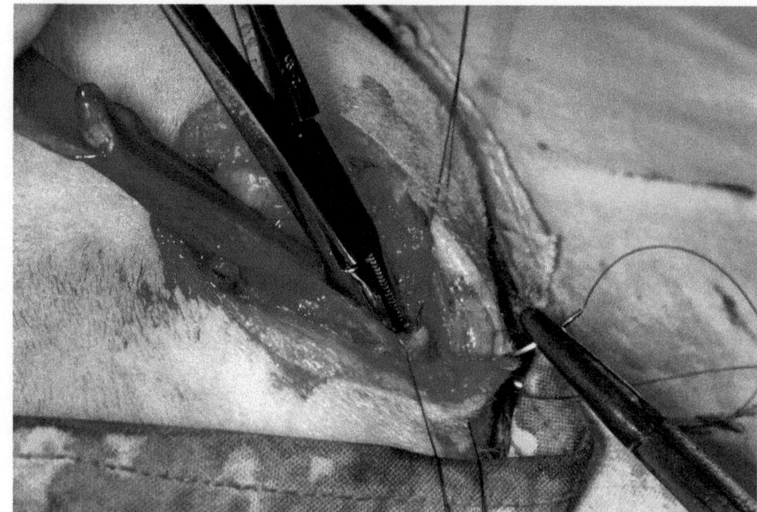

Figure 44-12 Insert a hemostat within the urethra while placing the 12 o'clock suture.

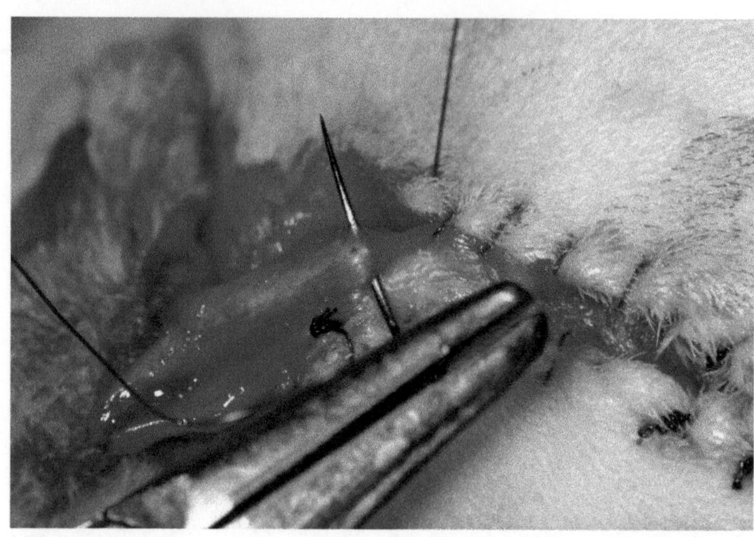

Figure 44-13 Appose the urethral mucosa to skin laterally with a simple continuous pattern along each side. Note how the mucosal bite is taken separately from the skin bite.

13. After tying the preplaced sutures, appose the urethral mucosa to the skin on each side with a simple continuous pattern of rapidly absorbable suture, working from dorsal (caudal) to ventral (cranial) and placing bites approximately 2 mm apart. (fig. 44-13). Continue the appositional pattern on the first side until the urethral "drain board" begins to narrow, then tie it off and start a new pattern on the opposite side.
14. Ligate the distal penile body with absorbable suture and amputate it with the attached preputial and scrotal skin before completing the skin closure (fig. 44-14). The final drain board is usually 1 to 2 cm long (fig. 44-15). Remove the anal purse string when finished.

Postoperative considerations

Cats should wear an Elizabethan collar for at least 7 days to prevent self-mutilation, which can increase the risk of strictures. Analgesics are recommended for several days after surgery, and cats that have undergone simultaneous

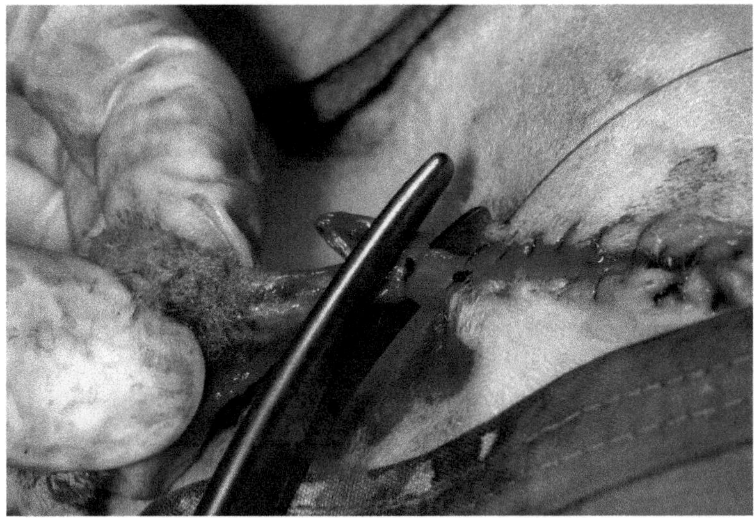

Figure 44-14 Ligate the distal penile body (prepuce still attached) before transecting.

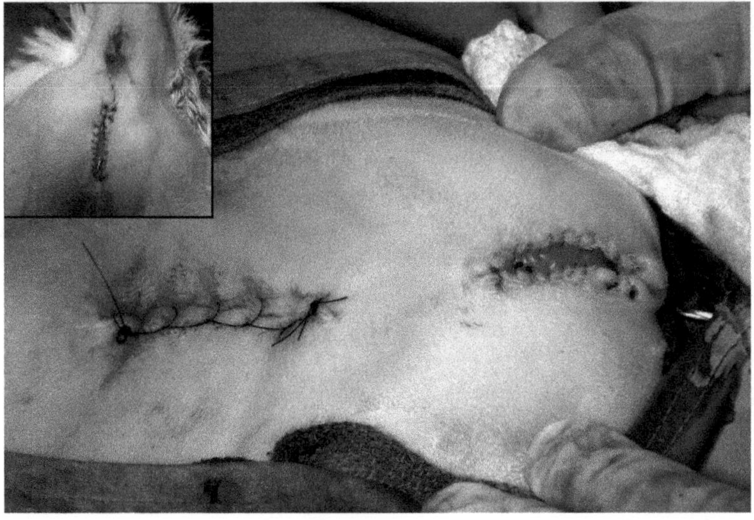

Figure 44-15 Ventral and caudal (inset) appearance after perineal urethrostomy with concurrent cystotomy.

cystotomy are kept on intravenous fluids during recovery to flush out any blood clots. Antibiotics are usually unnecessary, since bacterial cystitis is rare in cats. Absorbable monofilament sutures along the urethrostomy site are left in place and are usually extruded, covered with epithelium, or removed by the cat once the Elizabethan collar is removed. Paper litter is often recommended for the first week after surgery.

Common early complications include hemorrhage and swelling. Hemorrhage is reduced by using a continuous pattern, including the mucosa in each suture bite, preventing self-trauma, and keeping the cat sedated immediately after the procedure. Because it retracts away from the incision edge, urethral mucosa is easy to miss during urethrocutaneous apposition. Poor mucosal apposition and postoperative swelling may allow urine to travel through gaps in the suture line and into the subcutaneous tissues, increasing postoperative swelling and risk of subsequent stricture. Subcutaneous urine leakage may also occur with catheter-induced urethral lacerations or suture line inversion secondary to anastomotic tension (e.g., a short urethra from a high PU). Urine extravasation often appears as red and yellow bruising radiating away from the incision site. In cats predisposed to subcutaneous urine leakage, a 5 French

Foley catheter can be left in place for 2 to 3 days after surgery until the urethrocutaneous junction seals. Use of catheters is otherwise not routinely recommended because of ascending infection and urethral irritation.

Mortality rates in the first 2 weeks after surgery are 5%–9% and are most frequently a result of euthanasia because of re-occlusion, sepsis, or multisystem disease. Other complications include stricture, bacterial urinary tract infections, recurrence of clinical signs, and incontinence. Incontinence is uncommon as long as dissection is limited, as described above. Clinical signs may reoccur in cats that have persistent feline lower urinary tract disease, form calculi, or develop urinary tract infections. Cystitis (sterile or bacterial) occurs after perineal urethrostomy in 1% to 40% of cats with feline lower urinary tract disease; therefore, periodic urinalysis and culture are recommended.

Strictures usually occur within 6 months after surgery and most commonly result from failure to free the penile body from its pelvic attachments or incise the urethra to the level of the bulbourethral glands. They may also occur if urine leaks between the mucosa and skin edges. Strictures are corrected by incising carefully around the urethrostomy and dissecting the remaining urethra up to the pelvis, where its attachments are transected. If the urethra cannot be found, a cystotomy is performed simultaneously, and the urethra is catheterized antegrade. Because cystotomy may be required, the cat should be positioned in dorsal recumbency for the approach. After urethral attachments are freed ventrally, the urethral opening is widened and sutured as described for a traditional perineal urethrostomy, although there may only be room for interrupted sutures. The resulting drain board will be much shorter than the original perineal urethrostomy; however, urine scald does not seem to be a problem in these cats.

Bibliography

Agrodnia MD et al: A simple continuous pattern using absorbable suture for perineal urethrostomy in the cat: 18 cases (2000–2002). J Am Anim Hosp Assoc 2004;40:479–483.

Corgozinho KB et al: Catheter-induced urethral trauma in cats with urethral obstruction. J Feline Med Surg 2007;9:481–486.

Griffin DW and Gregory CR: Prevalence of bacterial urinary tract infection after perineal urethrostomy in cats. J Am Vet Med Assoc 1992;200:681–684.

Phillips H and Holt DE: Surgical revision of the urethral stoma following perineal urethrostomy in 11 cats: (1998–2004). J Am Anim Hosp Assoc 2006;42:218–222.

Ruda L, Heine R: Short- and long-term outcome after perineal urethrostomy in 86 cats with feline lower urinary tract disease. J Small Anim Pract 2012;53:693–698.

Segev G, LIvne H, Ranen E, et al: Urethral obstruction in cats: predisposing factors, clinical, clinicopathological characteristics and prognosis. J Feline Med Surg 2011;13" 101–108.

Tobias KM: Procedures pro: perineal urethrostomy in the cat. NAVC Clinician's Brief 2007;5:19–22.

Chapter 45
Urethral Prolapse

Urethral prolapse is an uncommon condition that occurs most often in young, intact, male brachycephalic dogs. The etiology is unknown but may be related to sexual excitation or genitourinary tract infection. Genetic factors and increased intra-abdominal pressure secondary to upper airway obstruction have also been proposed as underlying causes, since English bulldogs have a risk more than 300 times that of other dogs. Affected dogs have a reddish, irregular mass protruding from the tip of the penis (fig. 45-1). In some dogs, the prolapse may only be present during erection or may become more prominent at that time. Other clinical signs include hemorrhage and excessive self-grooming.

Preoperative management

The penile body and prepuce should be examined in affected dogs for inflammation and abnormal discharge (balanoposthitis). A hemogram is evaluated, since some dogs develop anemia secondary to hemorrhage from the prolapsed tissues. Prostatic disease, calculi, and structural bladder abnormalities can be ruled out with abdominal radiographs and ultrasound. If cystitis is suspected, antibiotic therapy is instituted once a urine sample has been obtained for culture and sensitivity.

Before surgery, the preputial cavity is flushed with an antiseptic solution. The prepuce does not need to be clipped, since this may cause skin irritation that leads to excessive grooming and recurrence of the prolapse. In dogs with stranguria, a urethral catheter can be advanced into the bladder under anesthesia to verify that the urethra is patent.

Surgery

Urethral prolapse is often repaired by resection and anastomosis of the protruding tissue or by urethropexy. Resection is performed in a "cut and sew" technique, similar to a rectal prolapse (p. 383). This prevents the urethral mucosa from retracting into the urethral lumen before it can be anastomosed to the penile mucosa. Anastomosis is performed with 4-0 or 5-0 rapidly absorbable monofilament suture material on a taper needle, while urethropexy usually employs larger suture material because of the need for a longer needle.

Manual of Small Animal Soft Tissue Surgery, Second Edition. Karen Tobias.
© 2017 John Wiley & Sons, Inc. Published 2017 by John Wiley & Sons, Inc.

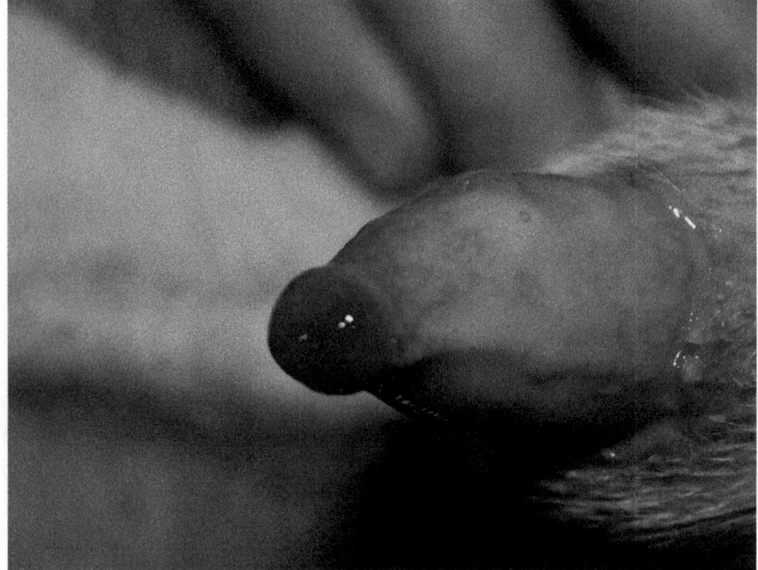

Figure 45-1 Urethral prolapse in a bulldog. This dog has concurrent inflammation of the internal preputial lamina and glans penis (balanoposthitis).

Because sexual excitement can result in recurrence, most surgeons recommend concurrent castration.

Surgical technique: urethropexy

1. To expose the penile body and provide hemostais, wrap a Penrose drain around the base of the penis, retracting the prepuce, and hold the drain firmly around the penis with a hemostat.
2. Insert a groove director into the urethra to reduce the prolapse and provide a platform for suture placement. If a groove director is not available, one can be manufactured out of a polypropylene catheter by making a longitudinal slit wide enough to accommodate the needle.
3. Using 3-0 absorbable monofilament suture on a taper needle, pass the needle through the penile body into the urethral lumen, along the groove director, and out the urethral opening (fig. 45-2).
4. Pull the needle out of the tissues and the suture through the penile body, leaving an end for tying.

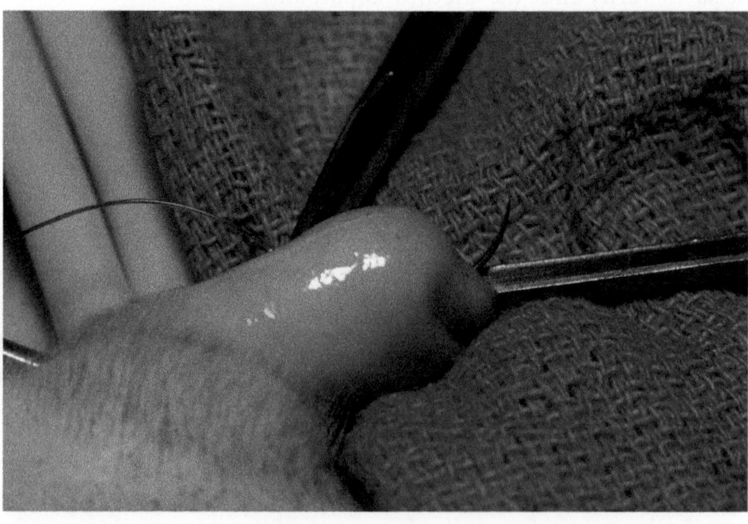

Figure 45-2 Urethropexy. Insert a groove director into the urethra and pass the needle and suture from the penile body out the urethral opening.

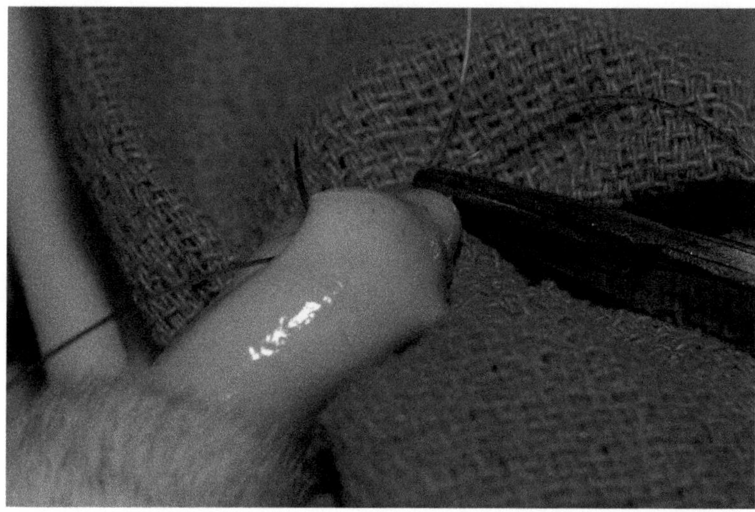

Figure 45-3 Urethropexy. Pass the needle back through the urethral lumen and out the penile body proximal to the first bite. Once the needle tip exits the penile body, remove the groove director to facilitate full needle passage.

5. Reverse the needle direction and pass the needle through the urethral opening, down the urethral lumen, through the penile body, and out the penis (fig. 45-3). Remove the groove director once the needle has exited the penile body.
6. Tie the suture on the penile body firmly so the penile epithelium indents slightly but the suture does not damage mucosa or penile body (fig. 45-4).
7. If desired, place a second suture similarly but on the opposite side of the penile body.
8. Release the tourniquet and examine the suture sites for bleeding before replacing the penile body into the prepuce.

Surgical technique: urethral prolapse resection

1. To expose the penile body, retract the prepuce with a Penrose drain (fig. 45-5) or gauze tie.
2. Using sterile technique, pass a lubricated red rubber urinary catheter into the penile urethra.

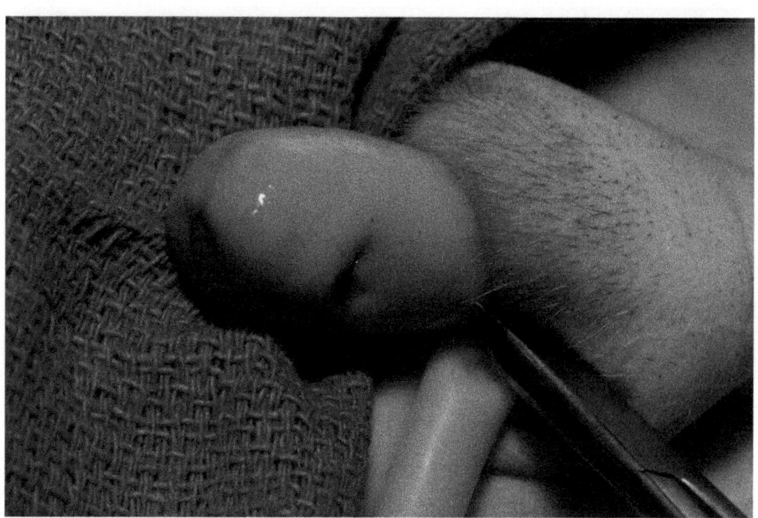

Figure 45-4 Completed urethropexy. Note penile tip inversion.

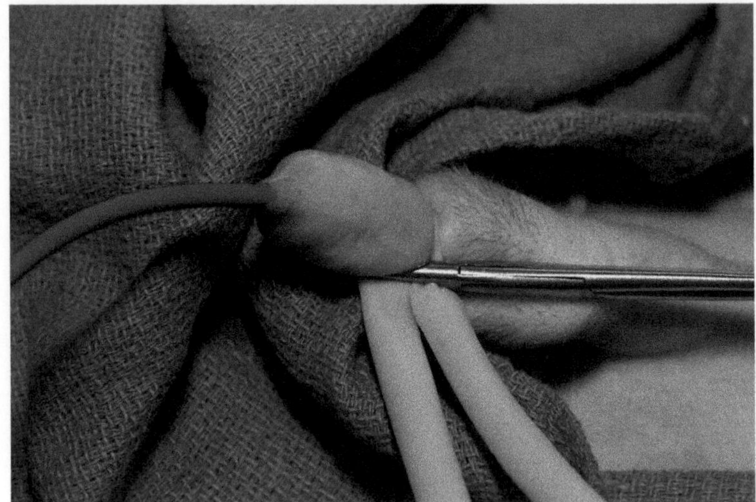

Figure 45-5 Retract the penis from the prepuce with a Penrose drain and catheterize the urethra.

3. With fine scissors, make an incision through the prolapsed mucosa toward the tip of the penis. This initial incision will be perpendicular to the edge of the prolapsed tissue.
4. Rotate the scissors so that they are parallel to the tip of the penis and prolapsed edge. Transect one-third to one-half of the base of the prolapsed tissue around the circumference of the prolapse (fig. 45-6). This cut will be immediately adjacent to the tip of the penis.
5. Start the anastomosis at one end of the transection, placing the knot on the external surface.
    a. Use 4-0 or 5-0 rapidly absorbable, monofilament suture on a taper needle.
    b. Take a 2–3 mm bite of penile mucosa, starting at one end of the transected edge.
    c. Take a 1.5–2 mm bite of the urethral mucosa and tie one or two knots, leaving the end long. Note: it is often necessary to use separate passes when taking bites of penile epithelium and urethral mucosa to better

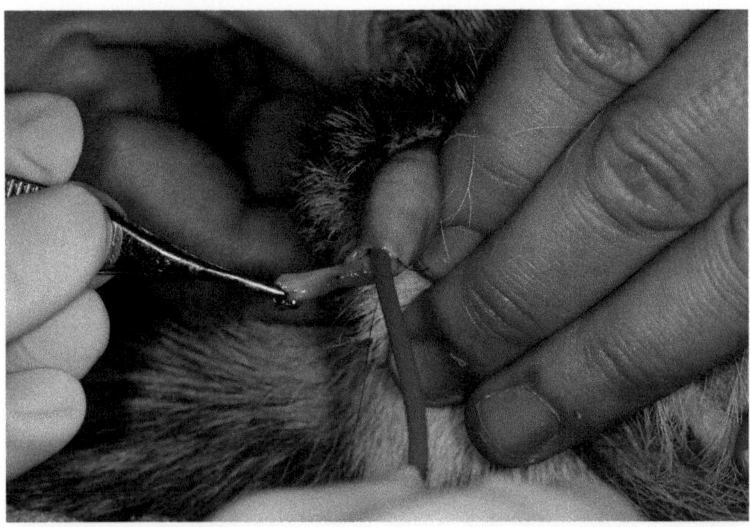

Figure 45-6 Transect a portion of the prolapsed urethral mucosa parallel to the penile tip.

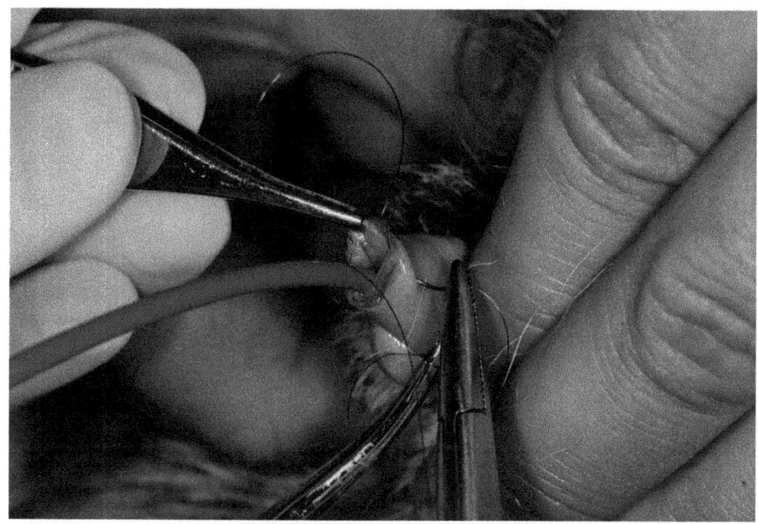

Figure 45-7 Suture urethral mucosa to penile mucosa with a simple continuous pattern.

align the tissues and avoid mucosal tearing. The needle should be pulled completely through each tissue before the subsequent tissue bite is taken.

d. Continue to appose the urethral and penile mucosa in a simple continuous pattern, placing sutures 1.5 to 2 mm apart.

6. Once several suture bites have been placed, continue to cut and sew the mucosa in stages until the entire circumference of prolapsed urethral mucosa is resected and anastomosed to the penile mucosa (fig. 45-7).
7. Tie the final suture bite to the original suture end, and remove the urinary catheter (fig. 45-8). If swelling is a concern, leave the catheter in for 24 hours.

Postoperative considerations

Treatment of underlying conditions such as cystitis should be continued after surgery. In dogs with balanoposthitis, a topical antibiotic/steroid cream can be

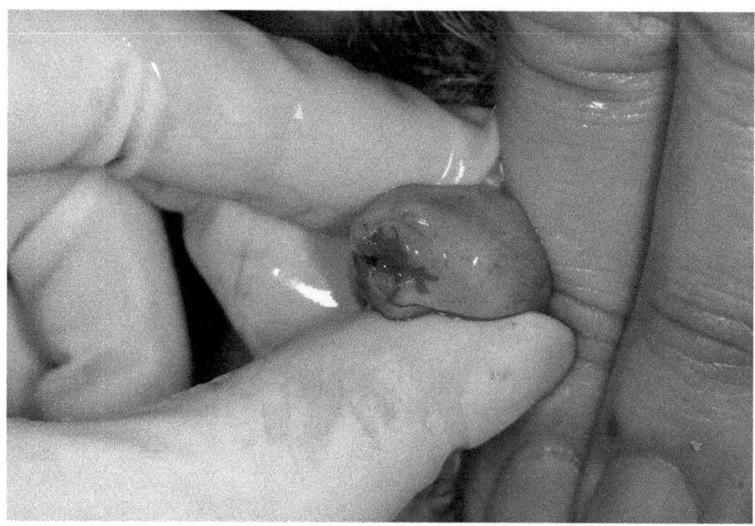

Figure 45-8 Final appearance after mucosal resection and anastomosis.

infused into the prepuce several times daily until inflammation has resolved. Dogs should wear an Elizabethan collar or other restraining device for at least 7 days and should be isolated from other dogs, particularly females in estrus. Sexual excitement increases postoperative swelling and hemorrhage; therefore, any triggers that incite self-stimulation should be removed from the environment. Many dogs will require sedatives, such as acepromazine or trazodone, until the site is healed. Sutures do not need to be removed.

Complications are common after surgery and include hemorrhage (39%) and recurrence (57%). Dogs undergoing urethropexy may also have urethral and penile swelling and local bruising. Hemorrhage from the anastomotic site may continue for up to 7 days after urethral prolapse resection, particularly if an interrupted pattern has been used. Recurrence is less common if dogs are sedated after the surgery. If the condition recurs after mucosal resection and anastomosis, a urethropexy can be attempted. Dogs with multiple recurrences may require penile amputation and scrotal urethrostomy.

Bibliography

Carr JG, Tobias KM, Smith L: Urethral prolapse in dogs: a retrospective study. Vet Surg 2014;43:574–580.

Kirsch JA et al: A urethropexy technique for surgical treatment of urethral prolapse in the male dog. J Am Anim Hosp Assoc 2002;38:381–384.

Lipscomb V: Surgery of the lower urinary tract in dogs: 2. Urethral surgery. In Pract 2004; January: 13–19.

Papazoglou LG and Kazakos GM: Surgical conditions of the canine penis and prepuce. Compend Contin Educ Pract Vet 2002;24:204–218.

Section 6 Perineal Procedures

Chapter 46
Anal Sacculectomy

Anal sacs produce a pasty, foul-smelling secretion that is normally expressed during defecation. Ducts from the sacs empty through openings at the 4 o'clock and 8 o'clock positions around the anus, just outside of the mucocutaneous junction. Inflammation within or around the sac or duct opening may change secretion characteristics or prevent emptying of the sacs, resulting in enlargement and discomfort. Anal sacculectomy is indicated for treatment of chronically infected or impacted anal sacs that do not respond to medical therapy or for removal of anal sac tumors. Dogs with perianal fistulas that have not resolved with immunosuppressive therapy may also benefit from the surgery.

Preoperative management

If an anal sac mass is detected on digital rectal examination, dogs should be evaluated for metastases. Anal sac tumors frequently spread to sublumbar lymph nodes and, less often, lungs. Paraneoplastic syndrome associated with some anal sac adenocarcinomas results in persistent hypercalcemia and secondary renal failure. Therefore, ionized or total calcium, phosphorous, BUN, and creatinine concentrations and urine specific gravity should be measured in dogs with anal sac masses. Dogs with anal sacculitis should be evaluated for allergies or other causes of dermatitis. Cellulitis from anal sac rupture should be treated with antibiotics and analgesics until inflammation is resolved. Focal abscesses should be drained and lavaged; anal sacculectomy is performed once swelling and infection have resolved.

Before surgery, a purse-string suture is placed in the anus craniomedial to the duct openings (see Chapter 48, pp. 382–383). The anal sacs are gently flushed with antiseptic solution or saline and the perineal region is clipped and prepped. The animal is placed in a perineal position over the padded end of a surgery table. The tail should be pulled up and forward with tape. Because of compression of the viscera on the diaphragm, respirations should be assisted while the animal is in the perineal position.

Surgery

Anal sacs can be removed by an open or closed technique. The closed technique, in which the sac is dissected out intact, should be performed in

Manual of Small Animal Soft Tissue Surgery, Second Edition. Karen Tobias.
© 2017 John Wiley & Sons, Inc. Published 2017 by John Wiley & Sons, Inc.

animals with anal sac tumors and in ferrets and other species that have particularly odoriferous secretions. Choice of technique is otherwise based on personal preference and experience. In dogs, the anal sacs are completely surrounded by a layer of external anal sphincter muscle fibers and are difficult to see during closed sacculectomy. If a mass is not present, identification of the sac can be facilitated by inserting something into the sac to make it larger and more firm. Options include umbilical tape, a Foley catheter, or a gel that hardens after infusion. Alternatively, an instrument or cotton-tipped applicator swab can be left in the duct and sac during dissection. In cats, the anal sacs are more readily apparent.

The open technique described below is easier to perform if the surgeon has small fingers or the anal sacs are large. With closed or open techniques, dissection should be as close to the sac as possible to reduce the chance of injury to the caudal rectal artery and nerve and to minimize trauma to the external anal sphincter. Resected tissue should be inspected to make sure the anal sac has been completely removed.

Surgical technique: closed anal sacculectomy

1. If the anal sac is not palpable, insert a groove director, cotton-tipped applicator swab, Kelly hemostatic forceps, or 5 or 6 French latex or silicone balloon-tipped (e.g., Foley) catheters down the duct and into the anal sac (fig. 46-1).
    a. If a Foley catheter is used, insert the catheter down the duct until the entire balloon is in the sac. Inflate the balloon with 1 to 2 mL of sterile saline until it is the size of the normal sac. If necessary, place a suture around the duct and catheter to prevent the catheter from backing out as the balloon is inflated.
    b. If a rigid instrument is used, angle the tip of the instrument so that the anal sac is forced caudally and superficially (toward the surgeon).
2. Make a 2- to 3-cm vertical curvilinear skin incision. The incision should be 1 to 2 cm lateral to the anus and centered over the tip of the probe or catheter balloon.

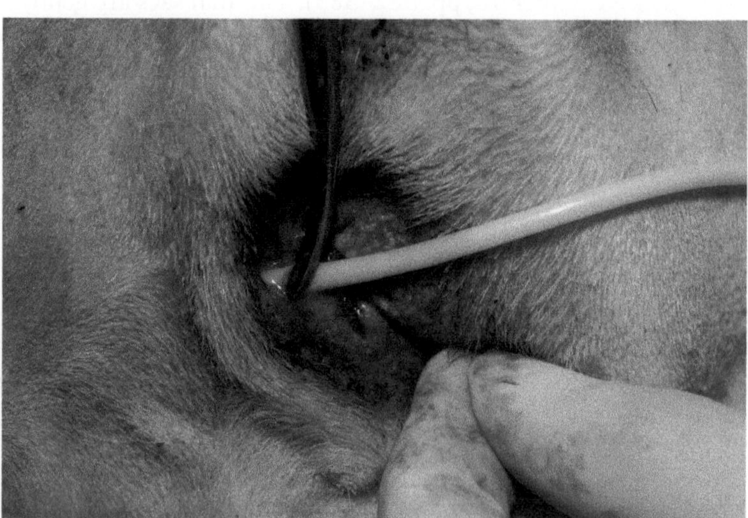

Figure 46-1 Insert a Foley catheter or rigid instrument down the duct and into the sac. If a Foley catheter is used, inflate the balloon with 1 to 2 mL of saline.

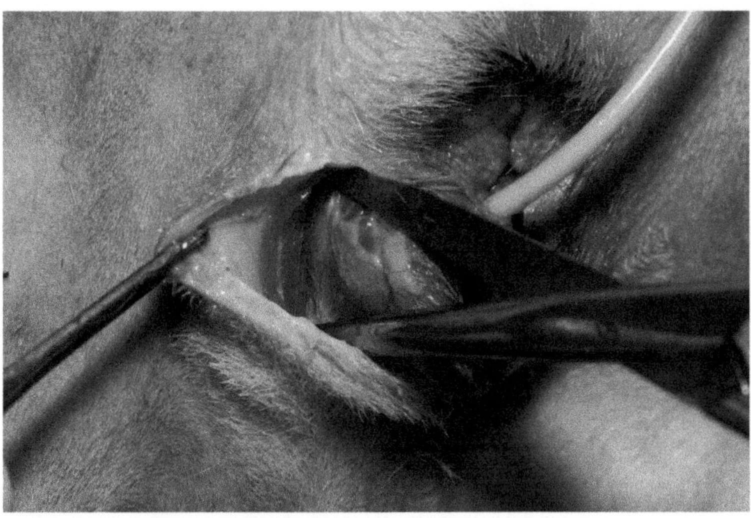

Figure 46-2 Remove overlying subcutaneous tissues and thin muscle fibers with scissors.

3. Dissect away the subcutaneous tissue and superficial muscle fibers overlying the sac (fig. 46-2).
4. Maintain caudal rotation and traction on the sac with the probe or another instrument.
   a. Grasp the exposed apex of the anal sac (and deflated Foley balloon, if one is in place) with an Allis tissue or Babcock forceps. Retract the sac caudally, pulling gently so that the tissues do not tear.
   b. Alternatively, continue to direct the tip of the forceps, groove director, or other inserted device caudally.
5. Using iris or Metzenbaum or blunt-tipped tenotomy scissors, dissect external anal sphincter muscle fibers off the sac, working from the sac apex toward the duct (fig. 46-3).
   a. Insert the scissors under the muscle fibers without penetrating the sac.
   b. Spread the fibers parallel to the sac wall so that the glistening, grayish white surface of the sac is exposed underneath.

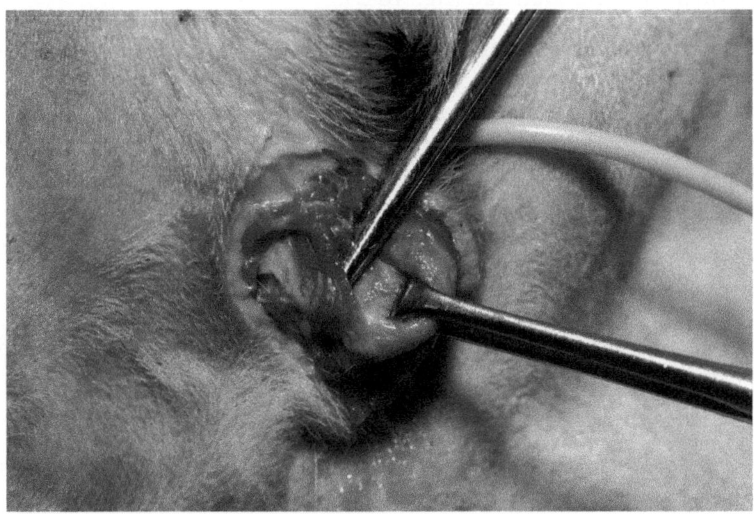

Figure 46-3 Remove external anal sphincter muscle fibers with blunt and sharp dissection, spreading the tissues parallel to the sac surface. If extra traction is needed during dissection, grasp the sac with Allis tissue or Babcock forceps.

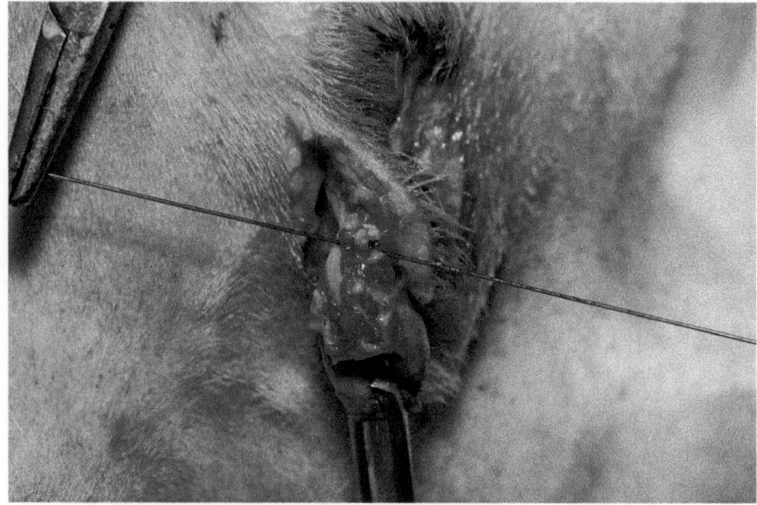

Figure 46-4 Remove the Foley catheter and ligate the duct before removing the sac.

c. Transect any large muscle fiber attachments, cutting close to the sac. Leave as much muscle as possible.

d. Alternately dissect along all sides of the sac until its entire surface is exposed.

6. Dissect the duct from the perianal tissues.
7. Pass a ligature around the duct and remove any inserted catheter or device. Ligate and transect the duct at its junction with the anus (fig. 46-4).
8. Flush the surgical site with sterile saline if contamination occurs.
9. Appose transected muscle and then subcutaneous tissues with interrupted sutures of 3-0 or 4-0 rapidly absorbable, monofilament suture.
10. If desired, place skin sutures or an intradermal pattern, or cover the incision with tissue glue.
11. Remove the purse-string suture.

Surgical technique: open anal sacculectomy

1. Insert one blade of a straight sharp/sharp or blunt/sharp scissors through the duct into the anal sac (fig. 46-5).
2. Tilt the scissors so the tips point caudally (toward the surgeon), forcing the anal sac superficially.
3. Close the scissors to cut skin, subcutis, external anal sphincter muscle, and anal sac wall simultaneously. Remove the scissors.
4. Identify the shiny, grayish white lining of the anal sac to determine its borders. Enlarge the sac opening as needed so the entire inner surface is visible.
5. Attach three or four mosquito hemostats to the edge of the sac (fig. 46-6). Space the hemostats evenly around the sac's circumference.
6. Insert the tip of your nondominant index finger into the open sac. Grasp one or two hemostats in the palm of the same hand to keep the sac on your finger.

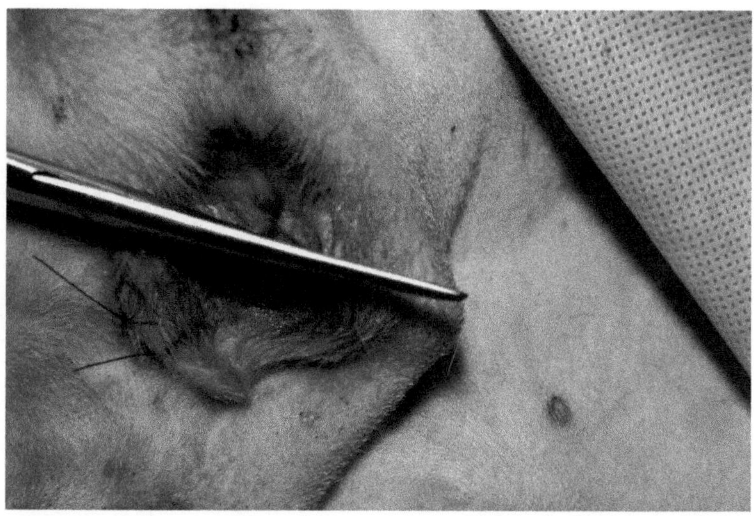

Figure 46-5 To perform an open sacculectomy, cut through the sac and overlying tissues with scissors.

7. Rotate the inserted finger and the apex of the sac caudally to expose the lateral surface of the anal sac and overlying muscle fibers.
8. With a no. 15 blade, gently transect the muscle fibers at their attachments to the sac (fig. 46-7).
   a. Hold the scalpel handle in a pencil grip.
   b. Use small "paint brush" strokes to transect the fibers at their sac attachments.
   c. Continue to rotate the sac caudomedially to expose and tense the muscle fibers.
   d. Alternately dissect along all sides of the gland until the entire sac wall has been freed.
9. With scissors or a blade, dissect along the duct and transect it at skin level.
10. Appose the tissues as described above (fig. 46-8), and remove the purse string suture.

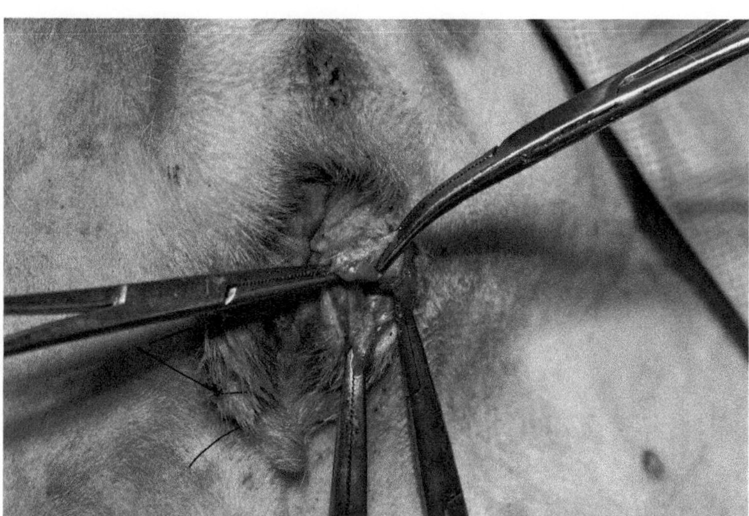

Figure 46-6 Grasp the edges of the sac with hemostats.

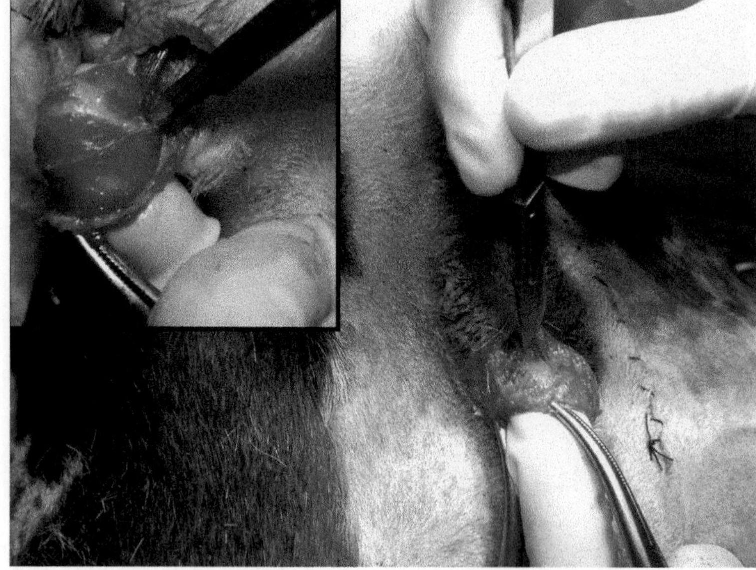

Figure 46-7 With a finger inserted in the sac, transect attached muscle fibers with a blade, gradually rotating the sac outward as you cut (inset).

Postoperative considerations

Elizabethan collars may be required to prevent self-trauma. Potential complications include hemorrhage, infection, dehiscence, draining tracts, stricture, fecal incontinence, and persistence of clinical signs. If the incision dehisces, the wound should be flushed, and the patient should be treated with systemic antibiotics. The open wound is allowed to heal by second intention. Draining sinus tracts may develop if secretory lining is left during dissection. Affected animals are treated with antibiotics and hotpacking until cellulitis and swelling resolve. The tract is then dissected to its origin, and the offending tissue is removed. Resected tissue can be submitted for histologic evaluation to verify that anal gland tissue was present.

In dogs with allergies or other generalized dermatologic conditions, clinical signs of scooting and excessive perineal grooming may persist unless the underlying etiology can be treated. Dogs with sublumbar lymphadenopathy

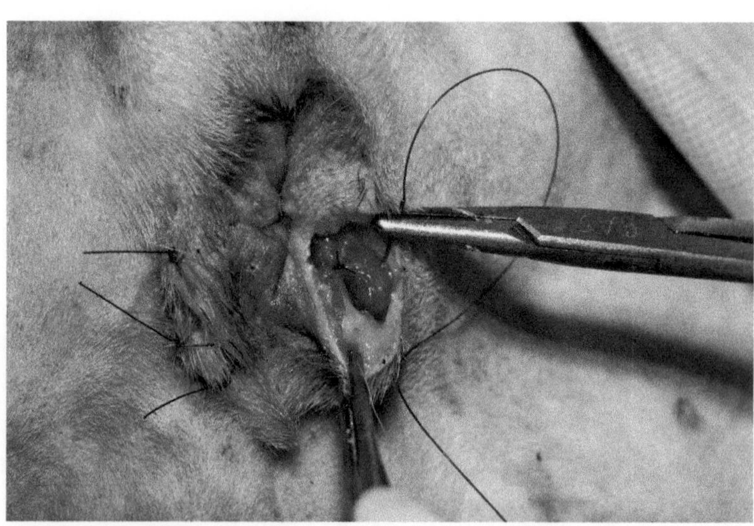

Figure 46-8 Close any muscle and subcutaneous defects with interrupted sutures.

secondary to metastatic disease may require lymph node removal to resolve hypercalcemia or constipation.

Although defecation problems (e.g., weak anal tone or perineal soiling) are noted in 15% of dogs within the first week after surgery, fecal incontinence from iatrogenic caudal rectal nerve damage is rare. If the damage is unilateral, the anal sphincter should reinnervate from the contralateral nerve in 4 to 6 weeks, restoring continence. Incontinence may also occur if the external anal sphincter is damaged from excessive dissection. Incontinence that persists longer than 4 months is unlikely to resolve.

Bibliography

Bennett PF et al: Canine anal sac adenocarcinomas: clinical presentation and response to therapy. J Vet Int Med 2002;16:100–104.

Bray J: Surgical management of perineal disease in the dog. In Pract 2001;23:82–97.

Bright RM: How to perform an anal sacculectomy. NAVC Clinician's Brief 2003; June: 36–38,40.

Charlesworth TM: Risk factors for postoperative complications following bilateral closed anal sacculectomy in the dog. J Small Anim Pract 2014;55:350–354.

Hill LN and Smeak DD: Open versus closed bilateral anal sacculectomy for treatment of non-neoplastic anal sac disease in dogs: 95 cases (1969–1994). J Am Vet Med Assoc 2002;221:662–665.

Ruffner E, Fancher MD, Sherman C, et al: Anal sacculectomy in cats. Procedures Pro. NAVC Clinician's Brief 2014;12:31–35.

Chapter 47
Perineal Hernia

The levator ani and coccygeal muscles form the pelvic diaphragm, which supports the rectal wall and helps to create a natural partition between the abdominal cavity and ischiorectal fossa. Muscular atrophy or stress from chronic straining can weaken the pelvic diaphragm, resulting in herniation of the rectal wall or abdominal organs into the perineal region.

Perineal hernias can be unilateral or bilateral. Most occur lateral to the anus; however, some are ventral. Contents usually include deviated rectal wall, serous or serosanguinous fluid, pelvic or retroperitoneal fat, and in 25% of dogs, the bladder and prostate. Prostatic cysts and intestine may also herniate into the space. Affected animals are most commonly male dogs, and many are breeds with cropped tails. Perineal urethrostomy may predispose male cats to perineal hernia formation. The most common clinical signs of perineal hernia include tenesmus, dyschezia, and perineal swelling. Animals with partial or complete urethral obstruction may have stranguria, anuria, or incontinence.

Perineal hernia can be diagnosed by digital rectal examination. During rectal palpation, the examiner's finger can easily be directed laterally and caudally when a hernia is present (fig. 47-1). Palpation may be more difficult if the rectum is packed with feces or a distended, entrapped bladder fills the hernia. Cats may need to be fully anesthetized to relax them sufficiently for rectal examination. Bladder retroflexion is diagnosed by urethral catheterization, contrast radiographs, ultrasound, or perineocentesis. Potassium and creatinine concentrations in the perineal fluid sample will be higher than in serum if the aspirated fluid is urine. Perineal hernia is considered a surgical emergency in animals with intestine or bladder obstruction or strangulation.

Preoperative management

Serum chemistries, complete blood count, and urinalysis are evaluated for metabolic abnormalities and evidence of sepsis or infection. Animals that are septic or in shock should be evaluated for coagulation abnormalities. If the urinary tract is obstructed, a urethral catheter should be passed into the bladder to keep it decompressed until surgery. Surgery can then be delayed until the patient is stable. Supportive care should be based on the patient's metabolic status. Hyperkalemic animals should be diuresed until potassium concentrations are normalized and BUN and creatinine have decreased. In cats, underlying diseases such as megacolon should be treated prior to

Manual of Small Animal Soft Tissue Surgery, Second Edition. Karen Tobias.
© 2017 John Wiley & Sons, Inc. Published 2017 by John Wiley & Sons, Inc.

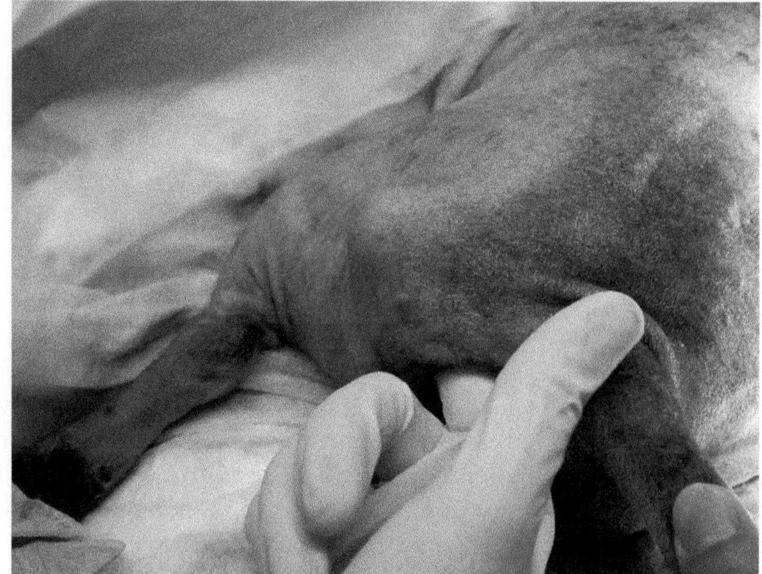

Figure 47-1 If a perineal hernia is present, the examiner's index finger can be rotated caudally into the subcutaneous perianal region during digital rectal examination.

herniorrhaphy. Enemas can be given to constipated animals but should be avoided within 12 hours of surgery, since liquefied feces are more likely to leak into the sterile field.

Animals undergoing perineal hernia repair are usually given prophylactic antibiotics at induction and again 90 minutes to 6 hours later. If possible, a caudal epidural nerve block is performed for intraoperative and postoperative analgesia. The perineum and base of the tail are clipped and prepped. Intact male dogs should also be prepped for caudal or prescrotal castration. The rectum is evacuated digitally, and a purse-string suture is placed in the anus. For herniorraphy, patients are usually placed in a perineal position with the tail pulled forward. If the tail is short, it can be grasped with a towel clamp, which can be pulled cranially with tape. The procedure can also be performed with the dog in dorsal recumbency with the rear legs pulled cranially, or in lateral recumbency. Some clinicians place a urethral catheter to facilitate identification during dissection.

Surgery

Techniques for perineal hernia repair include primary apposition, internal obturator muscle flap, synthetic or biologic implants (e.g., polypropylene mesh or porcine intestinal submucosa), and semitendinosus or superficial gluteal muscle flaps. Bilateral herniorrhaphies can be performed during the same anesthetic episode when hernias are closed with muscle flaps or implants. In addition to herniorrhaphy, colopexy is recommended in animals with concurrent rectal prolapse or recurrent hernias, and some surgeons will perform cystopexy in animals with bladder retroflexion.

Internal obturator flap herniorrhaphy provides excellent coverage of the hernia region. The internal obturator muscle is a fan-shaped structure that covers the dorsal surface of the obturator foramen. It arises medially along the pubis and caudally along the ischiatic arch and extends laterally under the sacrotuberous ligament. Its tendon often has three distinct bands that converge on the ventrolateral surface of the muscle. The tendons of the internal obturator and gemelli muscles run in the lesser sciatic notch and join with the tendon of the external obturator muscle before inserting in the trochanteric fossa. To improve coverage and relieve tension, the internal obturator tendon is transected just medial to the sacrotuberous ligament during perineal herniorrhaphy.

The internal pudendal artery and vein and the pudendal nerve run over the dorsal surface of the internal obturator muscle. At the caudal border of the levator ani, the caudal rectal nerve leaves the pudendal nerve and enters the external anal sphincter muscle a little below the middle of the sphincter. Within the pelvic canal, the sciatic nerve runs cranial to the internal obturator muscle. The extrapelvic portion of the sciatic nerve runs along the lateral surfaces of the internal obturator tendon. Damage to vessels and nerves is avoided during herniorrhaphy by limiting dissection dorsal to the internal obturator muscle and by transecting the tendon before it crosses over the lateral edge of the ischium.

Because intact males have higher recurrence rates, dogs should be castrated before or at the time of herniorrhaphy. Castration can be performed through a prescrotal incision or through a caudal scrotal approach. Caudal castration is more difficult but can be performed with the dog in a perineal position.

Surgery technique: internal obturator flap herniorrhaphy

1. Make a curvilinear skin incision 2 to 4 cm lateral and parallel to the anus (fig. 47-2). Start the incision dorsal to the level of the anus and extend it at least 2 to 3 cm ventral to the ischial tuberosity.
2. Break through the subcutaneous layer into the hernia cavity with scissors or fingers and extend the subcutaneous incision. Fluid may pour out of the hernia.
3. If necessary, empty the bladder by cystocentesis before pushing it back into the abdomen (fig. 47-3).
4. Reduce hernia contents with a "sponge-on-a-stick"—a gauze sponge folded in fourths and clamped firmly with an Allis tissue forceps (fig. 47-4). If needed, the instrument can be left in place during the initial part of the obturator muscle dissection.

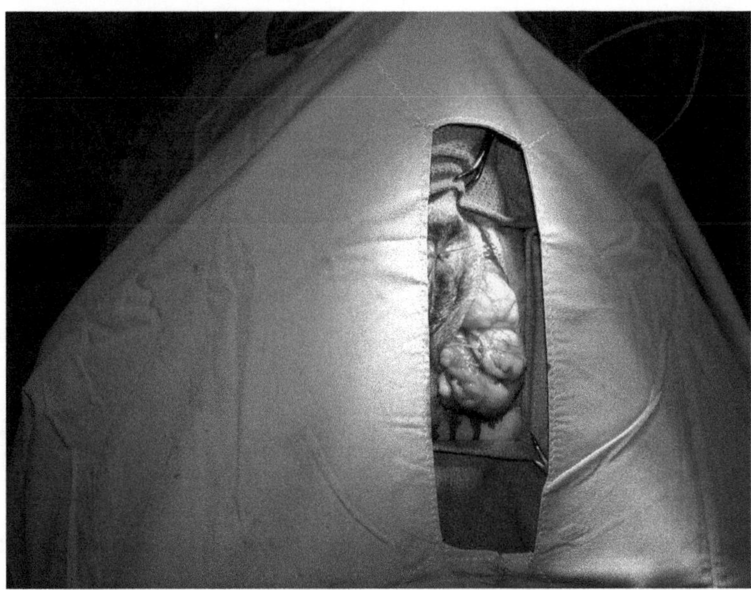

Figure 47-2 Expose the hernia contents through a curvilinear incision that extends ventral to the ischial tuberosity.

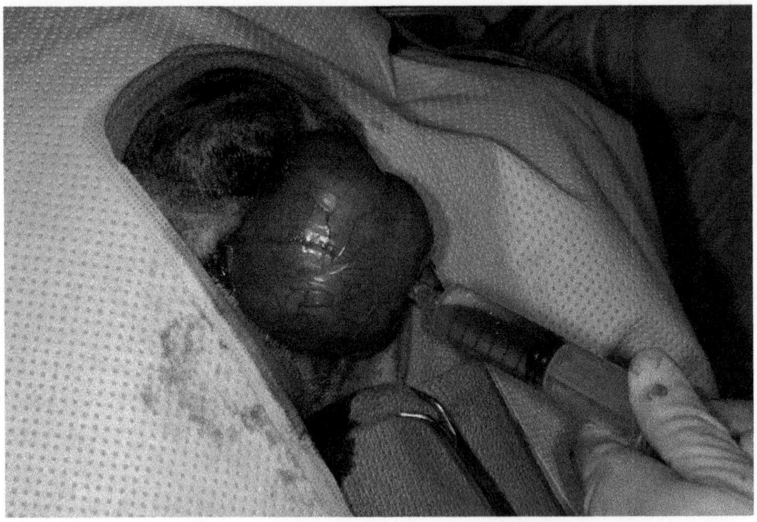

Figure 47-3 If the bladder is herniated and full, empty it by cystocentesis to facilitate reduction.

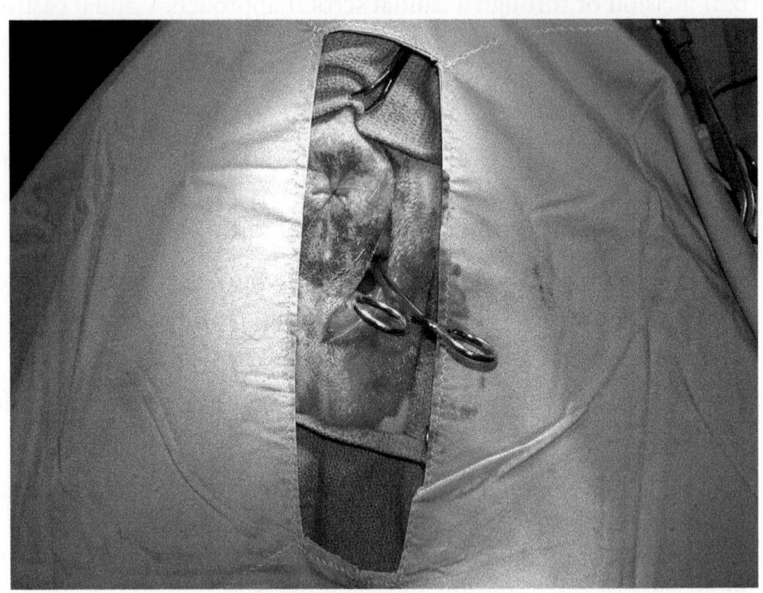

Figure 47-4 Reduce hernia contents with a "sponge-on-a-stick."

5. Identify the muscles and vessels within the ischiorectal fossa (fig. 47-5).
6. Place an index finger and middle finger on the medial and lateral borders of the ischial tuberosity to retract tissues and outline the area for the initial muscle incision. Incise the internal obturator muscle attachments along the dorsocaudal edge of the ischium, cutting down to the bone (fig. 47-6).
7. Insert a periosteal elevator under the internal obturator muscle and against the bone. Elevate the muscle off the ischium to a level just cranial to the caudal edge of the obturator foramen.
8. Insert an index finger under the muscle and palpate laterally and medially to verify that all caudal ischial attachments have been transected, especially along the lateral border of the muscle.
9. If desired, place a stay suture on the caudal edge of the muscle to help identify it.

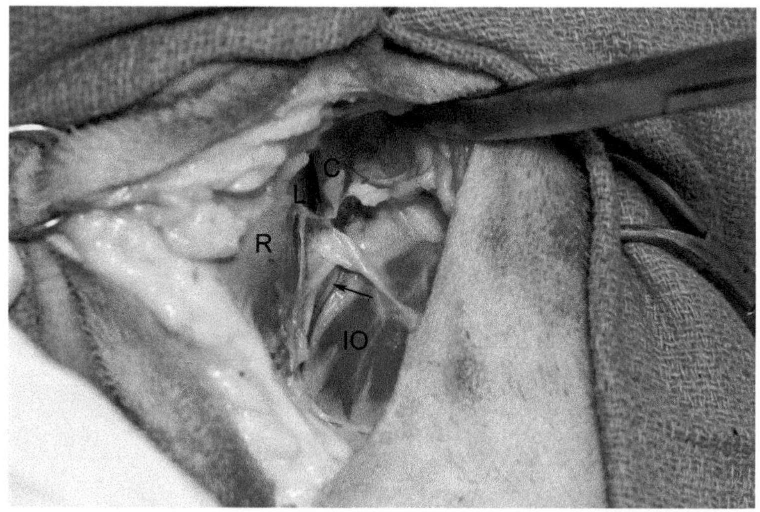

Figure 47-5 Anatomy of the perineal region. R, rectum; L, levator ani; C, coccygeus muscle; IO, internal obturator muscle. Arrow indicates internal pudendal artery and vein. The anal sphincter muscle is hidden under fat.

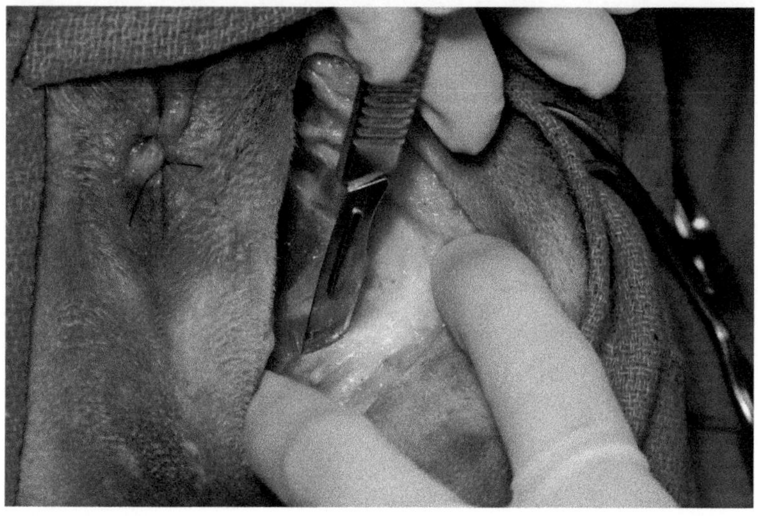

Figure 47-6 Place your index and middle fingers on the borders of the ischial tuberosity and incise the fascial attachments of the internal obturator muscle.

10. Insert a curved Kelly hemostat, tips down, over the internal obturator tendon and under the muscle fibers dorsal to the tendon.
11. Rotate the hemostat handles dorsocranially and tips caudally and ventrally to expose the three bands of the internal obturator tendon (fig. 47-7).
12. Incise the tendon over the hemostat with scissors or blade, medial to the sacrotuberous ligament. This will prevent damage to the sciatic nerve.
13. Palpate under the muscle flap with an index finger to verify that the flap is freed from its lateral and caudomedial attachments. If more cranial dissection is needed, use an index finger to gently lift the muscle from the ischium.
14. Preplace 4 to 6 sutures of 2-0 absorbable monofilament material between the external anal sphincter and internal obturator muscle, leaving each suture long and securing its ends with a hemostat.
    a. Identify the external anal sphincter by gently dragging a curved hemostat, with tips facing medially and caudally, from cranial to

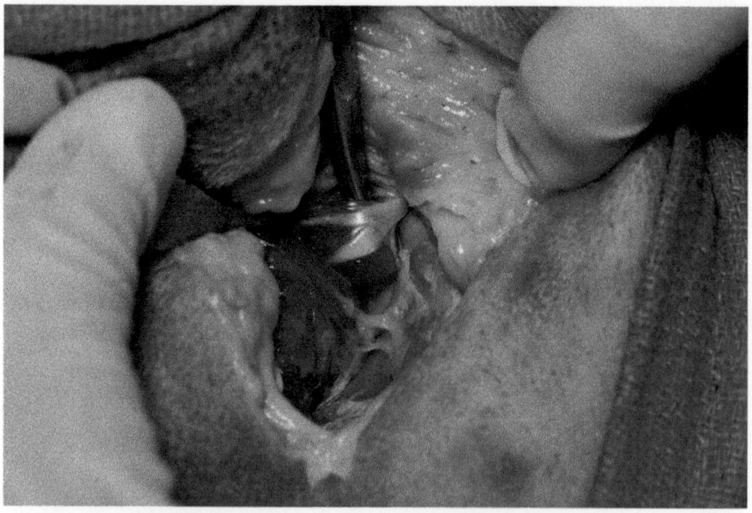

Figure 47-7 After elevating the muscle, expose the internal obturator tendon by hooking it with a curved Kelly hemostat.

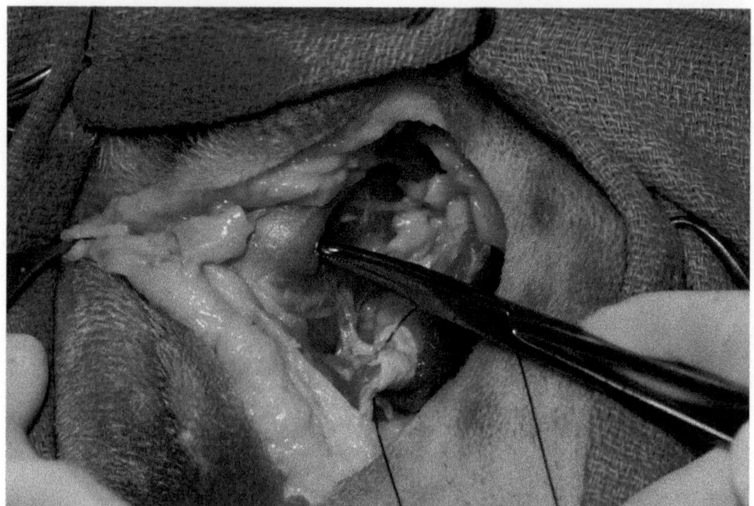

Figure 47-8 Preplace sutures between the internal obturator muscle and external anal sphincter. To identify the external anal sphincter, gently run the tips of a curved hemostat along the rectal wall until they hook on the sphincter.

caudal along the rectal wall until the tips "catch" on the perpendicularly oriented sphincter muscle (fig. 47-8). Sphincter fibers run in a dorsoventral direction.

b. Rotate the muscle flap to determine how far it will reach along the dorsolateral anal sphincter without excessive tension, then place the first suture from the lateral-most aspect of the internal obturator muscle (or its tendons) to the dorsolateral anal sphincter.

c. Place a hemostat on the suture ends. Pull on the suture to verify that the anus moves laterally and thus has been incorporated in the bite, then leave the suture loose to facilitate subsequent suture placement.

d. Continue to preplace sutures, working ventrally. Make sure to include internal obturator muscle fascia (on the dorsal surface of the muscle) in each bite.

e. Place the final suture at the ventromedial border of the internal obturator muscle and the ventral portion of the anal sphincter. The ventral portion of the anal sphincter is often difficult to identify; compare the position of the anus to your suture bite to determine if you are in the correct location.

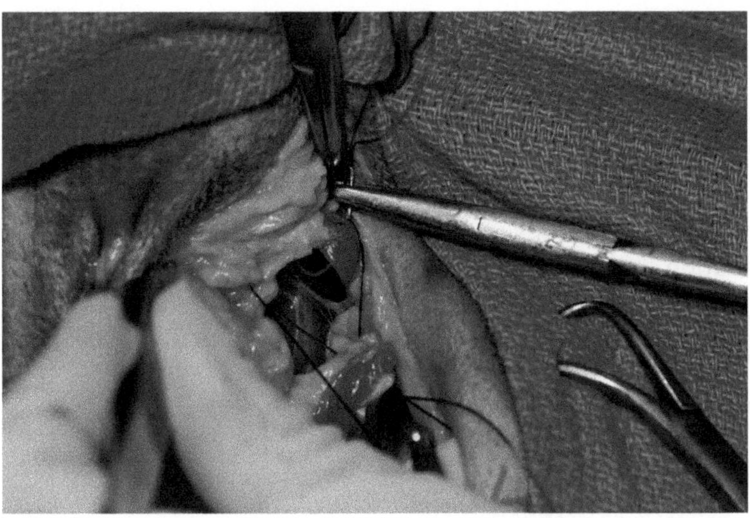

Figure 47-9 If possible, include the levator ani or coccygeus muscle in the dorsalmost sutures.

15. If the levator ani/coccygeal muscles can be identified, place one or more sutures from these muscles to the external anal sphincter dorsolaterally. If possible, include the end of the internal obturator muscle in the suture closest to that muscle (fig. 47-9).
16. Once the sutures are all preplaced, tie each one so that the tissues are apposed but not necrosed. If still in place, remove the sponge-on-a-stick after the first suture is tied.
17. Close subcutaneous tissues and skin with interrupted sutures.
18. In an intact male, expose the dorsal scrotal region for a caudal castration, or reposition the dog for a prescrotal or scrotal castration.

Surgical technique: caudal castration

1. Make a skin incision at the junction of the caudodorsal scrotum and perineal skin (fig. 47-10), staying superficial to the penile body.

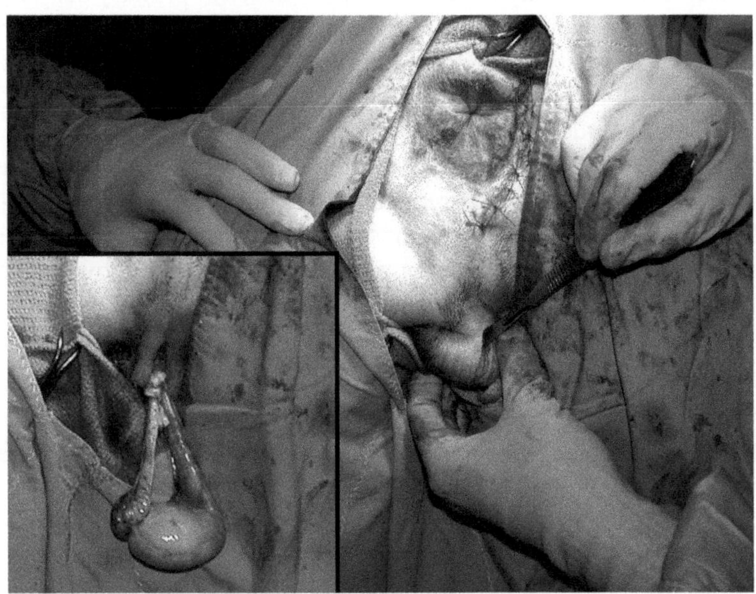

Figure 47-10 Incision for a caudal open castration. The testicle is easier to extrude from the incision if the castration is open (inset).

2. Push the testicle dorsally and extend the incision length and depth for an open castration.
3. Extrude the testicle from the incision. The cord will be shorter than in a routine castration, and more force will be needed to retract the testicle and free it from the scrotum.
4. Expose the testicular vessels and ligate and transect as with a routine castration (p. 244).
5. Remove the second testicle through the same incision, incising through the overlying tissues to perform an open castration.
6. Close the skin with interrupted sutures.

Postoperative considerations

Before the animal is recovered, the anal purse-string suture is removed, and a digital rectal exam is performed to confirm that the hernia is repaired. The rectal wall should feel solidly supported, as in a normal animal. Analgesics are administered for several days. A low-residue diet and a stool softener such as lactulose can be prescribed to reduce postoperative straining until the site is healed. Elizabethan collars are recommended for 1 week to prevent self-trauma.

Common complications of perineal herniorrhaphy include swelling, wound infection, tenesmus, rectal prolapse, fecal or urinary incontinence, and hernia recurrence. Wound infection rates can be reduced by use of perioperative antibiotics and strict asepsis during the procedure. Postoperative tenesmus can lead to rectal prolapse (see Chapter 48). Treatments include stool softeners, analgesics, and acepromazine to reduce straining; in some patients, colopexy may also be required. Fecal incontinence is uncommon and may be a result of the underlying condition or from damage to the caudal rectal nerve. The external anal sphincter can reinnervate from the contralateral side if nerve damage occurs during surgery. Urinary incontinence may occur after bladder entrapment and may be permanent if the detrussor muscle was severely damaged from ischemia or overdistension.

Recurrence of hernias may be related to persistence of primary disease, poor surgical technique, or atrophy of the internal obturator muscle. Recurrence rates are higher in intact male dogs and may be more common in cats with untreated megacolon. Internal obturator muscle herniorrhaphy will fail if the sutures do not include external anal sphincter muscle. The external anal sphincter is difficult to identify in obese animals, particularly along its ventral extent. Options for repair of recurrent hernias include colopexy (pp. 211–214), prosthetic mesh, or semitendinosus muscle flaps. Bladder retroflexion can be prevented temporarily by performing abdominal cystopexy; however, cystopexy alone may not prevent recurrence long-term.

Bibliography

Brissot HN et al: Use of laparotomy in a staged approach for resolution of bilateral or complicated perineal hernia in 41 dogs. Vet Surg 2004;33:412–421.

Grand JG, Bureau S, Monnet E: Effects of urinary bladder retroflexion and surgical technique on postoperative complication rates and long-term outcome in dogs with perineal hernia: 41 cases (2002–2009). J Am Vet Med Assoc 2013;243:1442–1447.

Morello E, Martano M, Zabarino S, et al: Modified semitendinosus muscle transposition to repair ventral perineal hernia in 14 dogs. J Small Anim Pract 2015;56:370–376.

Shaughnessy M, Monnet E: Internal obturator muscle transposition for treatment of perineal hernia in dogs: 34 cases (1988–2012). J Am Vet Med Assco 2015;246:321–326.

Snell WL, Orsher RJ, Larenza-Menzies MP, et al: Comparison of caudal and prescrotal castration for management of perineal hernia in dogs between 2004 and 2014. N Zealand Vet J 2015;63:272–275.

Stoll MR et al: The use of porcine small intestinal submucosa as a biomaterial for perineal herniorrhaphy in the dog. Vet Surg 2002;31:379–390.

Szabo S et al: Use of polypropylene mesh in addition to internal obturator transposition: a review of 59 cases (2000–2004). J Am Anim Hosp Assoc 2007;43:136–142.

Welches CD et al: Perineal hernia in the cat: a retrospective study of 40 cases. J Am Anim Hosp Assoc 1992;28:431–438.

Morello E, Martano M, Zabarino S et al. Modified semitendinosus muscle transposition to repair ventral perineal hernia in 14 dogs. J Small Anim Pract 2015;56:370–376.

Shaughnessy M, Monnet E. Internal obturator muscle transposition for treatment of perineal hernia in dogs: 34 cases (1998–2012). J Am Vet Med Assoc 2015;246:321–326.

Snell WL, Orsher RJ, Larenza-Menzies MP, et al. Comparison of caudal and pre-scrotal castration for management of perineal hernia in dogs between 2004 and 2014. N Z Vet J 2016;64:272–275.

Stoll MR et al. The use of porcine small intestinal submucosa as a biomaterial in perineal herniorrhaphy in the dog. Vet Surg 2002;31:379–390.

Szabo S et al. Use of polypropylene mesh in addition to internal obturator transposition: a review of 59 cases (2000–2004). J Am Anim Hosp Assoc 2007;43:136–142.

Welches CD et al. Perineal hernia in the cat: a retrospective study of 40 cases. J Am Anim Hosp Assoc 1992;28:431–438.

Chapter 48
Rectal Prolapse

Conditions that cause straining and rectal mucosal irritation may result in partial- or full-thickness prolapse of the rectal wall. Common etiologies include intestinal parasites, loss of anal tone, severe enteritis, rectal polyps, intestinal neoplasia, cystitis, prostatic disease, or dystocia. Rectal prolapse may also occur after perineal hernia repair.

Preoperative management

Affected animals should be evaluated for predisposing conditions, such as intestinal parasites, and a digital rectal examination should be performed to palpate for masses and to verify the prolapse is rectal in origin. In animals with rectal prolapse, the anal mucocutaneous junction is readily visible, and a lubricated finger or probe can only be passed into the intestinal lumen. In animals with prolapsed ileocolonic intussusception (fig. 48-1), a blunt probe can easily be passed into the anus lateral to the prolapsed tissue. If an ileocolonic intussusception is present, an abdominal approach will be required for repair and possible resection and anastomosis.

After anesthetic induction, epidural analgesia is recommended to further relax the anal sphincter and reduce straining in the immediate postoperative period. During surgery, patient positioning depends on the procedure to be performed. Purse-string sutures can easily be placed with the animal in lateral or dorsal recumbency. Rectal resection and anastomosis is usually performed with the animal in a perineal position: the animal is placed in sternal recumbency with the back legs hanging over the padded edge of the surgery table. Because the table is tilted with the animal in a head-down position, respiration should be assisted during a perineal approach.

Before attempting manual reduction of a simple rectal prolapse, edematous tissue should be gently lavaged with warm water or saline. Edema can be reduced by soaking the mucosal surface in 50% dextrose; this may cause further irritation in some animals. The prolapsed tissue is coated liberally with a sterile water-soluble lubricant and then reduced with a gloved finger.

Surgery

If the prolapse is secondary to polyps, the masses can be removed by mucosal resection and closure; in this case, the prolapse usually resolves without further

Manual of Small Animal Soft Tissue Surgery, Second Edition. Karen Tobias.
© 2017 John Wiley & Sons, Inc. Published 2017 by John Wiley & Sons, Inc.

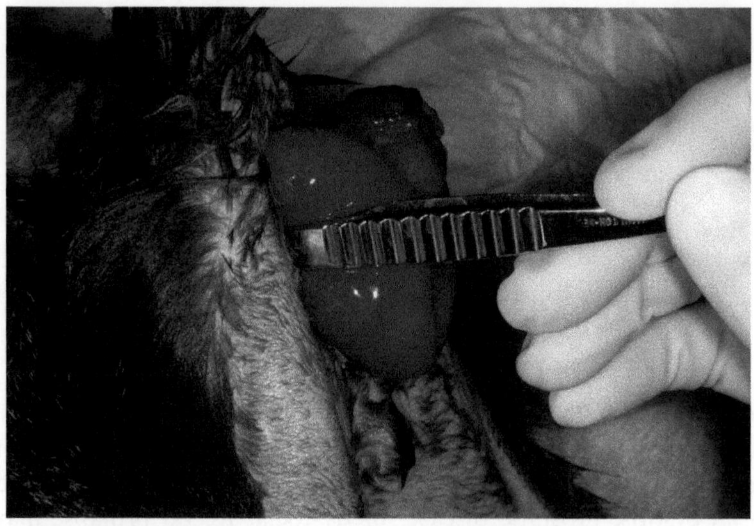

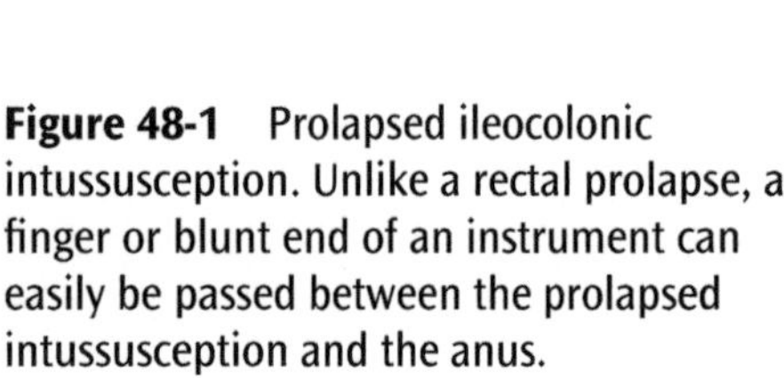

Figure 48-1 Prolapsed ileocolonic intussusception. Unlike a rectal prolapse, a finger or blunt end of an instrument can easily be passed between the prolapsed intussusception and the anus.

treatment. If the prolapse is acute and the tissue is still viable and not mutilated, manual reduction and fixation are recommended. A purse-string suture is placed to keep the tissues reduced. If the prolapse is extensive, an abdominal approach may be necessary to reduce healthy tissue. Devitalized prolapsed tissue will require rectal resection and anastomosis before reduction.

Surgical technique: purse-string suture

1. Use a curved or straight needle with 2-0 or 3-0 monofilament non-absorbable suture.
2. Insert the needle at the mucocutaneous junction, staying medial (deep) to the anal sac openings so they are not obstructed or damaged (fig. 48-2).
3. Take 1-cm bites around the circumference at the mucocutaneous junction (fig. 48-3).
4. Once the anus is completely encircled, insert a lubricated syringe case into the opening to approximate the final desired diameter, then tighten the suture and tie it (fig. 48-4). The final diameter should be large enough to permit passage of soft feces.

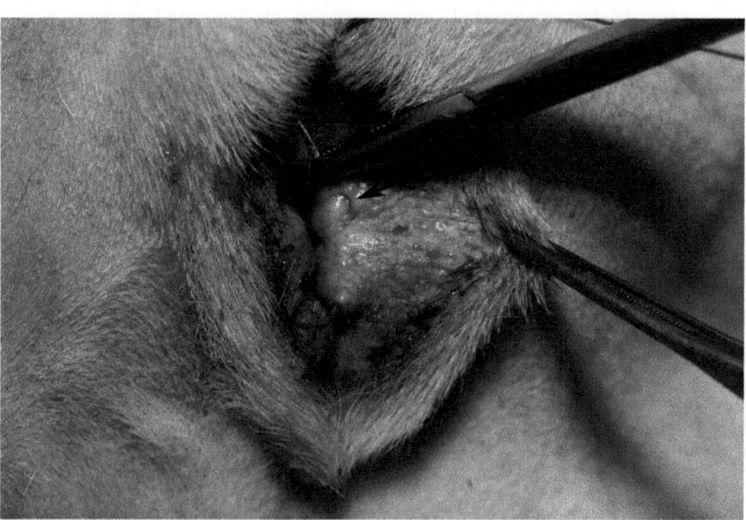

Figure 48-2 Take 1-cm bites at the mucocutaneous junction, staying medial to the anal sac duct opening (arrow).

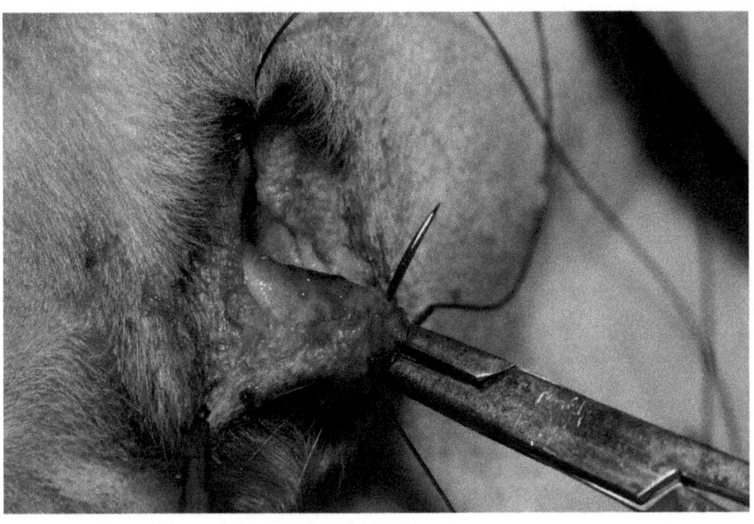

Figure 48-3 Continue taking bites around the circumference of the anus.

Surgical technique: rectal resection and anastomosis

1. Place the animal in a perineal position.
2. Insert a lubricated syringe case, flexible tubing, or red rubber catheter into the intestinal lumen.
3. To prevent retraction of the rectum, secure the two full-thickness layers of the prolapsed tissue.
   a. Place three to four full-thickness, interrupted, monofilament mattress sutures around the circumference of the prolapse 1 to 2 cm from the anus. The needle should hit the syringe case, tubing, or catheter as it is being passed through all the layers. Place hemostats on the sutures or tie them to gently appose the layers, and leave the suture ends long.
   b. Alternatively, place two long, straight needles perpendicular to each other through the prolapse and tubing or red rubber catheter to keep the tissues retracted (fig. 48-5).
4. Cut one-third to one-half of the way around the prolapse circumference (fig. 48-6).

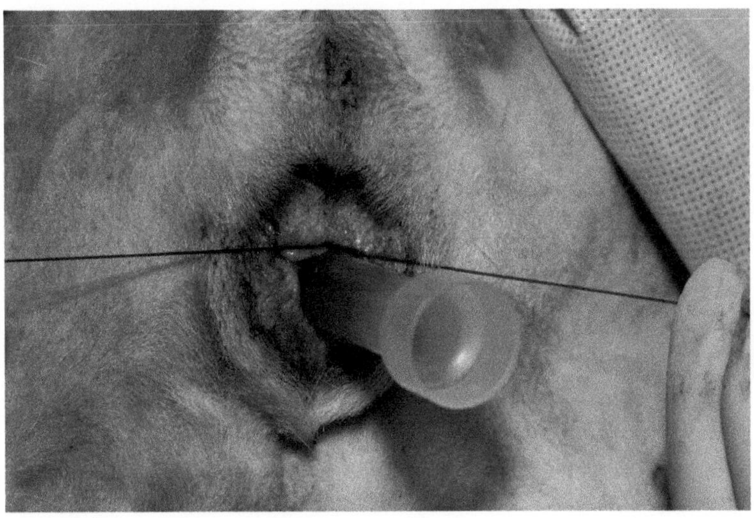

Figure 48-4 Tighten the purse-string suture around an appropriate-sized tube or cylinder so that the maximum anal opening is about one-third of the original diameter.

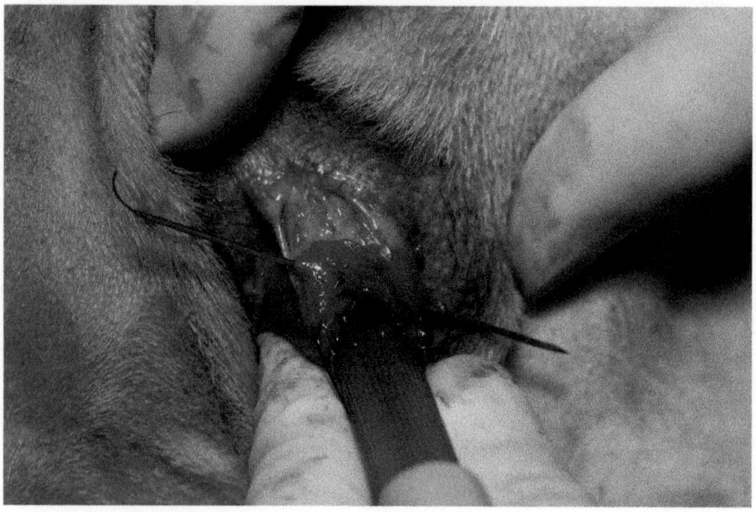

Figure 48-5 Straight needles can be placed through the prolapsed tissue and a soft tube to prevent rectal retraction.

a. With a scalpel blade, incise the rectum parallel to the anocutaneous junction, using the tubing or syringe case as a cutting board.

b. Alternatively, start your cut by incising the rectum with scissors along the length of the prolapse (perpendicular to the prolapse edge), then change their direction to cut around a portion of the circumference of the prolapsed tissue, parallel to the anocutaneous junction.

5. Sew the cut edges together with a full-thickness, simple continuous or simple interrupted pattern of 3-0 or 4-0 monofilament synthetic absorbable suture, placing sutures 2 to 3 mm apart and leaving knots in the rectal lumen (fig. 48-7). Make sure to identify serosa and muscularis, which tend to retract away from the cut edge of the mucosa, and include them in the suture bites.
6. Cut and sew the remaining tissue in sections.
7. Remove the stay sutures or needles to release the rectum (fig. 48-8).
8. With a well-lubricated finger, gently perform a digital rectal examination to verify that the rectal lumen is patent and no mucosal defects are palpable.

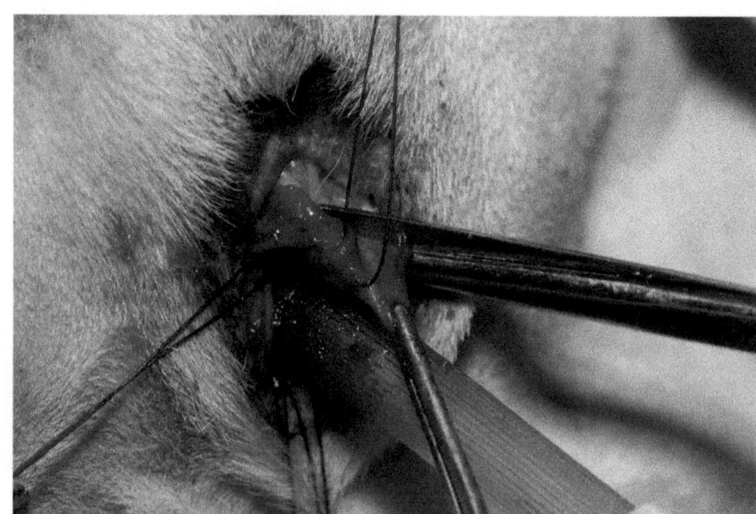

Figure 48-6 Cut one-third to one-half of the circumference of the prolapsed tissue. In this patient, the prolapsed tissue has been secured with stay sutures proximal and distal to the resection site.

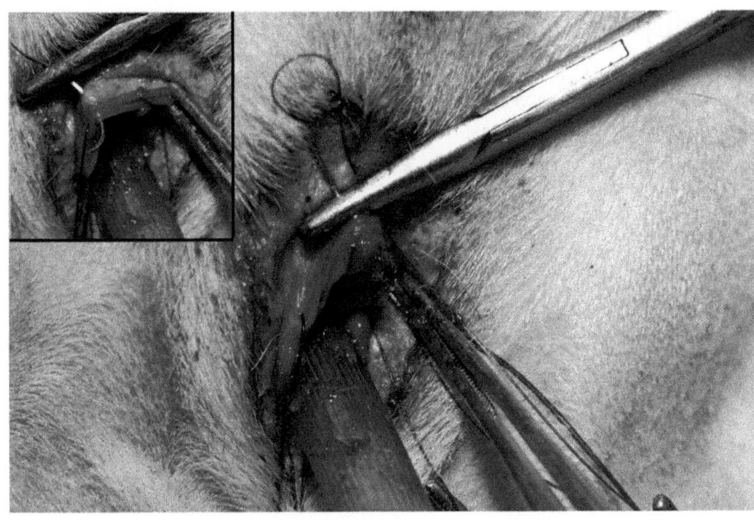

Figure 48-7 Appose the cut edges with a full-thickness continuous or interrupted pattern. Be sure to include the serosa, muscularis, and submucosa of both edges (inset).

Postoperative considerations

In animals undergoing resection and anastomosis, postoperative temperature should not be monitored rectally. Purse-string sutures in animals with rectal prolapse are left in place for 3 to 7 days while the animal's underlying condition is treated; the animals are fed a low-residue diet during that time. Stool softeners such as lactulose are administered as needed to keep the feces soft. Acepromazine and analgesics will reduce straining and discomfort. Some clinicians also apply topical lidocaine to the area to decrease tenesmus.

Postoperative complications include tenesmus, hematochezia, dyschezia, and prolapse recurrence. Fecal character and diameter of the anal stoma should be evaluated in animals that strain or are painful during defecation. Recurrent rectal prolapse is treated with colopexy (pp. 211–214). Dehiscence, local infection, stricture, fecal incontinence, or rectal prolapse may occur after resection and anastomosis. For patients that undergo transrectal ileocolonic resection and anastomosis (as in the cat in fig. 48-1), an abdominal exploratory can be performed after the anastomosis is complete to evaluate the security of the intestinal anastomosis and explore the abdomen for other issues.

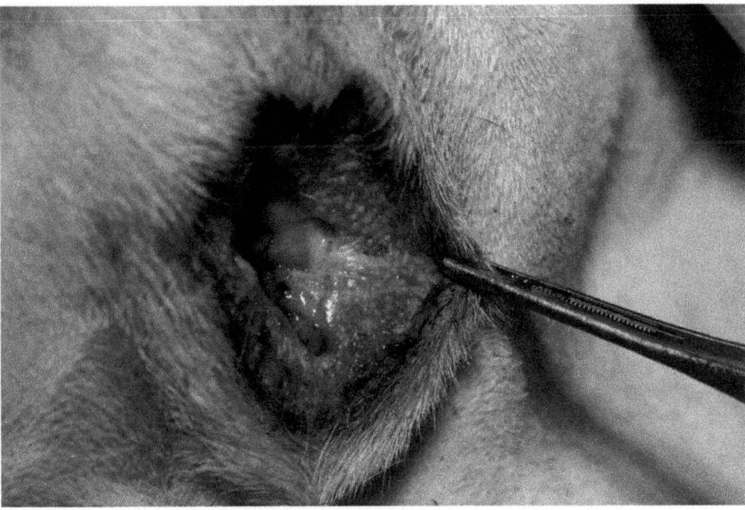

Figure 48-8 Final appearance after rectal resection and anastomosis.

Bibliography

Popovitch CA et al: Colopexy as a treatment for rectal prolapse in dogs and cats: a retrospective study of 14 cases. Vet Surg 1994;23:115–118.

Pratschke K: Surgical diseases of the colon and rectum in small animals. In Pract 2005;27:354–362.

Chapter 49
Tail Amputation

In mature dogs, tail amputation is most commonly performed for treatment of traumatic skin loss, ischemia, or denervation. Combined with other therapies, tail amputation may also improve outcome in dogs with perianal fistulas that do not resolve with immunosuppressive treatment. Pyoderma resulting from ingrown or "screw" tails will also improve after amputation of the tail and associated skin folds. Surgical resection for this latter condition can be complicated; therefore, referral is recommended.

Preoperative management

If the tail tip is to be amputated, the pet owner should be advised of the risk of dehiscence, which is common in greyhounds and other animals that continue to traumatize the tail as they hit it against hard surfaces. Animals with paralyzed tails should be evaluated for other neurologic abnormalities such as spinal fractures and urinary dysfunction. In dogs with ingrown tails, preoperative radiographs will provide a better understanding of the anatomy and surgical approach. Anal purse-string suture and prophylactic antibiotics are recommended for proximal and complete amputations. The surgical site can be blocked by epidural or by local instillation of bupivicaine. The tail is clipped for at least 10cm around the proposed incision, and the distal portion of longer tails is wrapped to cover any hair. A hanging prep can be performed, with sterile wrap placed over the initial bandage during surgery.

Surgery

To reduce intraoperative hemorrhage during partial caudectomy, a tourniquet (e.g., Penrose drain) can be placed several centimeters proximal to the amputation site. Tail amputation is usually performed at the intervertebral space. The joint space is identified by palpating the vertebral bodies while flexing and extending the tail near the proposed amputation site. The joint will be at the site of greatest motion and just cranial to the mammillary processes, which are located on the dorsolateral surfaces of the cranial vertebral bodies. The joint regions are palpably wider and thicker than the vertebral midbodies. The skin is incised distal to the joint space to leave a flap of tissue that can be rolled over the bone end. The flap should be long enough so that there is no

Manual of Small Animal Soft Tissue Surgery, Second Edition. Karen Tobias.
© 2017 John Wiley & Sons, Inc. Published 2017 by John Wiley & Sons, Inc.

tension on the skin closure. Tail skin adheres tightly to underlying structures and can be difficult to elevate; sharp transection of fibrous attachments is usually required to free the skin.

Major vessels of the tail include the lateral caudal arteries, which are near the transverse processes, and the median caudal artery ventral to the tail. Occasionally these vessels can be identified during dissection. More commonly, they are buried in muscle; hemostasis is then provided by mass ligation of the vessels and surrounding muscle bundles cranial to the level of the amputation. Smaller vessels are located dorsolaterally and ventrolaterally along the vertebra, anastomosing intermittently with the other vessels. These may be ligated or cauterized before or after transection.

Surgical technique: partial tail amputation

1. On the dorsal surface of the tail, make a U-shaped skin incision 1 to 2 cm distal to the joint space at the proposed amputation site. Incise the skin on the ventral surface in a similar fashion.
2. Alternatively, make a longitudinal incision along the right and left sides of the tail. Connect the cuts 1–2 cm below the desired level of amputation with transverse or curved incisions dorsally and ventrally (fig. 49-1). The corners of the constructed flaps can be trimmed as needed at closure.
3. Using curved Mayo scissors or a scalpel blade, transect attachments between the skin and vertebrae (fig. 49-2).
4. Elevate the skin and subcutaneous tissues to a point cranial to the intervertebral space.
5. Ligate the blood vessels lateral and ventral to the vertebral body cranial to the amputation site. For en bloc ligation, use 3-0 absorbable suture on a taper needle. Take a large bite of tissue in the area of the vessel, passing the needle down to the bone (fig. 49-3). When the suture is tied, the vessel will be encircled along with surrounding muscle.

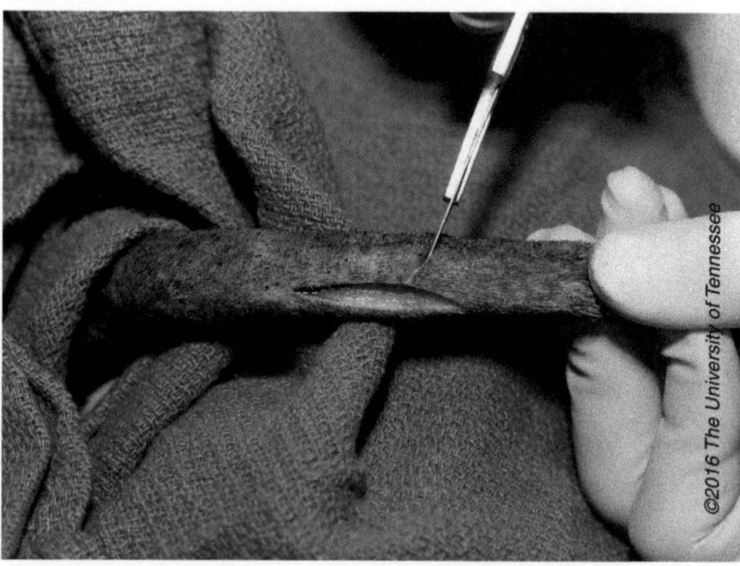

Figure 49-1 Make longitudinal incisions on each side of the tail and connect them dorsally and ventrally with transverse incisions below the proposed level of amputation. © 2016 The University of Tennessee.

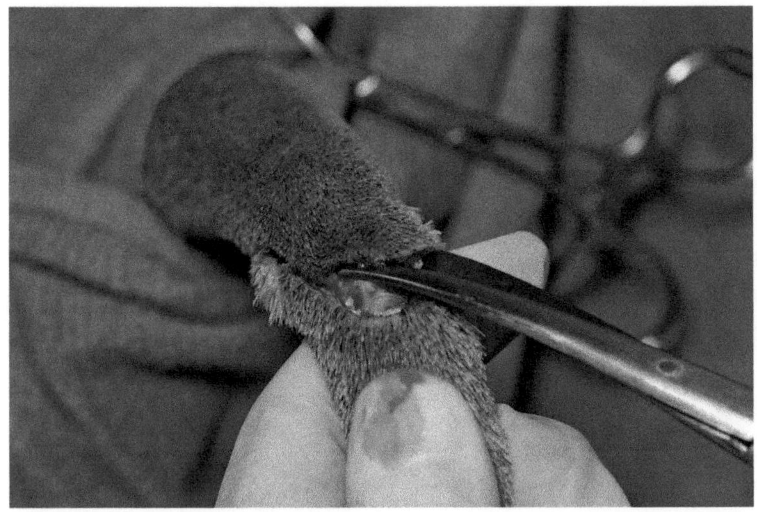

Figure 49-2 Transect attachments between the skin and underlying tissues with sharp dissection. In this dog, U-shaped skin incisions were made.

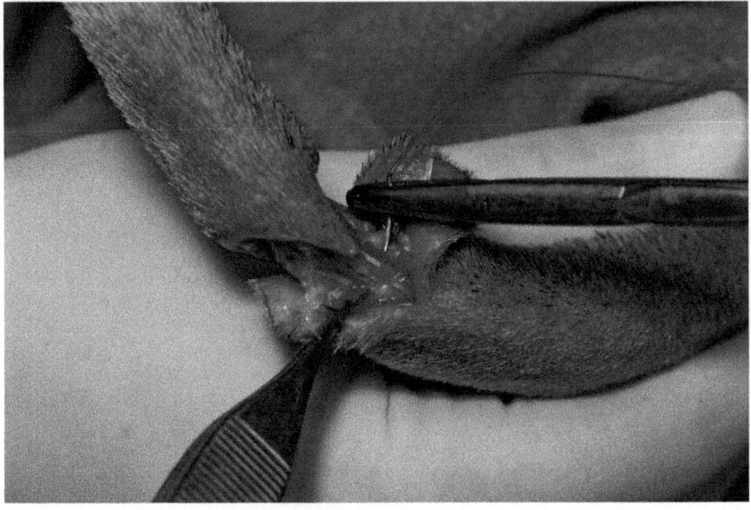

Figure 49-3 Ligate vessels en bloc by passing a needle around the muscles and down to the bone.

6. Amputate the tail cranial enough to the skin incision to provide a tension-free closure.
   a. With thumbnail and fingers, palpate the bone to find its thickest portion (the joint) or point of motion.
   b. Insert a scalpel blade perpendicular to the long axis of the tail into the ventral or dorsal joint space and cut the connecting ligaments and muscle (fig. 49-4). If the joint is difficult to find, slowly "walk" the blade cranially over the joint surface until it falls into the joint space.
   c. Alternatively, transect the caudal (coccygeal) vertebra midbody with bone cutters. Cut any remaining soft tissue attachments, and then smooth the bone end with a rongeur.
7. If a tourniquet was placed, remove it and evaluate the surgery site for bleeding. Ligate or cauterize any bleeding vessels (fig. 49-5).
8. Pull the skin over the bone end to evaluate flap length. If excessive, trim the ventral flap so that the dorsal flap can be pulled over the bone tip.
9. If possible, appose muscle and subcutaneous layers with interrupted buried sutures of 3-0 monofilament absorbable material (fig. 49-6).

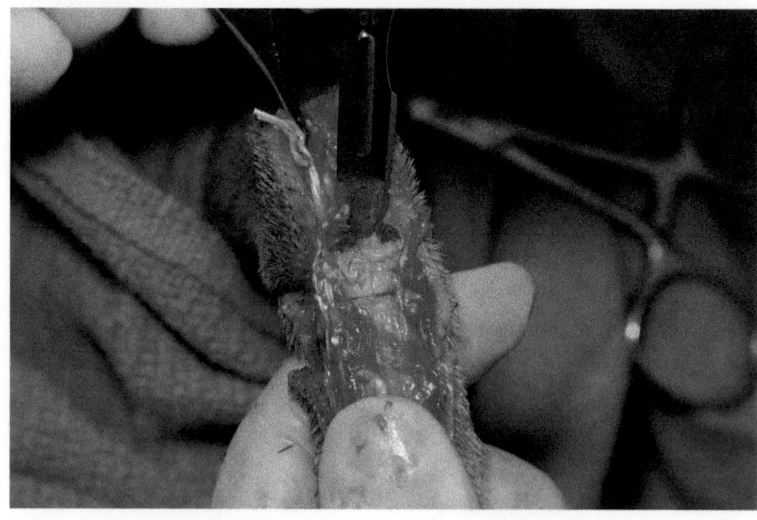

Figure 49-4 Retract the skin cranially and insert the blade perpendicular to the long axis of the tail to find the joint space. The space will be at the thickest part of the bone.

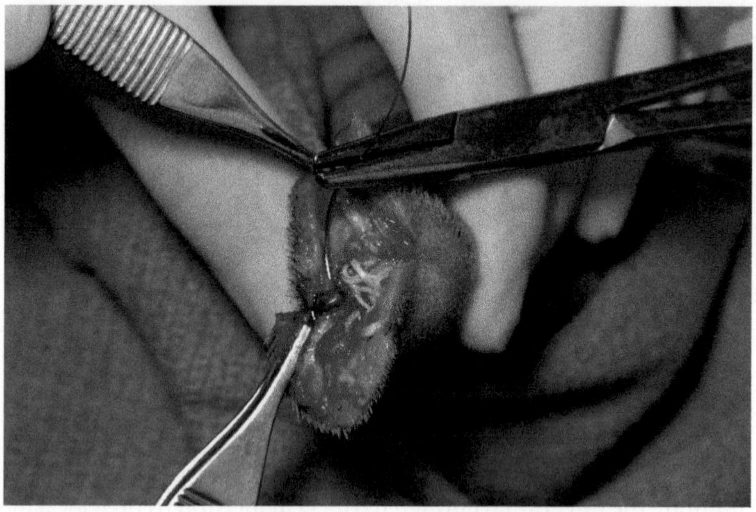

Figure 49-5 Remove the tourniquet and ligate or cauterize any bleeding vessels.

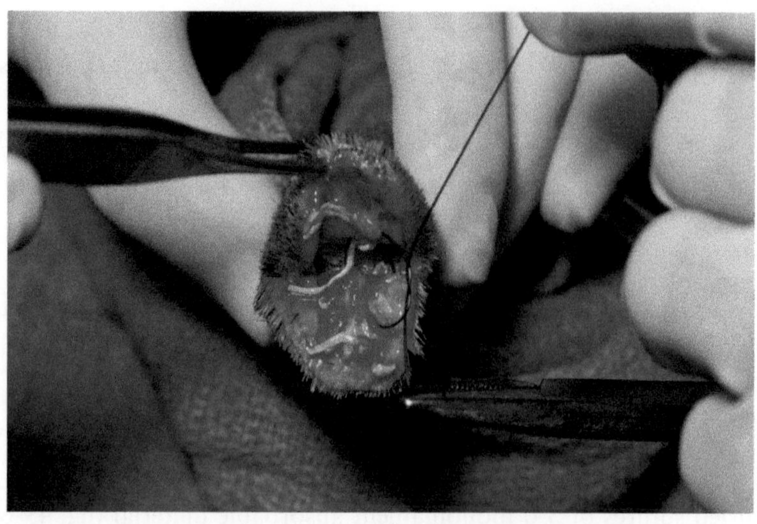

Figure 49-6 If possible, appose subcutaneous tissues with interrupted sutures before closing skin.

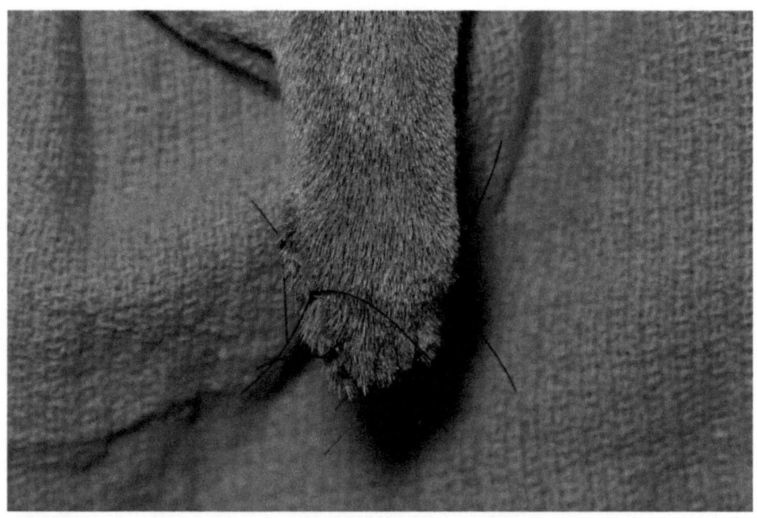

Figure 49-7 Final appearance after skin closure.

10. Close the skin with interrupted sutures (fig. 49-7).
    a. Take dorsal and ventral bites separately, positioning the needle parallel to the skin surface with each bite and pulling the needle and suture through the skin in the first bite before taking the second bite.
    b. Take bites only through the epidermis and dermis, so that the subcutaneous tissues are inverted and covered with skin.
    c. If tension is encountered during skin closure, remove excess bone with rongeurs or amputate the distal vertebra before completing the closure.

Surgical technique: caudectomy for screw tail

1. Position the dog in sternal recumbency and prep thoroughly, including the skin folds and recesses (fig. 49-8). Perform a final prep of all visible skin once the recesses have been cleaned out.

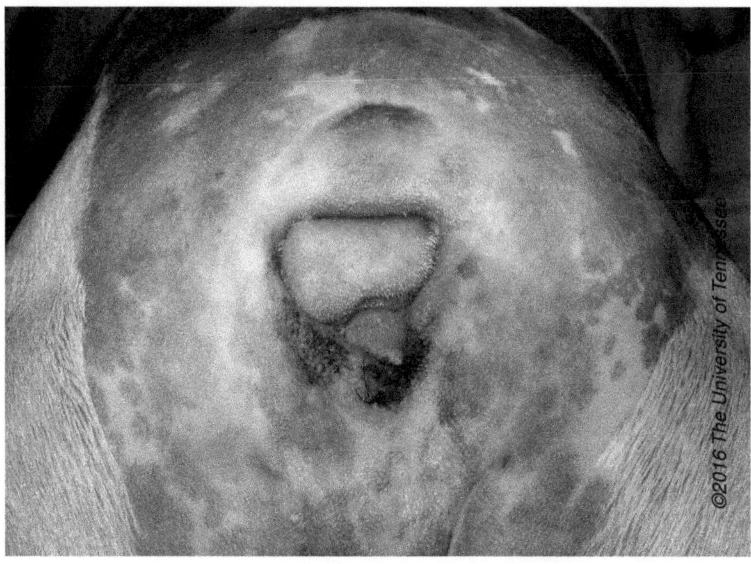

Figure 49-8 For caudectomy of ingrown tails, clip and prep the region around the tail widely. Make sure to clean the folds and crevices around and under the tail thoroughly; these areas are often infected, ulcerated, and contain feces. © 2016 The University of Tennessee.

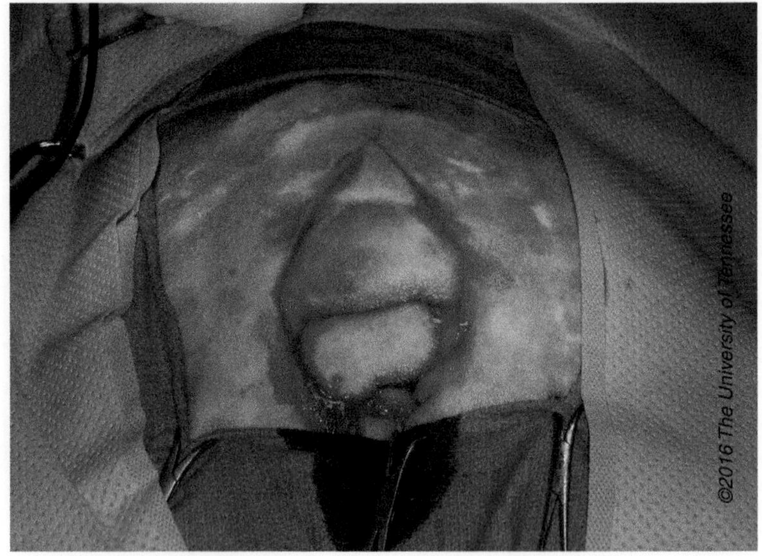

Figure 49-9 Make an elliptical incision around the tail. The cranial extent of the incision depends on the location of the cranial-most vertebral anomaly. The ventral portion of the incision must be dorsal to the anus. © 2016 The University of Tennessee.

2. Make an elliptical incision around the tail and cranially to the level of vertebral transection (fig. 49-9).
   a. The ventral edge of the incision must be dorsal to the anus, which is often hidden under the tail. If the anus is not visible, this portion of the incision can be made after the bone is transected.
   b. To facilitate manipulation of the tail during incision and dissection, place a towel clamp through the end of the tail.
3. Dissect the subcutaneous tissues and muscle down to the level of the deviated vertebra or the vertebra just cranial to it (fig. 49-10).
   a. To limit contamination, avoid penetrating through tail folds.
   b. Dissect attachments of the levator ani, rectococcygeus, and coccygeus muscles to the caudal (coccygeal) vertebrae destined to be removed.
   c. Ligate or cauterize the lateral, median, and ventral caudal arteries.

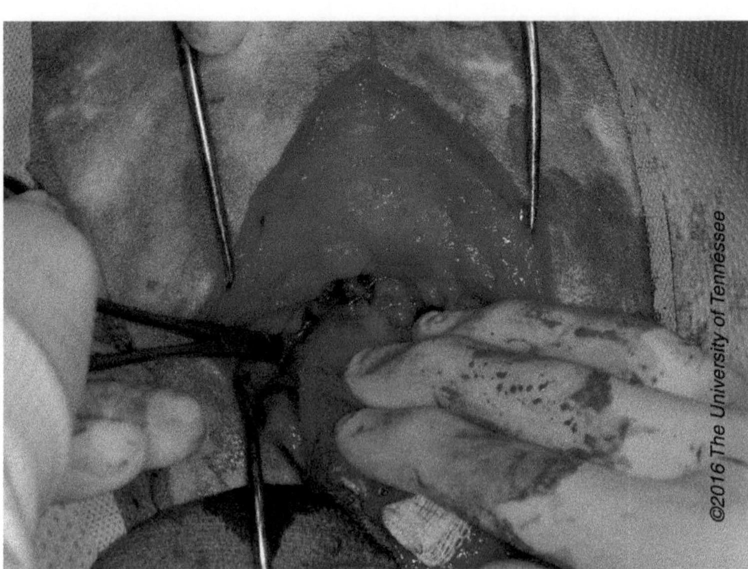

Figure 49-10 Dissect the subcutaneous tissues dorsally to expose the point of caudal vertebra deviation. © 2016 The University of Tennessee.

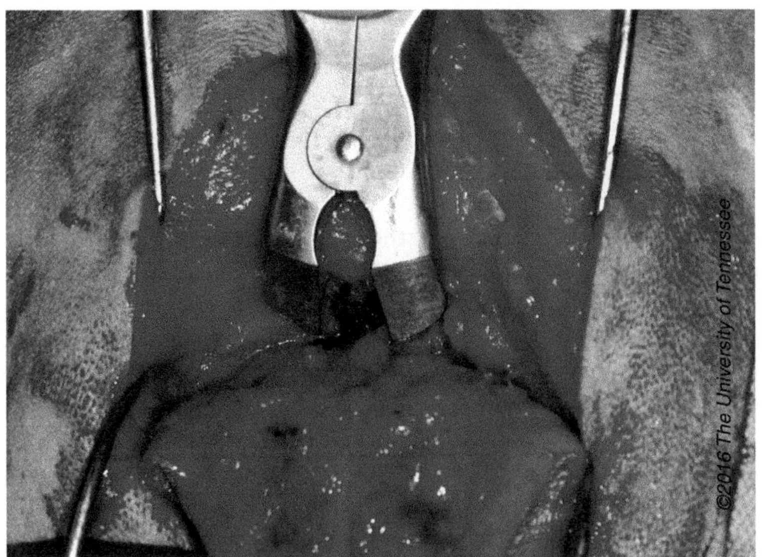

Figure 49-11 Transect the bone at the level of the deviation. © 2016 The University of Tennessee.

   d. If the ventral half of the soft tissues cannot be exposed, dissect around the dorsal half of the bone and complete the soft tissue dissection once the bone is transected.

4. Carefully transect the tail between vertebrae or through the bone.
   a. If the joint can be palpated, cut through the ligaments at the joint just above the deviation.
   b. If the joint cannot be palpated, transect the caudal (coccygeal) bone at or just above the level of the vertebral deviation with bone cutters (fig. 49-11). Trim off any sharp edges with a rongeur or smooth them with a bone rasp.
5. Complete the soft tissue dissection circumferentially to remove the tail.
6. Lavage the area with sterile saline, and place a continuous suction drain if dead space cannot be closed.
7. Appose the subcutis (fig. 49-12). If no suction drain is placed, close the subcutaneous tissue in 2 layers, tacking the fat down to close deadspace. Close the skin with interrupted sutures.

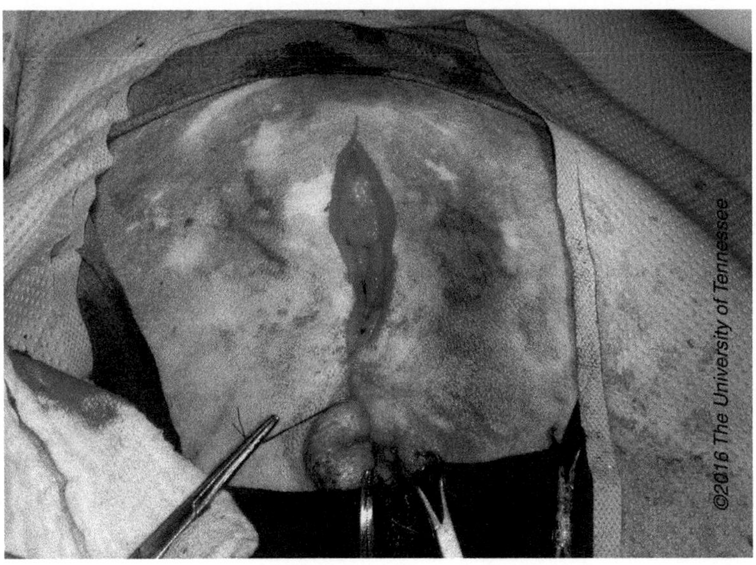

Figure 49-12 Close subcutaneous tissue in 2 layers, then appose skin. © 2016 The University of Tennessee.

Postoperative considerations

Elizabethan collars and bandages may be required to prevent self-trauma. Long tails can be protected by taping the tail to the side of the dog or to aluminum side bars attached to the dog. For dogs that tend to hit their tails frequently against objects, a padded cylinder of plastic, tubing, foam, or casting material can be placed over the tail and taped proximally to healthy skin or secured by straps to a harness to protect the amputation site until suture removal. Sutures are usually removed 10 to 14 days after surgery.

Potential complications include dehiscence, trauma, hemorrhage, and necrosis. Complications are more likely to occur in dogs that continue to traumatize the remaining tail or that had pre-existing infections. High amputations are less likely to dehisce or necrose because tissues are more vascular, the skin is more easily elevated during dissection, and the tail remnant does not get knocked against walls or caught in dog doors. Some dogs with screw tail may have temporary changes in defecation habits.

Bibliography

Knight SM, Radlinsky MAG, Cornell KK, et al: Postoperative complications associated with caudectomy in brachycephalic dogs with ingrown tails. J Am Anim Hosp Assoc 2013;49:237–242.

Rigg DL and Schwink KL: Tail amputation in the dog. Compend Contin Educ Pract Vet 1983;5:719–724.

Simons MC, Ben-Amotz R, Popovitch C: Post-operative complications and owner satisfaction following partial caudectomies: 22 cases (2008–2013). J Small Anim Pract 2014;55:509–514.

Van EE RT and Palminteri A: Tail amputation for treatment of perianal fistulas in dogs. J Am Anim Hosp Assoc 1987;23:95–100.

Section 7 Surgery of the Head and Neck

Chapter 50
Oronasal Fistulas

Oronasal fistulas are congenital or acquired connections between the mouth and nasal cavity. In young animals, they usually result from congenital secondary cleft palate (clefts of the hard and soft palate). Acquired oronasal fistulas most commonly occur after upper canine or canassial tooth extraction. Oronasal fistulas are classified as healed or nonhealed; healed fistulas have mucosal continuity between the oral and nasal cavity.

Clinical signs of oronasal fistulas include sneezing, nasal discharge, rhinitis, and fetid breath. Treatment depends on the size of the fistula and its chronicity. In older animals, acute fistulas from maxillary canine tooth extractions are usually closed with flaps and suture; in younger animals, fistulas from freshly removed teeth may heal on their own. Necrotic or infected fistulas are left open to drain and granulate. Patients with large necrotic fistulas are treated with antibiotics and esophageal or gastric feeding tubes until the mucosa and fibrous tissue are strong enough to tolerate surgical manipulation.

Many surgeons will delay repair of congenital oronasal fistula (cleft secondary palate) until the animal is at least 3 or 4 months of age. Delaying the surgery allows the palatal mucosa to thicken and the head to grow wider and improves the patient's tolerance to long anesthetic episode. In puppies, the relative size of the palatal cleft gradually decreases from weeks 5 to 12, and then gradually increases until week 20, after which it remains fairly constant in size.

Preoperative management

Thoracic radiographs should be obtained if aspiration pneumonia is suspected. Animals with pneumonia should be medically managed until the condition resolves. Skull radiographs or computed tomography may be useful in detecting tooth root abscesses, retained tooth roots, foreign bodies, and osseous changes from neoplasia or infection. To rule out tumor recurrence, biopsies of the fistula margin are recommended in patients that develop fistulas after maxillectomy for neoplasia. Culture and sensitivity of the nasal cavity should be obtained in animals with nonresponsive rhinitis. Antibiotics are usually administered in animals with rhinitis, abscesses, or gingivitis but may not be required in other patients.

Local nerve blocks provide excellent postoperative analgesia and may reduce intraoperative anesthetic requirements. The rostral maxilla, which is supplied

Manual of Small Animal Soft Tissue Surgery, Second Edition. Karen Tobias.
© 2017 John Wiley & Sons, Inc. Published 2017 by John Wiley & Sons, Inc.

by the infraorbital nerve, can be blocked at the palpable infraorbital foramen dorsal to the second or third premolar. The maxillary nerve can be blocked by injecting local anesthetic in the depression below the zygomatic arch, caudal to the maxilla and rostral to the ramus of the mandible. If dehiscence is a concern, an esophagostomy or gastrostomy tube can be placed for enteral nutrition. For patients with chronic, recurrent fistulas, additional repairs should be delayed for at least 1 month after the previous surgery to allow local tissues to revascularize and strengthen. During surgery, animals are usually placed in dorsal recumbency; an elbow attachment to the endotracheal tube will keep hoses out of the surgeon's way. If a cuffed endotracheal tube has been placed, the oral cavity can be flushed gently with an antiseptic solution.

Surgery

Most acute, nonhealed fistulas can be repaired with a single pedicle sliding or advancement flap of gingival mucosa and adjacent palatal, gingival, or labial mucosa (fig. 50-1). Chronic, healed fistulas are often closed with two layers to improve strength and provide immediate reconstruction of nasal and oral cavities. The nasal epithelium is re-formed with one or two inverting flaps of surrounding oral mucosa and then covered with a sliding or rotating flap of palatal or labial mucosa. Removal of healthy teeth may be required to prevent damage to the base of the labial pedicle.

Elevated tissues should be handled minimally and gently with stay sutures or fine-toothed thumb forceps. Flaps are sutured in place with 3-0 to 5-0 absorbable synthetic material in interrupted or continuous patterns with the knots in the nasal or oral cavity. Synthetic multifilament sutures have been recommended because they are soft, strong, and pliable; however, many

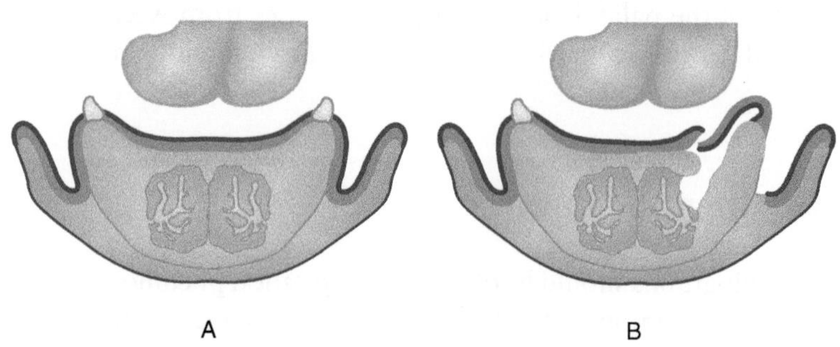

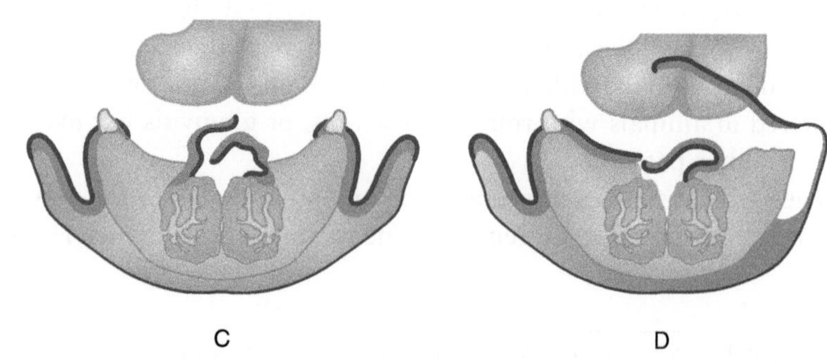

Figure 50-1 Techniques for oronasal fistula repair (animal positioned in dorsal recumbancy). **A:** Transverse section through maxilla and tongue (top of figure) in normal dog. **B:** Unilateral inverting gingival mucosa flap. **C:** Bilateral inverting palatal mucosa flaps. **D:** Two-layer closure with inverting palatal mucosa flap and labial advancement flap.

surgeons prefer absorbable monofilament materials for their handling characteristics.

Minor hemorrhage during surgery is usually controlled with digital pressure to prevent tissue damage. The major palatine artery exits the palatine foramen medial to the fourth upper premolar tooth and travels rostrally within the mucosa. In rare cases, ligation or bipolar cauterization of this artery may be required if it is lacerated.

Surgical technique: unilateral or bilateral inverting mucosal flap (fig. 50-1 B and C)

Note: Inverting mucosal flaps are used only for repair of healed fistulas because their blood supply relies on their attachments to nasal mucosa. Inverting flaps can be used alone or as the initial layer of a two-layer closure.

1. Measure the diameter of the fistula to determine the size of flap needed. For a unilateral inverting flap, add 4 to 5 mm to the diameter measurement. For bilateral inverting flaps, divide the diameter measurement in half and add 2 to 3 mm for each flap width.
2. Incise the mucosa and periosteum lateral and parallel to the border of the fistula (fig. 50-2).
3. Using a periosteal elevator, elevate the mucosa and underlying periosteum carefully toward the fistula.
    a. In laterally located fistulas, elevation of lateral flaps will initially include the mucosa and periosteum or fibrous tissue over the maxillary alveolar process.
    b. Proceed cautiously toward the healed base of the flap at the nasal and oral mucosal junction along the bone edge. Vigorous elevation here could accidentally damage the blood supply or transect the flap base along the fistula.
4. For bilateral pedicle flaps:
    a. Elevate and invert the flaps from each side so that the oral mucosa becomes the new nasal epithelium.

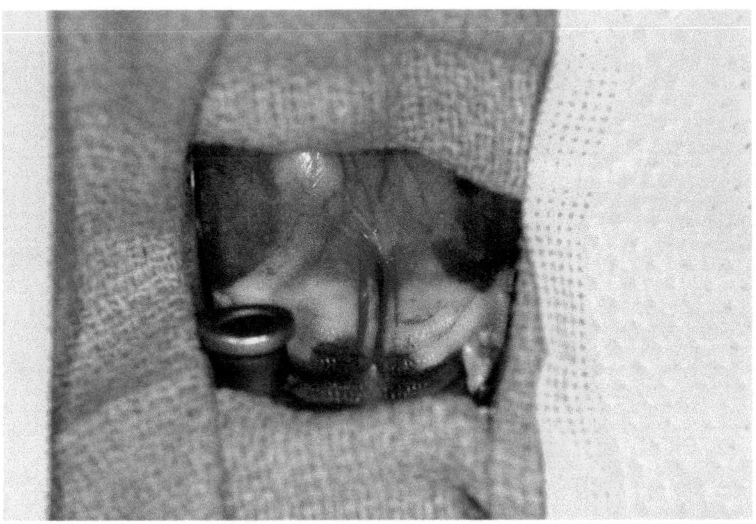

Figure 50-2 Bilateral inverting flaps. Incise the palatal mucosa and periosteum several millimeters lateral and parallel to each side of the fistula.

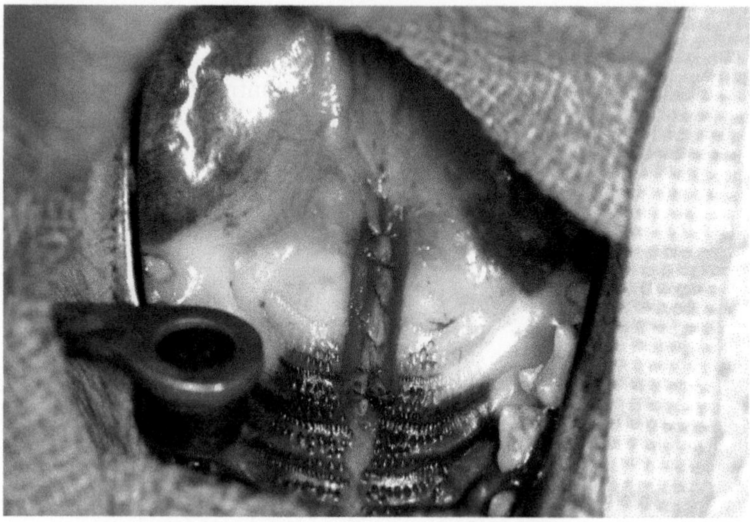

Figure 50-3 Once the mucoperiosteum is carefully elevated to the bone edge along the fistula, invert the flaps and suture together with a continuous pattern.

b. Appose the inverted flaps over the middle of the fistula with interrupted or continuous sutures (fig. 50-3).

5. For a unilateral flap, invert the flap and suture it to the oral mucosa on the opposite side:

   a. Incise and elevate tissues along one side of the fistula to make a single inverting flap based along one fistula margin.

   b. Make an incision along the remaining fistula margin (the side opposite the flap), and elevate the palatal mucosa laterally along this incision (fig. 50-4).

   c. Elevate the unilateral mucoperiosteal flap (fig. 50-5), invert it, and tuck it between the elevated mucoperiosteum and the bone of the hard palate on the contralateral side (fig. 50-6).

   d. Appose the tissues with mattress sutures of 3-0 or 4-0 absorbable material so that the knots will lie over bone.

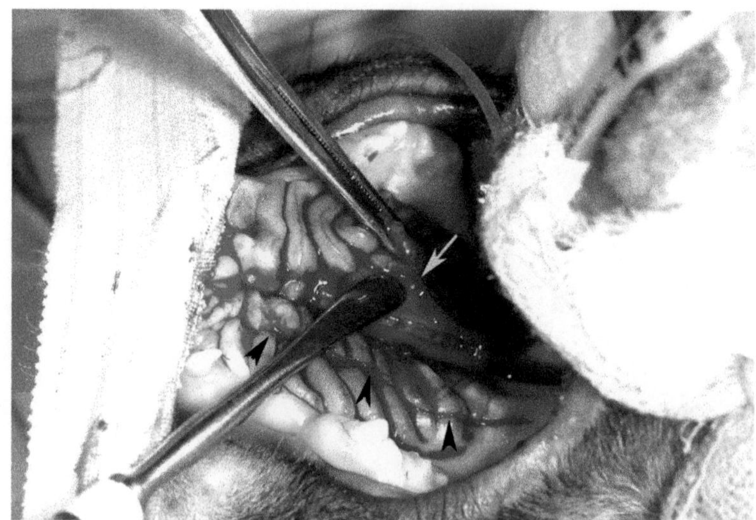

Figure 50-4 Unilateral inverting flap. Make an incision parallel to the fistula (arrowheads) to develop a flap that is 4 to 5 mm wider than the fistula. On the side opposite the developed flap, make an incision parallel and adjacent to the edge of the fistula, and elevate the mucoperiosteum laterally (yellow arrow) so that the contralateral inverting flap can be tucked under the mucoperiosteum.

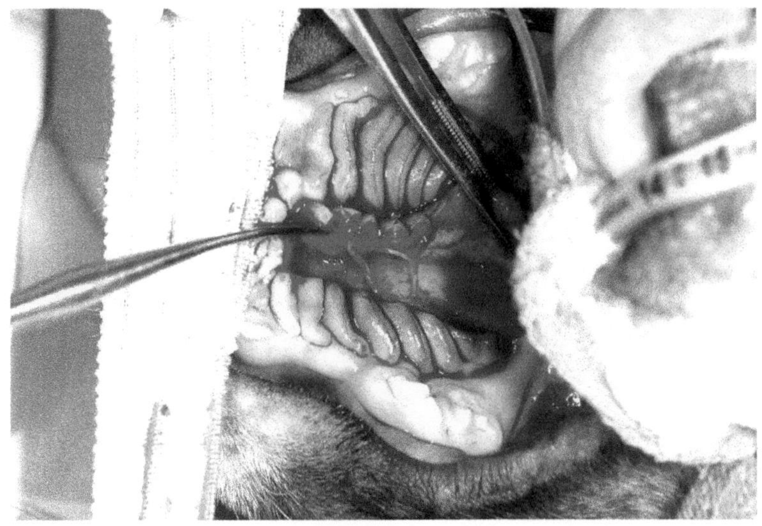

Figure 50-5 Elevate the unilateral inverting flap by working toward the fistula. Leave the flap base along the fistula intact. If possible, spare the major palatine arteries.

6. Close any remaining gaps (usually rostral and caudal) around the fistula with interrupted sutures. If possible, cover the inverted flap(s) with a labial advancement flap or bilateral bipedicle mucoperiosteal flaps.

Surgical technique: labial/buccal advancement flap (fig. 50-1 D)

Note: Labial or buccal advancement flaps can be used for single-layer closure of a nonhealed or healed fistula, or as a second layer over an inverted mucosal flap.

1. If the fistula is at the center of the palate, pull any teeth between the fistula and the flap donor site. Rongeur or file the rough edges of the maxillary alveolar process along the extraction sites; this will make a wide, smooth trough in which the flap can rest.
2. Make two incisions through the gingival and labial mucosa, starting at the rostral and caudal edges of the fistula and extending toward the lip margin (fig. 50-7). The incisions should diverge slightly so that the base of the flap (closer to the lip margin) is wider than the fistula.

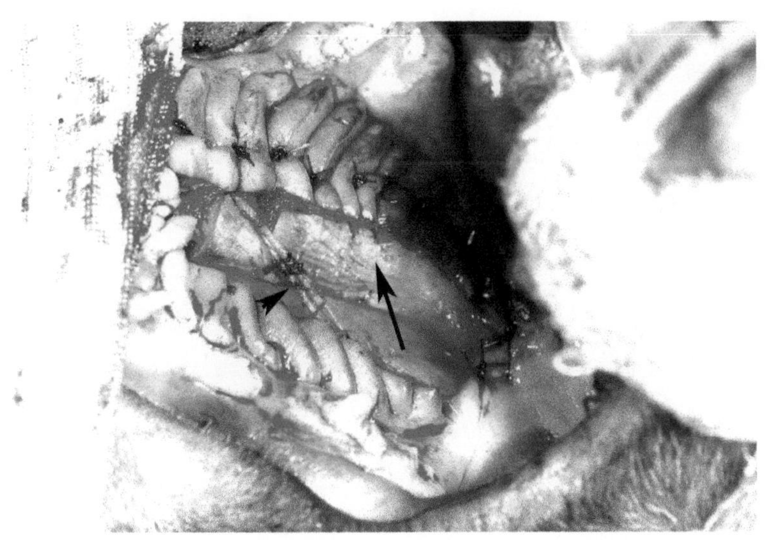

Figure 50-6 Invert the flap (arrow) so that its edge rests atop bone and under the elevated mucoperiosteum on the contralateral side, and suture it in place. If possible, leave the major palatine vessels (arrowhead) intact.

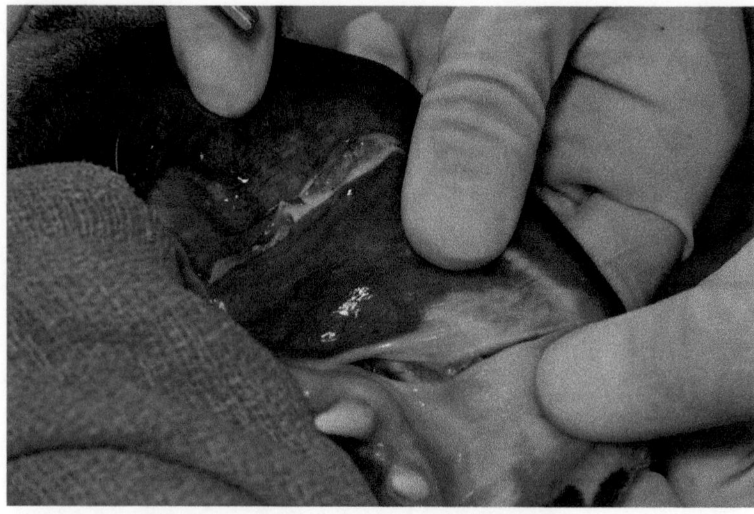

Figure 50-7 Labial advancement flap. Make two incisions perpendicular to the fistula margin and extending toward the lip margin.

3. Using Metzenbaum scissors, separate the labial mucosa and its thin, fibrous lamina propria from the remainder of the lip with blunt and sharp dissection.
   a. To make tissue elevation easier, start dissection along one side of the proposed flap, leaving the flap attached to the fistula edge (fig. 50-8). This will allow the flap to be elevated without excessive handling. Once it is freed from its bed, the attachments along the fistula margin can be transected and elevated (fig. 50-9).
   b. Undermine the flap far enough laterally so that it will reach across the fistula without tension and without causing severe inward lip deviation (fig. 50-10). If necessary, extend the parallel flap incisions to lengthen the flap.
4. With a Freer periosteal elevator, elevate the edge of the palatal mucosa and periosteum along the opposite side of the fistula. Incise around the edge of a healed fistula before elevating.
5. Suture the labial flap to the free edge of the palatal mucoperiosteum (fig. 50-11) with one or two layers of interrupted sutures, using synthetic

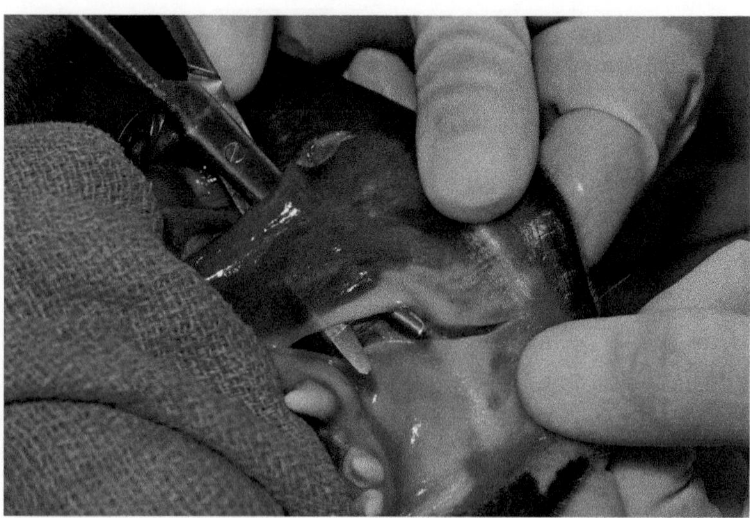

Figure 50-8 Elevate the labial and buccal mucosa with scissors, staying superficial to labial nerves.

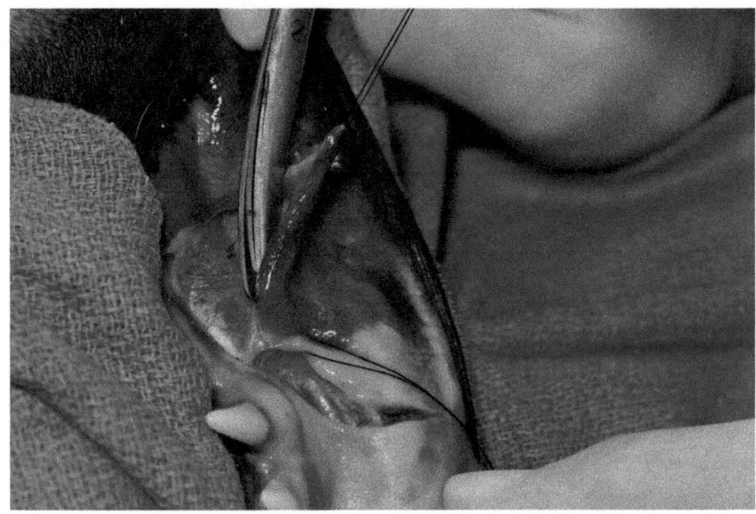

Figure 50-9 Incise the mucosal attachments of the flap along the fistula margin, and transect any remaining submucosal attachments with sharp and blunt dissection. Place stay sutures in the flap to facilitate manipulation.

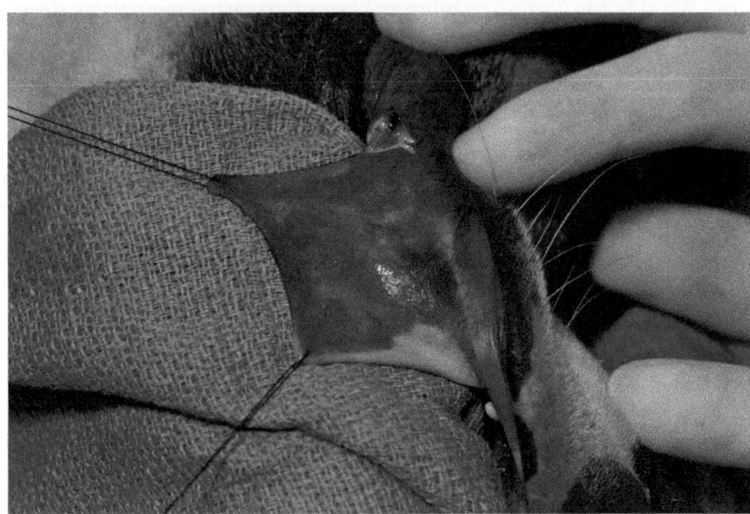

Figure 50-10 Elevate the flap toward the labial margin until the flap size is sufficient to cover the fistula without tension.

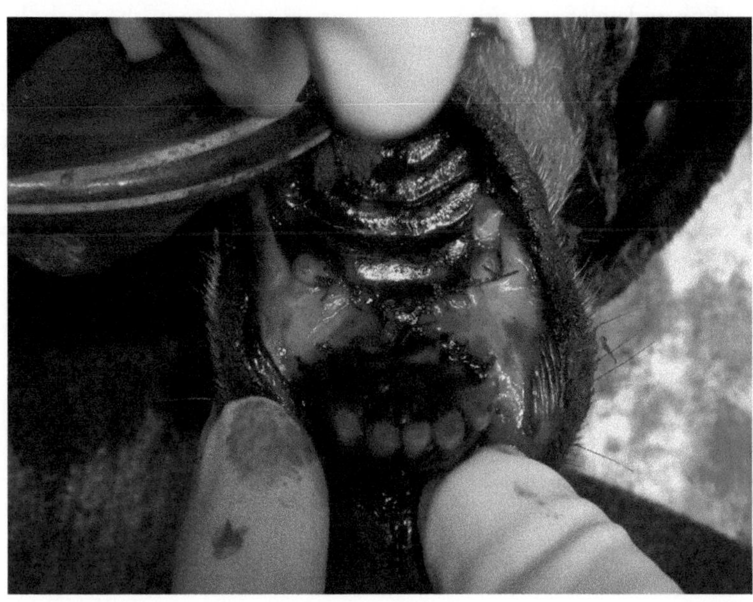

Figure 50-11 Suture the flaps to the free edge of the palatal, gingival, and labial mucosa.

absorbable suture on a reverse cutting or tapercut needle. Place sutures 3 to 4 mm apart.

   a. For a single-layer closure, use a simple interrupted appositional pattern with or without burying the knots.

   b. For closure with two layers of suture, place a few interrupted sutures in the mucoperiosteum of the hard palate (or nasal mucosa side of a healed fistula) and the lamina propria of the labial flap, and then a second layer of sutures along the oral surface between the free margins of the mucoperiosteal and labial flaps.

6. Close the labial mucosal defects along the sides of the pedicle base with simple interrupted sutures. To improve bite width and suture hold, elevate the mucosa off the bone along the incision edges and take wide, deep tissue bites.

7. Leave oral suture tags 2 to 3 mm long.

8. Large fistulas may require bilateral labial advancement flaps. In this case, perform steps 1 through 5 bilaterally; suture the flaps together on midline and close gaps along the sides as described above.

Surgical technique: bilateral sliding mucoperiosteal flap

Note: Bilateral sliding mucoperiosteal flaps are used for repair of central palatal oronasal fistula. If enough tissue is present, they can be used as a second layer over an inverted palatal flap.

1. If possible, cover the fistula first with unilateral or bilateral inverting mucosal flaps (fig. 50-2).

2. Make full-thickness releasing incisions in the palate, leaving the flaps attached rostrally and caudally.

   a. Make flaps wider and longer than the cleft so they will contact each other on midline and will overlap the defect and the bone.

   b. For wide clefts, incise near the lingual surfaces of the teeth, leaving a border of gingiva along the teeth.

3. Starting rostrally along the fistula edge, gently elevate laterally under the mucoperiosteum to separate the flap from the palatal bone. Try to spare the major palatine artery.

4. Once both flaps are elevated, slide them toward midline and suture them together with simple interrupted sutures (fig. 50-12).

5. Leave the palatal bone lateral to the flaps exposed; it will cover with granulation tissue within 24 to 48 hours.

Surgical technique: soft palate cleft repair

Note: Many puppies have an obvious point or corner on each side of the soft palate defect that indicates the caudal boundaries of the two sides of the palate. In brachycephalic breeds, it may be necessary to make the repair shorter (e.g.,

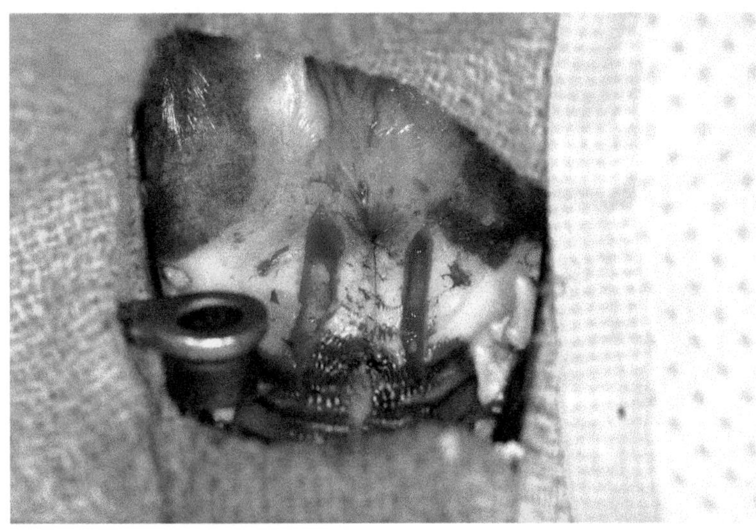

Figure 50-12 Bipedicle sliding mucoperiosteal flaps were used as a second layer over inverting palatal flaps in the cat in figures 50-2 and 50-3.

to the level of the caudal tonsillar borders) to avoid the elongated soft palate naturally occurring in so many of these animals.

1. Identify the proposed caudal extent of the soft palate.
   a. For most dogs this is a point level with the caudal edges of the tonsils.
   b. The tip of the palate does not have to overlap with the tip of the epiglottis in brachycephalic breeds.
2. On each side of the cleft, incise the edge of the palate at its oronasal junction with a no. 11 or no. 15 scalpel blade (fig. 50-13), ending at the proposed caudal extent of the repaired palate.
3. Starting at the caudal extent of the incision, appose the nasal mucosal margins of the palatal incisions with 3-0 or 4-0 rapidly absorbable monofilament suture in a simple continuous pattern (fig. 50-14).
4. Appose the oral mucosal margins of the palatal incisions with 3-0 or 4-0 rapidly absorbable monofilament suture in a simple continuous pattern.

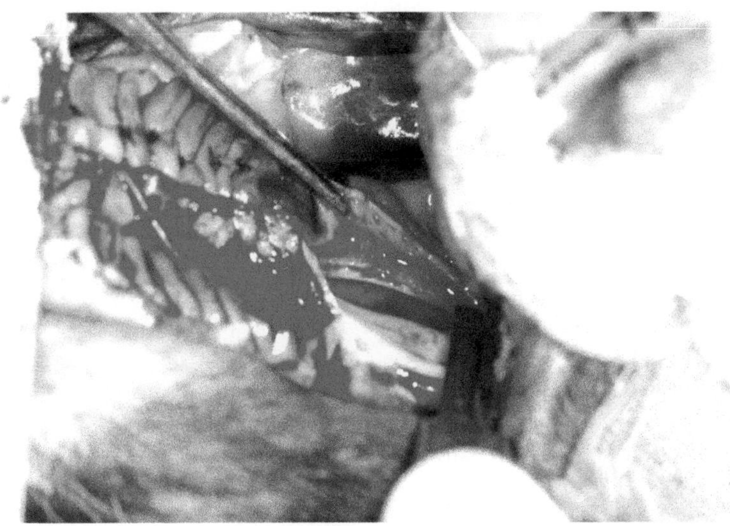

Figure 50-13 Incise the margin of the soft palate fistula on each side.

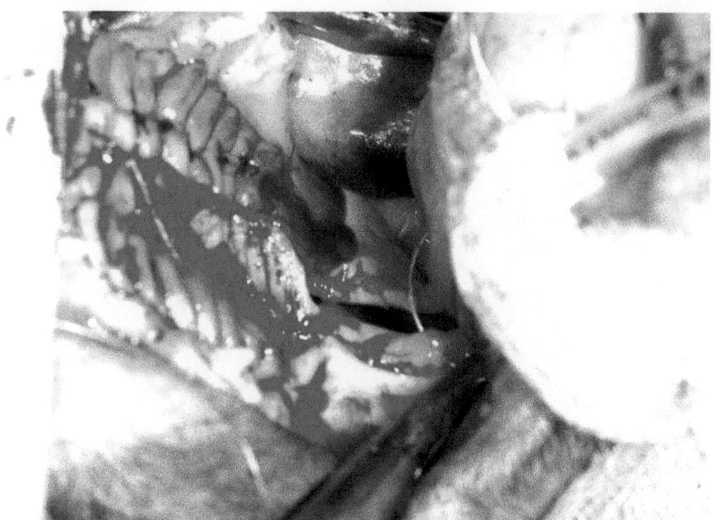

Figure 50-14 Appose the soft palate defect in 2 layers, starting with the nasal mucosal edges, with absorbable suture.

Postoperative management

Animals should be monitored for dyspnea postoperatively, since hemorrhage from the surgical site can obstruct the nasal cavity. Additionally, brachycephalic animals that have undergone repair of soft palate clefts may develop swelling that obstructs the airway. They should be monitored closely during anesthetic recovery, and the veterinarian should be prepared to administer sedation or flow by or nasal oxygen or even anesthetize and reintubate the animal.

To reduce trauma to hard palate repairs, use a feeding tube for 1 to 2 weeks or soft diet for up to 5 weeks. Canned food can be formed into meatballs to facilitate prehension and swallowing. Access to chew toys, bones, and other hard objects should be prevented for a month until the site is completely healed. Oral sutures do not need to be removed since they will be extruded from the tissues within 2 to 3 weeks after surgery.

Dehiscence is common with large fistulas and usually occurs within 3 to 5 days of the surgery. Traumatic surgical technique, tension on the repair, use of electrocautery during dissection, or previous irradiation of the area may increase the risk of dehiscence. Animals with recurrent oronasal fistulas are treated with antibiotics if purulent rhinitis is present and fed via a feeding tube if aspiration is a concern. After 1 month, the tissues are reevaluated and a second procedure is performed.

Bibliography

Maretta SM: Single mucoperiosteal flap for oronasal fistula repair. J Vet Dent 2005;22:200–205.

Paradas-Lara I, Casado-Gomez I, Martin C, et al: Maxillary growth in a congenital cleft palate canine model for surgical research. J Cranio-Maxilo-Facial Surg 2014;42:13–21.

Sivacolundhu RK: Use of local and axial pattern flaps for reconstruction of the hard and soft palate. Clin Tech Small Anim Pract 2007;22:61–69.

Smith MM: Oronasal fistula repair. Clin Tech Small Anim Pract 2000;15:243–250.

Chapter 51
Lateral Ear Canal Resection

Indications for lateral ear canal resection, also known as a lateral ear canal ablation or Zepp procedure, include correction of congenital lesions, removal of benign masses of the dorsolateral canal wall, and enlargement of inflamed canals to provide access for medical management. In animals with infantile stenosis (most commonly seen in Shar-Pei dogs) or excessive hair growth of the external canals, poor aeration and moisture entrapment may result in recurrent otitis externa. Improving the local microclimate of the canals by excising the lateral walls may be the only treatment necessary for these animals. In animals with inflamed canals, lateral ear canal resection improves drainage and facilitates application of topical medications. Surgery is often not required in these animals, however, if local medical management is appropriate and underlying dermatologic conditions are treated. Lateral ear canal resection is unlikely to be beneficial once canals become hyperplastic or calcified.

Preoperative management

A thorough dermatologic examination should be performed to rule out generalized skin diseases. Evaluation for systemic illness should include measurement of T4 and TSH, since hypothyroidism can predispose animals to otitis. Ear cytology and cultures are recommended in animals with recurrent infections or Gram-negative organisms. If yeast is present on ear or skin cytology, dogs may have underlying allergies that will need to be addressed. Skull radiographs or computed tomography are recommended to evaluate the bullae for evidence of otitis media. Chronic otitis media may require ventral bulla osteotomy or lavage through a myringotomy.

Under anesthesia, the side of the face is clipped ventrally to midline, rostrally to the lateral commissure of the eyelid, and for 5 to 8 cm caudal to the palpable ear canal. The haired, convex surface of the pinna can either be clipped or draped out of the field. The animal is positioned in lateral recumbency. A folded towel can be placed under the head to elevate it toward the surgeon. The ear is prepped with antiseptic solution and scrub. Because ototoxicity has been reported with antiseptics, some clinicians recommend using only sterile saline to flush the horizontal ear when the tympanic membrane is perforated.

Manual of Small Animal Soft Tissue Surgery, Second Edition. Karen Tobias.
© 2017 John Wiley & Sons, Inc. Published 2017 by John Wiley & Sons, Inc.

Antibiotics may be administered prophylactically if the animal is not already on therapeutic perioperative antimicrobials.

Surgery

The lateralmost portion of the vertical canal contains two notches: the tragohelicine, or pretragic, incisure rostrally and the intertragic incisure caudally. These notches mark the rostral and caudal boundaries of the resection. In some dogs, the parotid gland overlies the vertical ear canal and must be dissected away to expose the lateral wall. Transection of the gland at this site does not result in a salivary mucocele. Because the vertical canal spirals as it reaches the horizontal canal, it is easy to accidentally cut a flap that is too narrow or oriented too far caudally. The lateral wall flap can either be developed, starting dorsally, by making small cautious cuts on alternate sides, or can be started ventrally so that the base of the flap is automatically positioned at the desired site. Once the flap is made, the horizontal canal should be easily visible and there should be no ridge of tissue between the flap base and the floor of the horizontal canal.

Surgical technique: lateral ear canal resection

1. Make a U-shaped skin incision over the vertical ear canal, starting and ending at pretragic and intertragic incisures and continuing ventrally at least a centimeter below the ventralmost portion of the palpable canal (fig. 51-1).
2. Dissect the subcutaneous tissue away from the lateral wall of the vertical canal with blunt and sharp dissection until the canal wall is exposed (fig. 51-2).
3. Make two parallel incisions in the lateral wall of the vertical ear canal that extend from the pretragic and intertragic incisures to the lateral aspects of the junction between the vertical and horizontal canals, starting at the incisures or at the junction of the canals. *Note: From dorsal to ventral, the ear canal spirals slightly inward, so be aware of the change in canal orientation as you cut. Also, some dogs have an outpouching of the*

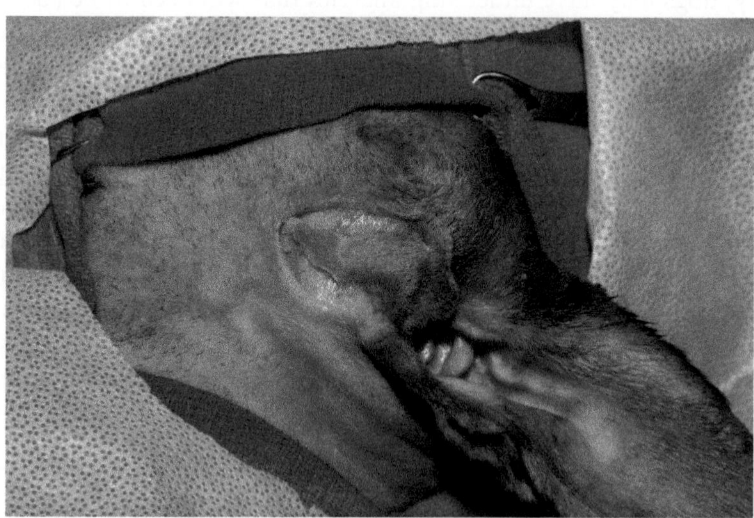

Figure 51-1 Make a U-shaped skin incision over the vertical ear canal.

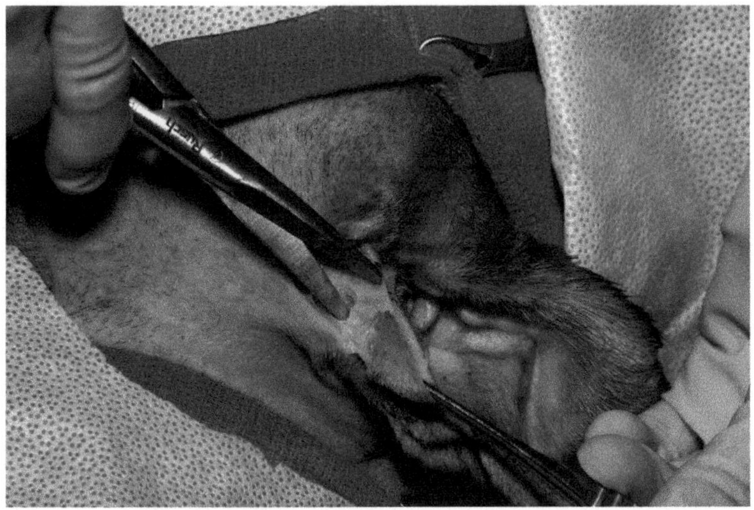

Figure 51-2 Expose the lateral wall of the vertical ear canal with blunt and sharp dissection.

vertical canal along its caudal aspect, which can be confusing during flap development.

a. If starting dorsally at the incisures (fig. 51-3):

   i. Stand on the dog's dorsal side and, with your nondominant hand, grasp the flap of skin or a pair of Allis tissue forceps attached to the dorsal edge of the lateral cartilage of the vertical canal.

   ii. With straight Mayo scissors, make a 1-cm cut down the vertical ear canal, starting at one incisure and angling toward the ventral aspect of the vertical canal (fig. 51-3).

   iii. Make a similar cut, starting at the opposite incisure.

   iv. Alternately extend each incision with short cuts, examining the interior of the canal before each cut to verify that the scissor blades are bisecting the canal along its length and following the gentle spiral of the canal. If necessary, insert a forceps down the canal to evaluate canal depth and position before continuing each cut.

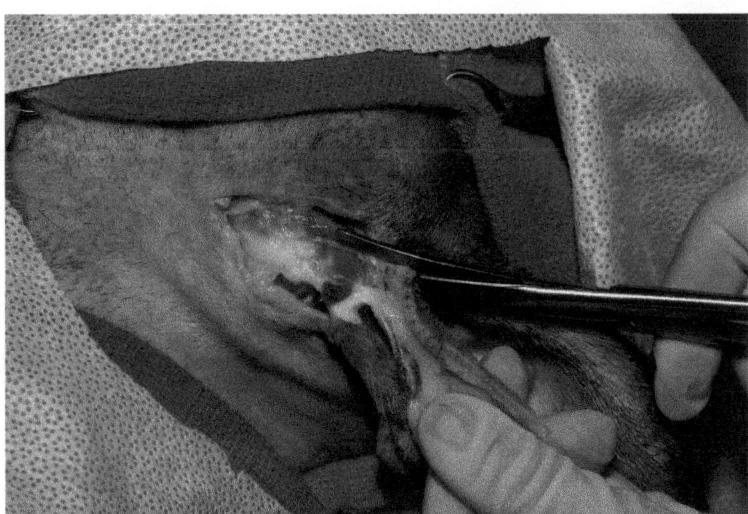

Figure 51-3 Standard technique: With Mayo scissors, make two parallel incisions through the lateral wall of the vertical canal, starting at the incisures and following the curve of the canal.

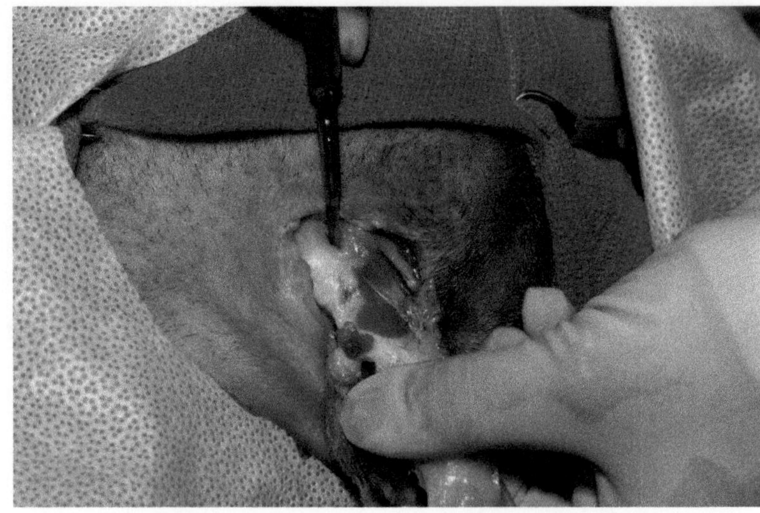

Figure 51-4 Alternate technique: Make two parallel stab incisions at the ventralmost aspect of the proposed flap to develop the flap base.

v. Continue the incisions until the bottom of the vertical canal is reached.

b. If starting ventrally at the junction of the horizontal and vertical canals:

i. Stand on the dog's ventral side.

ii. Make two parallel stab incisions (fig. 51-4) with a no. 11 blade at the ventralmost extent of the proposed flap (just dorsal to the junction of the horizontal and vertical canals).

iii. With Mayo scissors, extend each incision dorsally to the ipsilateral incisure (fig. 51-5).

4. Verify that the lateral wall of vertical canal has been cut sufficiently by pulling the flap ventrally (fig. 51-6). If the flap forms a fold that obstructs the ventral half of the horizontal canal opening, extend the cartilage cuts (figs. 51-7 and 51-8) toward the midpoints of the horizontal canal so that the opening is circular and unobstructed.

5. Resect half to two-thirds of the lateral cartilage flap length, with attached skin, leaving a 1- to 3-cm drain board below the horizontal canal opening (fig. 51-9).

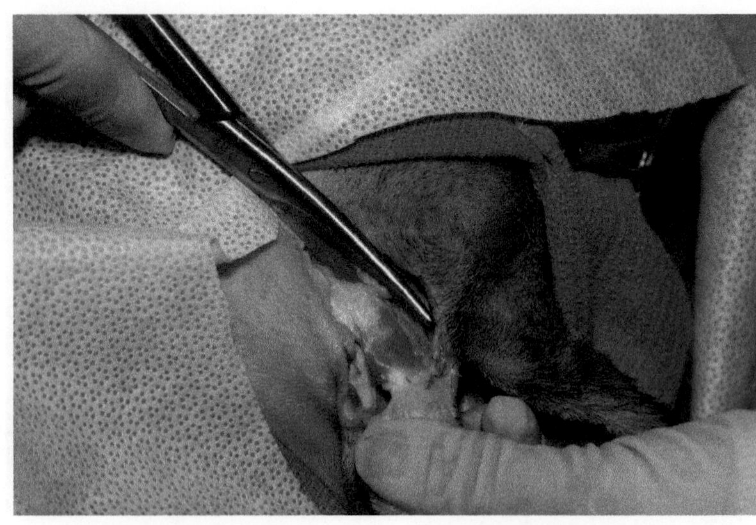

Figure 51-5 Alternate technique: Insert one blade of the Mayo scissors into one ventral stab incision and cut the lateral wall up through the ipsilateral incisure. Repeat on the opposite side.

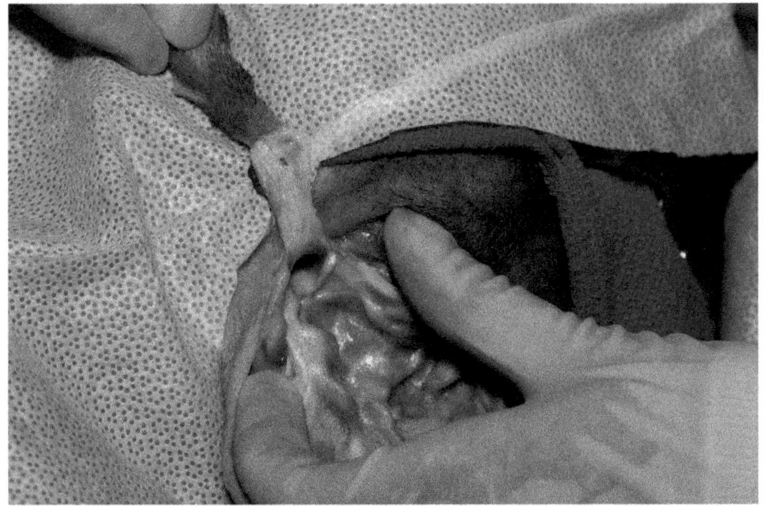

Figure 51-6 Examine the new ostium. The opening in this dog is crescent-shaped and partially obstructed by a fold at the rostral base of the flap.

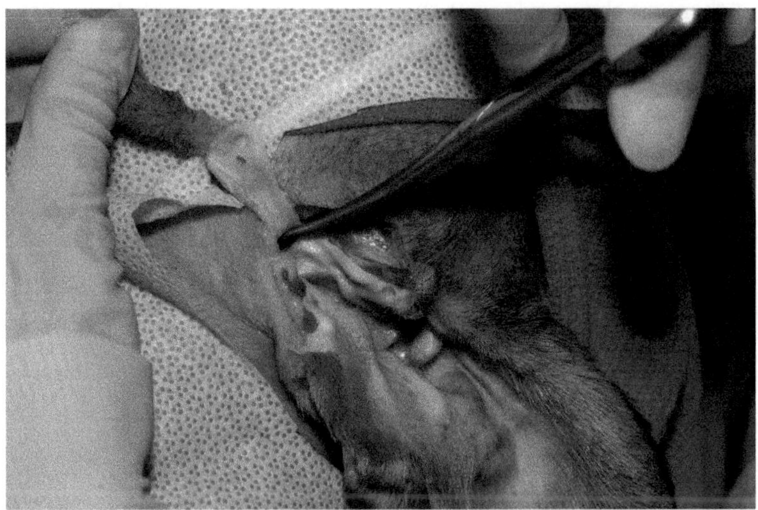

Figure 51-7 If the ostium is collapsed, make additional cuts, aiming for the midpoints along the horizontal canal ostium rostrally and caudally, to open the ostium and improve flap position.

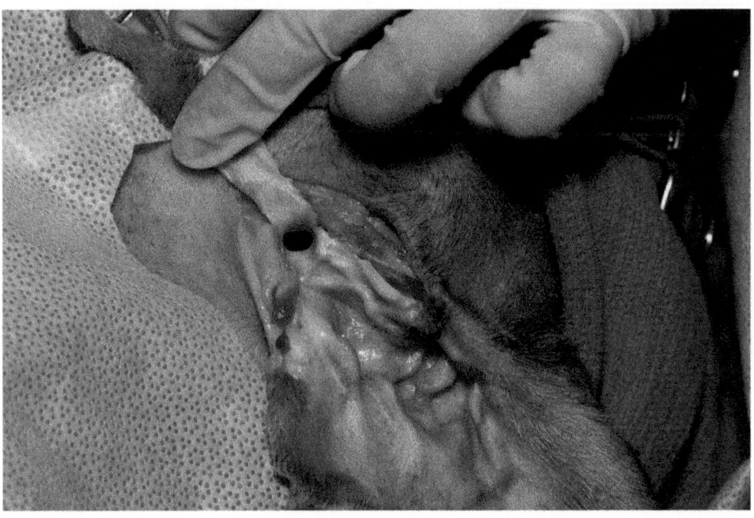

Figure 51-8 Final appearance of ostium. The opening is more circular, and the flap lies flat.

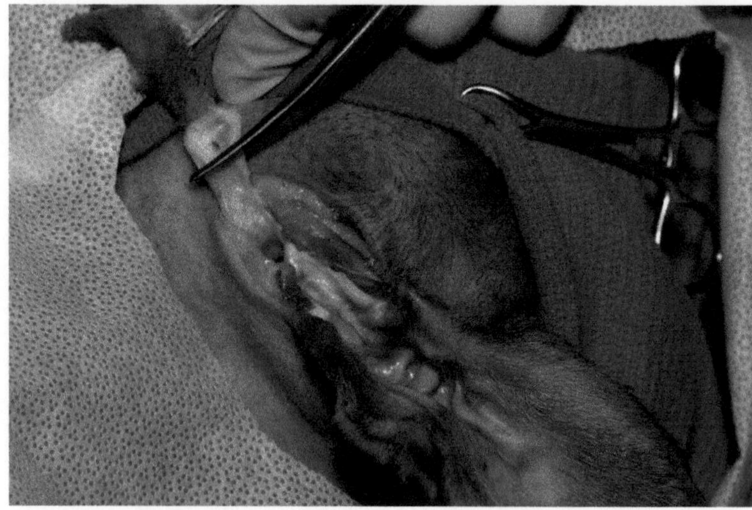

Figure 51-9 Transect the flap to shorten its length.

6. If the flap does not lie flat because the cartilage is too thick, dissect between the cartilage and inner epithelium at the desired hinge site with a hemostat and then cut the cartilage at that site, leaving the epithelium intact.
7. Remove additional facial skin as needed so that the flap is pulled ventrally away from the horizontal canal opening.
8. Appose canal epithelium to skin with 3-0 or 4-0 monofilament sutures.
   a. Initially, place a simple interrupted suture from flap epithelium to adjacent facial skin at each flap corner (fig. 51-10).
      i. If the epithelium is friable, include cartilage in each suture bite.
      ii. If the flap does not lie flat, remove additional facial skin along the ventral surgical margin to provide a small amount of ventral tension to the flap.
   b. Place a simple interrupted suture at the cartilage notch (fig. 51-11) on each side of the flap's base.
      i. Take cartilage and skin bites in separate passes to prevent tearing of the cartilage.

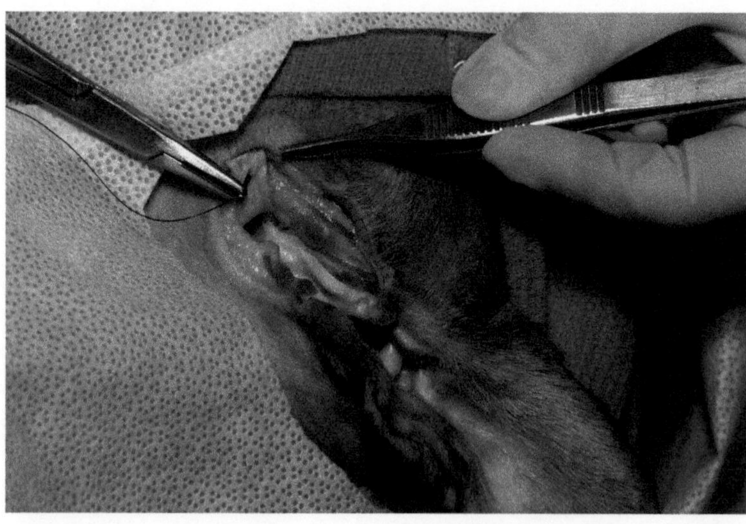

Figure 51-10 Place a simple interrupted suture between the epithelium at the corner of each flap and the ventrolateral margin of the adjacent skin incision.

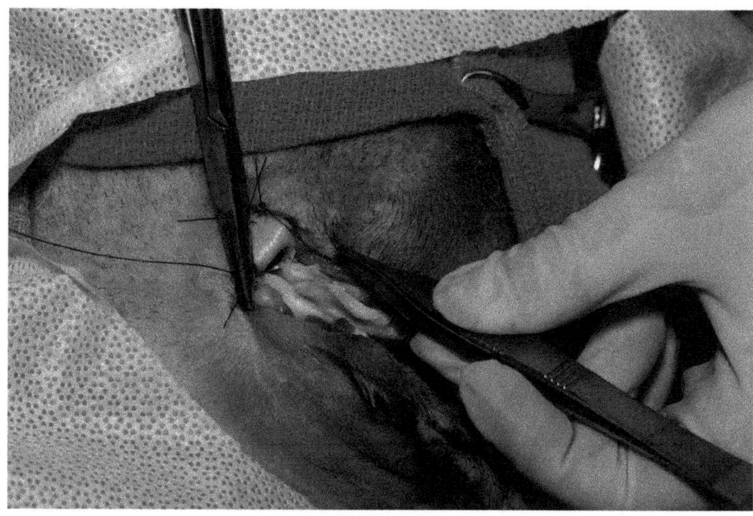

Figure 51-11 Take a full-thickness bite of the horizontal canal when placing interrupted sutures between the canal at the hinge notch and the adjacent skin.

ii. If the skin is thick, take partial thickness bites so the canal epithelium and skin surface are level when the suture is tied.

c. Suture the remaining margins of the drain board to the adjacent facial skin with simple interrupted sutures and the vertical canal walls to adjacent facial skin with simple interrupted or simple continuous sutures (fig. 51-12).

Postoperative considerations

Before recovery, a thin layer of petroleum-based antibiotic ointment can be applied to the suture line to prevent blood and other materials from adhering to the sutures. Analgesics should be continued for several days after surgery. Nonsteroidal anti-inflammatory drugs are contraindicated in animals that have received oral glucocorticoids. Animals should wear Elizabethan collars for at least 7 days after the surgery, since self-trauma is common. Dermatologic treatments should be continued as needed. Sutures are removed in 10 to 14 days.

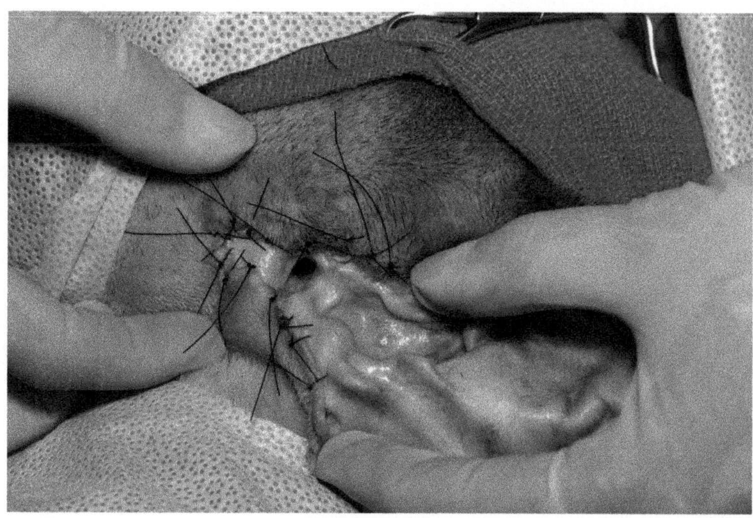

Figure 51-12 Add additional sutures to appose the remaining flap margins to the skin.

The most common complications after lateral ear canal resection are dehiscence of the surgery site and progression of disease. Dehiscence occurs in about one-fourth of patients because of self-trauma, tension, infection, or poor technique. Extensive flap dehiscence that is not repaired may result in stenosis of the canal opening. Stenosis can also occur with inadequate ventral reflection of the cartilage flap; this will require revision to prevent canal obstruction and subsequent otitis and draining sinus tracts. It may be necessary to clip the hair around the opening occasionally to improve ventilation and drainage. Animals that have congenital stenosis of the ear canal without hyperplastic changes usually have excellent outcomes. Ear disease will inevitably progress in cocker spaniels and in dogs in which the underlying cause of otitis has not been controlled, and many of these animals will require total ear canal ablations within a few years.

Bibliography

Doyle RS et al: Surgical management of 43 cases of chronic otitis externa in the dog. Irish Vet J 2004;57:22–30.

Lanz OI and Wood BC: Surgery of the ear and pinna. Vet Clin N Am Small Anim Pract 2004;34:567–599.

O'Neil T and Nuttal T: Ear surgery part 1: the vertical canal. UK Vet 2005;10:1–5.

Qahwash M, Tobias KM: Lateral ear canal resection in dogs (procedures pro). Clincian's Brief 2013;11:21–26.

Sylvestre AM: Potential factors affecting the outcomes of dogs with a resection of the lateral wall of the vertical ear canal. Can Vet J 1998;39:157–160.

Chapter 52
Vertical Ear Canal Resection

The most common indication for vertical ear canal resection is removal of tumors and polyps that extend beyond the lateral surface of the canal. Vertical ear canal resection has also been used to treat patients with persistent or recurrent otitis externa. Improvement is seen in these animals as long as the horizontal ear canal is patent and the underlying cause of otitis is controlled.

Dogs with traumatic avulsion of the ear canal can develop a stricture at the base of the vertical canal. Subsequently, the horizontal canal can become severely dilated with sebaceous or purulent material. In some dogs, traumatic vertical ear canal avulsion can be repaired with vertical ear canal resection. In these animals, the fibrous wall of the distended horizontal canal is sutured directly to the skin.

Compared with lateral ear canal resection, vertical ear canal resection removes more inflamed tissue and is associated with less postoperative discharge and pain, fewer complications, and better healing. Cosmesis is excellent in most animals; however, vertical ear canal resection may cause drooping of erect ears.

Preoperative management

Diagnostics and surgical-site preparation are similar to those for lateral ear canal resection (Chapter 51). The entire pinna should be clipped and prepped for surgery. Electrocautery may be necessary for hemostasis if canals are inflamed or well vascularized.

Surgery

If the horizontal canal cannot be thoroughly examined before surgery, veterinarians should be prepared to convert a vertical ear canal resection to a total ear canal ablation and lateral bulla osteotomy. Total ablation is much more complicated than vertical ear canal resection and is often referred to an experienced surgeon. Animals with otitis media that undergo vertical ear canal resection may require ventral bulla osteotomy or lavage through a myringotomy to resolve clinical signs.

Manual of Small Animal Soft Tissue Surgery, Second Edition. Karen Tobias.
© 2017 John Wiley & Sons, Inc. Published 2017 by John Wiley & Sons, Inc.

The dorsal vertical ear canal resection incision can be made above or below the antihelix, depending on the extent of canal pathology. The antihelix is the horizontal ridge of cartilage on the medial portion of the vertical canal. Drooping will be more evident in animals with upright ears if the antihelix is removed. Skin closure to the pinna margin can be more difficult if the antihelix remains.

During surgery the vertical ear canal, or conchal cartilage, is exposed to the level of the horizontal canal (annular cartilage). Use of Gelpi, Senn, or ring retractors can improve exposure during dissection of this area. The facial nerve and several large vessels circumnavigate the ventral half of the horizontal canal (fig. 52-1). Damage to the nerve during dissection or retraction may result in loss of palpebral function, which increases the risk for postoperative corneal ulceration.

A layer of fibrous tissue connects the conchal cartilage to the annular cartilage. When the vertical canal is amputated, a small portion of the conchal cartilage should be left intact to make cartilage flaps. These flaps are hinged at the fibrous tissue connection and sutured dorsally and ventrally to reduce the risk of canal stenosis. If the entire vertical canal must be removed, the circular opening of the annular cartilage is sutured directly to the skin.

Vertical canal epithelium is usually sutured to the surrounding skin with 3-0 nonabsorbable monofilament suture in an interrupted pattern. Some surgeons prefer to appose the skin around the canal opening with 3-0 rapidly absorbable monofilament suture in a continuous pattern to reduce the amount of debris collection. If possible, suture bites on the flap side should include only epithelium so that cartilage edges are covered by skin. If the canal epithelium tears easily, however, cartilage should be included in suture bites.

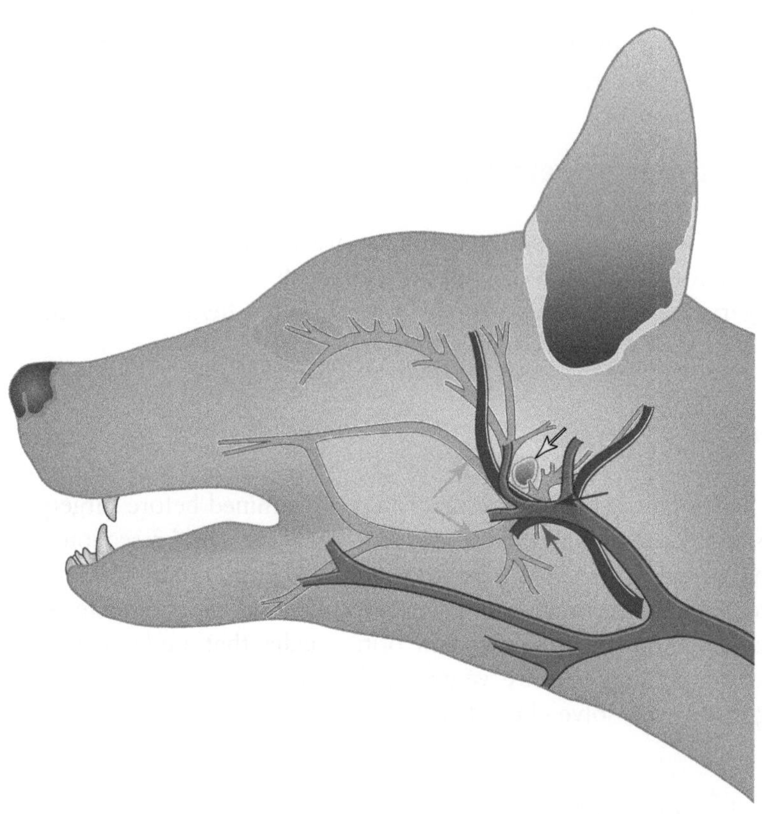

Figure 52-1 Anatomy of the nerves and vessels of the lateral head. The external carotid artery (red arrow) and maxillary vein (blue arrow) are ventral to the horizontal canal (yellow arrow), and the facial nerve (green arrows) wraps around the ventral two-thirds of the canal.

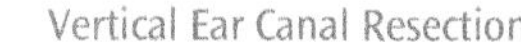

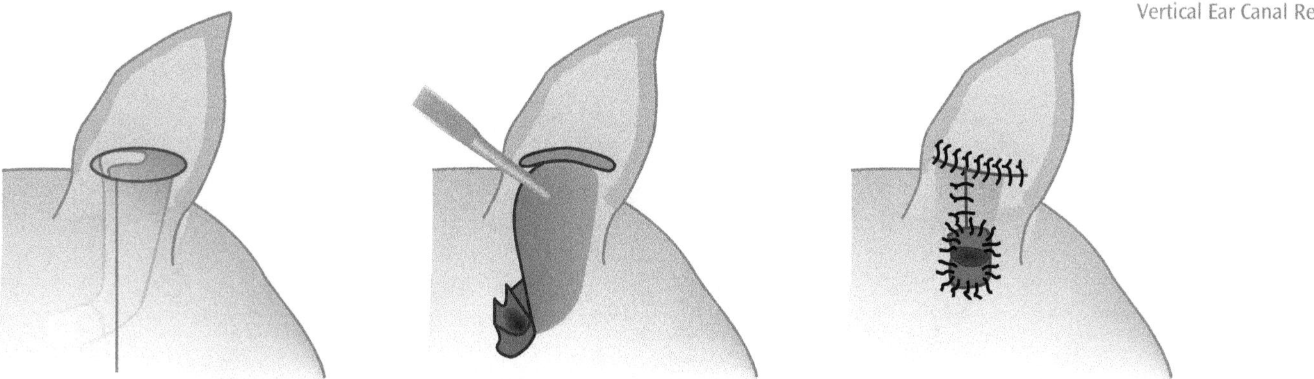

Figure 52-2 Vertical ear canal resection. **A.** A skin incision is made around and along the vertical ear canal. **B.** After the vertical ear canal cartilage has been resected, skin positioning is tested by pulling the caudal flap of skin rostrally over the site. More skin may need to be resected to allow exposure of the remaining canal. **C.** Final appearance. Courtesy of Samantha Elmurst.

When the vertical ear canal resection closure is complete, the remaining canal should lie in a horizontal orientation and the pinna should have minimal tension. To reduce tension on the closure, the vertical skin incision can be extended ventrally before suturing begins so that more free skin is available to close the gap along the medial pinna margin.

Surgical technique: vertical ear canal resection

1. Incise the skin around the entire circumference of the external ear canal opening at the level of the antihelix (fig. 52-2).
2. Insert a closed hemostat into the vertical canal to determine its ventral extent.
3. Incise the skin over the lateral surface of the vertical ear canal, starting at the circumferential skin incision and ending 1 to 4cm below (ventral to) the ventral extent of the canal.
4. Dissect the subcutaneous tissues away from the lateral surface of the vertical ear canal (fig. 52-3).

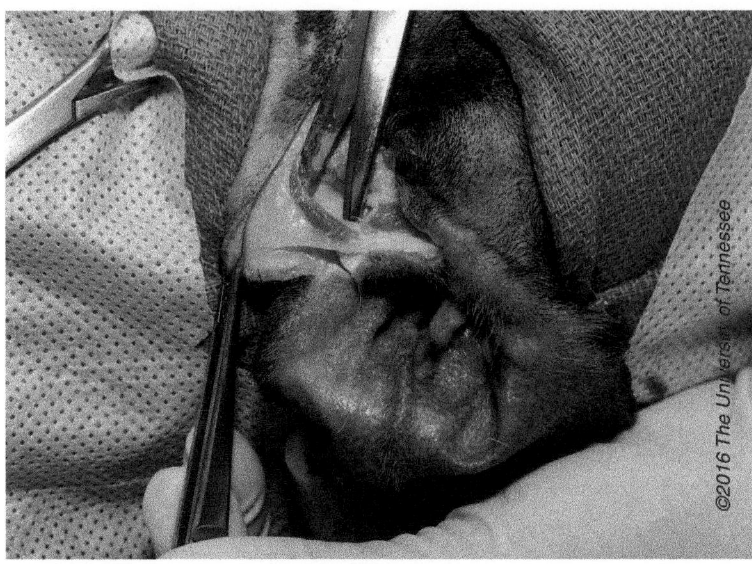

Figure 52-3 Dissect the subcutaneous tissues off of the vertical canal. © 2016 The University of Tennessee.

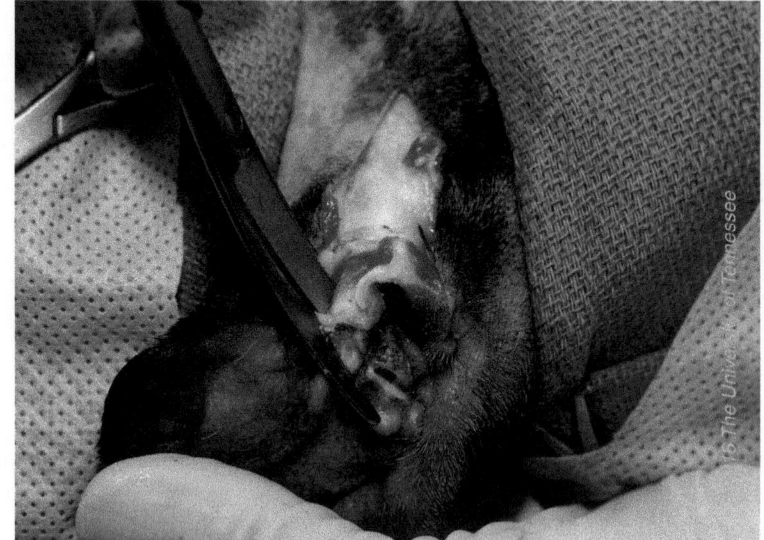

Figure 52-4 Transect the cartilage circumferentially at the level of the skin incision with Mayo scissors. © 2016 The University of Tennessee.

5. With Mayo or cartilage scissors, transect the cartilage around the vertical canal opening at the level of the circumferential skin incision (fig. 52-4). Note that the cartilage near the antitragus and pretragus is doubled over, requiring more force during cutting.
6. With a combination of blunt and sharp dissection, free the entire vertical canal to the level of the annular cartilage.
   a. Grasp the dorsal portion of the medial ear canal wall with an Allis tissue forceps and strip downward along the canal with a dry gauze sponge to remove any fascial attachments (fig. 52-5).
   b. Insert closed scissor tips under the muscles immediately adjacent to the canal, orienting the scissors perpendicular to the long axis of the vertical canal. Spread the scissor blades parallel to the long axis of the canal to elevate the muscle from the cartilage.

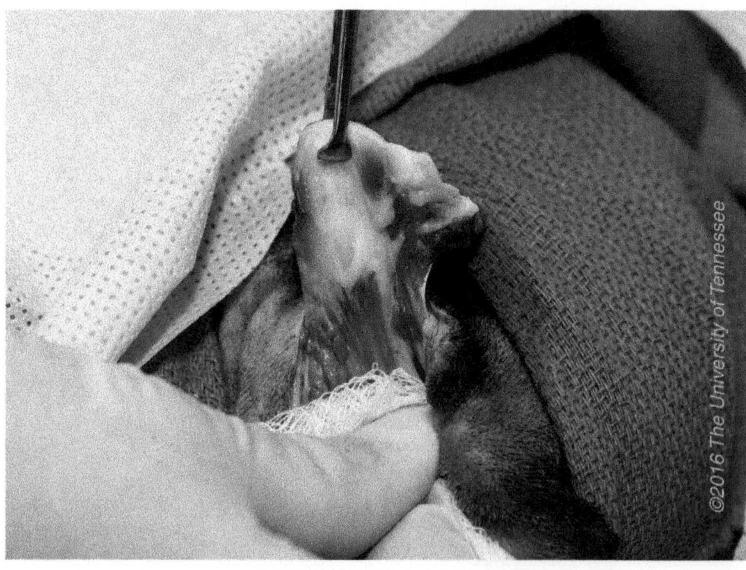

Figure 52-5 Retract the vertical canal with Allis tissue forceps and expose the cartilage and muscle attachments by stripping with a dry gauze sponge or dissecting with scissors. © 2016 The University of Tennessee.

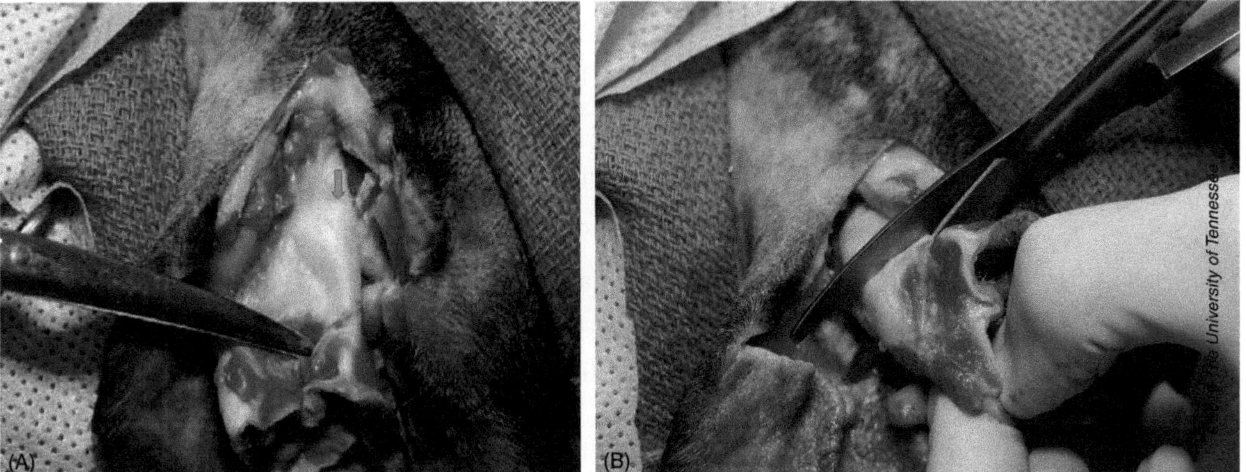

Figure 52-6 **A.** Identify the proximal end of the vertical canal (arrow). **B.** Transect the vertical canal, leaving at least 5 mm of vertical canal, if possible, to make cartilage flaps. © 2016 The University of Tennessee.

   c. Transect the muscles at their cartilaginous attachments with the scissors or electrocautery.

   d. Retract the parotid gland from the ventrolateral surface of the canal during lateral dissection.

7. Expose the vertical canal to its junction with the horizontal canal (fig. 52-6A). Retract and dissect the tissues near the horizontal canal cautiously to avoid damaging the facial nerve.

8. Transect the vertical canal cartilage at least 1 cm beyond any tumor margin. If possible, leave at least 5 mm of vertical canal to make cartilage flaps (fig. 52-6B).

9. Make paired cartilage flaps (fig. 52-7).

   a. Incise the remaining vertical ear canal midway along its rostral and caudal circumferences to make a dorsal and ventral flap.

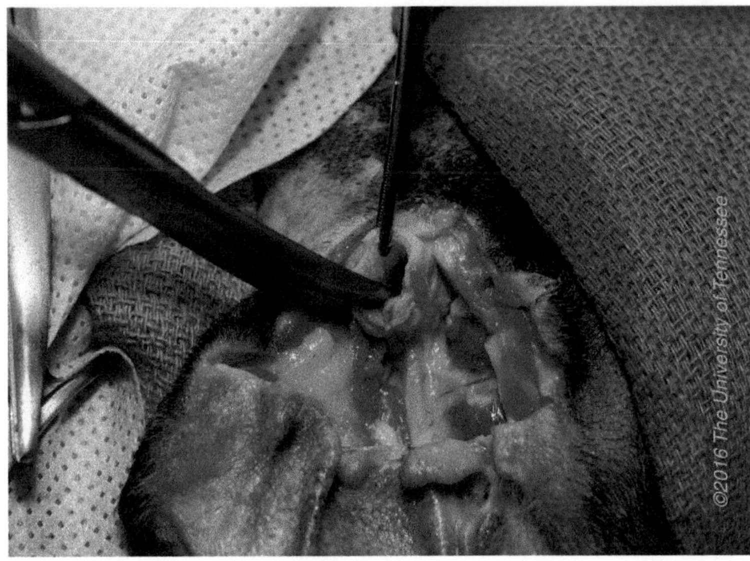

Figure 52-7 Incise the remaining vertical canal rostrally and caudally to make two cartilage flaps. © 2016 The University of Tennessee.

b. Reflect the flaps so that they are 180 degrees from each other.

c. If the new opening is obstructed ventrally by a cartilage fold, extend the flap incisions toward the rostral and caudal centers of the horizontal canal, or slightly ventrally, to relax the ventral flap so it will lay flat against the underlying tissues.

10. Appose the lateral facial skin flaps to the pinna.

a. Determine the final site for the lateral facial skin flaps (see fig. 52-2B).

i. Grasp the skin along the rostral margin of the facial incision and pull it up toward the skin incision along the pinna near the antihelix.

ii. Similarly grasp and move the skin on the caudal margin of the facial incision (fig. 52-8).

iii. Orient the flaps of skin so that the pinna will remain curved and upright to preserve its original position.

iv. If more loose skin is needed to reduce tension on the pinna and canal flaps, or if the horizontal canal is not visible when the flaps are in their final positions, extend the vertical portion of the skin incision caudoventrally for several centimeters to expose the canal.

b. Place the first two interrupted skin sutures from the corners of the skin flaps to the pinna to verify skin positioning is satisfactory and to hold the skin flaps in place.

11. Suture the ventral cartilage flap in place.

a. Grasp the ventral cartilage flap and pull it downward so that the new canal opening is properly positioned.

i. The horizontal canal should be level or angled slightly downward.

ii. The new opening should appear round or slightly ovoid.

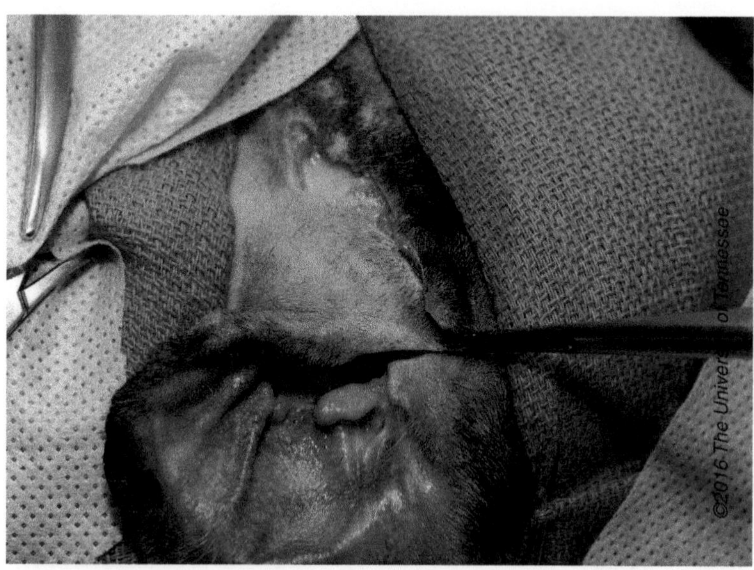

Figure 52-8 Test the final skin position by pulling the caudal skin rostrally. If the ear canal opening is no longer visible, extend the skin incision caudoventrally. © 2016 The University of Tennessee.

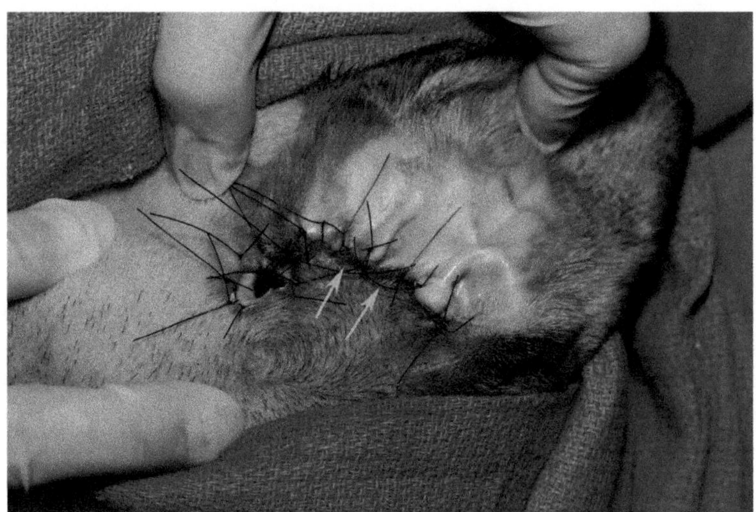

Figure 52-9 Final appearance. The caudal skin has been pulled forward as an advancement flap (arrows) to provide a tension free closure.

iii. The ventral flap may be directed cranioventrally in some animals.

iv. If necessary, remove additional skin ventrally to adjust the flap position.

b. Appose the skin at each corner of the ventral flap to the ventral margin of the lateral facial skin incision.

c. Place interrupted sutures rostrally and caudally between the facial skin margin and the junction (hinges) of the ventral and dorsal flaps.

d. Add additional sutures to appose the skin edges around the ventral flap.

12. Suture the dorsal cartilage flap in place and complete the skin closure (fig. 52-9).

a. Position the dorsal cartilage flap and surrounding skin so that the canal remains open and tension on the pinna is minimized.

b. If necessary, shorten the dorsal cartilage flap to reduce tension on the pinna.

Postoperative considerations

As with lateral ear canal resections, the surgical site must be protected from trauma with an Elizabethan collar. A thin layer of petroleum-based antibiotic ointment can be applied to the sutures to prevent accumulation of blood and debris. In dogs that vigorously shake their ears, the pinna can be taped to the head or enclosed in a stockinette to reduce trauma. Analgesics are usually administered for several days after surgery. Nonsteroidal anti-inflammatory drugs should be avoided if the animal is receiving glucocorticoids. Besides continued therapy for dermatologic conditions, the animal may also require intermittent clipping around the new stoma to maintain ventilation and drainage.

The most common complications after vertical ear canal resection are dehiscence and stenosis. Dehiscence may require primary repair to prevent stenosis, otitis media, or formation of draining sinus tracts, or the animal may need a total ear canal ablation and bulla osteotomy. Facial nerve paralysis and infection are uncommon after vertical ear canal resection. If palpebral function is absent after surgery, topical eye ointment should be applied 4 to 6 times daily to protect the cornea.

Excellent results have been reported in 72% to 95% of dogs and cats after vertical ear canal resection. In fact, 95% of dogs with end-stage otitis externa and patent horizontal canals reportedly were improved by the procedure, even when horizontal canals were hyperplastic. These patients will continue to have clinical signs and require therapy for otitis or its underlying causes, but they may require less frequent treatment. If the horizontal ear canal occludes completely, total ear canal ablation and bulla osteotomy will be required to resolve clinical signs.

Bibliography

Lanz OI and Wood BC: Surgery of the ear and pinna. Vet Clin N Am Small Anim Pract 2004;34:567–599.

McCarthy RJ and Caywood DD: Vertical ear canal resection for end-stage otitis externa in dogs. J Am Anim Hosp Assoc 1992;28:545–552.

O'Neil T and Nuttall T: Ear surgery part 1: The vertical canal. UK Vet 2005;10(4).

Chapter 53
Mandibular Lymph Node Excision

The primary indication for removal of a mandibular lymph node is for cancer staging, particularly in animals with tumors of the oral cavity. Regional metastases are more likely to be detected with histologic evaluation of lymph node biopsies than with cytology. Excisional biopsy of a lymph node is preferred over incisional biopsy because it provides more information on nodal architecture. In animals with periodontal disease, however, differentiation of neoplasia and reactive hyperplasia in mandibular lymph nodes may be difficult. Therefore, in animals suspected to have lymphoma, biopsy of prescapular and popliteal lymph nodes is preferred. Dogs with head and neck neoplasia may have metastases to lymph nodes on the contralateral side.

Preoperative management

Because animals undergoing unilateral mandibular lymph node excision usually have neoplasia, staging for metastases should be performed before surgery. In most patients, this includes blood work, thoracic radiographs, and possibly computed tomography of the head. Before surgery, the ventrolateral surface of the face and neck, centering over the palpable lymph node, is clipped and prepped. The area should be clipped widely, since the lymph node tends to retract into deeper tissues during the surgical approach. The animal is positioned in dorsolateral recumbency, and the head is elevated with a towel.

Surgery

The mandibular lymph nodes lie caudal to the angle of the mandible, caudoventral to the masseter muscle, and craniolateral to the basihyoid bone. Most commonly, there are two or three ovoid-shaped nodes on each side of the head, with at least one dorsal and one ventral to the facial branch of the linguofacial vein (fig. 53-1).

Location of the mandibular lymph node is usually determined by palpation. The tissues are grasped at the caudoventral edge of the mandible and steadily compressed between the fingers as the hand is pulled away. The larger,

Manual of Small Animal Soft Tissue Surgery, Second Edition. Karen Tobias.
© 2017 John Wiley & Sons, Inc. Published 2017 by John Wiley & Sons, Inc.

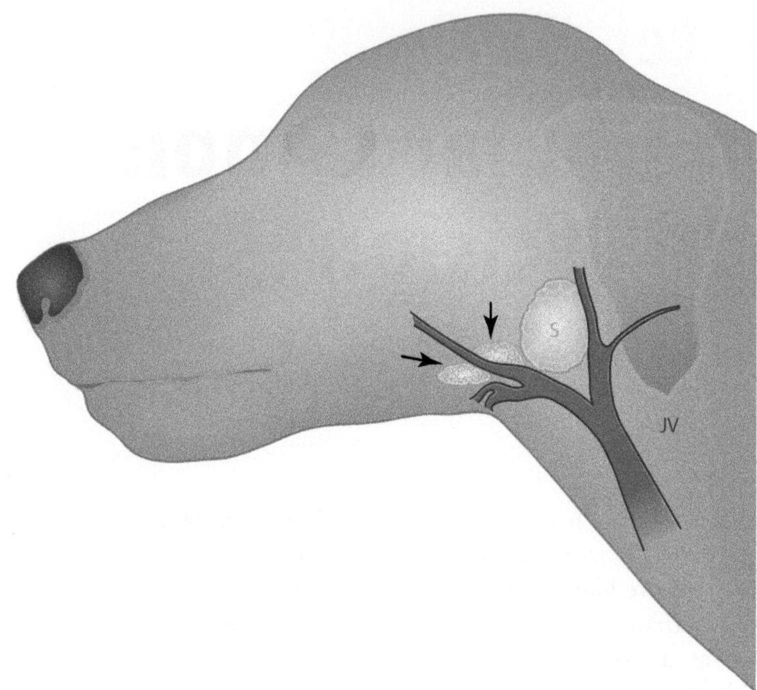

Figure 53-1 The mandibular lymph nodes (arrows) are located dorsal and ventral to the linguofacial vein, which bifurcates off the jugular vein (JV). The most easily palpable nodes are rostrolateral and slightly ventral to the salivary gland (S).

medially located mandibular and subligual salivary glands will slip through the examiner's hand first, followed by the lymph nodes, which are rostral and more superficial. In normal animals, mandibular lymph nodes will be firm and freely movable and feel 1 to 2 cm in diameter.

Before making an incision, the clinician should identify the jugular vein and its bifurcation so that accidental damage to these vessels can be avoided. During incision and dissection, the lymph node can be stabilized against the skin with thumb and middle finger, similar to the technique used for castration. This will keep the lymph node within the surgical field until it can be grasped with an instrument.

Surgical technique: unilateral mandibular lymph node removal

1. If desired, temporarily hold off the jugular vein and mark the location of the linguofacial vein with a sterile marker.
2. With thumb and forefingers of the nondominant hand, stabilize the lymph node against the overlying skin (fig. 53-2).
3. Incise the skin over the lymph node. Avoid going too deep at this point, especially if the linguofacial vein has not been identified.
4. As you continue to stabilize the lymph node, remove the subcutaneous tissues and platysma over the node with blunt or sharp dissection (figs. 53-3 and 53-4) until the node is visible. Dissect parallel to the linguofacial vein to prevent vessel damage.
5. Free the lymph node from remaining attachments with blunt dissection (fig. 53-5) until you identify its blood supply.
    a. If you lose your grip on the lymph node and it retracts away from you, you may need to extend the subcutaneous tissue dissection or place

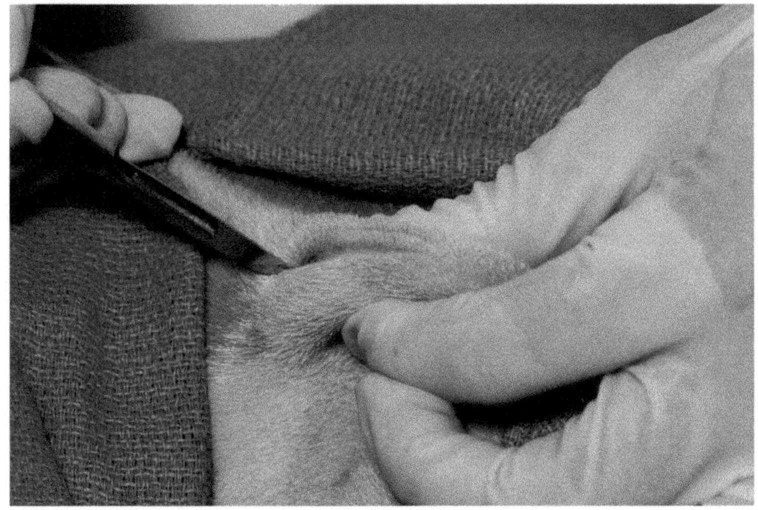

Figure 53-2 Grasp the lymph node and overlying tissue firmly between thumb and forefingers and incise the overlying skin.

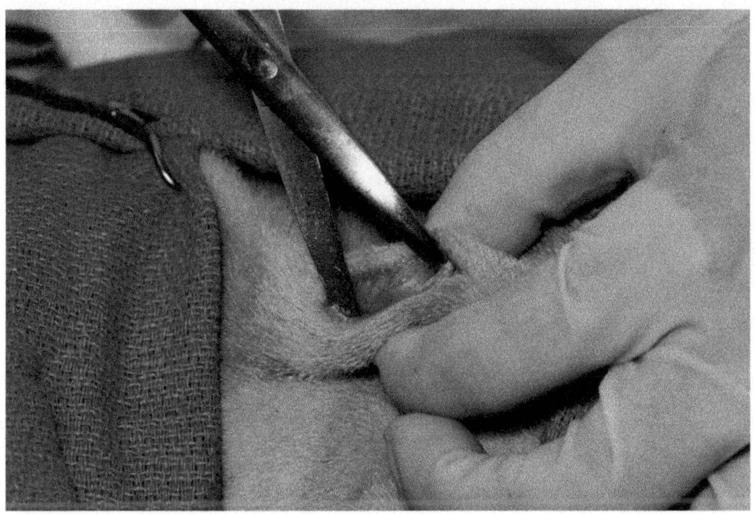

Figure 53-3 Bluntly dissect the subcutaneous fat from the surface of the lymph node, spreading parallel to the linguofacial vein.

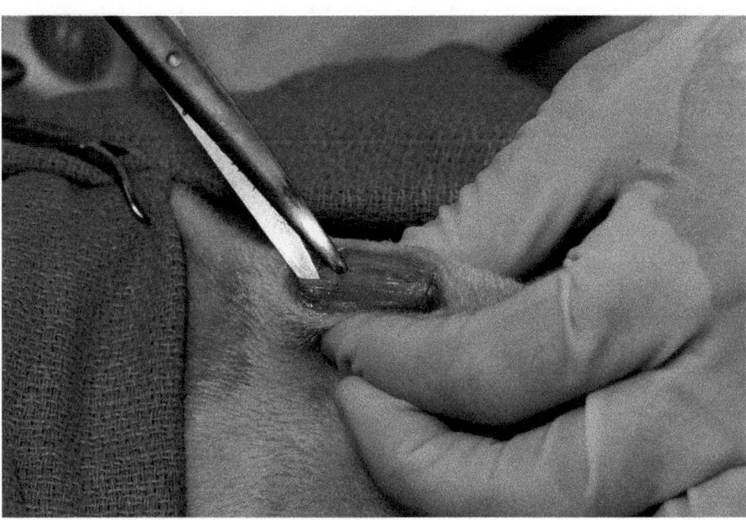

Figure 53-4 Separate the fibers of the platysma, dissecting parallel to the linguofacial vein.

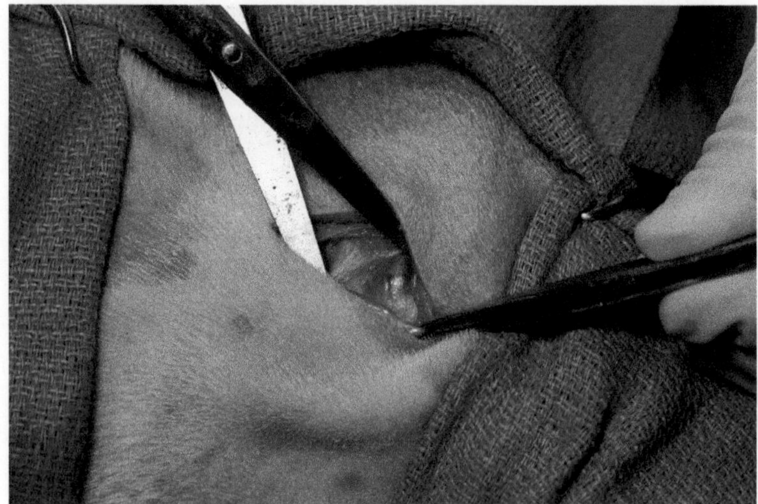

Figure 53-5 Bluntly dissect the remaining fascial attachments to the lymph node.

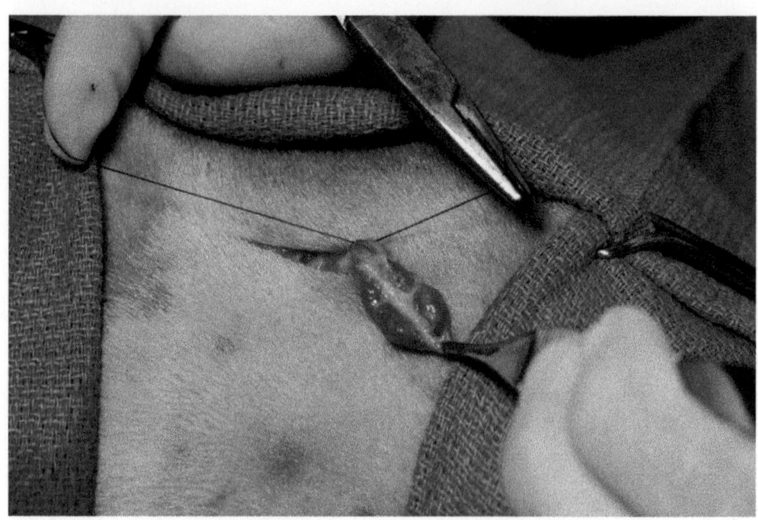

Figure 53-6 Ligate the vascular pedicle at the base of the lymph node before transecting.

Gelpi retractors to improve visibility. Small nodes often slip medial to the mandible.

b. Handle the lymph node with fingers, or use a forceps or stay suture on the capsule. Lymph nodes are friable and can be easily damaged.

6. If the lymph node can be retracted out of the incision, place a hemostat across the pedicle along its medial surface. If the lymph node cannot be easily retracted, extend the skin incision and continue dissection until the lymph node is only attached by its vascular pedicle.
7. Ligate the vascular pedicle with 3-0 absorbable suture (fig. 53-6). Transect the pedicle and remove the lymph node.
8. Close subcutaneous tissues and skin routinely.

Postoperative considerations

Samples are submitted for histologic evaluation, bacterial and fungal cultures, and cytology, depending on the suspected underlying disease. If lymphoma is suspected, samples of the lymph node can also be submitted for immunophenotyping.

Complications of mandibular lymph node resection are rare. Laceration of the linguofacial vein is the greatest intraoperative concern; if torn, the vessel can be ligated without consequence, however. A small amount of swelling may occur after surgery if dead space or hemorrhage is present. Dehiscence is uncommon; therefore, chemotherapy can often be initiated within 3 to 5 days after surgery.

Bibliography

Green K, Boston SE: Bilateral removal of the mandibular and medial retropharyngeal lymph nodes through a single ventral midline incision for staging of head and neck cancers in dogs: a description of surgical technique. Vet Compar Oncol 2014,1–7; doi 10.1111/vco.12154; downloaded 8/15/16.

Herring ES et al: Lymph node staging of oral and maxillofacial neoplasms in 31 dogs and cats. J Vet Dent 2002;19:122–126.

Skinner OT, Boston SE, de M. Souza CH: Patterns of lymph node metastasis identified following bilateral mandibular and medial retropharyngeal lymphadenectomy in 31 dogs with malignancies of the head. Vet Compar Oncol 2016,1–9; doi 10.1111/vco.12229.

Smith MM: Surgical approach for lymph node staging of oral and maxillofacial neoplasms in dogs. J Vet Dent 2002;19:170–174.

Sözmen M et al: Use of fine needle aspirates and flow cytometry for the diagnosis, classification, and immunophenotyping of canine lymphomas. J Vet Diagnost Invest 2005;17:323–329.

Wright T, Oblak ML: Lymphadenectomy: overview of surgical anatomy and removal of peripheral lymph nods. Today's Vet Pract 2016;6:24–32.

Chapter 54
Sialoceles

Sialoceles, or salivary mucoceles, are abnormal collections of saliva within tissues. Sialoceles are usually caused by subcutaneous leakage from the mandibular and sublingual salivary glands or ducts. Most affected dogs present with a fluctuant, nonpainful, subcutaneous swelling located in the intermandibular region or ventrally along the proximal cervical region. Occasionally the swelling may be inflamed and painful early in the disease process. Fluid can leak submucosally from the rostral portion of the salivary glands and ducts, resulting in a sublingual swelling, or ranula (fig. 54-1). Large ranulae can force the tongue out of the intermandibular space and cause dysphagia. Occasionally, fluid migrates dorsally into the retropharyngeal region. The resultant pharyngeal mucocele may cause dyspnea in affected animals (fig. 54-2).

Diagnosis is based on clinical signs and appearance of the fluid. Fluid obtained by aspirate is usually hypocellular; mucinous; and clear, slightly yellow, or blood tinged. Cervical sialoceles originating from the mandibular and sublingual salivary glands must be differentiated from parotid sialoceles, which often cause a firm, more lateralized swelling. Sialography will also differentiate mandibular and sublingual salivary glands from other causes of swelling but is rarely performed. Cannulation of the mandibular and sublingual salivary ducts for contrast injection can be very difficult, particularly if multiple ductal openings are present.

Recurrence of sialoceles is common after aspiration and drainage alone; therefore, surgical resection of the affected glands is recommended. Occasionally, ranulae can be treated by marsupialization. Sialadenectomy should be performed if the ranula reoccurs.

Preoperative management

Most dogs that present with cervical sialoceles are metabolically stable; therefore, minimal preoperative diagnostics and treatment are required. If the swelling is firm or painful, aspirates for cytology and culture are recommended to differentiate sialoceles from abscesses, granulomas, cellulitis, and neoplasia. If neoplasia or infection is suspected, blood work and cervical and thoracic radiographs should be evaluated. In animals with cervical mucoceles, the oral cavity should be thoroughly examined for ranulae and pharyngeal mucoceles. In dogs with pharyngeal mucoceles, swelling of the caudodorsal

Manual of Small Animal Soft Tissue Surgery, Second Edition. Karen Tobias.
© 2017 John Wiley & Sons, Inc. Published 2017 by John Wiley & Sons, Inc.

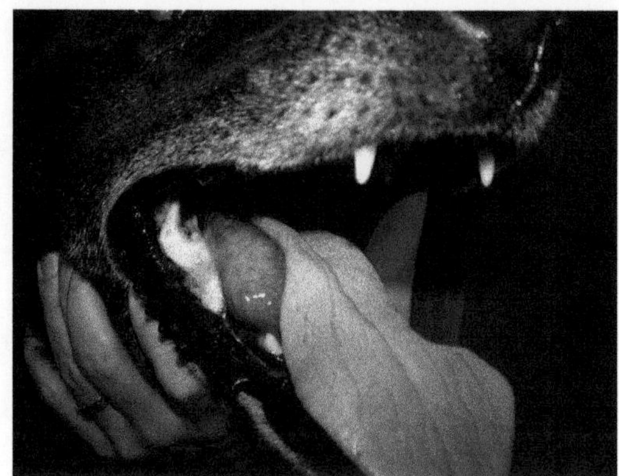

Figure 54-1 Ranula.

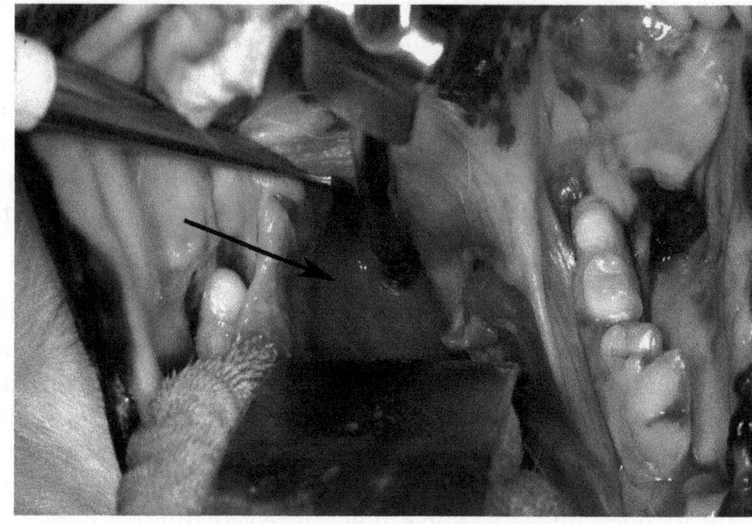

Figure 54-2 Pharyngeal mucocele (arrow). The tongue, epiglottis, and endotracheal tube are being retracted ventrally with a malleable retractor. To drain the mucocele, make a stab incision in the dorsal wall of the mucocele and suction out the fluid with a small Poole suction tip.

pharyngeal wall may make intubation difficult. If a pharyngeal mucocele is present, it can be drained through an intraoral stab incision and suctioned before the affected salivary glands are removed (fig. 54-2).

Cervical sialoceles are usually unilateral. To determine the affected side, the dog is placed on its back with its head and neck straight (fig. 54-3). In this position, the fluid pocket will usually lateralize to the affected side, unless the condition is bilateral. Affected glands can also be identified with ultrasound or computed tomography. If the affected side cannot be determined, mandibular and sublingual salivary glands can be removed bilaterally without negatively affecting salivary production.

Dogs undergoing unilateral sialadenectomy are clipped from the midmandible to midcervical region and from the base of the pinna to ventral midline. Unilateral sialadenectomy is usually performed with the dog in lateral or dorsolateral recumbency. A towel can be placed under the neck to elevate the affected side. Some surgeons prefer a ventral approach that permits incision and dissection, parallel and just medial to the mandible, from the level of the salivary glands caudally to the level of the sublingual caruncle rostrally. This permits exposure of the entire salivary gland-duct complex.

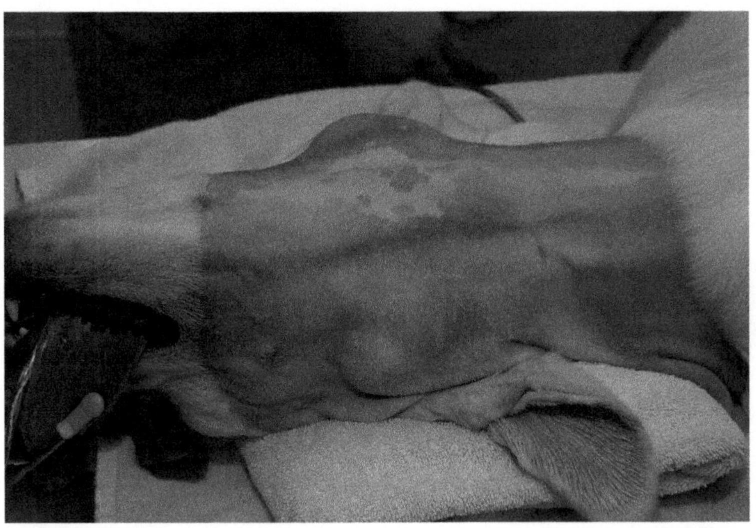

Figure 54-3 To identify the affected side, place the dog in dorsal recumbency with its head and neck extended so that fluid in the sialocele will lateralize. This dog had bilateral cervical sialoceles.

Surgery

The mandibular and sublingual salivary glands are located at the bifurcation of the jugular vein (see fig. 53-1, p. 424). The mandibular lymph nodes lie rostral and ventrolateral to the mandibular salivary gland. The mandibular and sublingual salivary glands are enclosed within the same capsule, which is deep to the maxillary and linguofacial veins. Their ducts run adjacent to one another, passing between the masseter and digastricus muscles and over the dorsomedial surface of the mylohyoid muscle. The lingual branch of the trigeminal nerve crosses their lateral surfaces before the ducts reach the oral cavity.

The sublingual salivary gland consists of several lobulated masses. The larger portion sits on the rostral surface of the mandibular gland and drains into the main sublingual duct. Rostrally, a 1 × 3 cm cluster of lobules lies under the oral mucosa. These lobules also drain into the main sublingual duct via four to six smaller ducts. During sialadenectomy, both of these monostomatic portions of the sublingual salivary gland are removed. The polystomatic portion of the sublingual salivary gland consists of 6 to 12 small lobules that drain directly into the oral cavity. These are usually left in place during surgery.

Surgical technique: unilateral mandibular and sublingual sialadenectomy from a lateral approach

1. To identify the location of the glands, hold off the jugular vein temporarily to visualize its bifurcation.
2. Incise the skin over the mandibular and sublingual salivary glands, starting just caudal to the angle of the mandible and extending over the jugular bifurcation (fig. 54-4). The incision should lie between the maxillary and linguofacial veins.
3. Spread, transect, and retract the subcutaneous tissues and platysma muscle to expose the capsule of the cystic cavity and salivary glands (fig. 54-5).
4. Incise the capsule and suction out the entrapped fluid (fig. 54-6).

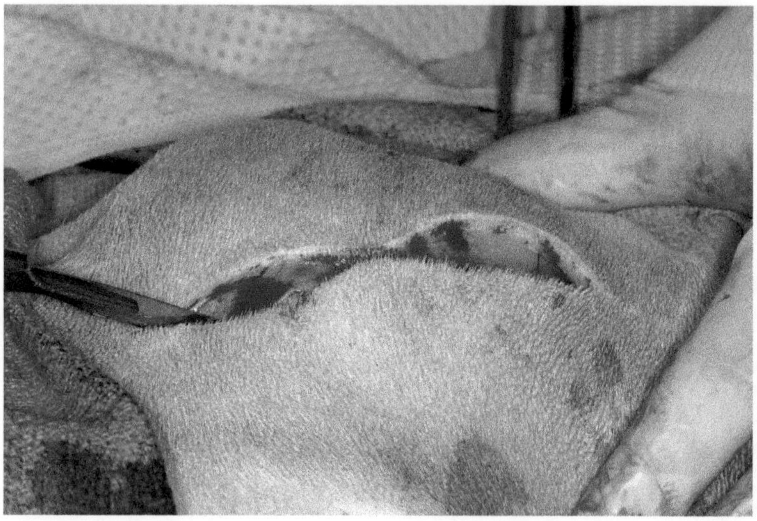

Figure 54-4 With the dog in lateral recumbency, incise the skin over the mucocele between the linguofacial and maxillary veins.

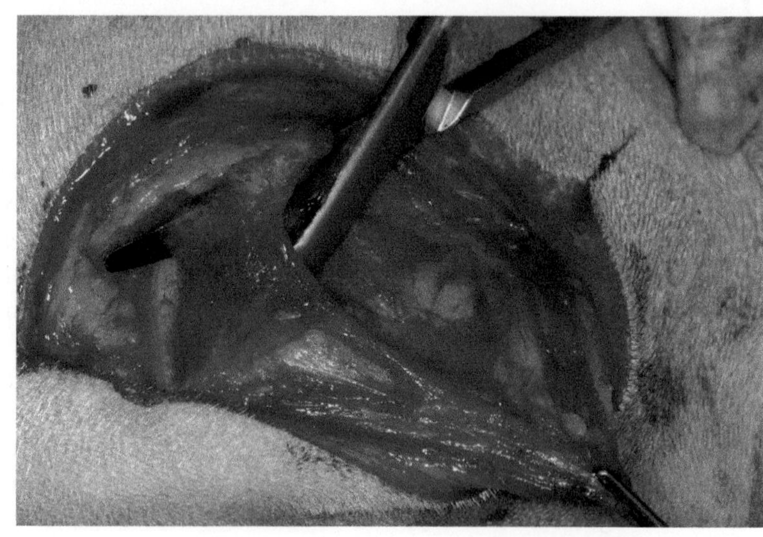

Figure 54-5 Transect overlying subcutaneous tissues and the platysma muscle. Before cutting the tissues, spread them with the scissor blades so that they are semitransparent. This will prevent accidental transection of large vessels.

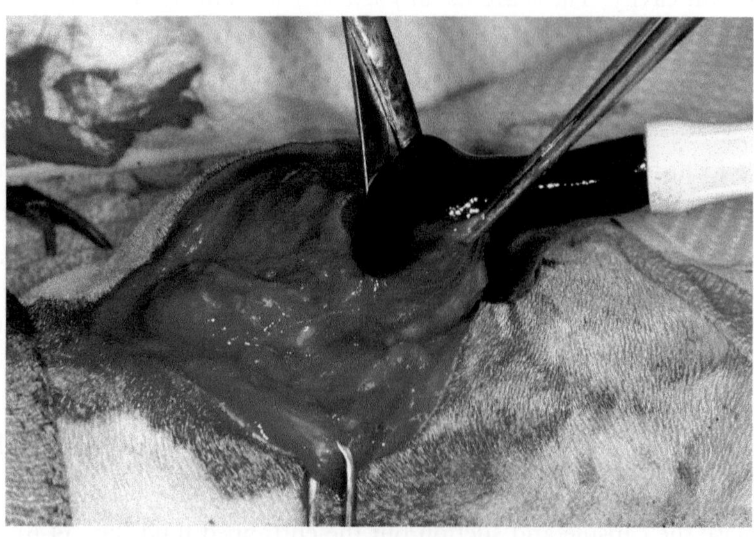

Figure 54-6 Incise the capsule and suction the contents. In this dog, the saliva was mucoid and hemorrhagic.

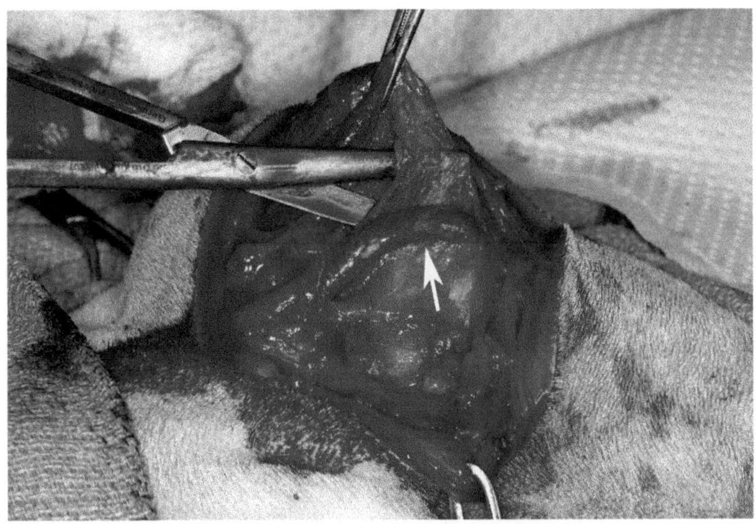

Figure 54-7 Grasp the gland with forceps and dissect it free from surrounding tissues, avoiding damage to the maxillary vein and linguofacial vein (arrow).

5. Extend the capsular incision rostrally over the mandibular and sublingual salivary glands, avoiding branches of the second cervical nerve and facial nerve. Retract the maxillary and linguofacial veins with the subcutaneous tissues and capsule.
6. Grasp the mandibular salivary gland with an Allis tissue or Babcock forceps to facilitate retraction.
7. Working rostrally, bluntly dissect the mandibular and monostomatic sublingual glands from their capsular attachments, taking care not to damage the ducts (fig. 54-7). Use electrocautery to control hemorrhage from small vessels. Ligate the glandular branch of the facial artery where it enters the medial surface of the glands.
8. Using fingers or scissors, bluntly dissect rostrally along the ducts and sublingual glands' lobules toward the mouth to separate them from the digastricus muscle medially. Stay close to the salivary tissue and ducts as you dissect.
9. With army-navy or Senn retractors, retract the digastricus muscle caudoventrally and the masseter muscle laterally (fig. 54-8).

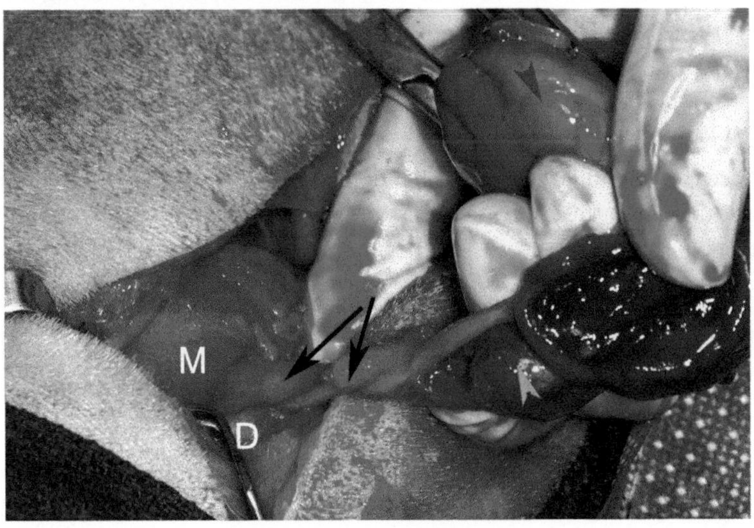

Figure 54-8 Bluntly dissect along the glands and ducts (arrows) to the level of the masseter muscle (M). In this dog the mandibular salivary gland (blue arrowhead) appeared normal; however, the sublingual gland (green arrowhead) was swollen and discolored and its duct remained dilated (left arrow) rostral to the digastricus muscle (D).

10. Expose the ducts to the level of the lingual branch of the trigeminal nerve by bluntly separating them from the surrounding tissue. Separate the lingual nerve (which carries sensory information from the tongue) away from the duct with blunt dissection.
    a. Retract caudally on the ducts to improve exposure of their rostral extent.
    b. To orient yourself, have a nonsterile assistant insert a finger or blunt probe into the oral cavity and medial to the caudal border of the mandible. The probe should be palpable under pharyngeal mucosa in your surgery site.
11. Dissect as far rostrally as possible, removing small clumps of sublingual salivary gland with the duct, then detach the rostral end of the duct and remove the salivary gland-duct complex using one of the following options:.
    a. Option 1: Pull the ducts caudally with steady retraction on the hemostats until the ducts tear from their sublingual attachments.
    b. Option 2: Clamp the ducts with a hemostat and ligate and transect them at their most rostral exposure.
    c. Option 3: Tunneling technique.
        i. Dissect along the caudoventral margin of the digastricus muscle to free the duct, then pass a curved hemostatic forceps under the muscle from caudoventral to rostrodorsal, avoiding damage to the hypoglossal nerve, lingual artery, internal carotid artery, and hyoid apparatus.
        ii. Grasp the ducts and any associated salivary tissue in the forceps tips, then transect the ducts beyond the forceps tips and remove them with the attached gland.
        iii. Pull the remaining ducts medial to the digastricus muscle with forceps tips, then continue the dissection rostrally, transecting the mylohyoideus muscle as needed, until the ducts can be transected or pulled from their sublingual mucosal attachments.
12. Place a continuous suction drain in the sialocele cavity, exiting the tubing out of a separate skin incision. Close subcutaneous tissues and skin.

Surgical technique: ranula marsupialization

1. Place the dog in lateral recumbency, with the affected side up, and insert a mouth gag on the contralateral side. The tongue should fall medially away from the ranula.
2. Grasp the dorsolateral surface of the ranula with thumb forceps or stay sutures. With scissors, open the ranula (fig. 54-9) and drain the contents.
3. Transect a portion of the wall and the inner folds of tissue to produce a 1- to 3-cm stoma.
4. Fold the edges of the remaining wall inward upon themselves, inverting the oral mucosal surface of the ranula into the cystic cavity (fig. 54-10).

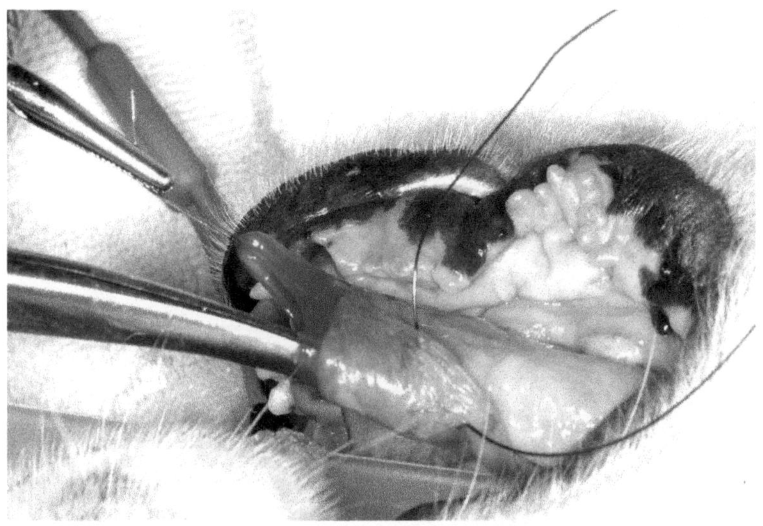

Figure 54-9 Stabilize the ranula with thumb forceps or stay sutures. Incise the wall and remove the contents.

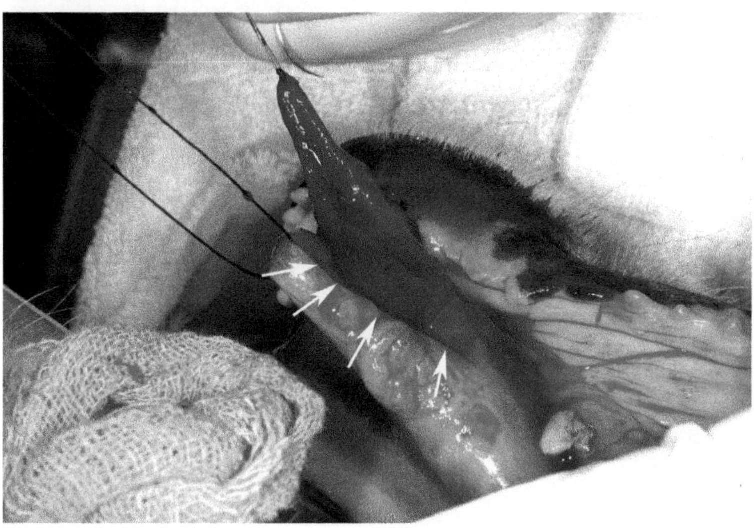

Figure 54-10 After removing a section of the ranula wall and its contents, fold the mucosa inward along one incision edge (arrows show folded mucosa).

5. Suture the folded edge to itself with a simple continuous pattern of 4-0 rapidly absorbable suture (fig. 54-11). The final appearance will be similar to a hemmed sleeve or pant leg.

Postoperative considerations

Do not place a padded bandage around the neck because it may cause respiratory distress if postoperative swelling occurs. Instead, drain exit sites can be covered with a small adhesive bandage square or a stockinette. Drains can usually be removed 1 to 3 days after surgery, depending on the amount of fluid production. Dogs undergoing ranula resection usually have blood-tinged saliva immediately after surgery.

Complications of sialadenectomy are rare. Seromas may occur early in the postoperative period if dead space has not been obliterated with subcutaneous tissue closure or drain placement. Recurrence of cervical sialocele is unlikely as long as the ducts and affected glands, including the small globules of

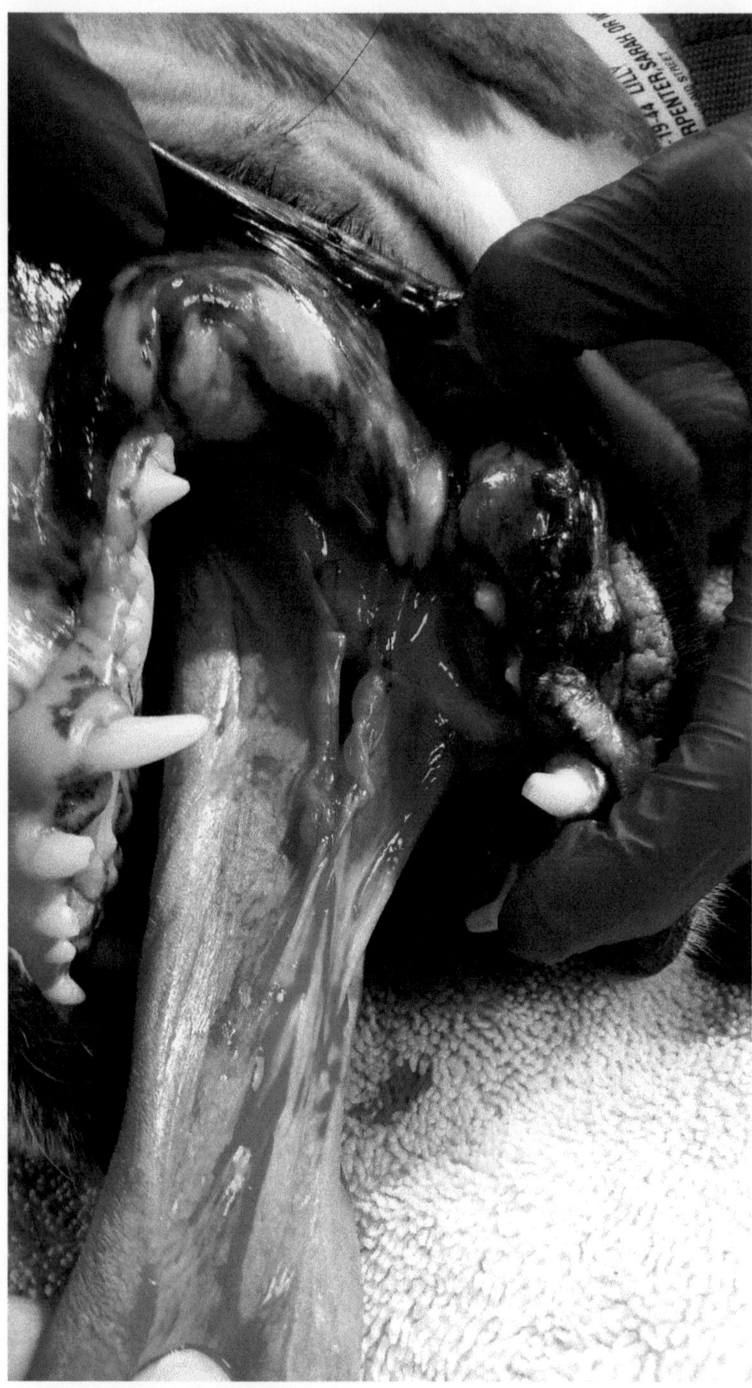

Figure 54-11 Final appearance after ranula marsupialization.

periductual sublingual gland tissue, have been removed. Recurrence may require removal of the contralateral glands or the ipsilateral parotid gland, or resection of any remaining sublingual glands rostral to the digastricus on the ipsilateral side. Computed tomography is useful for evaluating the remaining glands.

Bibliography

Benjamino KP, Birchard SJ, Niles JD, et al: Pharyngeal mucoceles in dogs: 14 cases. J Am Anim Hosp Assoc 2012;48:31–35.

Kiefer KM and Davis GJ: Salivary mucoceles in cats: a retrospective study of seven cases. Vet Med 2007;102:582–585.

Marsh A, Adin C: Tunneling under the digastricus muscle increases salivary duct exposure and completeness of excision in mandibular and sublingual sialoadenectomy in dogs. Vet Surg 2013;42:238–242.

Ritter MJ et al: Mandibular and sublingual sialocoeles in the dog: a retrospective evaluation of 41 cases, using the ventral approach for treatment. New Zealand Vet J 2006;54:333–337.

Torrad FA, Hassan EA: Clinical and ultrasonographic characteristics of salilvary mucoceles in 13 dogs. Vet Radiol Ultrasound 2013;54:293–298.

Chapter 55 Stenotic Nares

The dorsolateral borders of the nares, or nostrils, are formed by the dorsal lateral and accessory nasal cartilages. Contraction of attached muscle fibers abducts these cartilages, widening the nares. The free end of the dorsal lateral cartilage, which is thick and vascular, merges with the rostral extremity of the ventral nasal concha. The bulbous portion of this concha forms the alar fold. In brachycephalic dogs and cats, the alar folds may be short and thick and can collapse inward from cartilaginous or muscular weakness (fig. 55-1). Subsequent stenosis of the nares leads to inspiratory dyspnea. Stenotic nares, which are reported in 40% to 50% of dogs with brachycephalic syndrome, significantly inhibit inward air flow. Early correction is recommended so that elongated soft palate and laryngeal collapse are not exacerbated in these animals.

In some brachycephalic animals, stenotic nares have been associated with nasal cavity and turbinate malformation. On CT, affected dogs will have a short, narrow nasal cavity that is oriented more vertically. Obstruction of the caudal nasal cavity and choanae by the deformed turbinates is visible on CT and sometimes with retroflexed rhinoscopy. In these animals, resolution of inspiratory dyspnea requires turbinectomy as well as alar fold resection.

Brachycephalic dogs are also predisposed to gastrointestinal issues such as distal esophagitis, gastroenteritis, hiatal hernia, and pyloric hyperplasia, which can result in vomiting, regurgitation, and ptyalism. Dogs may need to be treated with omeprazole (1 mg/kg q12h PO), sucralfate, and other medications before or after the procedure. In some cases correction of the airway issues may assist in resolution of gastrointestinal signs.

Preoperative management

Severely dyspneic animals may present with cyanosis, hyperthermia, or collapse. Immediate therapy should include oxygen, sedatives, and fluids. Intubation may be required in extreme cases. Thoracic radiographs are recommended to rule out tracheal hypoplasia, which is common in brachycephalic breeds, and pulmonary pathology, including aspiration pneumonia. Cytology and culture of fluid can be obtained via transtracheal wash if pneumonia is suspected; however, many clinicians prefer to attempt treatment with a broad spectrum antibiotic first, unless the animal is to be intubated. In

Manual of Small Animal Soft Tissue Surgery, Second Edition. Karen Tobias.
© 2017 John Wiley & Sons, Inc. Published 2017 by John Wiley & Sons, Inc.

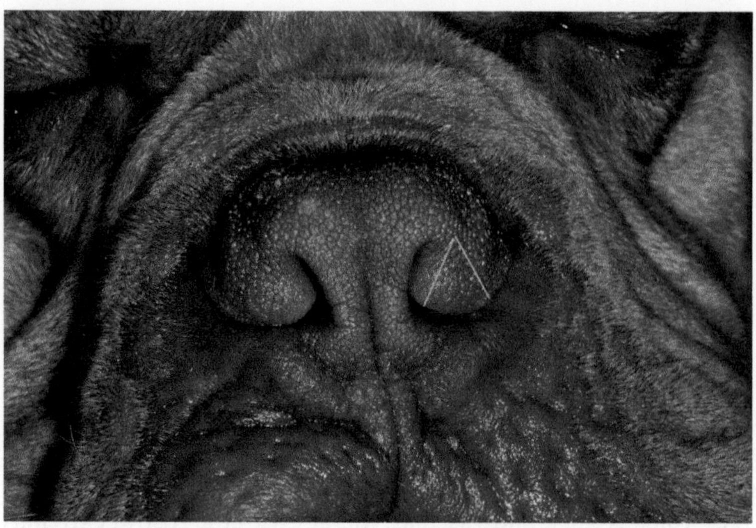

Figure 55-1 Stenotic nares in a mastiff. The proposed wedge resection is outlined in green. The first incision starts level with the dorsalmost opening of the nares and parallels the medial border of the alar fold. The second incision angles 40 to 60 degrees laterally.

that case, intubation can be performed with a sterile endotracheal tube so that the wash can be performed through the tube.

Brachycephalic animals should be preoxygenated before anesthetic induction. Induction and intubation should be rapid to avoid hypoxia. Since affected breeds are predisposed to elongated soft palate (Chapter 56), everted laryngeal saccules, and laryngeal collapse, the larynx and palate should be thoroughly evaluated at the time of anesthesia. Resection of elongated soft palates is performed concurrently with nares reconstruction.

Surgery

Options for correction of stenotic nares include alar fold wedge resection, punch resection alaplasty, alar fold amputation (Trader technique), and alapexy. Wedge resection provides immediate cosmetic results and is successful in most animals. The resection must go deep enough to include a portion of the ventral nasal concha to open up the entire nares. In immature animals, amputation of the folds (including a portion of the dorsolateral nasal cartilage) with a laser, blade, scissors, or electrocautery is easier than wedge resection. Scars that develop after amputation may remain white for several months. In patients with muscular weakness, the alar folds can be sutured to the face in an abducted position (alapexy) to prevent inward collapse. With alapexy, the skin along both sides of the midlateral slit of the nostrils is resected, and the remaining tissue is apposed primarily. This technique is not effective for animals with stenosis from caudal alar fold thickening.

Surgical technique: alar fold wedge resection

1. Position the animal in sternal recumbency, with its head resting on a towel or foam block.
2. Identify the wedge of tissue to be removed (fig. 55-1). There should be at least 2 mm of tissue to either side of the excised wedge to permit suturing.
3. Grasp the middle of the ventral portion of the alar fold parallel to the medial border of the fold with Brown Adson thumb forceps (fig. 55-2).

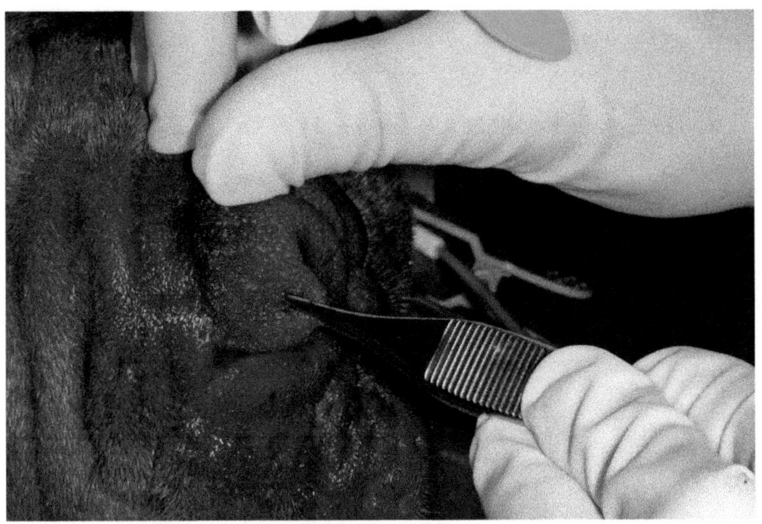

Figure 55-2 Grasp the ventral alar fold firmly with Brown Adson thumb forceps.

   a. A portion of the fold should remain visible medial to the thumb forceps.
   b. The tips of the thumb forceps should rest just below the level of the dorsal limit of the nasal opening.
4. With a no. 11 blade, incise parallel to the medial edge of the forceps and alar fold (fig. 55-3).
   a. Begin the incision at a point level with the dorsal boundary of the nares, leaving the dorsomedial attachment of the alar fold intact.
   b. Insert the blade deeply into the fold and cut downward until the blade exits the ventral edge of the fold. In some large bulldogs, this cut may be ≥10 mm deep. Bleeding is usually profuse, unless the nose is thickened, but will stop once sutures are in place.
5. While continuing to hold the fold securely with the thumb forceps, make the lateral cut.
   a. Begin the cut dorsally as before, starting at the previous incision.

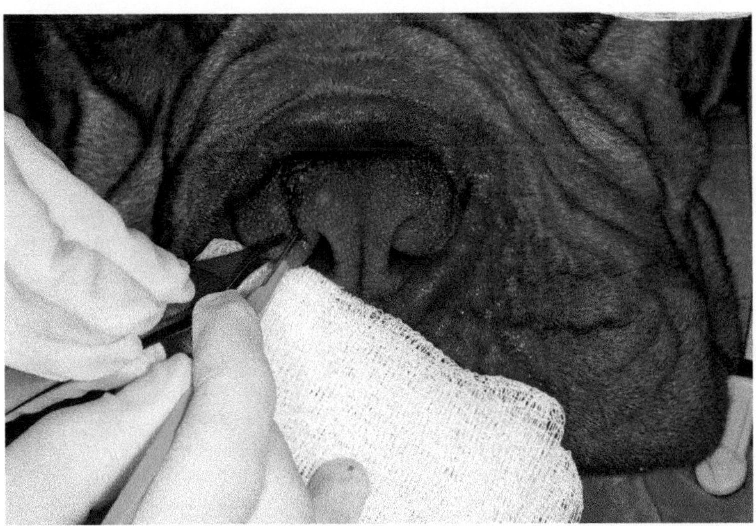

Figure 55-3 Incise parallel to the medial border of the alar fold, starting level with the dorsal limit of the nasal opening and angling inward. Incise deeply to include tissue caudally.

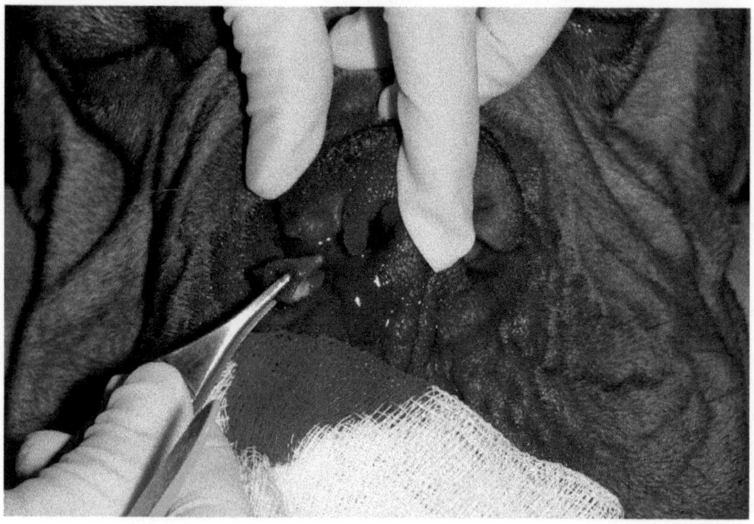

Figure 55-4 Angle the second incision laterally and slightly inward so that the final wedge is pyramidal in shape.

b. Cut outward from dorsal to ventrolateral, angling the tip of the blade inward (toward midline) at the deepest site to meet the caudal margin of the previous incision. In other words, the blade will be cutting from a dorsomedial to ventrolateral angle from a front view and from lateral to medial from a top view.

c. Complete the cut through the base of the tissue and ventral edge of the alar fold. The resultant wedge will often appear pyramidal in shape (fig. 55-4).

6. Using 4-0 monofilament rapidly absorbable material, place a simple interrupted suture to align the rostroventral margins of the remaining tissue of the alar fold (fig. 55-5). Take each tissue bite separately, pulling the needle through between each, and tie the suture firmly. Leave the suture ends long and secure them with a hemostat.

7. Retract the first suture dorsally to view the ventral defect (fig. 55-6). Place a simple interrupted suture across the middle of the ventral defect (fig. 55-7); tie it tightly and cut the ends short.

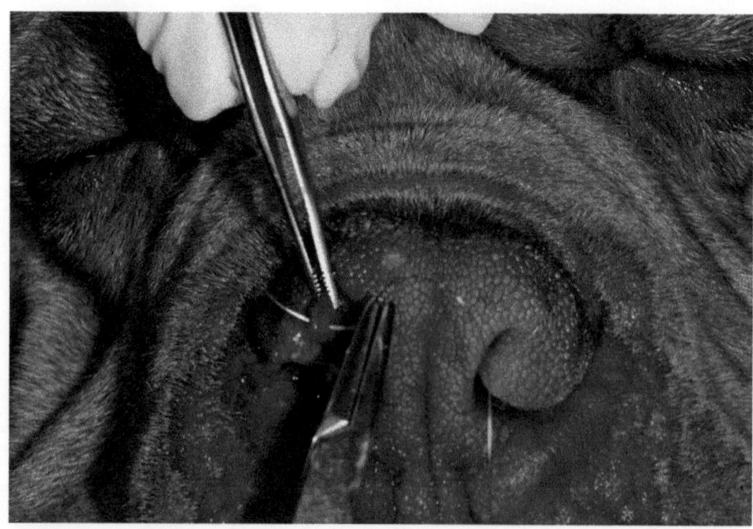

Figure 55-5 Place the first suture to appose the rostroventral margins of the incision.

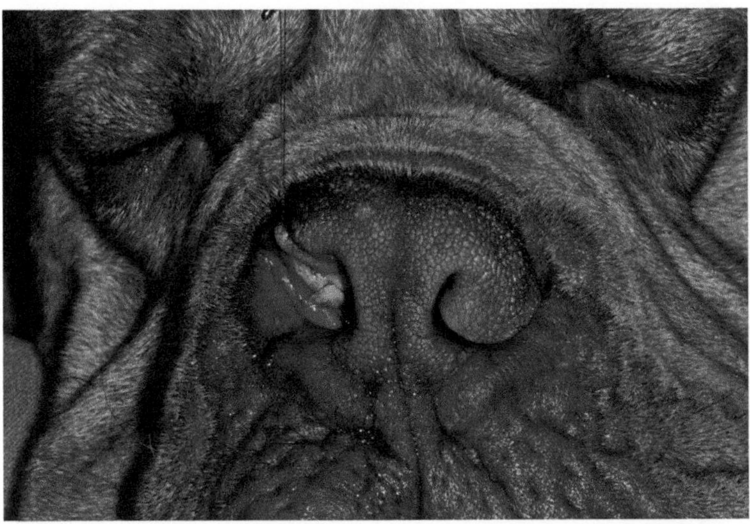

Figure 55-6 Retract the ends of the first suture dorsally to expose the ventral margin of the cut.

8. Release your retraction on the initial suture, and place a third suture across the dorsal half of the defect. Cut all suture ends short.
9. Repeat the procedure on the opposite side, removing the same amount of tissue so that the final nares diameter will match (fig. 55-8).

Surgical technique: alar fold amputation

1. Position the dog in sternal recumbency with its head resting on a towel.
2. With a no. 11 scalpel blade, transect each alar fold (fig. 55-9).
   a. Start the cut at the dorsalmost extent of the nares.
   b. Angle the blade so that it cuts from dorsomedial to ventrolateral at 15° to 20° degrees from the horizontal (dorsal) plane, about 40° from the vertical (sagittal) plane, and about 45° from the cross-sectional (transverse) plane,
   c. The cut should result in a pyramidal-shaped wedge that is narrower at its dorsal, caudal, and lateral aspects.

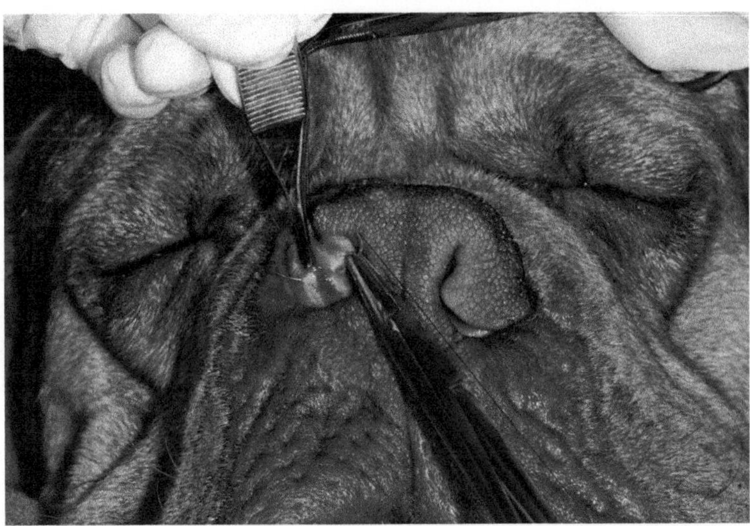

Figure 55-7 Appose the ventral incision margins with one or more interrupted sutures.

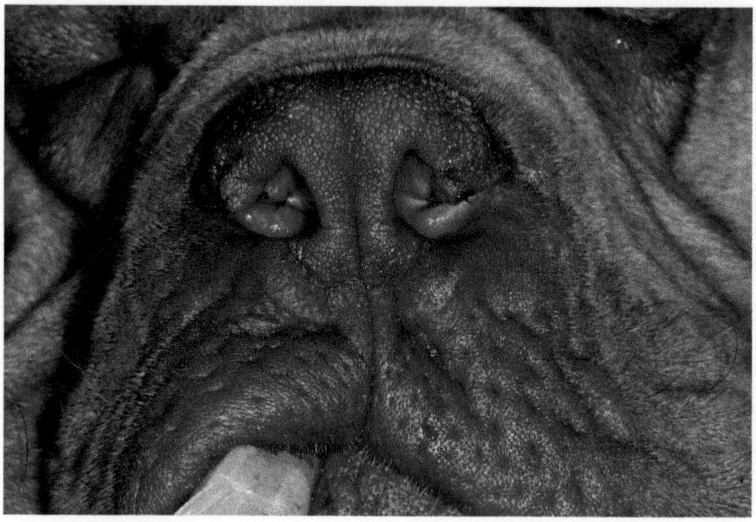

Figure 55-8 Add additional sutures to close any remaining gaps, and cut suture ends short.

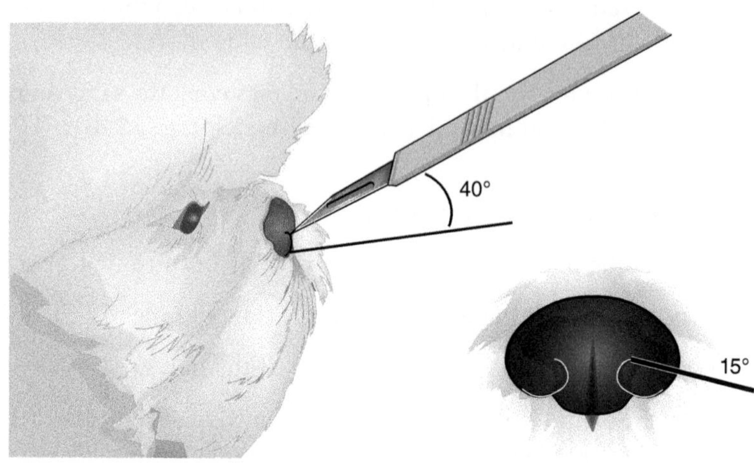

Figure 55-9 Amputation of the alar fold. The line of transection angles approximately 15° downward from the horizontal plane, about 45° inward from a top view and 40° downward from a side view.

3. Apply pressure to the open wound firmly with a cotton tipped applicator for 5 to 10 minutes.
4. Leave the wounds open to heal by second intention.

Postoperative considerations

Hemorrhage usually resolves once the sutures are in place (wedge resection) or with pressure (alar fold amputation). Occasionally, animals may require Elizabethan collars if they paw or rub at their noses. Absorbable sutures used to close the wounds after wedge resection will usually fall out on their own in 2 to 4 weeks. For dogs undergoing alar fold amputation, the scars from second intention healing often appear white for 2 to 3 months after the procedure (fig. 55-10) but will eventually repigment.

In brachycephalic dogs, complications associated with stenotic nares correction are rare unless other conditions such as elongated soft palate, hypoplastic trachea, and laryngeal collapse are present. Anecdotally, animals undergoing alar fold amputation may develop ocular discharge if the opening to the nasolacrimal duct is damaged. In dogs with medium or long muzzles, the ducts

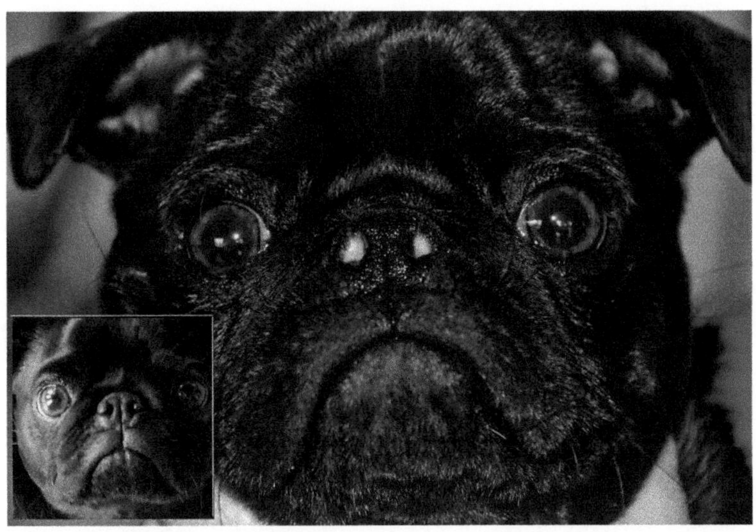

Figure 55-10 White scars visible 6 weeks after amputation of alar folds with a laser. Within 6 months, the dog's nose was repigmented (inset).

open at the ventromedial attachments of the alar fold. The opening is more variable in brachycephalic breeds.

Bibliography

Ellison GW: Alapexy: an alternative technique for repair of stenotic nares in dogs. J Am Anim Hosp Assoc 2004;40:484–489.

Huck JL et al: Technique and outcomes of nares amputation (Trader's technique) in immature shih tzus. J Am Anim Hosp Assoc 2008;44:82–85.

Meola SD: Brachycephalic airway syndrome. Topics in Compan An Med 2013;29:91–96.

Oechtering GU et al: New aspects of brachycephalia in dogs and cats. ACVIM Proc 2008; pp. 11–17.

Riecks TW et al: Surgical correction of brachycephalic syndrome in dogs: 62 cases (1991–2004). J Am Vet Med Assoc 2007;230:1324–1328.

Torrez CV and Hunt GB: Results of surgical correction of abnormalities associated with brachycephalic airway obstruction syndrome in dogs in Australia. J Small Anim Pract 2006;47:150–154.

Trostel CT, Frankel DJ: Punch resection alaplasty technique in dogs and cats with stenotic nares: 14 cases. J Am Anim Hosp Assoc 2010;46:5–11.

Chapter 56
Elongated Soft Palate

Elongated soft palate is most commonly reported in brachycephalic dog breeds such as English bulldogs and pugs (fig. 56-1). Palates may also elongate with increased negative inspiratory pressure secondary to upper respiratory tract obstruction such as with stenotic nares, laryngeal paralysis, or tracheal collapse. Initially, clinical signs of elongated soft palate may be limited to stertorous breathing, snoring during sleep, and mild exercise intolerance. Gastrointestinal signs such as vomiting, retching, gagging, and regurgitation are also common. With time, elongated soft palates become chronically thickened. Trauma to thickened palates during tachypnea may cause palate edema and ulceration. Animals that are tachypneic from stress, heat, or overexertion can present with cyanosis, collapse, and hyperthermia. Severely affected animals may require emergency intubation or tracheostomy.

Diagnosis of elongated soft palate is based on evaluation of palate length under anesthesia. Palate thickening and elongation are also noticeable on lateral cervical radiographs and computed tomography. Brachycephalic dogs suspected to have elongated soft palates should also be evaluated for associated respiratory anomalies, including everted laryngeal saccules, stenotic nares, hypoplastic trachea, laryngeal collapse, and abnormal conchal (turbinate) growth with subsequent obstruction of the choanae. Most dogs with elongated soft palates also have one or more of these conditions. Chronic gastritis and pyloric mucosal hyperplasia are reported in over 75% of brachycephalic dogs with upper airway syndrome. Other digestive anomalies that may occur concurrently include cardial atony, gastroesophageal reflux, gastric retention, pyloric stenosis, pyloric atony, duodenitis, gastroduodenal reflux, and hiatal hernia.

Preoperative management

Thoracic radiographs are recommended, since animals with elongated soft palates are predisposed to tracheal hypoplasia, bronchial collapse, and aspiration pneumonia. Hiatal hernia may also be visible on thoracic films. If aspiration pneumonia is present, a transtracheal wash can be performed to retrieve samples for cytology and cultures, or the animal can be treated empirically with broad spectrum antibiotics and monitored for response to treatment. If possible, surgery is delayed until pneumonia has resolved. If abnormal conchal development is suspected, computed tomography or

Manual of Small Animal Soft Tissue Surgery, Second Edition. Karen Tobias.
© 2017 John Wiley & Sons, Inc. Published 2017 by John Wiley & Sons, Inc.

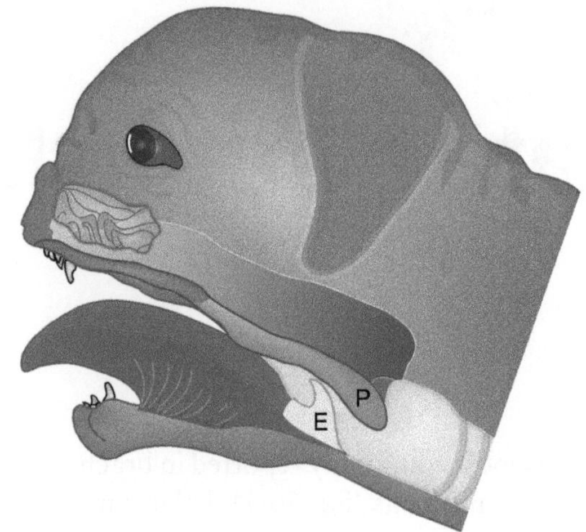

Figure 56-1 Elongated soft palate. The soft palate (P) is thickened and extends caudal to the tip of the epiglottis (E). During inspiration, the elongated palate is pulled into the laryngeal ostium.

retroflexed choanal endoscopy should be performed. Obstruction from abnormal conchal development is treated with laser turbinectomy.

Hydromorphone and morphine should be avoided as preanesthetic agents, since they will prolong recovery and potentially increase the risk of aspiration. Animals are preoxygenated before anesthetic induction. Induction should be as rapid as possible to permit immediate intubation with a cuffed endotracheal tube. The tube is secured to the lower jaw to keep it out of the way during surgery. Because aspiration is common in English bulldogs, some clinicians will administer metoclopramide perioperatively, although its effectiveness in reducing intraoperative reflux at clinical doses is questionable. Most clinicians will also administer an anti-inflammatory dose of glucocorticoids (e.g., dexamethasone SP, 0.25 mg/kg IV) after induction to reduce postoperative swelling, unless nonsteroidal anti-inflammatory administration is planned or ongoing. For the procedure, the patient is positioned in sternal recumbency. The mouth is held open by resting the maxilla on an aluminium bar stand (fig. 56-2) or suspending it between two fluid stands with tape or gauze ties. The mandible can be retracted ventrally with tape or gauze.

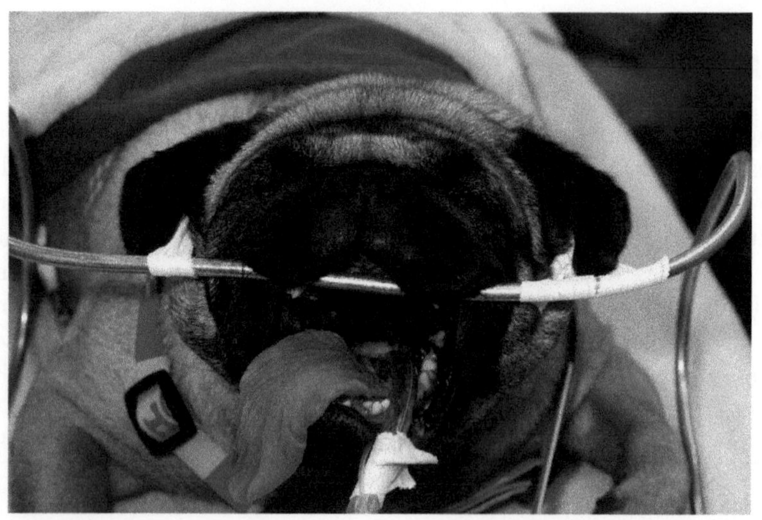

Figure 56-2 Place the dog in sternal recumbency with the upper jaw resting on an aluminum bar "ether" stand. Secure the dog's head to the crossbar by wrapping tape around the bar on one side of the head, around the back of the head below the ears, and around the bar on the opposite side of the head. The endotracheal tube can be tied around the lower jaw behind the canines or, as in this dog, sutured to the lower jaw.

Surgery

In dogs with elongated palates, determining the appropriate palate length can be difficult. Normal palate length is thought to be to the caudal end of the tonsillar crypts (not the tonsils themselves!) or just slightly overlapping the tip of the epiglottis, but this varies with breed conformation. Fortunately, brachycephalic dogs with palatal thickening can tolerate shorter palates, as long as nasopharyngeal constrictor muscles are still present and functional, and some may obstruct with postoperative swelling if normal standards are used. Appropriate palate length is therefore usually based on the breed and the clinician's judgment. The author prefers to shorten bulldog palates so the caudal border is even with the caudal aspect of the tonsillar crypts; the palate is not expected to overlap the tip of the epiglottis when the procedure is complete

Palatal resection ("staphylectomy") can be performed with a carbon dioxide (CO_2) laser, radiosurgical scalpel, or cut-and-sew technique. Laser resection provides immediate hemostasis and a comfortable recovery. Proper safety equipment (e.g., specialized eyewear) is required, and the endotracheal tube must be protected from laser damage and potential ignition of delivered oxygen. The CO_2 laser will not cut through black tissue, so char that develops during palatal incision must be removed frequently. If the laser tip comes in contact with the palate during cutting, the tissues will immediately swell. No additional safety equipment is needed for radiosurgical scalpel resection of the tissues. The technique is very similar to laser resection. The surgeon must cut slowly with the radiosurgical scalpel, however, or hemostasis will be inadequate, and suture closure is often required. With the cut-and-sew technique, excess palatal tissue is excised and oversewn in stages. Long-handled scissors, thumb forceps, and needle holders may be required in large dogs. Reported outcomes for laser and cut-and-sew techniques are similar.

Another alternative to traditional staphylectomy is a "folded flap" palatoplasty, in which the soft palate is resected partial thickness, and the caudal edge (nasopharyngeal border) is pulled forward (making the folded flap) and sutured to the cranial edge of the resection (oral mucosa). This technique is used for brachycephalic dogs with thick palates and results in sutures that are placed more rostrally and away from the caudal border of the reconstructed palate. It is much more technically demanding than the traditional technique, however.

Stenotic nares, if present, are repaired at the time of staphylectomy (see Chapter 55). Tonsilectomy is usually not required, unless enlargement is severe enough to obstruct the airways. Everted laryngeal saccules causing airway obstruction can be amputated at their bases with scissors after the palate is resected. Extubation may be required for laryngeal saccule resection.

Surgical technique: laser staphylectomy

1. Prepare the laser.
   a. Insert a 0.4-mm tip into the CO_2 laser handle.
   b. Set the laser in a continuous mode at a power of 5 to 7 watts (7 W for thicker palates).
   c. Test the laser beam on a tongue depressor to verify that a narrow, well-defined score mark is produced when the tip is held several millimeters from the wood surface.

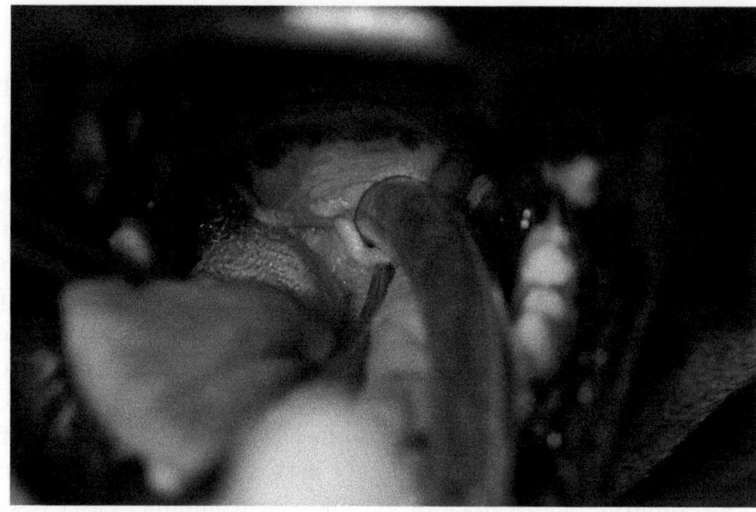

Figure 56-3 Locate the tip of the epiglottis (resting on thumb forceps) or the caudal edge of the tonsillar crypts. The palate should be resected approximately level with or just rostral to those points, depending on breed.

2. Position the dog in sternal recumbency with the mouth propped open (fig. 56-2).
3. Determine the final palate length, usually at the caudal border of the tonsillar crypts or level with tip of the epiglottis, depending on breed (fig. 56-3). Mark the site.
4. Place a full-thickness monofilament stay suture at each side (or "corner") of the palate caudal (distal) to the proposed line of resection. Be sure to include any palate that has everted into the nasopharynx. Secure the stay suture ends with hemostats.
5. Pull the palate rostrally with the stay sutures (fig. 56-4). Place a moistened gauze sponge between the palate and endotracheal tube to protect the tube (and the flammable oxygen inside!) from laser damage.
6. With the laser tip several millimeters from the tissue surface, apply the laser beam to mark the palate superficially at several sites along the proposed line of resection (fig. 56-4). Do not let the laser touch the tissues, or they will inflate and swell.

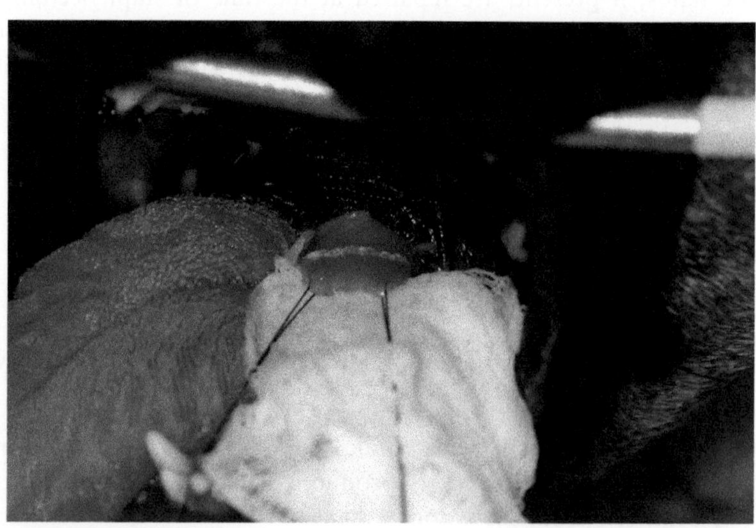

Figure 56-4 Retract the palate rostrally and ventrally with full-thickness stay sutures placed near the lateral margins of the palate and place a moistened gauze sponge between the everted palate and the endotracheal tube. Mark the palate by scoring it lightly with the laser beam at the proposed level of transection, then return the palate to its normal position to check the proposed length.

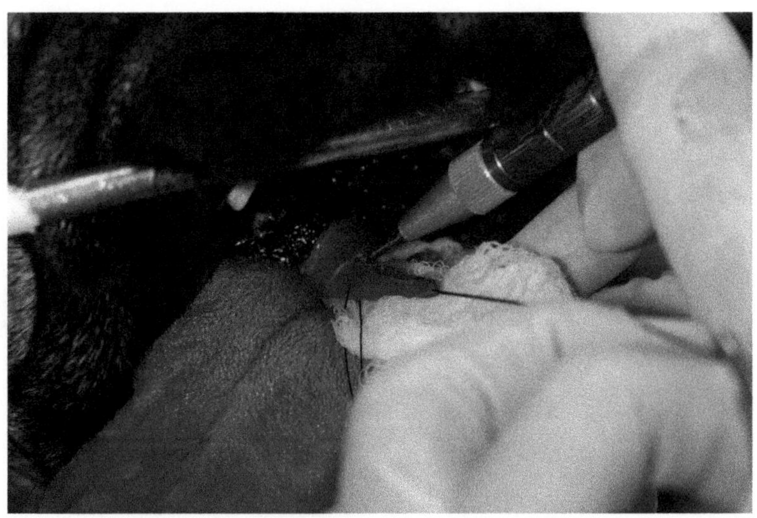

Figure 56-5 Retract one stay suture rostroventrally and cut along the marked line with the laser tip positioned 1 to 2 mm above the tissue.

7. Remove the moistened sponge and return the palate to its normal position. Check the proposed line of resection a final time.
8. Pull the palate tip rostrally with the stay sutures and replace the moistened sponge.
9. Retract one stay suture rostroventrally. On the same side, begin to cut the width of the palate with the laser by slowly passing the beam back and forth over the lateral portion of the proposed incision site. Keep the tip 1 to 2 mm above the tissues.
   a. If you are right-handed, use your left hand to retract rostroventrally on the stay suture on the dog's left (your right).
   b. Begin the cut along the dog's left side of the palate (your right) while keeping continuous traction on the stay suture.
10. From a lateral direction, continue to apply the laser beam along the width of the palate and across its center until the tissue is cut full thickness and the incision edges separate (fig. 56-5).
    a. Retract firmly on the stay suture while cutting. This will pull the partially amputated piece forward, constantly exposing fresh pink surfaces that will cut more easily.
    b. With moistened cotton-tipped applicator swabs, remove char as it develops.
11. Once at least half the palate is transected, retract the opposite stay suture. Use the laser to make a partial-thickness cut along the remaining incision line, now aiming the laser from the opposite direction (e.g., the dog's right).
12. Continue to apply the laser beam to transect the remainder of the palate, either from the right or the left.
13. Once the resection is complete, remove the moistened sponge and check the palate position to determine whether further resection is needed (fig. 56-6).
14. Thick palates may require suture closure after laser staphylectomy.

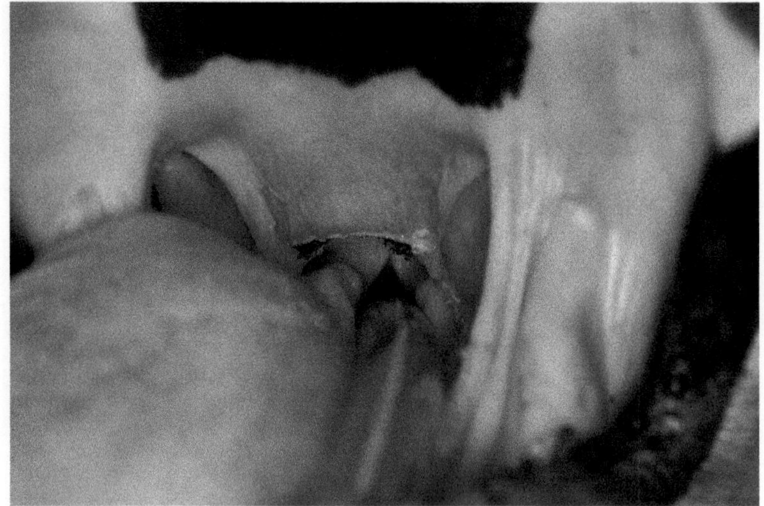

Figure 56-6 Final appearance after laser staphylectomy. In this dog the tonsils are enlarged, so the caudal aspects of the crypts are not visible.

Surgical technique: cut-and-sew staphylectomy

1. If desired, mark the proposed site of resection by drawing a line with electrocautery or a marker or by crushing small areas along the site with thumb forceps or a hemostat.
2. Place full-thickness monofilament stay sutures on the right and left margins of the palate, or grasp the palate edge with hemostats or thumb forceps (fig. 56-7).
    a. Stay sutures can be placed on the section of tissue to be resected, with the cut made just rostral (proximal) to the suture.
    b. Alternatively, stay sutures can be placed on the corner of the tissue that will remain. In that case, the stay suture on one side can be tied and used for simple continuous closure of the transected edges.
3. Retract the palate tip rostrally so that the ventral surface of the palate is visible.
4. Cut one-third to one-half of the width of the palate at the proposed resection site with curved Metzenbaum scissors (fig. 56-7).

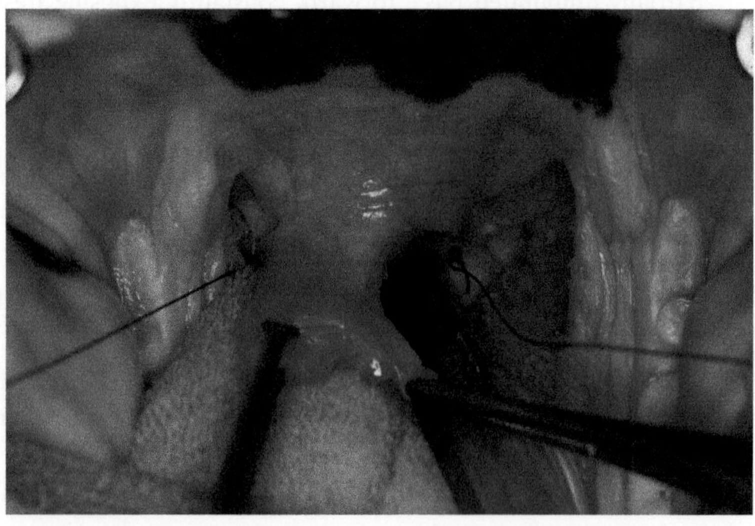

Figure 56-7 Cut-and-sew staphylectomy. Retract the palate tip rostrally and cut one-third to one-half of the width of the palate. In this dog, a suture has been secured at the beginning of the incision line.

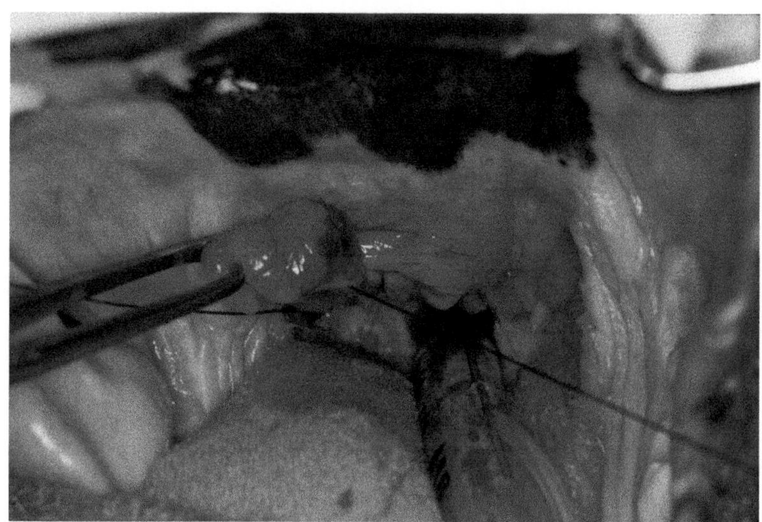

Figure 56-8 Appose the cut edges of the nasopharyngeal and oral mucosa of the soft palate with a simple continuous pattern.

5. With 4-0 monofilament rapidly absorbable suture, sew nasal mucosa to oral mucosa in a simple continuous pattern.
   a. Take a bite across the lateral border of the incision and tie two knots (fig. 56-7).
   b. Cut the suture end short, or place a hemostat on it to use for retraction.
   c. Evert the palate with long Debakey thumb forceps to expose the retracted edge of the nasal mucosa.
   d. Take bites of nasal mucosa and oral mucosa to appose them over the edge of transected palatal muscle (fig. 56-8).
   e. Appose mucosal edges with a continuous pattern, spacing sutures 3 to 4 mm apart.
6. Continue the cut-and sew-technique in one or two more steps (fig. 56-9).
7. After tying the final knots, cut all knot ends very short to prevent vomiting and gagging from pharyngeal irritation by the suture ends. The cuneiform

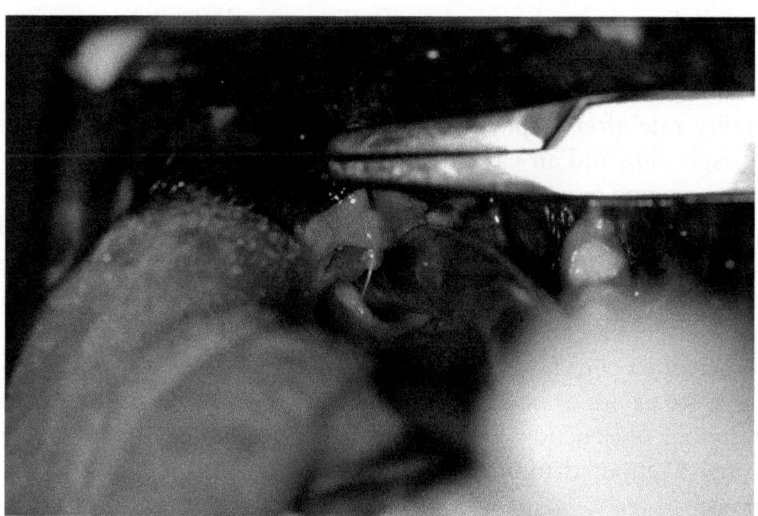

Figure 56-9 Continue to cut and sew, including nasal and oral mucosa surfaces of the palate in each suture bite.

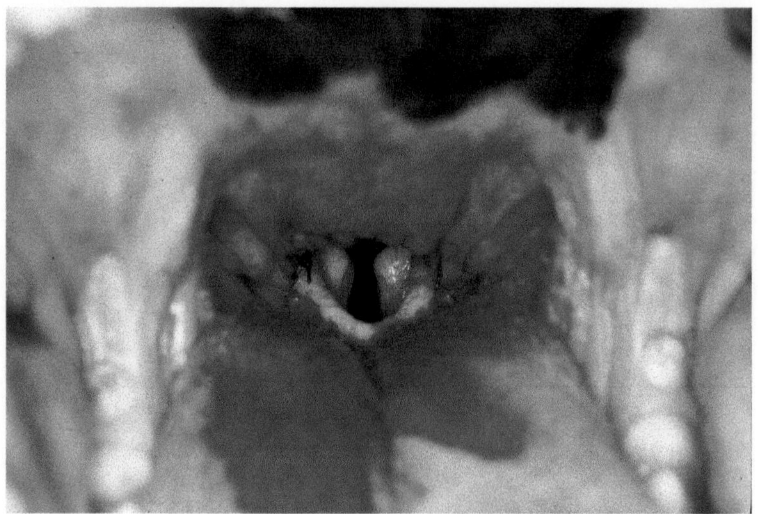

Figure 56-10 Final appearance of a cut-and-sew staphylectomy.

processes of the arytenoids should be visible when the staphylectomy is complete (fig. 56-10).

Postoperative considerations

Some animals may require mild sedation (e.g., dexmedetomidine or acepromazine) and analgesics (e.g., buprenorphine) after the procedure. Heavy sedation may limit the animal's ability to protect its airway, however. If mild respiratory signs are present (e.g., snoring), the patient is administered oxygen by nasal catheters, mask, or other means to reduced respiratory effort so that swelling is not promoted by high negative airway pressures. If severe swelling develops, tracheal intubation (under light anesthesia until swelling decreases) or temporary tracheostomy may be required. Dyspnea and cyanosis can also occur as a result of aspiration pneumonia. Brachycephalic dogs are predisposed to corneal ulcerations, so artificial tears or eye lubricant should be applied frequently during anesthesia and recovery.

Because gastrointestinal disease is common in dogs with brachycephalic syndrome, prokinetic agents and antacids are often continued for several weeks. Duration of therapy is based on clinical response or endoscopic appearance of the esophageal, gastric, and duodenal mucosa. Correction of brachycephalic airway disease may facilitate resolution of gastrointestinal signs. Obese animals should be placed on a weight reduction diet to further reduce stress on the airways.

Mortality rate after staphylectomy is less than 5%. Major complications include aspiration and airway obstruction from postoperative swelling. Postoperative vomiting or regurgitation is reported in up to 18% of animals. If the palate resection was inadequate, clinical signs will likely reoccur. If the resection was excessive, the animal will reflux water and food through the nose and develop coughing and rhinitis. Laryngeal collapse, which has been reported in over half of dogs with elongated soft palates, will continue to cause mild to moderate clinical signs in affected animals. Besides laryngeal collapse or inadequate palate or nares correction, recurrence of respiratory signs may be a result of obstruction by nasopharyngeal turbinates or chronic palate thickening. Computed tomography is recommended for diagnosis of these conditions.

Bibliography

Davidson EB et al: Evaluation of carbon dioxide laser and conventional incisional techniques for resection of soft palates in brachycephalic dogs. J Am Vet Med Assoc 2001;219:776–781.

Dunie-Merigot A, Bouvy B, Poncet C: Comparative use of CO_2 laser, diode laser and monopolar electrocautery for resection of the soft palate in dogs with brachycephalic airway obstructive syndrome. Vet Rec 2010;167:700–704.

Fasanella FJ, Shivley JM, Wardlaw JL, et al: Brachycephalic airway obstructive syndrome in dogs: 90 cases (1991–2008). J Am Vet Med Assoc 2010;237:1048–1051.

Findji L, Dupre G: Brachycephalic syndrome: innovative surgical techniques. Clinician's Brief 2013;11:79–85.

Oechtering GU, Pohl S, Schlueter C, et al: A novel approach to brachycephalic syndrome. 1. Evaluation of anatomical intranasal airway obstruction; and 2. Laser assisted turbinectomy (LATE) Vet Surg 2016;165–181.

Poncet CM et al: Long-term results of upper respiratory syndrome surgery and gastrointestinal tract medical treatment in 51 brachycephalic dogs. J Small Anim Pract 2006;47:137–142.

Riecks TW et al: Surgical correction of brachycephalic syndrome in dogs: 62 cases (1991–2004). J Am Vet Med Assoc 2007;230:1324–1328.

Torrez DV and Hunt GB: Results of surgical correction of abnormalities associated with brachycephalic airway obstruction syndrome in dogs in Australia. J Small Anim Pract 2006;47:150–154.

Chapter 57
Feline Thyroidectomy

Hyperthyroidism is a common endocrine disease in middle-aged to older cats. It is most frequently caused by benign adenomatous hyperplasia of the thyroid glands, and, in 70% to 91% of affected cats, the condition is bilateral. Additionally, about 9% of cats have hyperactive ectopic thyroid tissue. Classic clinical signs of hyperthyroidism include weight loss, polyphagia, behavior changes, poor hair coat, hyperactivity, polydypsia, pollakiuria, vomiting, and a palpable neck mass. However, with the inclusion of T4 measurement in geriatric panels, more cats are being diagnosed with subclinical hyperthyroidism. In 95% of cats, diagnosis is based on persistent increases in thyroid hormone concentrations. In cats with normal T4 concentrations and clinical signs suggestive of hyperthyroidism, the condition can be confirmed by repeating a T4 measurement several weeks later or through a free T4 measurement or thyroid scintigraphy. Cats with hyperthyroidism should be evaluated for common comorbidities such as thyrotoxic heart disease, hypertension, retinopathy, chronic kidney disease, gastrointestinal disease, and insulin resistance.

Treatments for feline hyperthyroidism include antithyroid drugs, such as methimazole or carbimazole; radioactive iodine (I-131); an iodine-restricted diet; or surgical removal of affected glands. Radioactive iodine has minimal side effects and destroys all hyperplastic thyroid tissue, regardless of location. Disadvantages of radioactive iodine therapy include limited availability and, depending on state and local radiation safety laws, the need for prolonged hospitalization. About 5% of cats fail to respond to radioactive iodine and require retreatment.

Surgery is readily available to most practitioners; however, care must be taken to preserve the parathyroid glands during bilateral thyroidectomy to prevent occurrence of iatrogenic hypoparathyroidism. Thyroid adenocarcinoma, which is diagnosed in 2% to 3% of cats with hyperthyroidism, can be treated by surgical resection, radioiodine therapy, or a combination of both modalities. Surgery and radioactive iodine therapy are contraindicated in cats with renal dysfunction, since reduction in thyroid function will decrease glomerular filtration rate. In some cats, renal dysfunction becomes apparent only after 2 to 3 weeks of methimazole administration. Side effects of methimazole occur in 10% of cats within 3 months of initiating methimazole therapy and include anorexia, vomiting, lethargy, pruritus, hepatotoxicity, neutropenia, and thrombocytopenia. Methimazole must be administered for the remainder of the cat's life if it is the sole therapy.

Manual of Small Animal Soft Tissue Surgery, Second Edition. Karen Tobias.
© 2017 John Wiley & Sons, Inc. Published 2017 by John Wiley & Sons, Inc.

Preoperative management

Tachycardia, hypertension, and heart murmurs are often noted in cats with hyperthyroidism; up to 50% of affected cats will develop hypertrophic cardiomyopathy, and 10% to 15% can develop congestive heart failure. Blood pressure measurements and echocardiography are recommended before anesthesia is considered. Most clinicians will treat hyperthyroid cats with methimazole or carbimazole, with or without a beta adrenergic blocking agent (propranolol, atenolol), for several weeks before surgery to restore euthyroidism, decrease occurrence of arrhythmias and tachycardia, and reduce the anesthetic risk and to verify that renal function remains unaffected once thyroid hormone concentrations normalize. If hypertension does not resolve with medical control of hyperthyroidism, other etiologies (e.g., chronic renal disease, diabetes mellitus, and hyperaldosteronism) should be investigated. If renal disease manifests with medical treatment, surgery should be abandoned.

Scintigraphy is often performed to determine whether the condition is unilateral or bilateral and to detect ectopic hyperplastic thyroid tissue, which can be found in the cervical region, thoracic inlet, or cranial thorax. Before surgery, serum chemistries should be evaluated for hypokalemia, which occurs in one-third of affected cats, and for renal dysfunction. Hemorrhage from jugular venipuncture sites can discolor and obscure the parathyroid glands and should therefore be avoided within the week prior to surgery.

The ventral cervical region should be clipped and prepped from the angle of the mandible to 4 cm caudal to the thoracic inlet. Surgery is performed with the cat in dorsal recumbency, with forelegs pulled caudally and the head and neck hyperextended. The cat should be positioned on towels or sandbags so that the neck is perfectly straight. Towel clamps should penetrate only through the skin to avoid trauma to the jugular veins. Bipolar cautery, fine scissors and thumb forceps, sterile cotton-tipped applicator swabs, and magnification are useful during dissection.

Surgery

If a scintigraphy is not available, then presence of disease is determined by gland size, shape, and color during surgery. Adenomatous glands are usually plump and liver-colored, while unaffected glands are small, thin, and pale because of atrophy. If the contralateral gland is normal in size in a cat with a hyperactive thyroid gland, it is most likely affected. External parathyroid glands are normally 1 to 3 mm in diameter, paler than the thyroid tissue (assuming no one has performed a jugular venipuncture), and located on the ventral surface of the cranial pole of the thyroid gland. In some cats, the external parathyroid glands are located on the caudal pole. If local hemorrhage occurs, parathyroid glands may appear pink or red. The parathyroid glands must be differentiated from fat deposits on the capsule. Under magnification, they will have a small vessel that bifurcates at the gland and surrounds it.

In cats with unilateral hyperthyroidism, the thyroid gland can be removed with an extracapsular procedure. With this technique, the vessels are ligated cranial and caudal to the thyroid gland, and the entire gland is removed along with the associated parathyroid glands. However, because most cats have bilateral disease, a modified extracapsular or intracapsular technique is recommended to preserve the external parathyroid glands and their associated blood supply. With the modified extracapsular technique, the external parathyroid gland and its artery are dissected free from the capsule before the thyroid gland is removed. With the modified intracapsular technique, the thyroid tissue is removed through a capsular incision; the remaining capsule is then excised, except for where the parathyroid gland and its blood supply are attached. Both procedures have potential complications: with the modified intracapsular technique, thyroid tissue can inadvertently be left within the capsule, while the parathyroid gland could be accidentally removed or devascularized during dissection with the modified extracapsular technique.

If parathyroid blood supply is disrupted during surgery, the parathyroid gland can be transplanted into local muscle. Autotransplanted parathyroid glands will revascularize and resume function within 14 to 21 days. Some clinicians will stage thyroidectomy procedures 3 to 4 weeks apart so that any parathyroid gland damaged during the initial thyroidectomy will be revascularized by the time of the second procedure.

Surgical technique: modified extracapsular thyroidectomy

1. Position the cat in dorsal recumbancy with the head and neck extended and perfectly straight and the front limbs pulled caudally. Make sure the cat is not tilted to one side.
2. Make a midline skin incision from the thyroid cartilage to the midcervical region.
3. Transect the transverse fibers of the thin sphincter colli muscle (fig. 57-1) with a blade to expose the underlying sternohyoideus muscles.
4. With a finger, press firmly on the paired sternohyoideus muscles and roll them back and forth until the median raphe can be identified (fig. 57-2).
5. Incise and separate the paired sternohyoideus muscles on the midline and retract them laterally with Gelpi retractors.
6. Use bipolar cautery to coagulate small vessels crossing the median raphe.
7. Staying close to the trachea, gently spread any fascia between the muscles and trachea with blunt dissection until you can identify the thyroid gland

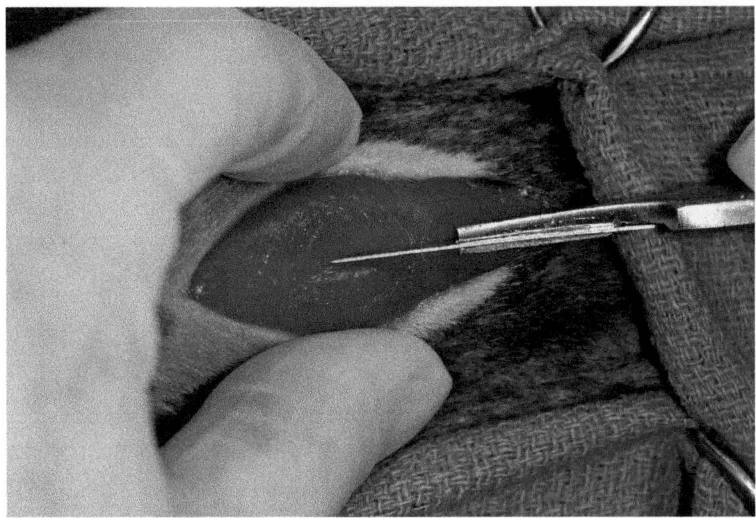

Figure 57-1 Incise the skin and the sphincter colli muscle along the ventral midline in the midcervical region.

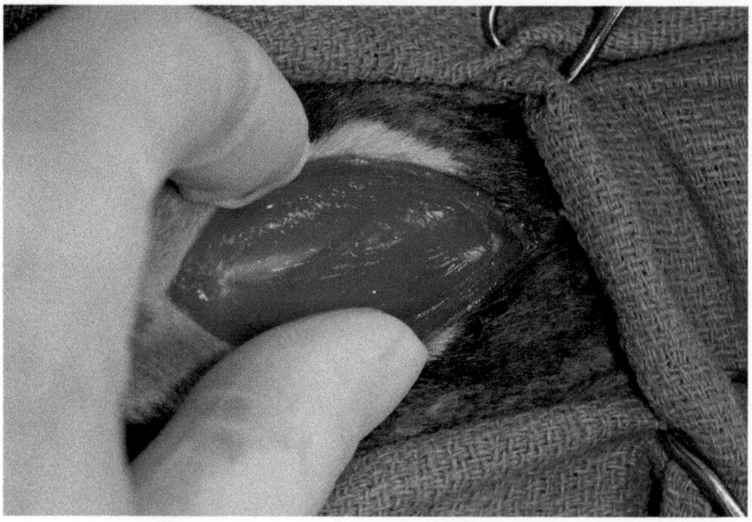

Figure 57-2 Compress and retract the tissues to expose the septum between the paired sternohyoideus muscles. Small vessels are often visible in the septal fascia.

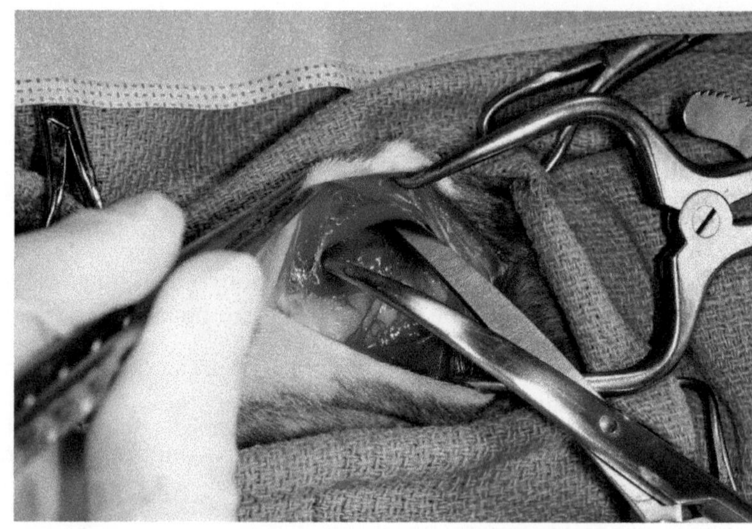

Figure 57-3 Once the sternohyoideus muscles are separated and retracted, expose the thyroid dorsolateral to the trachea. If the thyroid is not readily visible, use blunt dissection to gently free any fascial attachments between the muscles and the trachea or thyroid gland.

on the lateral or dorsolateral surface of the trachea, ventromedial to the common carotid artery (fig. 57-3). The thyroid gland may be located near the thyroid cartilage.

8. Identify the recurrent laryngeal nerves. They may be running along the trachea medial to the gland or in the fascia just dorsal to the gland. Avoid damaging the nerves during dissection and retraction of the thyroid gland.
9. Identify the external parathyroid gland (fig. 57-4).
10. If possible, identify the parathyroid branch of the thyroid artery (magnifying glasses help). With a no. 11, no. 15, or Beaver blade, incise the thyroid capsule around the parathyroid gland (fig. 57-5), except where the artery travels to the parathyroid gland. Alternatively, make a small incision in the capsule with a blade and then extend it with iris scissors.

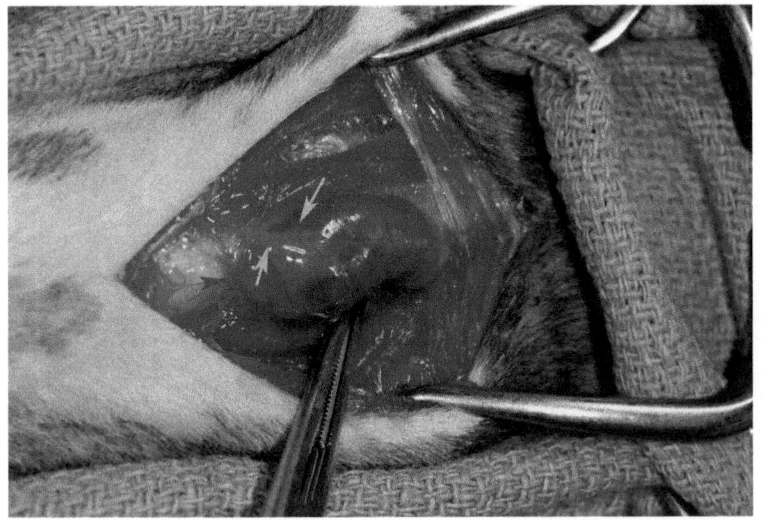

Figure 57-4 Exposed thyroid and external parathyroid gland. Two small arterial branches (green arrows) travel from the cranial thyroid artery (blue arrowheads) to the parathyroid gland. These vessels should be spared during dissection.

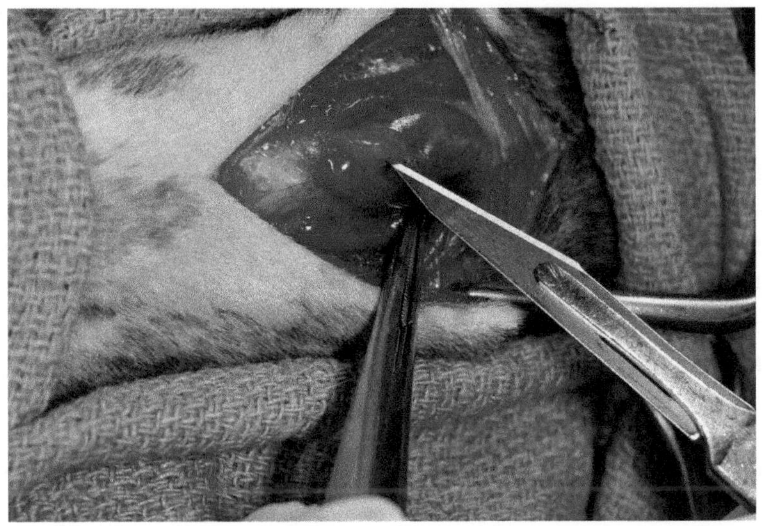

Figure 57-5 With a fine-tipped blade, incise the capsule around the parathyroid gland, except for where the parathyroid arteries lie.

11. With a blade or iris scissors, gently free the parathyroid gland and attached capsule from the thyroid gland, being careful not to disturb the parathyroid artery (fig. 57-6).
12. Free any remaining fascial attachments to the thyroid gland and ligate its blood supply.
    a. With fine hemoclips or absorbable 4-0 synthetic suture, ligate the thyroid artery distal to the bifurcation of the parathyroid branch. Transect the tissues distal to the ligature. Excise the thyroid gland in its remaining capsule, ligating any thyroid vessels at the opposite pole.
    b. Alternatively, begin vessel ligation and fascial dissection of the thyroid gland at the pole opposite to the visible external parathyroid

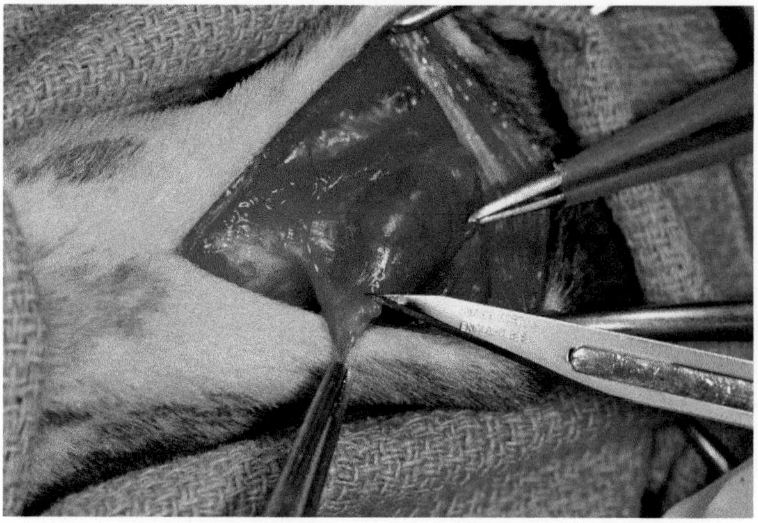

Figure 57-6 Gently separate the parathyroid gland, with its attached blood supply, from the thyroid gland and reflect it dorsally.

gland (usually the caudal pole). While elevating the caudal pole of the thyroid gland by its transected tissue, gradually dissect cranially to free the gland from surrounding fascia (fig. 57-7). Then ligate (fig. 57-8 inset) and transect the cranial thyroid artery distal to its parathyroid branch.

13. If ectopic thyroid tissue is present in the cervical region on scintigraphy, extend the skin incision cranially or caudally to locate and remove the tissue. The sternocephalicus muscles cover the caudal third of the sternohyoideus muscles; separate them on midline and retract them to expose the trachea near the thoracic inlet.

14. If the parathyroid gland is detached from its blood supply accidentally, free it from all thyroid tissue. Make an incision in the sternothyroideus or sternohyoideus muscle. Insert the parathyroid gland into the muscle pocket (fig. 57-9) and close the muscle pocket over it with 3-0 or 4-0 absorbable suture.

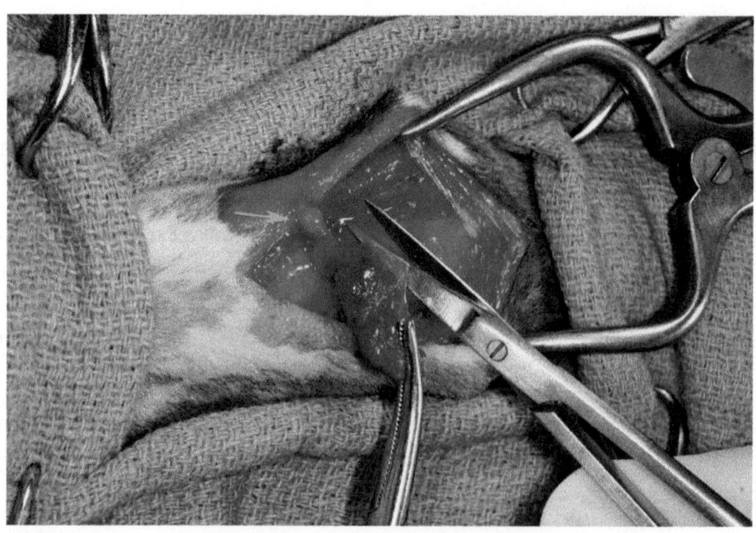

Figure 57-7 Ligate the caudal thyroid vessels and gently free the thyroid from the trachea, working toward the reflected parathyroid gland (arrow).

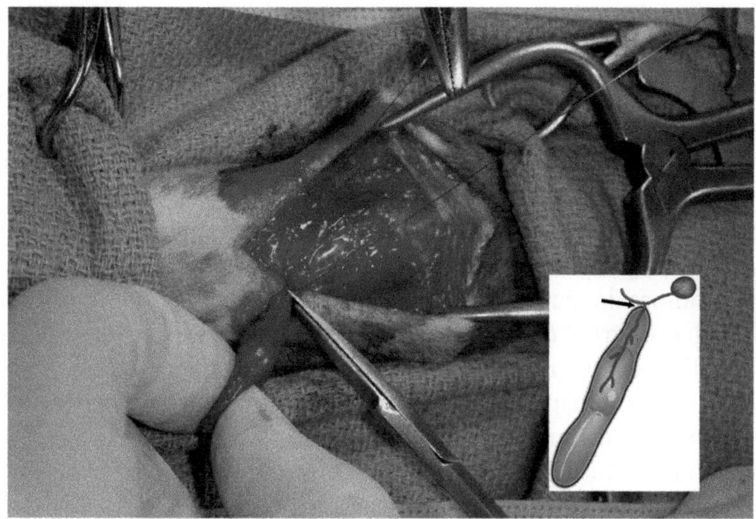

Figure 57-8 Ligate the cranial thyroid artery between the thyroid gland and the parathyroid artery branches (arrow, inset illustration) before transecting the pedicle.

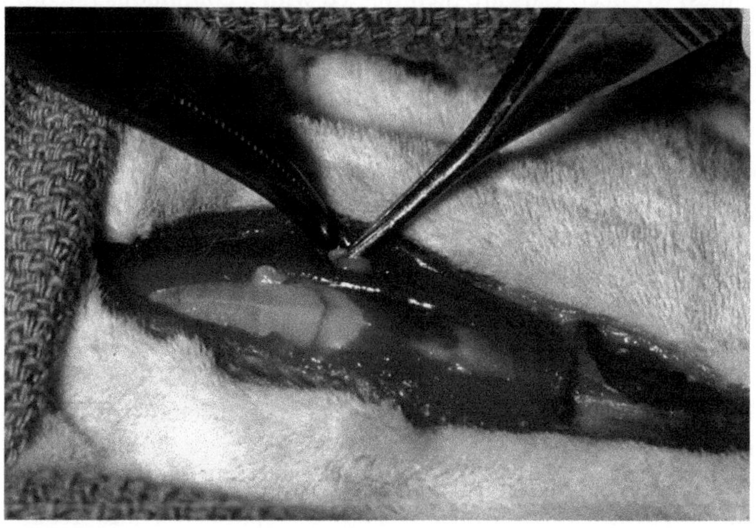

Figure 57-9 If the blood supply to the parathyroid is damaged, insert the gland into a pocket in the sternothyroideus or sternohyoideus muscle.

15. If a unilateral thyroidectomy is performed, examine the contralateral thyroid before closure. The thyroid should be small, thin, and pale. If the thyroid gland is normal in size, then it is most likely hyperplastic and should be removed simultaneously or in the future.
16. Appose the musculature along midline with 3-0 absorbable suture. Close the subcutaneous tissue and skin routinely.

Postoperative considerations

After surgery, cats are monitored for hemorrhage, arrhythmias, laryngeal dysfunction, and evidence of hypocalcemia. If parathyroid glands are left in situ, hypocalcemia usually occurs in ≤6% of cats when the procedure is performed by an experienced surgeon. Permanent hypothyroidism is possible after bilateral thyroidectomy, and thyroid hormone supplementation may be necessary in clinically affected animals. Restoration of euthyroidism is critical for managing cats with renal dysfunction. Thyrotoxic cardiac disease will resolve after thyroid function normalizes; persistent cardiac abnormalities may indicate other primary cardiac disease.

Hypocalcemia is the greatest immediate concern after bilateral thyroidectomy. Clinical signs include restlessness, facial or generalized muscle twitching, weakness, anorexia, panting, tetany, or seizures and may occur 12 hours to 6 days after parathyroid disruption. Only 60% of cats with severe hypocalcemia (<6.5 mg/dL) demonstrate clinical signs. Cats that have undergone bilateral parathyroid autotransplantation will become hypocalcemic within 24 hours but are usually normocalcemic within 14 days; 87% do not need calcium supplementation during the postoperative period. In cats that have undergone removal of all parathyroid glands, hypocalcemia can persist for 2 to 3 months, despite oral calcium supplementation.

In cats with acute signs of hypocalcemia, intravenous calcium gluconate (0.25–1.5 mL/kg of 10% calcium gluconate) is administered slowly (over 10 to 20 minutes) to effect. Cats are then treated with a continuous rate infusion of calcium gluconate (5–15 mg/kg/h IV). Alternatively, the IV dose of calcium gluconate can be diluted 1:3 or 1:4 with saline and administered subcutaneously in two or three sites two to four times daily. The electrocardiogram should be monitored during intravenous administration and treatment stopped if arrhythmias occur. Oral calcium carbonate (0.25–0.5 g calcium PO q12h) and calcitriol (0.25 μg/kg/day for 2 days, then taper over 5 days to 0.25 μg total q 24 h–48 h) are initiated once the cat is stable. Duration of oral supplementation depends on the extent of parathyroid damage and should be based on results of weekly calcium measurements. Tapering of all drugs can be attempted after 1 to 2 months. Cats that have lost all parathyroid tissue may be able to maintain normal serum calcium concentrations without supplementation 3 months after surgery but may become hypocalcemic in times of stress or with anorexia.

Other potential complications include anesthetic death, hemorrhage, development of Horner's syndrome or laryngeal paralysis, and recurrence of hyperthyroidism. Recurrence is seen in 10% of cats 1.5 to 2 years after surgery. Potential sources of recurrence include incomplete removal of a hyperplastic gland (e.g., leaving capsular remnants with attached thyroid tissue), disease in the contralateral thyroid gland, or hyperplastic ectopic tissue. Scintigraphy should be performed to determine the site of the remaining hyperplastic tissue; treatment may include radioactive iodine or additional surgery.

Bibliography

Birchard SJ: Thyroidectomy in the cat. Clin Tech Small Anim Pract 2006;21:29–33.

Carney HC, Ward CR, Bailey SJ, et al: 2016 AAFP guidelines for the management of Feline Hyperthyroidism. J Feline Med Surg 2016;18:400–416.

Naan EC et al: Results of thyroidectomy in 101 cats with hyperthyroidism. Vet Surg 2006;35:287–293.

Padgett SL et al: Efficacy of parathyroid gland autotransplantation in maintaining serum calcium concentrations after bilateral thyroparathyroidectomy in cats. J Am Anim Hosp Assoc 1998;34:219–224.
Peterson ME, Broome MR: Thyroid scintigraphy findings in 2096 cats with hyperthyroidism. Vet Radiol Ultrasound 2015;56:84–95.

Padgett SL et al. Efficacy of parathyroid gland autotransplantation in maintaining serum calcium concentrations after bilateral thyroparathyroidectomy in cats. J Am Anim Hosp Assoc 1998;34(3):219–224.
Peterson ME, Broome MR. Thyroid scintigraphy findings in 2096 cats with hyperthyroidism. Vet Radiol Ultrasound 2015;56:84–95.

Section 8 Tube Placement

Chapter 58
Esophagostomy Tube Placement

For animals with anorexia or lesions of the oral cavity or that are difficult to medicate, esophagostomy tubes provide an excellent avenue for administering enteral nutrition and medications. Esophagostomy tubes are quick, easy, and inexpensive to place. Unlike placement of gastrostomy tubes, esophagostomy tube placement requires no special equipment, and tubes can be removed at any time after insertion. Compared to pharyngostomy tubes, they will not cause upper airway obstruction, dysphagia, or pharyngeal irritation that stimulates vomiting. Large-bore tubes can be inserted in most patients, permitting infusion of a canned recovery diet. Although esophagostomy tubes are usually avoided in patients with persistent or frequent vomiting, patients with intermittent vomiting can often be fed successfully by slow continuous rate infusion through an esophagostomy tube. In fact, dogs with severe pancreatitis have fewer episodes of vomiting and regurgitation when fed via esophagostomy tube, as compared with parenteral nutrition.

Preoperative management

Animals should be fully anesthetized during placement because lightly anesthetized animals may awaken or reflexively bite down when the instrument or tube passes through the pharyngeal area, potentially injuring the veterinarian. Many veterinarians intubate the patients so that the trachea will be protected during the procedure; the endotracheal tube should be tied to the lower jaw, if possible, to keep it out of the way during esophagostomy tube placement. Some veterinarians place mouth gags; however, these tend to make tube placement more difficult.

Surgery

Esophagostomy tube size is based on the size of the patient. In a cat, a 12 or 14 French tube may be sufficient; in dogs, tube sizes may range up to 28 French. Commercial tubes of soft, flexible silicone are easy to place and are premade with a capped proximal end and an open distal end. Tubes with blind ends may

Manual of Small Animal Soft Tissue Surgery, Second Edition. Karen Tobias.
© 2017 John Wiley & Sons, Inc. Published 2017 by John Wiley & Sons, Inc.

clog more easily; therefore, if a red rubber catheter is used, the tube tip is usually removed. Tubes are advanced in the esophagus to the level of fifth to eighth intercostal space. Long tubes should be cut off to an appropriate length so that they won't inadvertently be advanced across the lower esophageal sphincter, which could result in gastric reflux with subsequent esophagitis.

Although often inserted in the left side of the esophagus, esophagostomy tubes can also be placed through the right side. The surgeon can determine the side on which the esophagus is most superficial during initial placement of the forceps.

Tubes are usually secured to the skin with a finger-trap suture. In animals with loose, stretchy skin, the tube can be inadvertently pulled part way out of the esophagus. In those animals, the attachment suture may need to include deeper muscle or even periosteum. Tube placement may need to be adjusted based on postoperative radiographs. If this is a concern, a separate suture loop should be placed in the skin while the animal is under anesthesia. That way, if repositioning must be performed when the animal is awake, the original finger trap can be cut, and the new finger trap secured to the skin via the suture loop.

Surgical technique: esophagostomy tube placement

1. Cut off any blind tube end, and shorten long tubes to an appropriate length (fig. 58-1). For larger tubes, cut the tip at an angle so that it will be easier to pull through the tissues.
2. Premeasure and mark the esophagostomy tube so that the designated length extends from the proposed (midcervical) skin insertion site to a point level with the fifth to eighth intercostal space.
3. Insert a closed curved Kelly, right angle, or regular or long narrow-tipped Carmalt forceps through the mouth and pharynx into the esophagus.
    a. Choose a forceps length that will reach several cm caudal to the level of the hyoid apparatus.
    b. Choose the narrowest tipped, longest forceps possible.
    c. Palpate the neck region for the forceps tips while angling the forceps tips toward one side of the neck and then the other to determine where the esophagus will be most superficial.

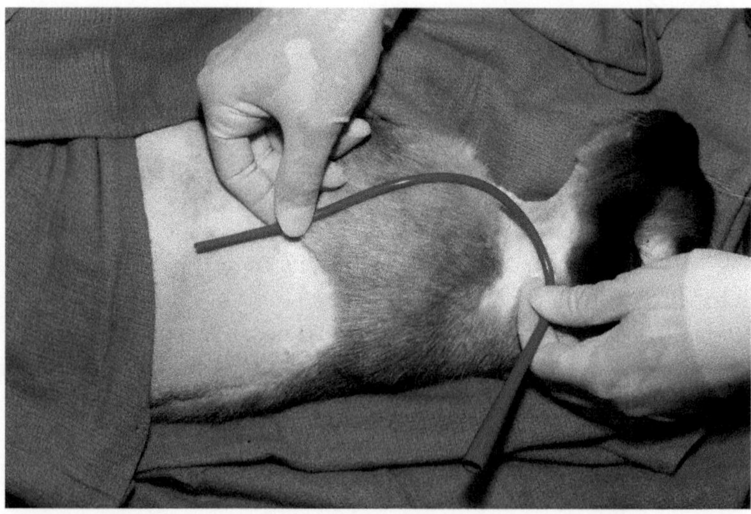

Figure 58-1 Cut the tube end off so that the tip will be level with the fifth to eighth intercostal space after placement.

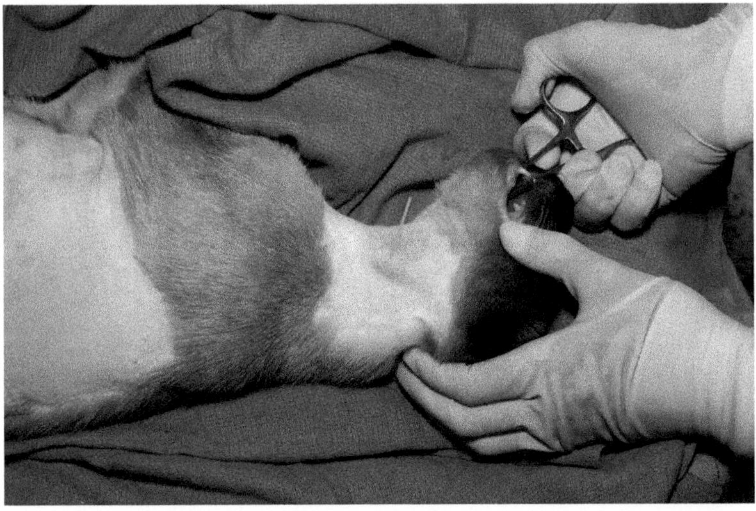

Figure 58-2 Insert a closed curved forceps through the mouth into the esophagus. Stabilize the forceps by placing the rings against the palm of your hand and angle the tips outward so that they visibly deviate the esophagus and overlying tissues (arrow).

4. Place the animal in lateral recumbency and clip, scrub, and drape the lateral cervical region where the esophagus is most superficial.
5. With handle rings grasped in your palm, insert the closed forceps through the mouth and down the esophagus into the midcervical region.
   a. Angle the forceps laterally so that the tips are palpable under the skin (fig. 58-2), dorsal to the jugular furrow.
   b. Stabilize the forceps by placing the rings against the palm of your dominant hand. Do not insert your fingers in the rings as this could result in inadvertent opening of the tips.
6. Make a loose fist with your nondominant hand, and press the medial side of your fist against the neck over the tips of the forceps (fig. 58-3). Keep your fist slightly opened so that the forceps tips, when pushed through the esophagus and muscle, will fall into the gap of your fist.
7. With your dominant hand, press firmly against the forceps rings with your palm. Simultaneously press your nondominant fist against the neck and around the forceps tips to force them through the esophageal wall,

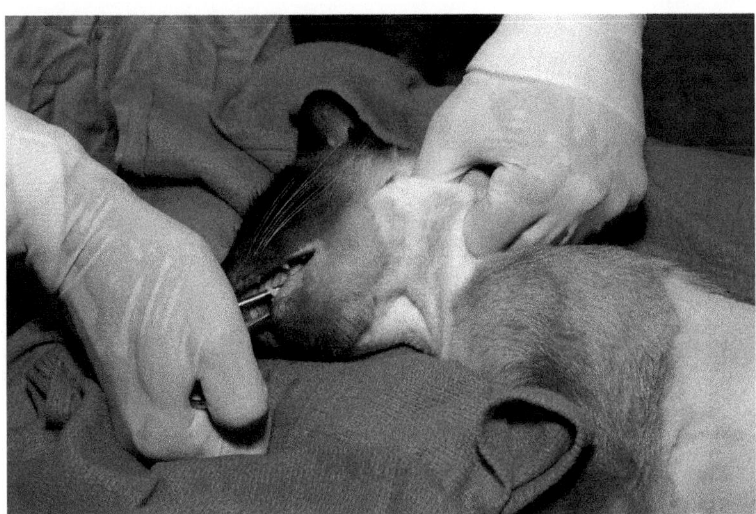

Figure 58-3 Force the forceps through the esophagus and subcutaneous tissues by pushing against the handle rings with the palm of one hand and applying pressure on the neck with the opposite fist.

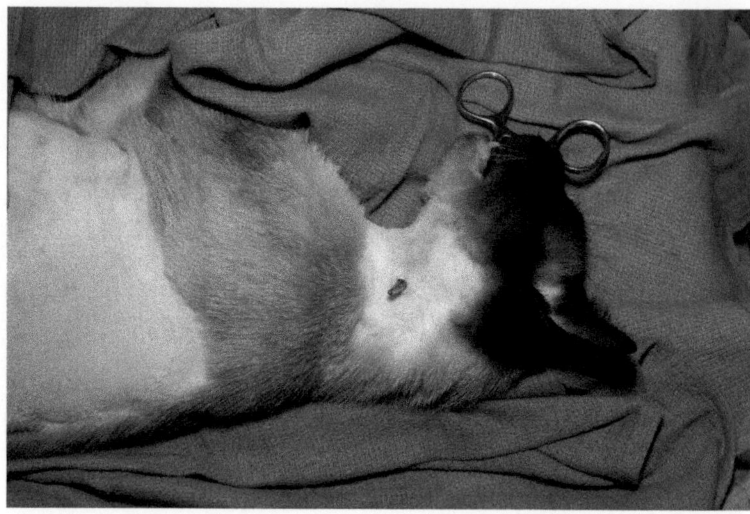

Figure 58-4 Incise the skin over the forceps to expose the tips.

cervical musculature, and subcutaneous tissue (fig. 58-3). Note: Before the forceps pass through esophagus and muscle, their tips will be indistinct. After they have pushed through, the tips are easily palpable through the skin and well defined.

8. Incise the skin over the tips of the forceps, and push the forceps through the incision (fig. 58-4).
9. Open the forceps slightly and insert the distal end of the tube into the forceps. Grasp the tube securely with the forceps tips and pull it through the skin incision, muscle, and esophageal perforation and then out the mouth (fig. 58-5).
10. Pull the tube through the neck as much as possible, while leaving several centimeters of the wide, proximal end extending from the neck incision. At this point, the proximal (syringe adaptor) end of the tube will be facing caudally and the distal end (tip) rostrally.
11. Redirect the distal end of the tube back into the oropharynx and esophagus (fig. 58-6) and, using fingers or forceps, feed the tube aborally as far as possible into the esophagus. Make sure the tube end is not entangled in the endotracheal tube cuff or tie.

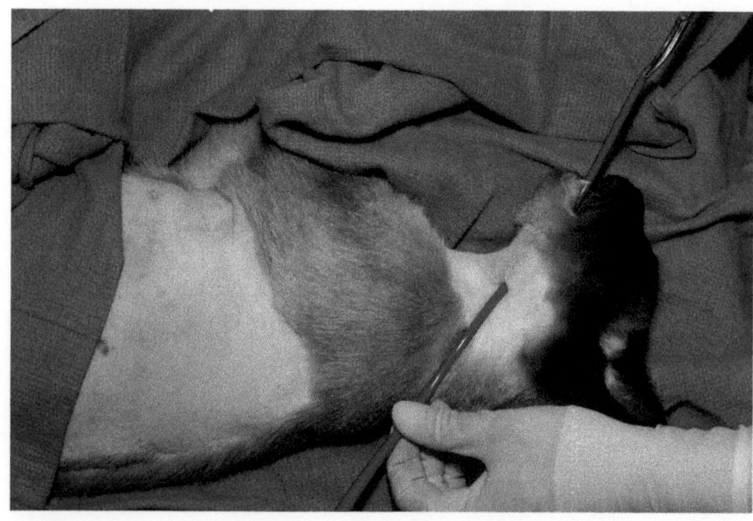

Figure 58-5 Grasp the tip of the tube with the forceps and pull it through the neck and out the mouth.

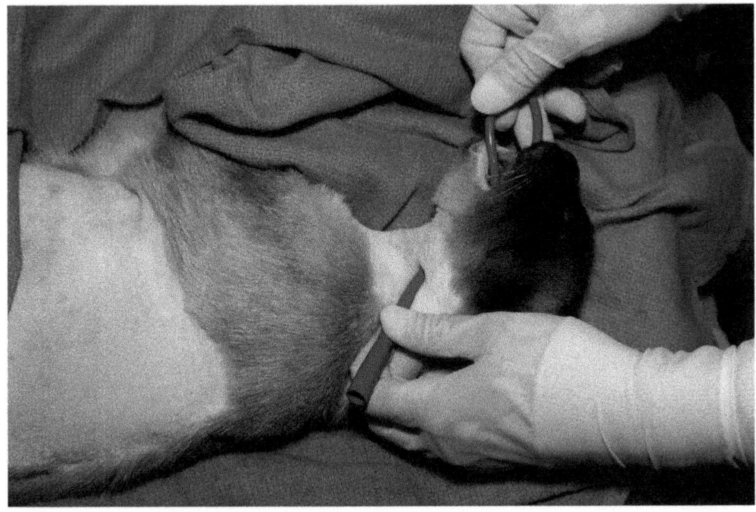

Figure 58-6 Redirect the tip of the tube down the esophagus. Note that the proximal portion of the tube is still oriented in a caudal-to-rostral position at this point.

12. The tube will usually be kinked or folded in the oropharynx or esophagus at this point. To remove the kink and reorient the tube direction, gently retract the proximal (syringe adaptor) end of the tube out through the skin incision while continuing to force the intraoral portion of the tube into the pharynx with fingers or an instrument (fig. 58-7). When the kinked region appears through the skin incision, allow the tube to straighten out, and feed it aborally (fig. 58-8). If the kink has been successfully removed, the tube will automatically be oriented with the proximal (syringe adaptor) end directed rostrally.
13. Advance the tube down the esophagus until the premeasured mark on the tube is at the level of the skin, and cap the tube. The tube tip should not extend beyond the ninth rib.
14. Do not place a purse-string suture around the tube stoma. Secure the tubing to the skin locally with a finger-trap pattern (see pp. 497–501) attached directly to the skin or to a suture loop in the skin. In cats, include underlying muscle or periosteum of the atlas wing in the skin bite to prevent tube migration with skin movement.

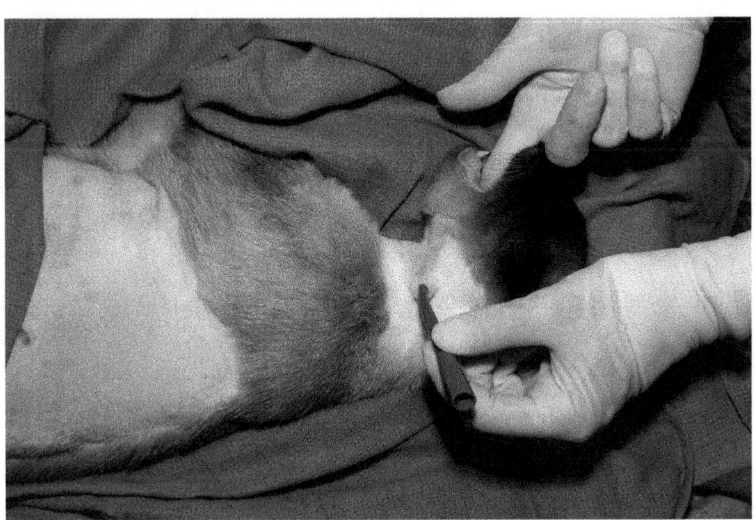

Figure 58-7 Retract the proximal, syringe adaptor end of the tube out of the neck while pushing the oral portion of the tube into the pharynx until the tube unkinks and its position changes to a rostral-to-caudal orientation.

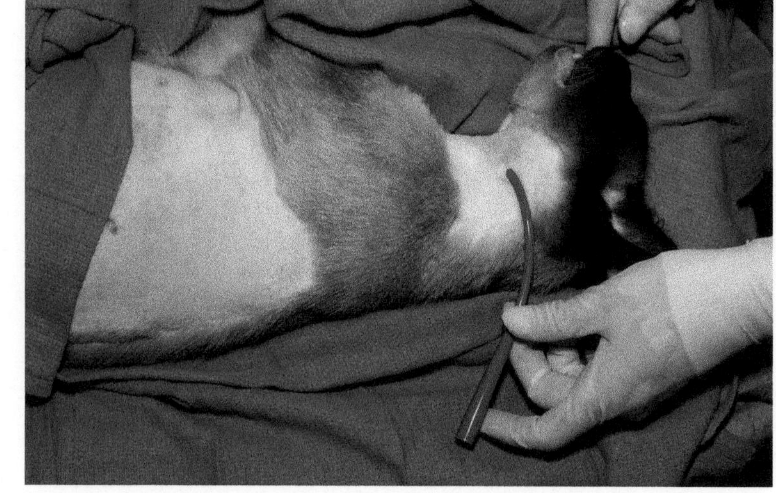

Figure 58-8 Adjust the tube to the predetermined length so that the tip will be level with a point between the fifth and eighth intercostal spaces

15. Cover the stoma with a thin layer of antibacterial dressing and non-adhesive pad, and bandage the neck loosely, with the esophagostomy tube exiting dorsally behind the head.

Postoperative considerations

Tube placement can be evaluated with a postoperative lateral thoracic radiograph. During placement, tubes can occasionally get wrapped around the endotracheal tube or its tie, which may affect the esophagostomy tube's position or even the ability to extubate the animal. Affected animals should be reanesthetized and the tube position examined and adjusted.

The tube can be protected from self-trauma by use of an Elizabethan collar or a customized, commercial fabric neck wrap to prevent premature removal. The nonadhesive dressing over the tube exit site should be changed daily to allow evaluation and cleansing of the stoma. Feedings can be started once the patient is awake and able to maintain a sitting position. Canned recovery diets are easiest to use because they are unlikely to clog the tube. Depending on caloric needs, cats are usually fed 180 to 250 mL/day, divided into four feedings (approximately 60 mL/feeding), once maintenance supplementation is feasible. Volumes fed to dogs vary with the size of the animal (maximum bolus, 15 mL/kg). Calculated volumes should include any water used to meet fluid requirements or to flush the tube. Initially, small meals (5–15 mL in cats; 1–4 mL/kg in dogs) are given every 3 to 4 hours until the animal has acclimated to the diet and volume; the volume is gradually increased over 4 days. Constant infusions of liquid diet can also be used, starting at 1 to 2 mL/kg/hour, and increasing to 4 mL/kg/hour. If patients show any signs of nausea, feedings are discontinued and a reduced volume of dilute, warm, liquid diet is infused more slowly at the next feeding.

Tubes should be flushed with 5 to 10 mL water before and after each use to prevent clogging. If the tube clogs, it can often be unblocked by filling the tube with water, then suctioning, flushing, and refilling the tube several times over an hour to soften the clog.

Once the animal is eating voluntarily and can maintain adequate nutrition, the tube is pulled. The finger-trap suture is cut, and the tube is occluded and gently pulled from the stoma. The wound is cleaned and bandaged daily until it has healed by second intention. Tubes can be removed immediately after placement or left in for months. Tubes left in long term may degrade or become brittle, especially those of red rubber; because a fibrous fistula is present after several weeks, the old tube can be pulled and a new one inserted immediately through the fistula.

Complications include local inflammation and pyoderma, swelling of the head from overly tight bandages, peristomal cellulitis from subcutaneous leakage, and clogging of the tube. Cellulitus is more common when the stoma has been sutured with a purse string. Inflammation and infection around the stoma site will resolve with tube removal and local therapy. Hemorrhage is rare as long as the tips of the forceps have been forced through esophagus, muscle, and subcutis before the skin incision is made. Animals can vomit smaller, soft tubes out of their mouths, so that the tube simultaneously extends from the neck, through the pharynx, and out the oral cavity. This is unlikely to occur with larger, stiffer tubes. Tubes are difficult to place in some large dogs because of limitations in forceps length. Percutaneous feeding tube applicators can also be used in place of forceps.

Rarely, the esophagus is torn during tube placement, resulting in esophageal leakage, abscessation, and possible sepsis. Tears may occur because the tissues are friable (e.g., in very young animals), the forceps are opened too wide while attempting to grasp the tube, the tube is stiff, or multiple attempts are made to pass the forceps through the esophagus or pull the tube through the neck. Some tears will heal with tube removal, while others require surgical closure and open wound management.

Bibliography

Devitt CM and Seim HB: Clinical evaluation of tube esophagostomy in small animals. J Am Anim Hosp 1997;33:55–60.

Han E: Esophageal and gastric feeding tubes in ICU patients. Clin Tech Small Anim Pract 2004;19:22–31.

Ireland LM et al: A comparison of owner management and complications in 67 cats with esophagostomy and percutaneous endoscopic gastrostomy feeding tubes. J Am Anim Hosp Assoc 2003;39:241–246.

Mansfield CS, James FE, Steiner JM, et al: A pilot study to assess tolerability of early enteral nutrition via esophagostomy tube feeding in dogs with severe acute pancreatitis. J Vet Intern Med 2011;25:419–425.

Mazzaferro EM: Esophagostomy tubes: don't underutilize them! J Vet Emerg Crit Care 2001;11:153–156.

Chapter 59
Tracheostomy Tube Placement

The primary indication for temporary tube tracheostomy is emergency relief of upper airway obstruction from oral, nasal, pharyngeal, or laryngeal disease. Tracheostomy tubes are occasionally placed to facilitate surgery of the oral cavity, pharynx, or larynx or anesthetic recovery after those procedures. Ideally, animals are initially intubated with a small endotracheal tube, so that the tracheostomy site can be clipped, aseptically prepared, and approached using appropriate surgical techniques. Unfortunately, some patients arrive in respiratory distress and require tracheostomy under less than ideal conditions. A pack specifically prepared for tracheostomy should therefore always be available for emergency situations.

Preoperative management

Oxygen is administered by face mask or nasal catheter until intubation. If the obstruction is severe and acute, a 20 gauge needle, attached to an extension set, is inserted through the cricothyroid ligament. The extension set is hooked to a 3-ml syringe barrel with the flange end cut off; the cut end can be fitted into oxygen tubing. The oxygen source is set at a flow rate of 150–200 mL/kg/min, and the needle is held in place manually by one team member while another gathers materials for intravenous catheter placement, anesthesia, and tracheostomy.

If possible, an intravenous catheter should be placed for administration of fluids and drugs. Sedatives and analgesics are administered to patients with respiratory distress, since tachypnea from stress and pain will increase negative airway pressure, exacerbating upper airway swelling and collapse. Opioids and reversible drugs (e.g., dexmedetomidine) are suitable as preanesthetic agents. Glucocorticoids and furosemide may reduce local edema. In intubated animals, anesthetic gas leakage may occur once the trachea is opened, unless the cuff can be inflated distal to the site; therefore, intravenous anesthetics (e.g., fentanyl or propofol) should be available. If the animal can be intubated transorally, further diagnostics (e.g., thoracic radiographs, blood gases, serum chemistries, oral examination) can be performed before surgery. In some animals a stylet (e.g., a rigid polypropylene catheter) can be placed in the

Manual of Small Animal Soft Tissue Surgery, Second Edition. Karen Tobias.
© 2017 John Wiley & Sons, Inc. Published 2017 by John Wiley & Sons, Inc.

trachea first to serve as a guide for the endotracheal tube, which is fed over the stylet into the trachea. If the patient cannot be intubated, then surgery should proceed quickly.

Surgery is performed with the animal in dorsal recumbency and the neck extended. A rolled towel is placed under the neck to elevate it, and the front legs are pulled caudally. If there is time, the ventral neck should be clipped and prepped from the intermandibular space to the thoracic inlet. If the animal is in imminent danger of respiratory arrest, the hair is soaked with chlorhexidine solution and parted on midline before incision. The hair can be clipped and the area cleaned once the tracheostomy tube is in place.

Surgery

Tracheal incisions for tube placement can be made transversely or vertically and as a linear, U-, I-, or H-shaped incision. Transverse tracheostomy is easiest, can be performed quickly with a blade, and does not cause any clinically significant postoperative stenosis.

Tracheostomy tubes should be approximately one-half of the diameter of the trachea so that the animal can breathe around it if the tube becomes clogged. For patients in which the tracheostomy tube will remain in place after recovery, tubes with inner cannulas (double lumen tubes) are preferred because the inner cannula can be removed, cleaned, and reinserted without disrupting the tracheostomy site. Double-lumen tubes are usually 5 mm or more in inner diameter (≥8 mm outer diameter) and are not available for smaller patients. If a single-lumen tube is used, it should be replaced once or twice daily. Cuffed tubes are only necessary in patients that require mechanical ventilation or gas anesthesia or are at risk for aspiration pneumonia. Cuffs should be high volume and low pressure to reduce the risk of tracheal inflammation and necrosis.

If tracheostomy tubes are not immediately available, one can be fashioned from a regular endotracheal tube. These "homemade" tracheostomy tubes are also useful in dogs with necks too thick for commercial tracheostomy tubes (e.g., English bulldogs). The connector is removed from the tube end, and the tube is cut vertically on both sides (avoiding the cuff tubing) to make two flaps. The connector is inserted back into the shortened tube, and each flap is perforated and threaded with umbilical tape to make ties for securing the tube in place.

Surgical technique: tracheostomy tube placement

1. Make a 4- to 10-cm ventral midline skin incision, starting over the cricoid cartilage and extending caudally.
2. Dissect through the subcutaneous tissues and sphincter colli muscle to expose the paired sternohyoideus muscles (fig. 59-1). The sphincter colli muscle fibers decussate and therefore must be transected (see fig. 57-1) rather than separated.
3. Separate the sternohyoideus muscles on midline with a blade or scissors (fig. 59-2) and retract them with Gelpi or Weitlaner retractors. During emergency tracheostomy, use the thumb and index finger of your free hand to grasp the trachea and simultaneously force the muscles laterally.

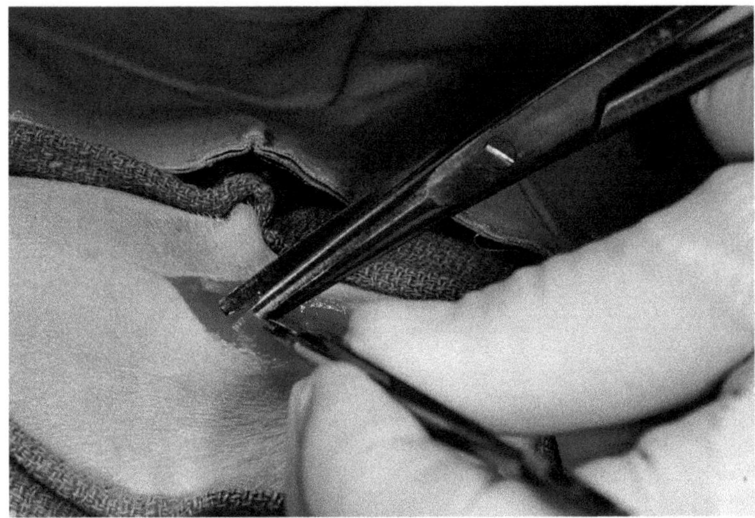

Figure 59-1 Incise the skin, subcutaneous fat, and sphincter colli muscle caudal to the thyroid cartilage.

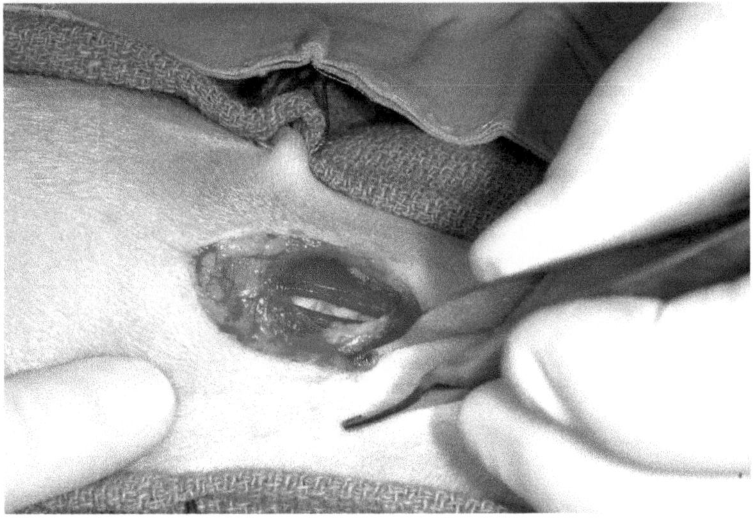

Figure 59-2 The sternohyoideus muscles have been bluntly separated along the midline.

4. With a scalpel blade, make a transverse incision through the annular ligament of the trachea between the third and fourth or fourth and fifth cartilage rings (fig. 59-3).
   a. If the animal is intubated with the endotracheal cuff inflated, deflate the cuff temporarily and make the incision carefully to avoid damaging the cuff.
   b. To avoid damaging the recurrent laryngeal nerves, do not extend the incision more than halfway around the circumference of the trachea.
5. Place 0 nylon or polypropylene stay sutures through the opening and around the cartilage ring above and below the incision (fig. 59-4). Temporarily secure the ends of each suture with a hemostat.
   a. These stay sutures will be left in place after surgery until the tracheostomy tube is removed.
   b. If emergency tracheostomy is required, place stay sutures after the tracheostomy tube is inserted.

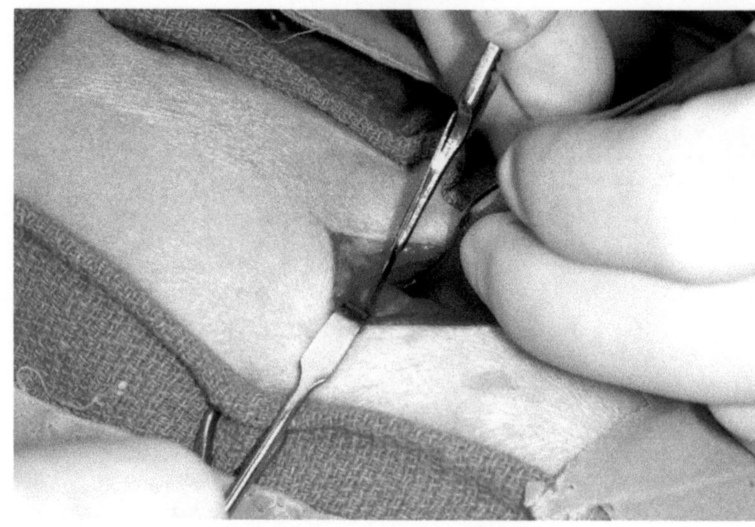

Figure 59-3 Incise the ventral aspect of the annular ligament between the third and fourth or fourth and fifth cartilage rings of the trachea.

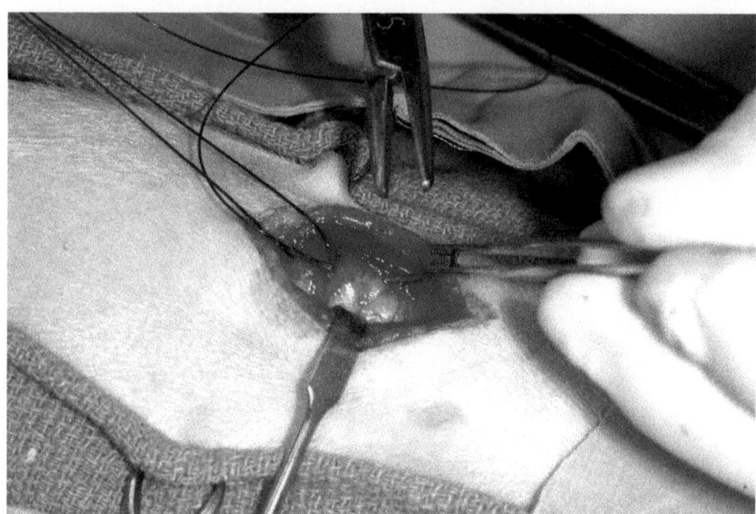

Figure 59-4 If the animal is already intubated, place stay sutures around the rings adjacent to the incision. If the animal is not intubated, place the tracheostomy tube first before placing stay sutures.

6. Open the tracheal incision.
   a. If stay sutures have been placed, pull the sutures up and away from each other to expose the tracheal lumen (fig. 59-5). Extend the tracheal incision as needed to accommodate the tube.
   b. If the animal must be intubated before stay sutures are placed, hold the tracheal incision open with the jaws of a hemostat or the blunt end of a scalpel handle during tube insertion.
7. If necessary, suction any blood or mucus from the trachea.
8. Insert the tracheostomy tube.
   a. If present, remove the transoral endotracheal tube.
   b. If available, place the plastic obturator into the tracheostomy tube, and insert the tube into the tracheal lumen.
   c. Remove the obturator and, if one is included, insert the inner tube cannula and lock it in place.

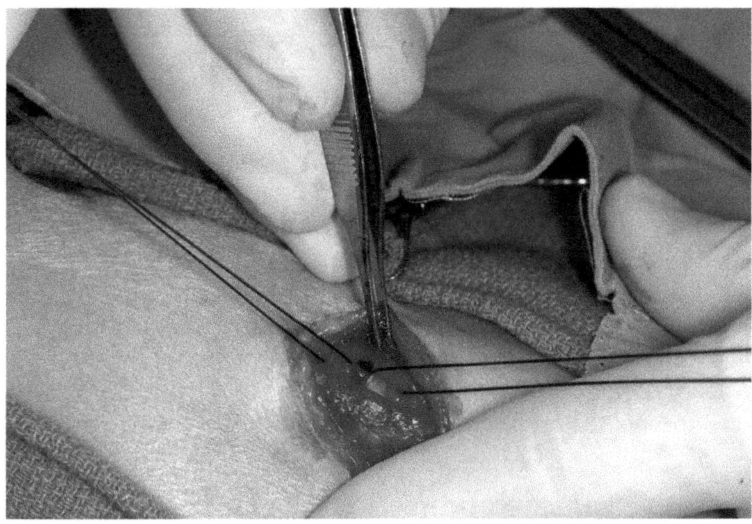

Figure 59-5 Retract the stay sutures and extend the annular ligament incision to permit passage of the tracheostomy tube.

   d. Resect a semicircular portion of the cartilage rings if tube insertion is difficult.
   e. If gas anesthetic is being administered or ventilation is needed, inflate the tracheostomy tube cuff gently until a peak inspiratory pressure of 15–20 mL/kg can be achieved.

9. Attach the oxygen hose to the tracheostomy tube (fig. 59-6). An elbow attachment will reduce the amount of torque placed by the hose. Make sure the tube does not become dislodged at this point.
10. Secure the tube to the patient by tying a piece of umbilical tape to each side of the fenestrated collar or flange on the tube, wrap the ends around the neck, and tie them in a double bow.
11. Leave the skin incision around the trachesotomy open for at least 3 cm in both directions to facilitate future access. If the skin incision is long, suture the skin cranial and caudal to the tracheostomy site with interrupted sutures.

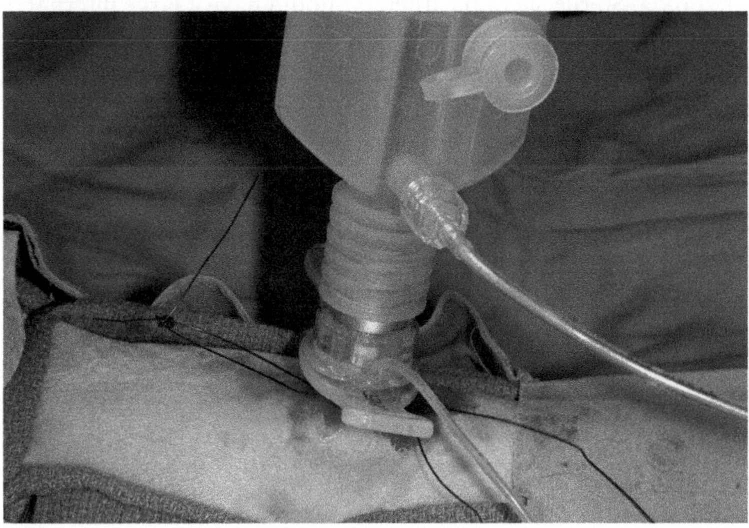

Figure 59-6 Transfer any oxygen source to the tracheostomy tube. Tie knots in the stay suture ends and secure them with tape so that they are available for later use.

12. In dogs with loose cervical skin, pull the skin folds away from the tracheostomy site and tack them with interrupted sutures laterally or dorsally to keep the folds tied back.
13. Secure each stay suture by taping the two ends together, and label the tapes "up" or "down." These sutures can be used later to hold the tracheotomy open if the tube needs to be replaced.
14. Place a thin layer of antimicrobial dressing over any open wounds and around the tracheostomy site, leaving the stay sutures exposed.
15. Place a loose, lint-free, thin wrap around the neck to hold the dressing in place, leaving the tracheostomy tube opening, cuff inflation port, and stay sutures exposed.

Postoperative considerations

After recovery, the animal must be monitored carefully for tube obstruction or dislodgement. In awake animals that are not being ventilated, the tube cuff is kept deflated to reduce the chance of tracheal obstruction or damage (fig. 59-7). Skin around the tracheostomy tube should be cleaned daily to remove debris, reduce bacterial load, and make the patient more comfortable. Initially the tracheostomy tube may need to be cleaned every 15 minutes to 3 hours, depending on the amount of secretions produced. Patients with minimal secretions can be suctioned and cleaned every 4 to 6 hours. Animals should be monitored for evidence of distress, such as dyspnea, coughing, or pawing at the tube, that may indicate irritation or partial obstruction necessitating more frequent tube maintenance.

To clean a double lumen tube, the inner cannula is removed, soaked in an antiseptic bath, and rinsed. The outer tube is instilled with saline and suctioned, and then the clean inner cannula is reinserted and locked in place. Single-lumen tubes must be sterilely suctioned in situ to remove secretions and are usually replaced every 12 to 24 hours. Infusion of 0.5 to 5 mL of sterile saline several minutes prior to suctioning will loosen secretions and humidify the airway. If secretions become thick, a few drops of dilute acetylcysteine (1:10) can be dripped into the tube. Animals should be preoxygenated for 3–5 minutes before suctioning, which should last less than 15 seconds to reduce the risk of hypoxia. Sterile suction catheters should have a large internal diameter and an external diameter that is less than half of the tracheostomy tube. Suction catheters should not be forced through obstructed tubes, since the clogging material could be ejected into the airway. If the tracheostomy tube lumen becomes narrowed by hardened secretions, the tube should be replaced under sedation. Suctioning the patient soon after it has eaten may induce vomiting.

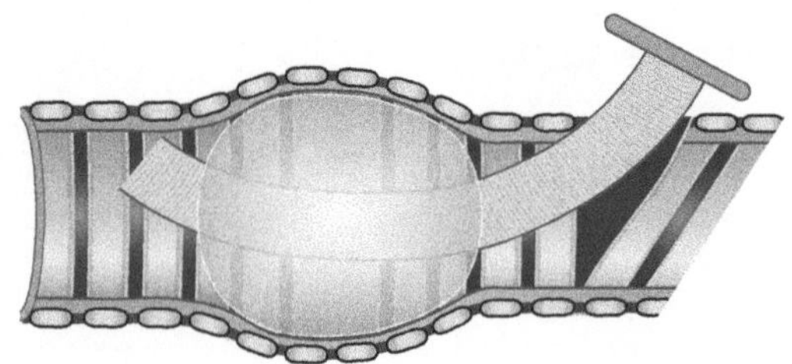

Figure 59-7 This animal is at risk for obstruction because the tube is too long and curved excessively. The external flange on the tube should lie parallel to the trachea so that the distal tube opening is parallel to the tracheal rings. Cuff overinflation can damage the trachea; the cuff is not inflated unless the animal is being ventilated or receiving anesthetic gas.

Humidification of inspired air reduces lung damage from dry air and loosens secretions, making tube maintenance easier. Because animals with tracheostomy tubes have greater fluid needs, intravenous fluids may be required to prevent dehydration. The patient should be weighed once or twice daily to monitor hydration status.

To reduce the risk of obstruction or other complications, tubes should be removed as soon as the upper airway obstruction has resolved. If the tube does not completely fill the airway, then presence of oral or nasal air movement may be evaluated by obstructing the tube. Some clinicians will remove the tube, replace it with one of smaller diameter, and then monitor the patient for dyspnea. During tube removal, a clean replacement tube and induction agents should be available and the taped ends of the tracheal stay sutures easily reachable. The tube should be immediately replaced if the patient shows any distress after extubation, and a permanent tracheostomy should be considered if the animal is still tube dependent after 5 days. After tube removal, the stoma will usually heal by second intention. The stomal site should be covered with a light wrap of loosely woven gauze until airway obstruction is no longer a concern. After that it can be covered more securely with a nonadhesive dressing and padded bandage. Patients should not be bathed or allowed to swim until the wound has healed.

Complications are expected in most animals with tracheostomy tubes, either because of the tube or the underlying disease, and close monitoring is required. Reported complications include tube obstruction or dislodgement (each reported in approximately 20% of dogs), pneumomediastinum, pneumothorax, aspiration pneumonia, stoma swelling, subcutaneous emphysema, hemorrhage, infection, and laryngeal paralysis. Large tubes may cause pressure necrosis with subsequent tracheal stenosis once the tube is removed. Tubes with necks that are too long for the patient may tilt within the tracheal lumen, obstructing the distal opening of the tube as it is tilted cranially and against the tracheal wall (fig. 59-7). Rarely, the tracheostomy site will form a tracheal fistula that requires resection and closure.

Bibliography

Mazzaferro EM: Temporary tracheostomy. Topics Compan An Med 2013;28:74–78.

Nicholson I, Baines S: Complications associated with temporary tracheostomy tubes in 42 dogs (1998 to 2007). J Small Anim Pract 2012;53:108–114.

Rozansk E and Chan DL: Approach to the patient with respiratory distress. Vet Clin N Am Small Anim Pract 2005;35:307–317.

Tillson M: Tracheostomy. NAVC Clinician's Brief 2008;6:21–24.

Chapter 60
Thoracostomy Tube Placement

The most common indication for thoracostomy or "chest" tube placement is for repeated removal of intrapleural air or fluid. Thoracostomy tubes also provide an avenue for pleural lavage in animals with pyothorax and for postoperative administration of regional analgesics after thoracotomy.

An alternative to a thoracostomy tube is a small-bore (10 to 14 French) multifenestrated drainage tube; these tubes have been used successfully to manage animals with pyothorax, pneumothorax, and chylothorax. Small-bore tubes are placed with a modified Seldinger technique, similar to a jugular catheter. The animal is placed in sternal or lateral recumbency, and the local skin is clipped and prepped. An introducer catheter is placed under the skin over the 9th intercostal space and tunnelled to the caudal aspect of the 7th or 8th intercostal space, where it is inserted into the pleural cavity. The catheter is directed into the dorsal half of the lateral thorax for a pneumothorax and the ventral half of thorax for pleural effusion. The introducer stylet is removed and replaced with a J-wire that is threaded cranially for 12 to 20 cm; the introducer catheter is removed from the guide wire, and the small-bore drainage tube is advanced over the guidewire into the pleural cavity. The tube is secured to the skin, and the chest is drained. For patients with pyothorax, the tubes can also be used for intermittent pleural lavage, which likely helps to keep them patent.

Preoperative management

Thoracic radiographs should be examined for masses or pleural adhesions; thoracostomy tubes should be placed away from those structures. A pleural fluid sample should be submitted for cytology, culture, and chemical analysis. For example, chylous fluid will have a triglyceride content greater than that of peripheral blood.

Appropriate connectors, syringes, clamps, and suture should be available before tube placement. A second tube, the same length as the one to be inserted, should be available to check the final tube position. Thoracostomy tubes are most easily placed under general anesthesia; if placed under sedation, opioids are administered for analgesia, and skin and intercostal blocks are performed at the proposed sites of skin incision and tube insertion. Animals should be

Manual of Small Animal Soft Tissue Surgery, Second Edition. Karen Tobias.
© 2017 John Wiley & Sons, Inc. Published 2017 by John Wiley & Sons, Inc.

preoxygenated before anesthetic induction. In animals with significant fluid accumulation and respiratory compromise, pleural effusion should be drained by thoracocentesis before anesthesia is induced. The lateral thorax should be clipped and prepped from the scapula to the thirteenth rib. The thorax is draped so that the skin is visible over the sixth through tenth intercostal spaces. During anesthesia, the patient is manually ventilated six to eight times per minute, except when the chest tube is being inserted and advanced through the intercostal space.

Surgery

Red rubber catheters or commercial trocar tubes are commonly used for thoracic drainage. Commercial thoracostomy tubes contain a trocar-tipped metal stylet that facilitates rapid placement and reduces the risk of air leakage; however, the stylet is sharp and can potentially puncture the lungs during insertion. Commercial thoracostomy tubes are stiffer than red rubber catheters and less prone to kinking as they cross the rib caudal to the intercostal perforation. Because of their stiffness, however, they may cause more post-operative discomfort and can be more easily dislodged.

Thoracostomy tube size is based on patient size and expected use. For thick effusions, tube size should be roughly comparable to the diameter of the mainstem bronchus and must be narrower than the width of the intercostal space. In cats and small dogs, 14 or 16 French tubes are often placed. In large dogs, tube size may be 24 to 36 French. Patients with pyothorax may need bilateral, large-diameter tubes if the exudate is tenacious. A smaller tube diameter may be sufficient in animals with pneumothorax.

In animals undergoing thoracotomy, multifenestrated continuous suction (e.g., Jackson Pratt) drains can be placed for postoperative drainage and analgesic administration. These drains are less likely to clog, kink, or dislodge than stiff, cylindrical tubes. The soft, narrow, flexible tubing extending from the drain passes easily within the intercostal space and over the ribs, reducing discomfort.

When placing a thoracostomy tube, the skin incision should be located several centimeters caudal and dorsal to the site of intercostal perforation. This will limit passage of atmospheric air or intrapleural fluid into or out of the thorax, respectively. If available, an assistant can pull the lateral thoracic skin cranioventrally. The thoracostomy tube can then be inserted directly through the skin overlying the proposed site of intercostal perforation. Once the tube is in place, the skin is returned to its normal position so that it covers several centimeters of the tube.

Surgical technique: trocar tube

1. Preplace a clamp on the tube; leave the clamp open. Verify that the stylet is inserted fully into the tube so that its trocar tip protrudes beyond the tube end.

2. Make a 1-cm skin incision over the ninth or tenth intercostal space (fig. 60-1). The incision should be located at the junction of the dorsal and middle two-thirds of the thoracic height.

3. Insert the tube with trocar stylet into the skin incision and direct it cranioventrally.

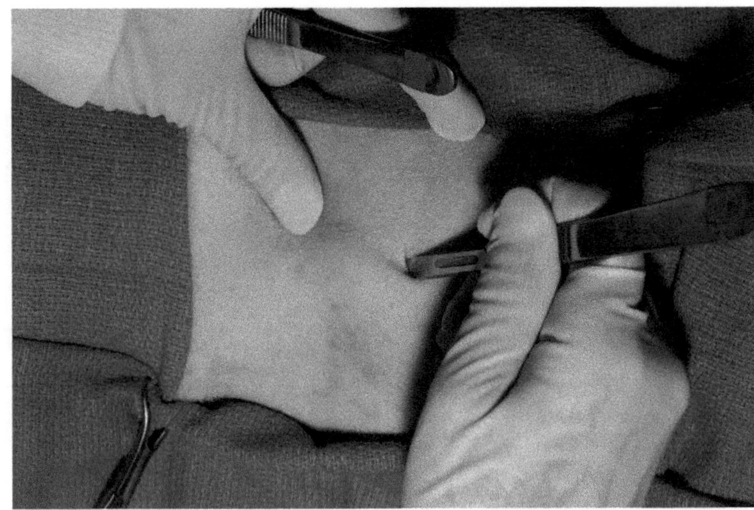

Figure 60-1 Make an incision over the dorsal third of a ninth or tenth intercostal space.

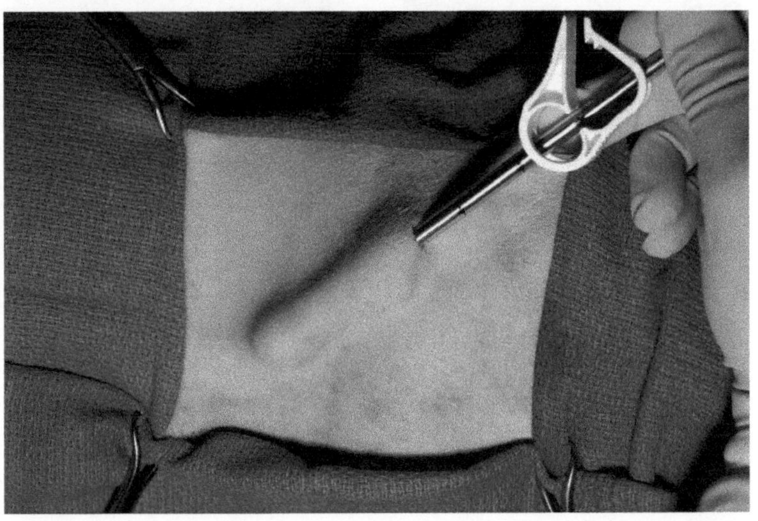

Figure 60-2 After the clamp is placed on the tube, tunnel the tube with trocar-tipped stylet cranioventrally to the seventh or eighth intercostal space. In this dog, the head is to the left.

4. Tunnel the tube under the skin to the caudal half of the seventh or eighth intercostal space, at a level midway between the dorsal and ventral borders of the thorax (fig. 60-2). The nerves and vessels run along the caudal aspects of the ribs.
5. Tilt the tube upright so it is perpendicular to the thoracic wall and table (fig. 60-3).
   a. This will position the tube for intercostal perforation and will simultaneously retract the skin.
   b. Alternatively, have an assistant pull the skin of the cranial half of the thorax forward.
6. Tightly grip the tube in the fist of your nondominant hand (fig. 60-3) at a distance from the skin slightly greater than the anticipated thickness of the thoracic wall. Your fist will act as a stopper to prevent the tube from penetrating the thorax too deeply.

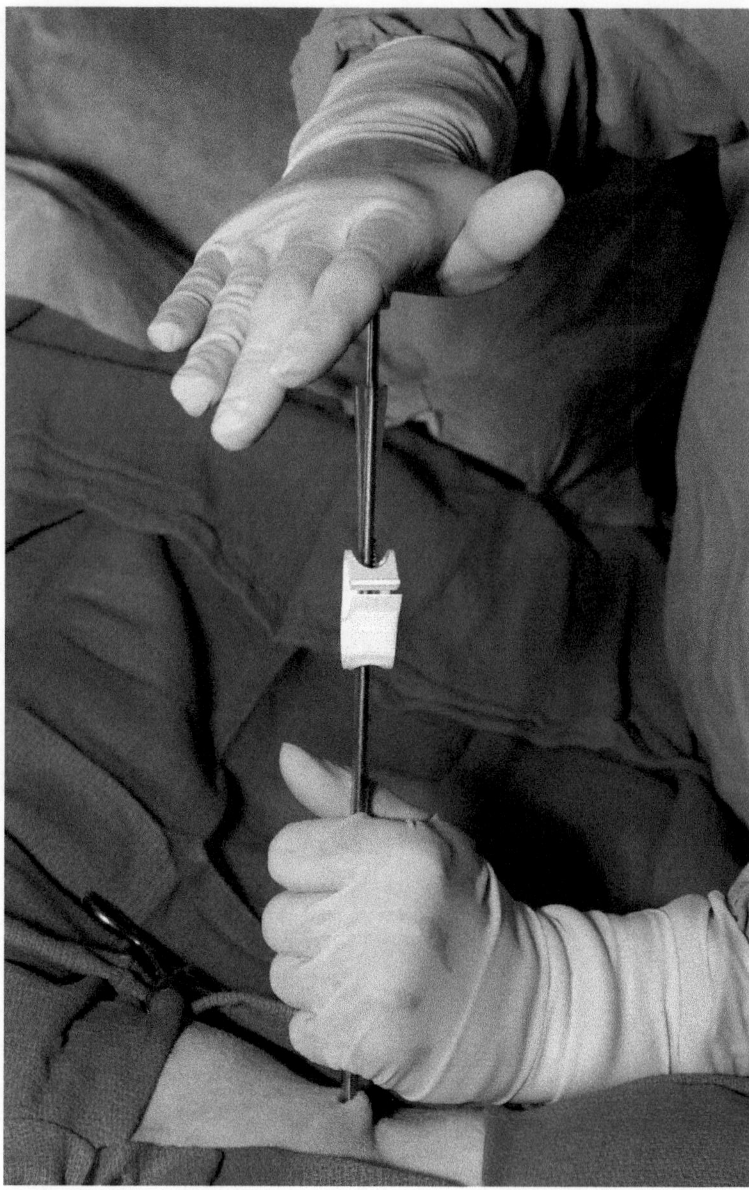

Figure 60-3 Tilt the tube perpendicular to the thoracic wall, and grasp the tube in your nondominant fist 2 to 3 cm above the skin. Press or hit the end of the tube to pop it through the intercostal space and pleura, using your nondominant fist to stop the tube from penetrating too deeply.

7. Press firmly on, or hit, the end of the tube with your dominant hand to push or pop the tube through the intercostal space into the chest (fig. 60-3).
8. Tilt the external portion of the tube caudally so that it is more parallel to the thoracic wall; this will point the trocar stylet tip more toward the ribs and away from the lungs. Advance the tube and stylet 1 cm into the pleural space between the lungs and thoracic wall. If the tube will not advance, then you are not completely through the pleura.
9. Hold the stylet stable with one hand and, with the other hand, advance the tube off the stylet and several centimeters farther into the thoracic cavity (fig. 60-4).
10. Retract the stylet out of the intrapleural portion of the chest tube. Leave the stylet temporarily in the extrathoracic portion of the tube.

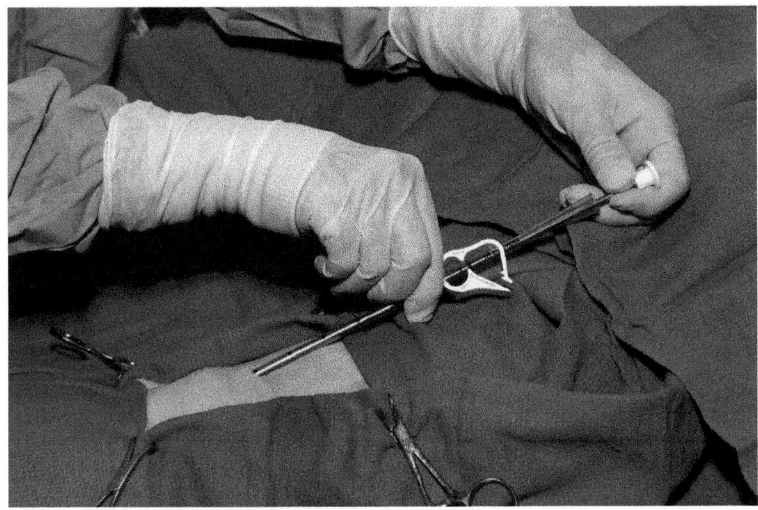

Figure 60-4 Lower the tube toward the thoracic wall, and advance the tube cranially off the stylet and into the thoracic cavity.

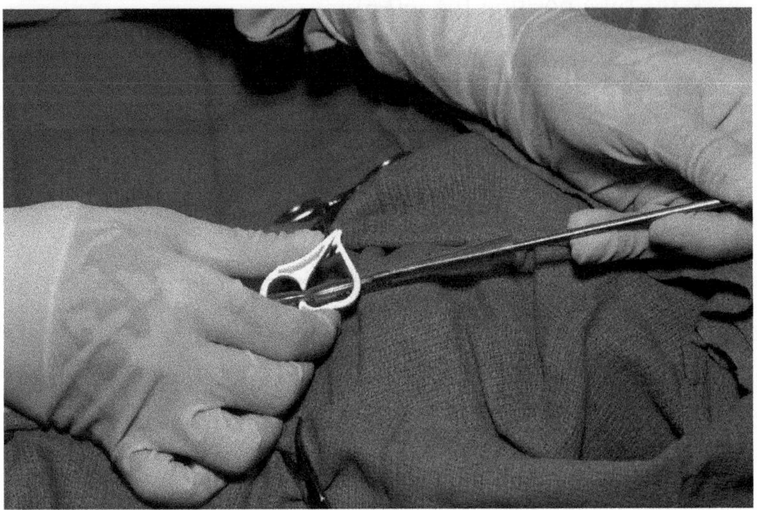

Figure 60-5 Clamp the tube once the stylet is partially retracted.

11. Clamp the tube between the skin incision and stylet before completely removing the stylet (fig. 60-5).
12. Attach the connector, three-way stopcock, and syringe to the tube end.
13. Release the clamp and suction out the pleural space.
    a. To suction out the chest, turn the long end of the three-way stopcock lever toward the open port (the port perpendicular to the tube and syringe) and apply suction with the syringe. To empty the syringe, turn the long end of the three-way stopcock lever toward the tube and away from the syringe and apply pressure to the syringe to blow the contents out the open port. Place a sterile container under the open port to collect any fluid.
    b. Suction until retraction on the syringe plunger produces 2 to 3 cm of negative pressure.
    c. Clamp the tube. Remove the syringe, and cap the open ports on the stopcock or connector.

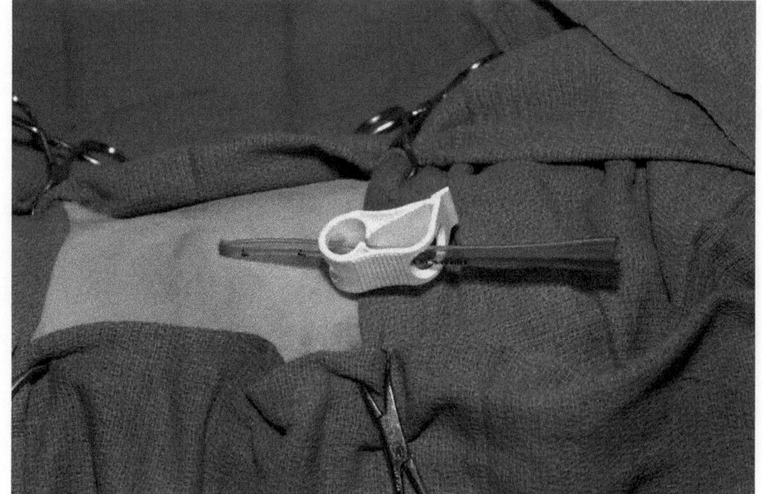

Figure 60-6 Adjust the tube position so that the tip is at the level of the second intercostal space before securing it in place.

14. Check the tube position (fig. 60-6).
    a. Compare the inserted tube to a tube of similar length (or to the stylet).
    b. Adjust the tube position as needed so that at least 8 cm of the tube are within the chest cavity (unless limited by small patient size). The tube should extend to the level of the second intercostal space but should not be advanced into the cranial mediastinum or thoracic inlet. If no fluid is obtained on suction, the tube tip may be too far cranial.
    c. Make sure that all tube fenestrations are within the pleural space.
15. Place a purse-string suture around the tube and secure the tube as described below.

Surgical technique: red rubber catheter placement

1. Add additional fenestrations to the end of the red rubber catheter (fig. 60-7).
    a. Fold the tube over 2 cm from the tip.

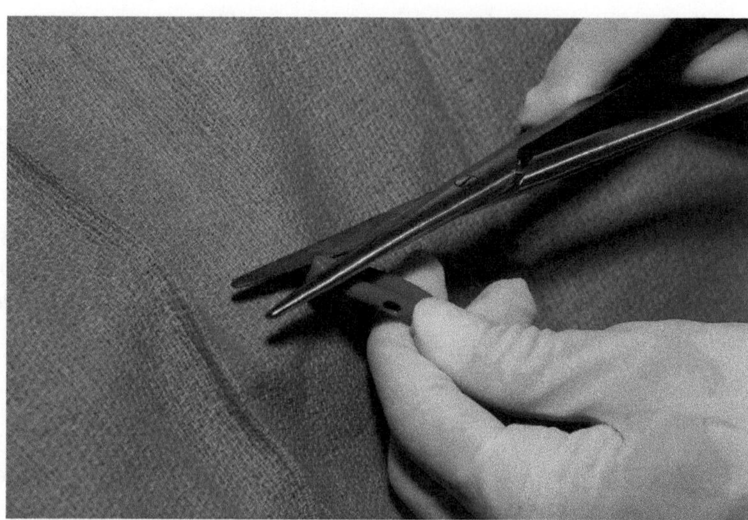

Figure 60-7 Add additional fenestrations to red rubber tubes by folding the tube over and snipping off the corner.

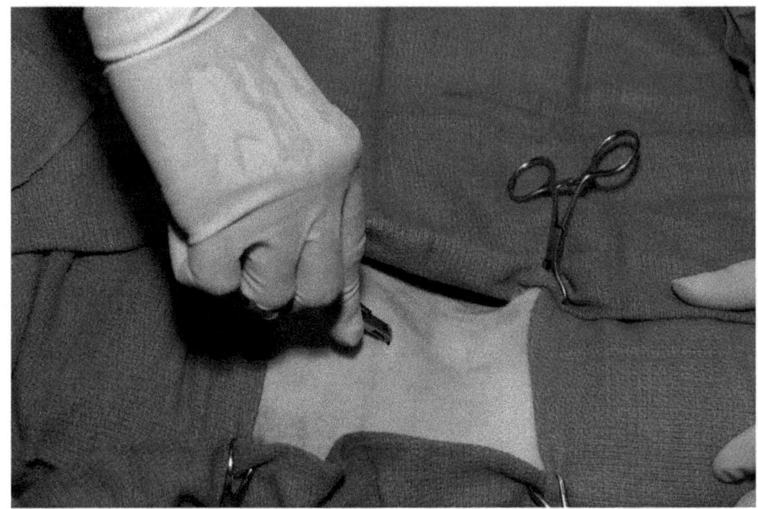

Figure 60-8 With a closed Kelly forceps, tunnel cranioventrally, then force the tips of the forceps through the seventh or eighth intercostal space. In this dog, the head is to the right.

   b. Cut off one corner of the fold to make a new opening in the tube. The opening should be no more than one-third of the tube diameter.
   c. Repeat as needed so that the tube has three to five openings in the last 4 to 6 cm of its tip.
2. Preplace a clamp on the tube. Close the clamp.
3. Make a 1- to 2-cm skin incision over the ninth or tenth intercostal space. The incision should be located at the junction of the dorsal and middle two-thirds of the thoracic height.
4. Insert the tube by tunneling it through the subcutis and intercostal space within the jaws of a Carmalt or Kelly forceps.
   a. Tunnel a closed Kelly forceps cranioventrally through the subcutaneous tissues to the seventh or eighth intercostal space (fig. 60-8).
   b. Force the tips of the Kelly forceps through the intercostal muscles and into the pleural cavity to make a small opening. Remove the Kelly forceps while keeping a finger or marker over the intercostal perforation site so that you can find it again.
   c. Secure the red rubber tube in the jaws of the Kelly forceps so that the tube tip is even with the forceps tips.
   d. Insert the forceps with enclosed tube through the subcutaneous tunnel and intercostal perforation made by the Kelly forceps (fig. 60-9).
      i. If you cannot find the intercostal perforation, proceed as for a trocar tube placement (fig. 60-10) or insert the tube by direct visualization, as described in step 5 below.
   e. Open the jaws of the forceps and advance the tube into the pleural space (fig. 60-11).
5. Alternatively, insert the tube by direct visualization.
   a. Have an assistant pull the lateral thoracic skin cranioventrally so that skin incision lies over the seventh intercostal space at a level midway between the dorsal and ventral borders of the thorax.

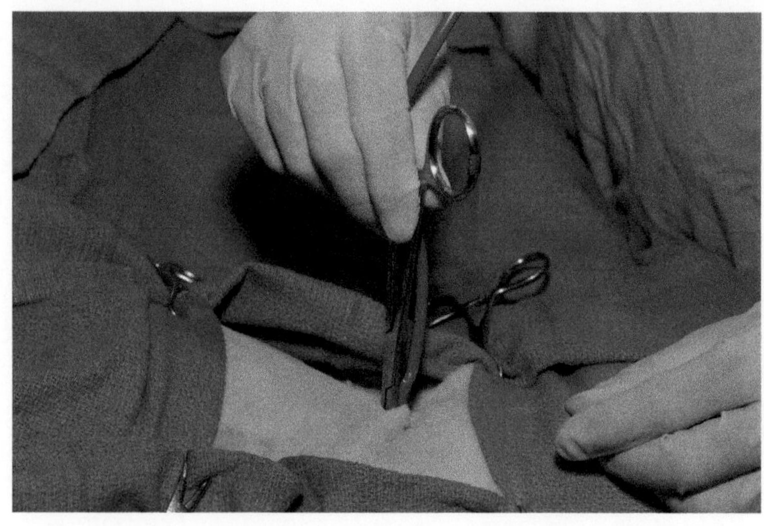

Figure 60-9 Grasp the catheter in the jaws of the Kelly forceps. Tunnel forward and insert the Kelly forceps and tube through the intercostal perforation into the pleural cavity.

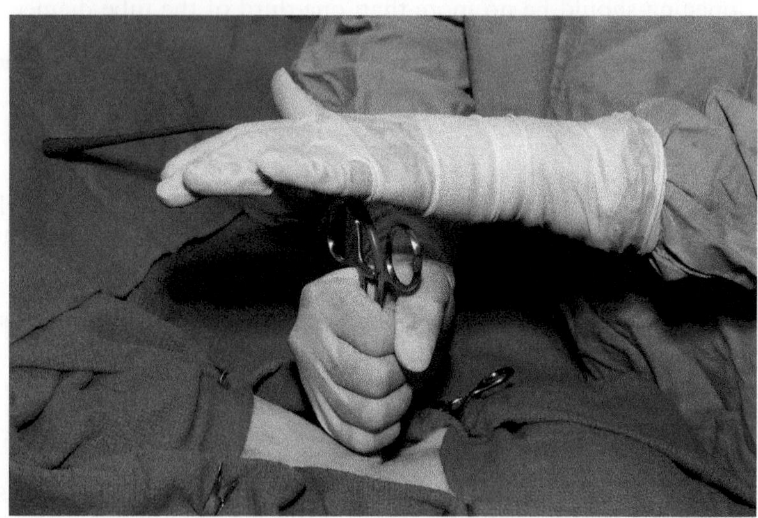

Figure 60-10 If you cannot find the intercostal perforation, force the tube and Kelly forceps through the intercostals using the same technique as for a trocar-tipped tube. Grip the Kelly forceps firmly in your fist to prevent penetrating too deeply.

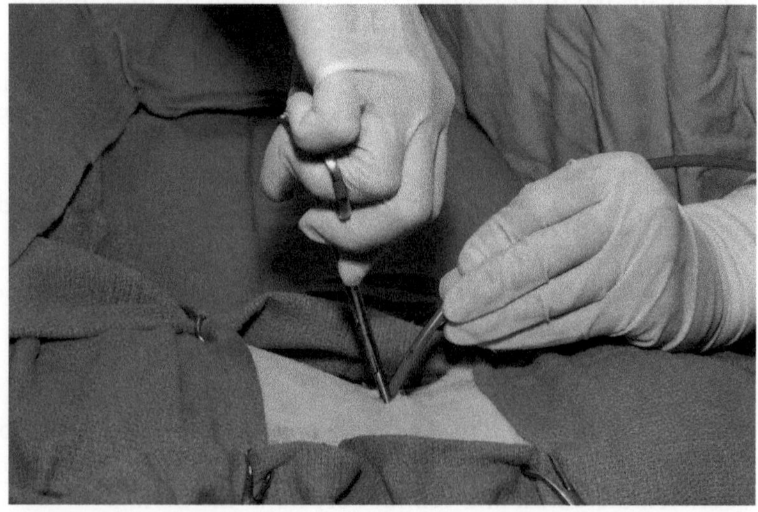

Figure 60-11 Once the Kelly forceps has been inserted through the intercostal muscles and pleura, open the jaws and feed the thoracostomy tube through the opening.

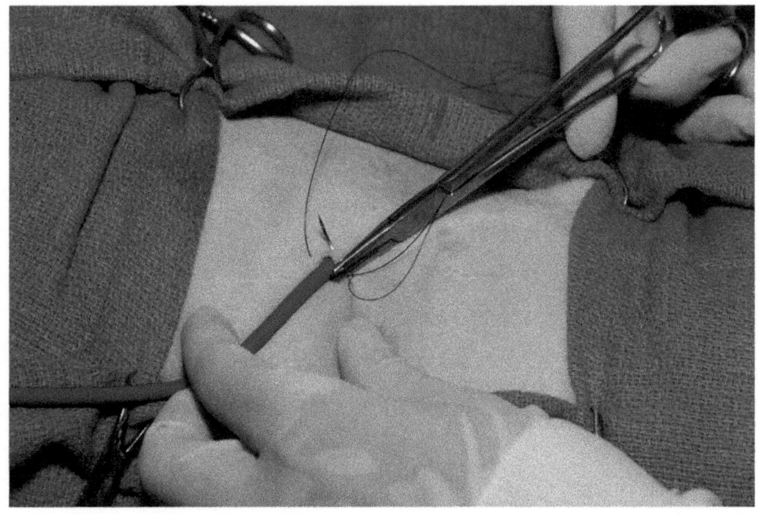

Figure 60-12 Place a purse-string suture of nonabsorbable monofilament material in the skin around the tube exit site.

b. Insert the tips of a Kelly forceps through the intercostal muscles and pleura.

c. Open the jaws of the forceps. Feed the tube between the jaws and into the pleural space.

6. Have the assistant release the skin so the tube exit site is covered. Suction the chest, check the tube position, and secure the tube.

Surgical technique: securing thoracostomy tubes

1. Place a purse-string suture in the skin around the tube exit site (fig. 60-12).

   a. With 2-0 or 3-0 monofilament nylon, take three to five full-thickness bites of skin around the tube until the suture encircles most of the tube.

   b. Tighten the suture snugly around the tube without necrosing the skin.

2. If a wide subcutaneous tunnel was inadvertently made during tube advancement, place a deep mattress suture of 2-0 nylon around the tunnel and tube (fig. 60-13).

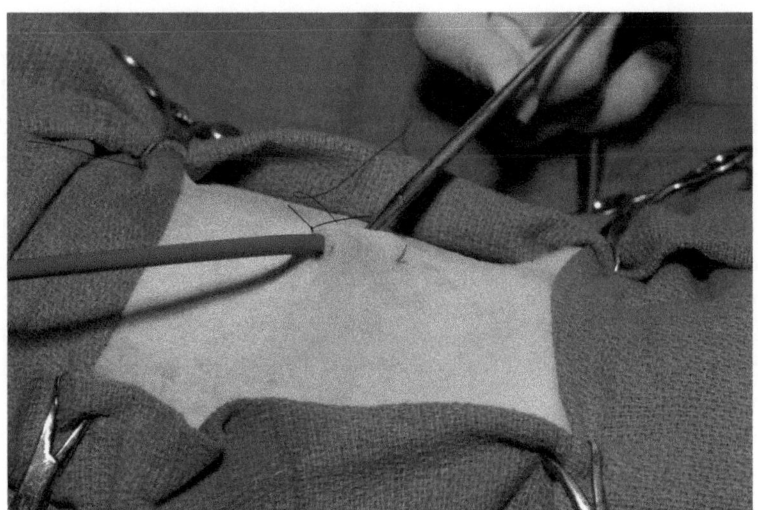

Figure 60-13 Close the subcutaneous tunnel around the tube with a suture by taking a deep bite below the tube and around it.

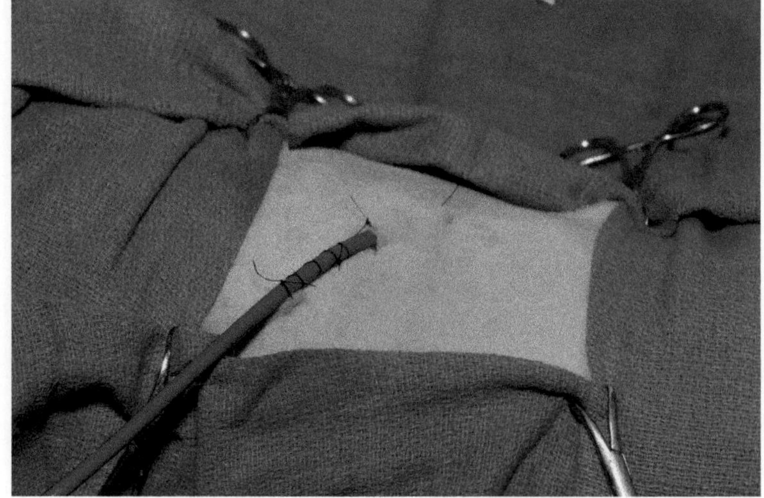

Figure 60-14 Secure the tube to the thoracic skin or muscle or around the last rib with a finger-trap suture.

a. Insert the needle into the skin dorsal to the tube and midway between the skin incision and intercostal perforation.

b. Pass the needle under the tube, catching underlying subcutis or muscle.

c. Pass the needle out of the skin ventral to the tube.

d. Tie the suture securely to compress the tissues around the tube without necrosing them.

3. Secure the tube (fig. 60-14) with a finger-trap pattern (pp. 497–501). In cats, take a bite of muscle or go around a rib while placing the finger trap to prevent tube migration with skin movement.

   a. If tube positioning is a concern, place an interrupted skin suture and secure the finger trap to that suture. If the tube location needs to be readjusted, the finger trap suture can be cut and a new one attached to the skin suture.

Postoperative considerations

Thoracic radiographs are recommended to verify tube position after placement. The animal should wear an Elizabethan collar to prevent self-trauma, and the tube exit site is covered with an adhesive dressing or bandage to decrease contamination and leakage. If a three-way stopcock is attached to the tube, it should also be covered to prevent it from catching on cage doors or floor grates. Some clinicians wire or suture stopcocks or connectors to thoracostomy tubes to prevent accidental dislodgement. Animals with thoracostomy tubes should be monitored continuously until the tube is removed. Antibiotics are not routinely administered unless the animal has a preexisting infection. Those with pyothorax are often started on combination therapy (a fluoroquinolone plus sulbactam-potentiated ampicillin) until culture results are available.

Patients with persistent pneumothorax may require continuous suction with an underwater seal. Negative pressure should be limited to 10 to 20 cm H_2O. In patients with pyothorax and tenacious pleural exudate, the pleural space can be flushed with 10 to 20 mL/kg of warm saline one to four times per day. Fluid is infused slowly over 10 to 15 minutes. Lavage solutions can be removed immediately or left in place for 30 to 60 minutes to loosen debris. Patients with persistent pyothorax or pneumothorax may require further diagnostics (e.g., computed tomography) and thoracotomy.

Thoracic aspiration is painful, and animals will require analgesics until the tube is removed. In dogs, bupivicaine intrapleural infusion provides excellent analgesia, particularly when combined with intravenous opioids. Bupivicaine (0.25–1 mg/kg q6h) is diluted in saline to a total of 10 mL. After the pleural space has been suctioned, the diluted bupivicaine is infused through the thoracostomy tube. The tube is flushed with 5 mL of air or of saline before clamping. Because lidocaine can cause cardiac dysfunction in cats, intrapleural analgesic infusion is usually avoided in this species.

Animals should be radiographed before thoracostomy tube removal to verify resolution of pleural fluid or air accumulation. Tubes are usually removed by cutting the finger-trap suture and pulling firmly. Purse-string and mattress sutures can be left in place unless they interfere with tube removal. The wound at the thoracostomy tube site is covered with a bandage, and the animal is observed for dyspnea. Intercostal and skin stomas usually seal in 1 to 2 days. Animals with significant pleural fluid accumulation may leak fluid subcutaneously or from the skin incision.

The most common complications of thoracostomy tube placement are tube obstruction and pneumothorax. Both can be fatal if resultant fluid or air accumulation causes respiratory compromise. Pneumothorax may occur from iatrogenic lung damage, inadvertent dislodgement of the adaptors or tube, insufficient tube advancement, air leakage around the tube, or operator error. If negative pressure cannot be obtained during tube aspiration, the clinician should check all connections to make sure they are secure. The tube should be then clamped and aspirated. If pressure is not negative when the tube is clamped, then air is leaking around or through the connectors or a defect in the tube. If the pressure is negative, the thoracic bandage should be removed and the tube exit site evaluated. A sterile dressing coated with antibiotic ointment should be pressed firmly over the tube exit site and the thoracostomy tube aspirated again. If negative pressure is obtained at this point, then most likely air is leaking around the tube, either from an excessively large or short subcutaneous tunnel or because the tube has partially backed out so that a fenestration is in the subcutis. The tube should be repositioned as needed, and the stoma and distal tube covered with a dressing and an iodine-impregnated sticky drape to seal the wound around the tube. Alternatively, the thorax can be radiographed; if no pneumothorax is present, then the leakage is from atmospheric air, and the easiest solution is to remove the tube.

Other complications include nosocomial infection, subcutaneous emphysema, and seroma formation. Damage to the heart or intercostal vessels may occur during tube placement. Occasionally, the tube is inadvertently inserted into the abdominal cavity or retracts completely into the subcutaneous space.

Because of local inflammation and irritation, thoracostomy tubes will stimulate production of 2.2 mL/kg/day of thoracic fluid. If no fluid is obtained from the tube, the thorax should be radiographed. If pleural effusion is present, the tube may be kinked or blocked by clots or debris. The tube can also be obstructed by local tissues, particularly if it is advanced too far cranially. Obstructed tubes can be flushed with sterile saline or repositioned. In some patients, tube replacement is required.

Bibliography

Moores AL: Indications, outcomes and complications following lateral thoracotomy in dogs and cats. J Small Anim Pract 2007;48:695–698.

Murphy K, Papasouliotis K: Pleural effusions in dogs and cats. 2. Placement of tubes and treatment. In Pract 2011;33:462–469.

Stillion JR, Letendre JA: A clinical review of the pathophysiology, diagnosis, and treatment of pyothorax in dogs and cats. J Vet Emerg Crit Care 2015;25:113–129.

Valtolina C, Adamantos S: Evaluation of small-bore wire-guided chest drains for management of pleural space disease. 2009;50:290–297.

Yoon HY, Mann FA, Lee S: Comparison of the amounts of air leakage into the thoracic cavity associated with four thoracostomy tube placement techniques in canine cadavers. Am J Vet Res 2009;70:1161–1167.

Chapter 61
Finger-Trap Suture

Several techniques are available to prevent inadvertent removal of tubes and drains. Adhesive tape, attached to a tube in a "butterfly" configuration (overlapping itself on both sides of the tube), can be sutured directly to the skin. This technique is excellent for small tubes because the tape will not inadvertently compress the tube and obstruct the lumen. The tube may slide within the tape if the adhesive is weak or becomes damp, however, and foreign material and moisture may collect around the tape. A finger-trap suture is preferred for securing a larger or less flexible tube. This technique permits cleansing around the tube exit site and, if properly placed, will tighten as it lengthens, reducing the risk of tube migration or loss.

Finger-trap sutures move with the skin. In animals with excessively loose or mobile skin (e.g., cats), a tube that is well secured to the skin can still be retracted several centimeters from its original site. This could result in infection, leakage, and other serious complications, particularly if the tube enters the thoracic cavity or gastrointestinal tract. In these animals, the finger-trap suture can be attached to deeper muscles or periosteum or around bone (e.g., the last rib in cats) to prevent tube migration.

Preoperative management

The skin should be clipped and prepped around the proposed sites for tube and suture placement.

Surgery

If negative pressure needs to be maintained (e.g., for a thoracostomy tube or continuous suction drain), a purse-string suture should be placed in the skin around the tube exit site. The finger-trap suture should be started separately from the purse-string suture. Tension on a finger-trap suture that is a continuation of the purse string may cause skin necrosis at the exit wound. Some clinicians prefer to place a separate suture loop in the skin and secure the finger trap to that suture. That way, if an esophagostomy or thoracostomy tube needs to be readjusted when the animal is awake, the finger trap suture can be cut and replaced, using that same suture loop to secure it to the skin.

Manual of Small Animal Soft Tissue Surgery, Second Edition. Karen Tobias.
© 2017 John Wiley & Sons, Inc. Published 2017 by John Wiley & Sons, Inc.

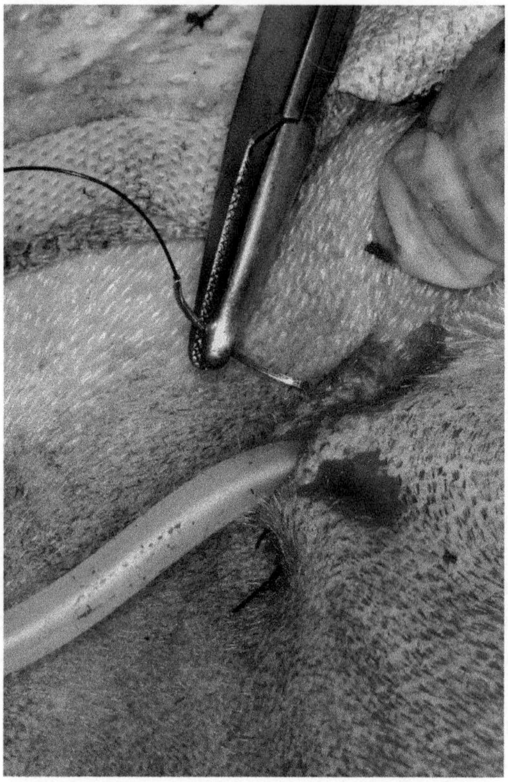

Figure 61-1 After determining the site at which the tube will rest most naturally, flip the tube away from the site and take a bite of skin in the designated area, 1 to 2 cm from the tube exit site. In this patient, the tube exit site has been narrowed with a separate purse-string suture.

Surgical technique: finger-trap suture

1. Place a purse-string suture in the skin around thoracostomy tubes or any tube that will be used for continuous suction of wounds. Tie it and cut the ends short.
2. Lay the external portion of the tube against the skin to determine in which direction the tube will rest most comfortably.
3. Flip the tube away from the area of suture placement. With a 40- to 60-cm strand of swaged-on, 2-0 or 0 monofilament suture, take a 1-cm bite in the skin (+/– underlying deep tissues), 1 to 2 cm away from the tube exit site (fig. 61-1).
4. Tie one or two knots (two or four simple throws) in the center of the suture strand, loosely apposing them to the skin. When the knots are tied, the needle end and free end of the suture should each be at least 15 cm long.
5. Flip the tube back into place. Wrap the suture ends around the tube from opposite directions so that the tube is encircled with the suture, then tie a surgeon's throw firmly on top of the tube (the surface closest to you; fig. 61-2). When tightening the surgeon's throw, indent the tube slightly but do not kink or crush it.
6. From opposite directions, pass the suture ends 360 degrees around the tube (fig. 61-3) so that the tube is once again fully encircled by each suture end, and firmly tie another surgeon's throw on top of the tube 3 to 6 mm distal to the previous throw.
7. Continue suture passage and surgeon's throws so that the tube is encircled at least five times.

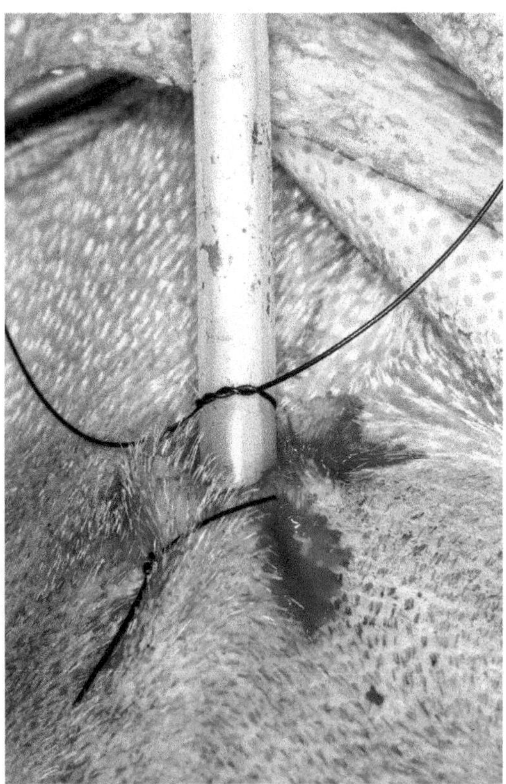

Figure 61-2 After tying one or two knots, bring both suture ends around the tube, and tie them firmly over the top of the tube with a surgeon's throw.

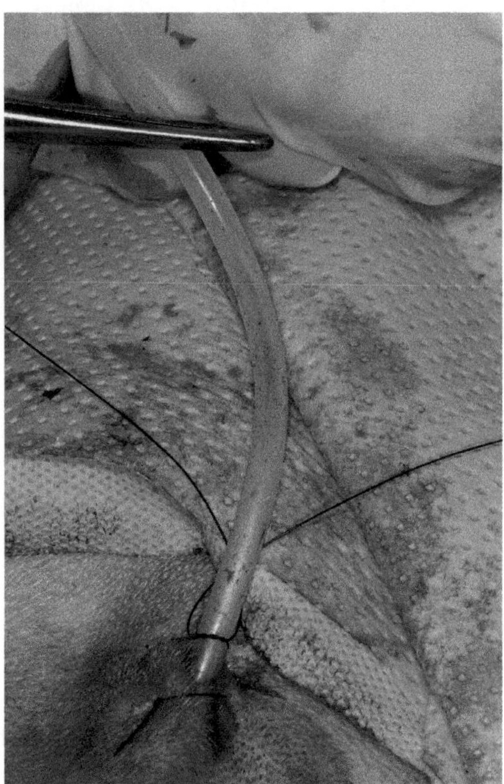

Figure 61-3 Pass the suture ends in opposite directions around the tube and back to the top side, then tie a surgeon's throw 3 to 6 mm distal to the previous throw.

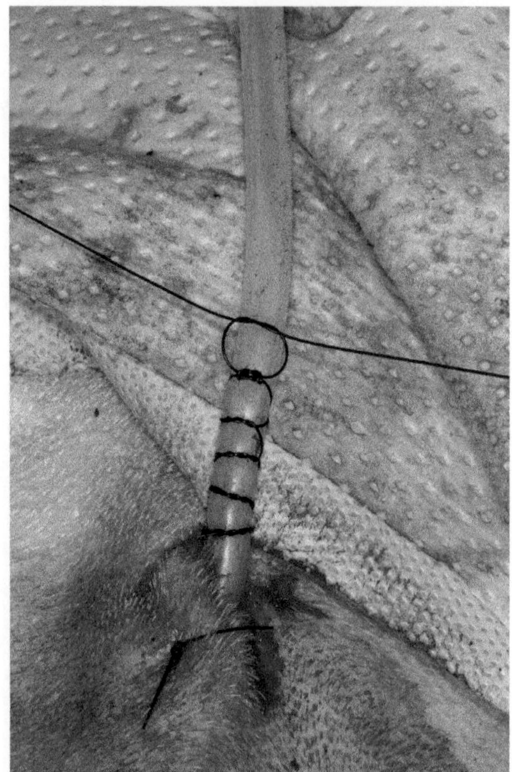

Figure 61-4 Repeat the process so that the tube is encircled at least five times; then tie two knots. Leave the suture ends long.

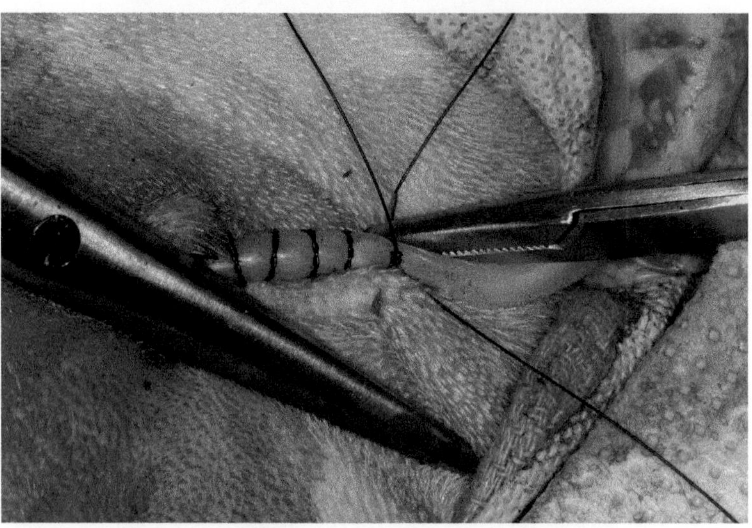

Figure 61-5 Take another bite of the skin under the tube and tie two more knots.

8. Tie two knots at the final throw (fig. 61-4). If desired, take a second bite of skin under the tube (fig. 61-5). Tie two more knots and cut off the ends (fig. 61-6).
9. Place a bandage over the tube exit site.

Postoperative management

Radiographs are recommended to evaluate esophagostomy and thoracostomy tube placement. If the tube position needs to be altered, the finger trap sutures are cut distal to the first knot, leaving a suture loop in the skin. Once the tube is

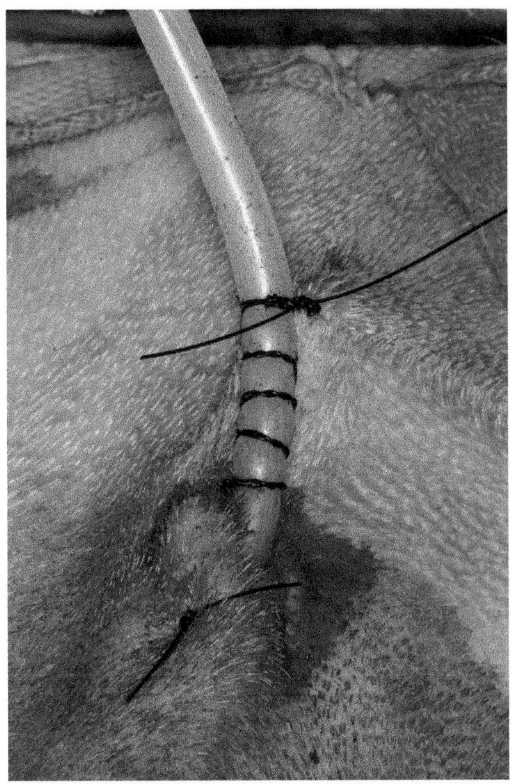

Figure 61-6 Final appearance. This finger trap suture is secured twice to the skin.

positioned appropriately, a new finger trap suture can be attached to the skin suture. Tubes are easily removed by cutting any skin attachments of the finger-trap pattern. The purse-string suture can be left in place as needed. Bupivicaine can be administered through the tube 20 minutes before removal to provide analgesia. Tubes are clamped before pulling to prevent leakage of contents, and the tube exit site is cleaned and bandaged after tube removal.

Complications are most likely to occur because of poor technique. Finger-trap sutures pulled too tightly around soft or narrow tubes can kink or obstruct the tube. If single throws or knots are tied instead of surgeon's throws, the finger trap may not tighten with traction on the tube. Surgeon's throws that are placed too close together on the top of the tube will result in a finger-trap suture that is too loose.

Bibliography

Smeak DD: The Chinese finger trap suture technique for fastening tubes and catheters. J Am Anim Hosp Assoc 1990;26:215–218.

Song EK, Mann FA, Wagner Mann CC: Comparison of different tube materials and use of Chinese finger trap or four friction suture technique for securing gastrostomy, jejunostomy, and thoracostomy tubes in dogs. Vet Surg 2008;37:212–221.

Section 9 Limb and Digit Procedures

Chapter 62
Onychectomy

Cats use their claws for a variety of purposes, including protection, climbing, hunting, and escape. Scratching is a natural behavior in cats; however, many owners object when their property or skin becomes damaged. Inappropriate scratching may be controlled or reduced in many cats by providing appropriate surfaces for exercising claws and by trimming the cat's toenails weekly. Occasionally, onychectomy ("declawing") may be necessary to protect owners with fragile skin, clotting disorders, or poor immunity or to prevent euthanasia of cats for behavioral reasons.

During onychectomy, the third phalanx of each digit is completely removed (fig. 62-1). The procedure can be performed with a scalpel blade, sterile guillotine-type Rescoe shears, CO_2 laser, or radiosurgical scalpel. When performed by veterinary students, onychectomy performed with a scalpel blade took longer and resulted in more acute postoperative pain and complications than onychectomy performed with shears. Onychectomy with shears, however, resulted in more chronic complications such as lameness and claw regrowth. Laser onychectomy can reduce postoperative pain, possibly because intraoperative tourniquets and postoperative bandages are not required.

Elective declawing of cats is illegal in several countries and U.S. cities, and several U.S. states have introduced legislation to ban feline declaws statewide. Persons performing the procedure in those areas could be subject to fines and incarceration. Therefore, it is critical that veterinarians be aware of regional laws governing the procedure.

Preoperative management

Since onychectomy is usually performed on young healthy animals, minimal preoperative diagnostics are required. While some surgeons clip and surgically prep the feet, most simply scrub the surgical area or soak the paws and antebrachium in a chlorhexidine antiseptic solution. Alcohol is flammable and should not be used for prep before laser onychectomy. Pre-emptive analgesia, including injectable opioids and local or regional nerve blocks, should be administered to limit postoperative discomfort. If a nerve block is performed, injections are made proximal to the carpus over the dorsomedial surface to block the superficial branches of the radial nerve (adjacent to the cephalic vein), dorsolateral and proximal to the carpal pad to block the dorsal and palmar branches of the ulnar nerve, respectively, and the palmar medial surface of the carpus to block the median nerve.

Manual of Small Animal Soft Tissue Surgery, Second Edition. Karen Tobias.
© 2017 John Wiley & Sons, Inc. Published 2017 by John Wiley & Sons, Inc.

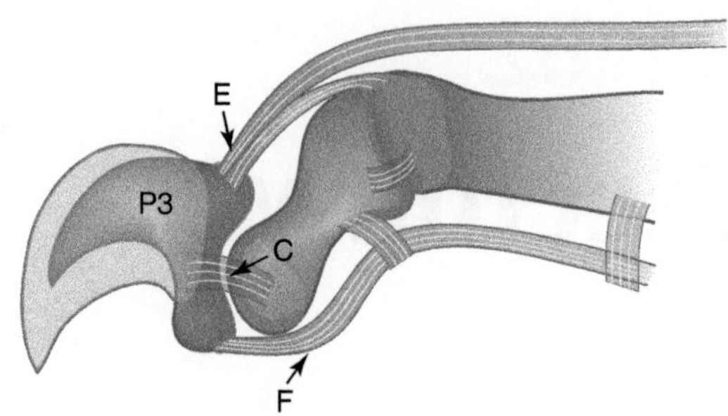

Figure 62-1 The third phalanx (P3) is secured to the foot dorsally by an extensor tendon (E) and an elastic ligament, ventrally by a flexor tendon (F), and laterally by collateral ligaments (C).

Surgery

If a shears or blade technique is performed, hemorrhage is limited by placing a tourniquet just above or below the elbow. A folded half-inch Penrose drain can be wrapped around the limb. The drain ends are inserted through the loop of the fold and pulled upward (like cinching a saddle), and a hemostat is placed across the drain ends near the fold to keep the tourniquet tight. Tourniquets placed below the elbow may not occlude the interosseous arteries; tourniquets placed above the elbow may cause nerve damage if left in place too long.

During onychectomy, all of P3 should be removed to prevent claw regrowth. The excision should include the "palmar tubercle"—the ventral boney process where the deep digital flexor tendon attaches. The digital pads are closely adherent to the tissues over the palmar tubercle and can be accidentally transected during dissection. This may increase postoperative discomfort.

After amputation of P3, the surgical site is usually closed primarily with a single interrupted skin suture or topical tissue adhesive. Occasionally, onychectomy sites are allowed to heal by second intention. Primary closure is often performed to control postoperative hemorrhage and reduce the risk of P2 exposure. Tissue glue should be placed on the surface of the apposed wound edges, or sparingly within the superficial tissues as described below. Tissue glue is not absorbable and can act as a source of irritation or nidus for infection if placed within the deep tissues.

A variety of methods have been described for bandaging after onychectomy. Bandages increase pain and stress in cats postoperatively and can cause lameness or ischemia if placed too tightly.

Surgery technique: Rescoe shears onychectomy

1. If the nails are long and curved, clip the tips off so they will not get caught in the small hole in the shear's blade. Leave enough length to allow digit manipulation.
2. With your dominant hand, press on the digital pad to extend the claw.
3. With your nondominant hand, place the Rescoe shears in the dorsal joint space between P2 and P3 with the blade facing upward and the handle toward you (fig. 62-2).
   a. To keep the shears in the joint space, lift your nondominant elbow up and pull the shears toward you. In this position, the shears should stay in the dorsal joint space, even when the blade is in the open position.

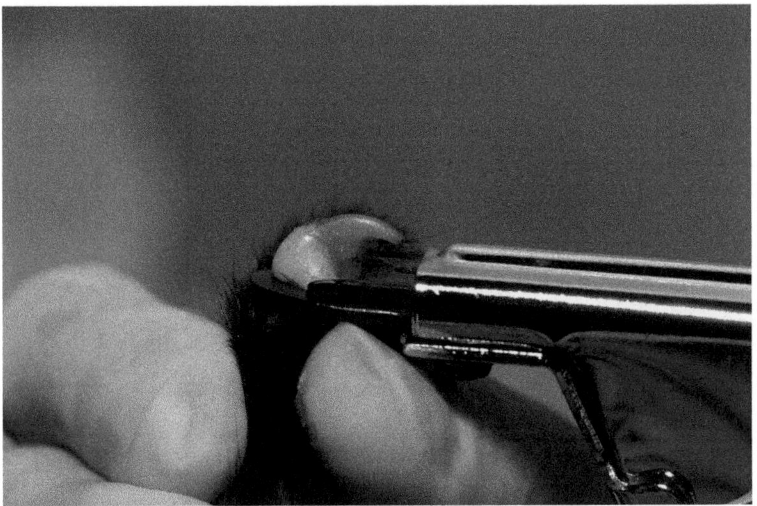

Figure 62-2 Expose the claw by pressing the pad against underlying bone. Place the Rescoe shears around the joint with the blade facing up and the handle toward the surgeon. The arch of the shear should rest within the dorsal joint space.

4. With the Rescoe shears seated firmly in the dorsal joint space, close the blade so that it is abutting the palmar surface of the claw.
5. With your dominant hand, use a sturdy forceps or your thumbnail to manipulate P3.
   a. Thumbnail technique: Insert your thumbnail under the tip of the toenail (fig. 62-3).
   b. Forceps technique: Clamp the nail across its dorsal surface with meniscus forceps, Kelly hemostat, or an old needle holder so that the forceps handle is away from you (fig. 62-4). The jaws of the forceps should lie parallel to the skin attachments along the claw and perpendicular to the long axis of the claw.
6. Pull the claw backwards (dorsally, in extension) and away from you over the rim of the shears. Simultaneously relax the blade enough to shift it under the palmar tubercle while keeping the pad retracted out of the surgery field (fig. 60-3).

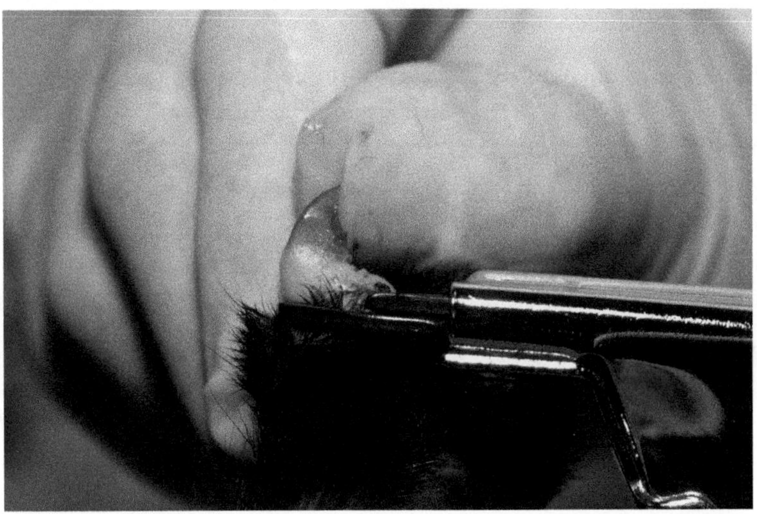

Figure 62-3 Using your thumb nail under the claw, force P3 dorsally (in extension) over the arch of the shears. Open the blade slightly to allow the palmar tubercle to rise above the blade while leaving the pad below it.

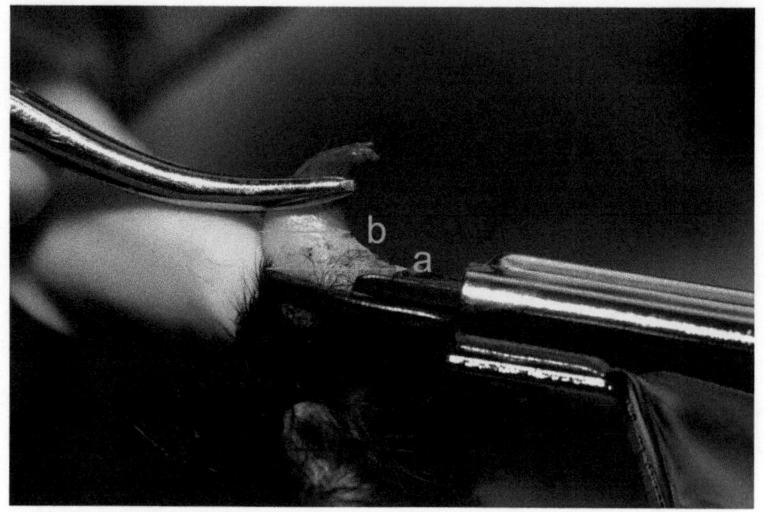

Figure 62-4 Alternatively, grasp the claw with forceps and pull dorsally (hyperextending the joint). Note that once the blade is properly positioned under the palmar tubercle, the amount of the bone (ungual crest) resting above the blade (line a) will be twice the thickness of the claw (line b).

   a. If the clamp slips off during this maneuver, you need to relax the shears handle more to open them enough so the tubercle slips through the space.

   b. If the pad is visible in front of (above) the blade, the shears were relaxed too much and will have to be repositioned.

   c. If the entire nail slips down and away from you, then the shears are no longer resting in the dorsal joint space and need to be repositioned.

7. Check the positioning of the blade to make sure it is under the palmar tubercle.

   a. The palmar tubercle will be evident as a slight bulge in front of (above) the blade.

   b. If the blade is in the correct place, the distance between the blade edge and dorsal rim of the shears will be about twice that of the nail base (fig. 62-4).

   c. If the shears are beyond the joint space, the pad will be visible in front of the blade.

8. Once the blade reaches the level of the interphalangeal joint (under the palmar tubercle where the deep digital flexor tendon attaches), close it slightly.

9. Close the shears gradually with your nondominant hand, while rotating the nail around its long axis with your dominant hand to force the blade into the joint space. Other than closing the shears, keep your non-dominant hand quiet: do not rock, lift, twist, or rotate the shears.

   a. Forceps technique: With your dominant hand, grasp the body of the clamp with the palm facing down. Rotate the clamp clockwise and counter clockwise around the long axis of the claw (fig. 62-5), keeping the forceps perpendicular to the claw and parallel to the joint space.

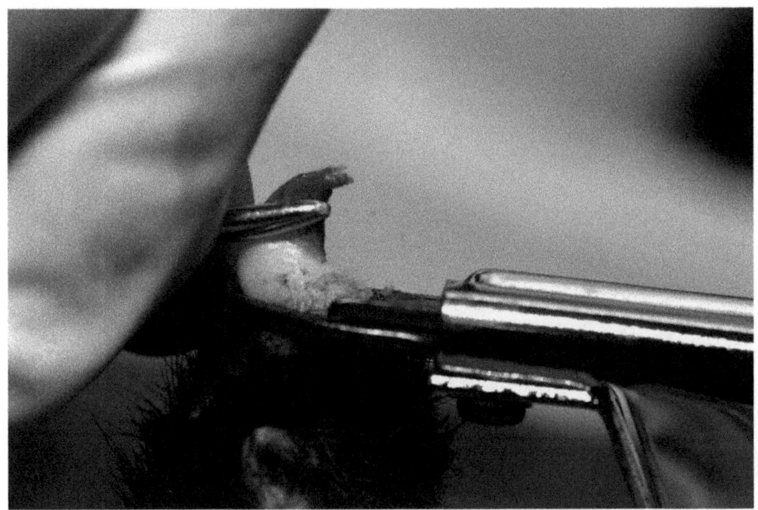

Figure 62-5 If rotating the claw with forceps, hold the forceps in an overhand grasp and rotate the claw clockwise and counterclockwise around its base while slowly closing the blade through the joint space.

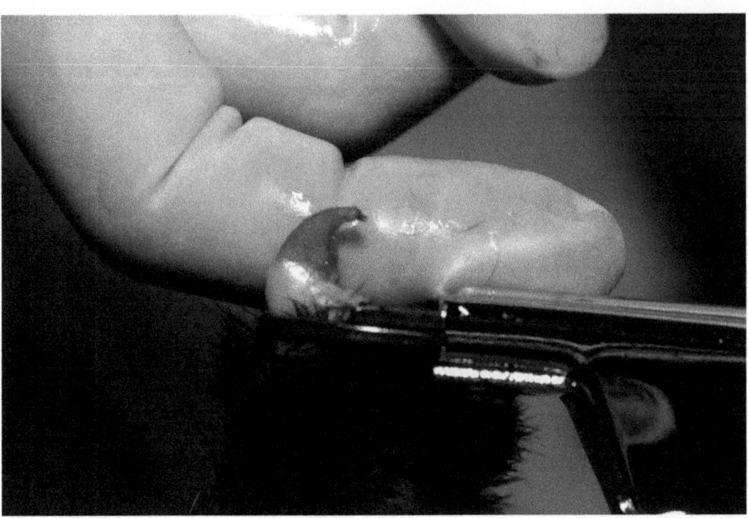

Figure 62-6 If rotating the claw with fingers, lay an index finger alongside the claw and secure the claw between the thumb pad and side of the index finger.

b. Thumbnail technique: Grasp the claw between the pad of your thumb and the side of your index finger (fig. 62-6). Rotate the claw around its long axis in a "screwdriver" motion (fig. 62-7).

c. If the shears are difficult to close or do not cut easily, check their position to make sure the blade is still at the level of the interphalangeal joint and within the dorsal joint space.

10. Once the blade is completely closed, pull the closed shears off the digit to transect any soft tissue attachments.

11. Press on the digital pad to examine the amputation site. The end of P2 should appear rounded (fig. 62-8). Remove any remnants of P3 by grasping the bone with forceps and transecting any soft tissue attachments with a no. 11 blade.

12. Close the wound side-to-side with a single simple interrupted suture of rapidly absorbable material (fig. 62-9), cutting the ends short, or with topically applied tissue adhesive (see below).

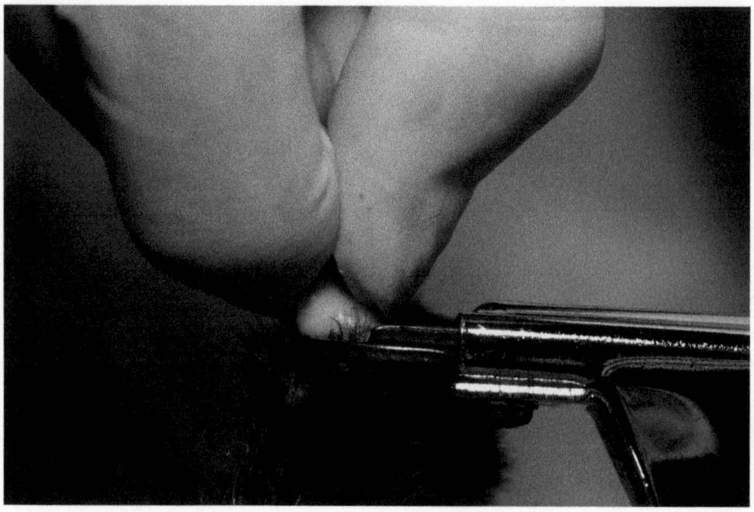

Figure 62-7 Rotate the claw around its base (as if turning a screwdriver) while gradually closing the blade.

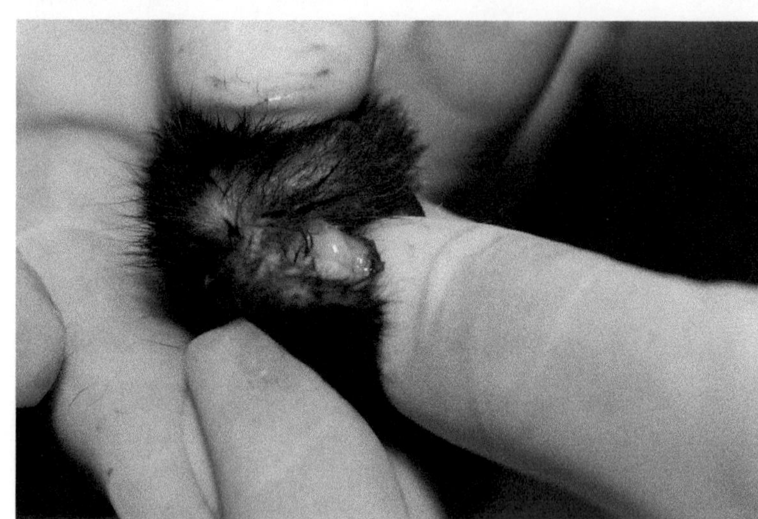

Figure 62-8 Compress the pad to expose and examine the smooth condyle of P2.

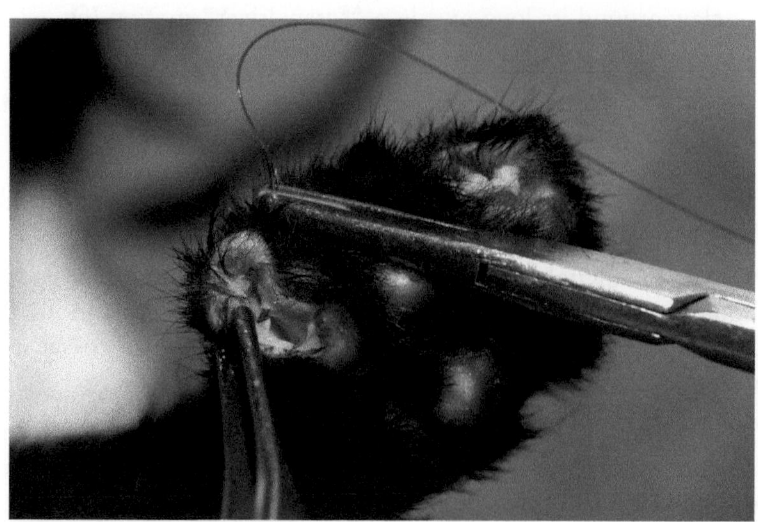

Figure 62-9 Appose wound edges on each toe with a simple interrupted skin suture of rapidly absorbable monofilament.

Surgical technique: blade onychectomy

1. Push the antiseptic-soaked hair away from the surgical site.
2. Grasp the claw with a hemostat placed from the claw's dorsal surface (the side away from you) and across its base. Hold the body of the hemostats in an overhand position with the handle toward you. This will help open the joint dorsally.
3. Using a no. 12 or no. 11 blade, incise the hairless skin circumferentially just proximal to its attachment with the claw, leaving as much skin as possible (fig. 62-10).
4. Push the skin proximally away from the claw to expose the extensor tendons over the dorsal joint space and the collateral ligaments laterally.
5. Use the blade to carefully transect the extensor tendon (fig. 62-11) and dorsal elastic ligaments.
   a. The blade will be pointed downward and will cut until it reaches the ventral prominence of P3.

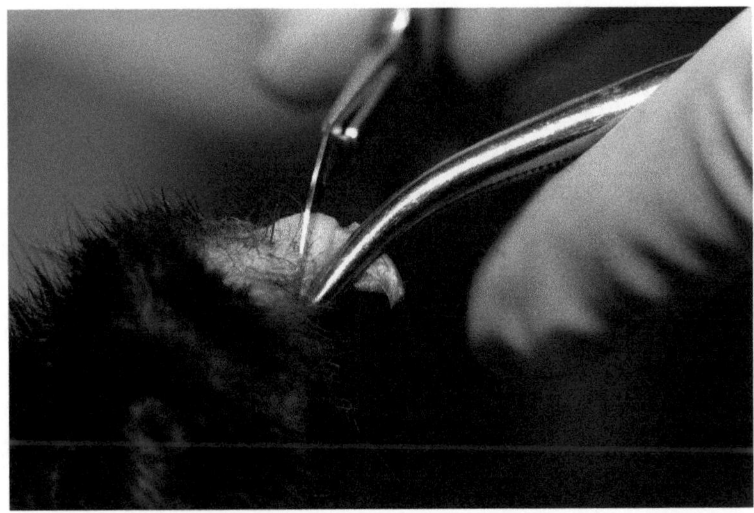

Figure 62-10 Grasp the claw with a hemostat and incise the skin circumferentially near its attachment to the claw.

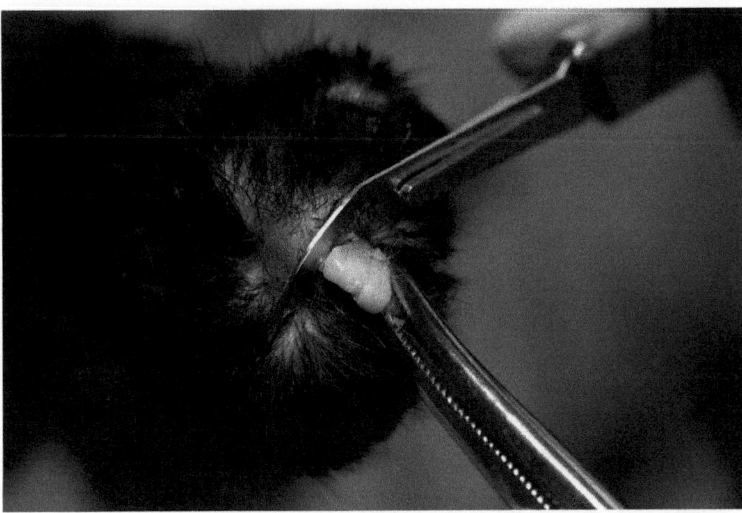

Figure 62-11 Transect the extensor tendon and dorsal elastic ligaments by cutting through the joint space in a dorsopalmar direction while rotating the claw clockwise and counterclockwise.

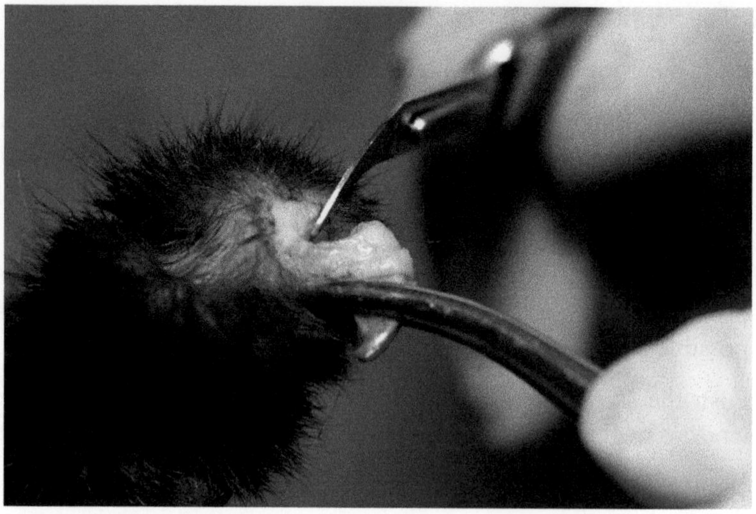

Figure 62-12 Flex the joint maximally and cut the collateral ligaments. Move the claw medially and laterally as you cut.

   b. With the hemostat, rotate the claw clockwise and counterclockwise along its long axis (in other words, use a screwdriver motion) to cut all parts of the extensor tendon.

6. Flex the claw to open the joint space and expose the collateral ligaments, and cut them carefully with the blade (fig. 62-12).
   a. To facilitate cutting, move the hemostat side to side (medially and laterally) to open up each side of the joint.
   b. If using a curved blade, make sure the tip does not damage any healthy skin.
7. Once the extensor tendon and lateral ligaments are cut, flex the joint maximally to open the space and identify the flexor tendon from a dorsal approach.
8. Cut the flexor tendon carefully with the blade in a vertical position (fig. 62-13). Stop once the tendon is severed.

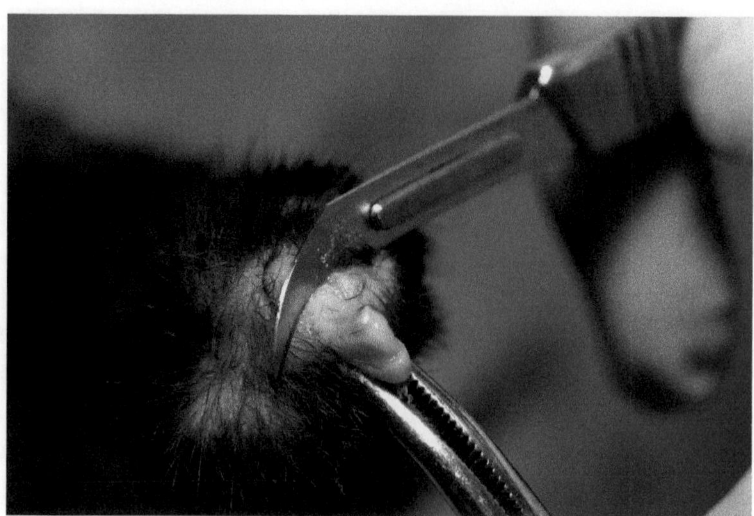

Figure 62-13 With the joint flexed maximally, place the blade on the flexor tendon between P2 and the proximal aspect of P3. Cut downward through the tendon while carefully rotating the claw clockwise and counterclockwise. Do not cut off the pad.

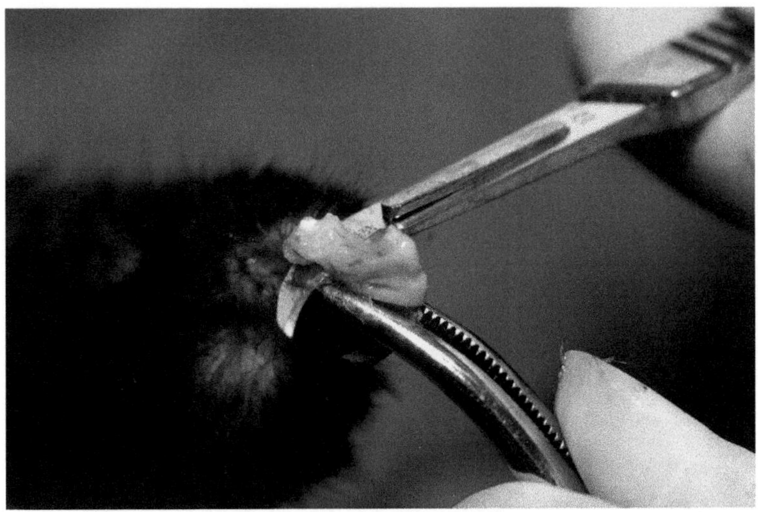

Figure 62-14 Place the blade flat between the palmar tubercle and pad and cut the pad attachments off the bone, following the curve of the palmar tubercle upward and toward yourself to avoid cutting the pad.

9. Angle the blade horizontally and slightly upward, and cut around the boney prominence of P3, following its surface as you sever the remaining attachments (fig. 62-14). To keep the pad intact, the cutting edge of the blade should be angling upward toward the claw and the surgeon's face during the final cut.
10. Close the wounds with suture or tissue adhesive once onychectomy is completed.

Surgical technique: laser onychectomy

1. Use a nonflammable antiseptic to prep the feet. All personnel should wear safety glasses, and the cat's eyes should be covered, to protect against damage from any reflected beam.
2. Insert a new 0.4-mm tip and set the CO_2 laser on 5 to 8 watts of power in a continuous wave mode. Adjust the power setting as needed, depending on how easily the tissues are incised or charred.
3. Grasp the nail from its dorsal surface with a forceps (see fig. 62-10).
4. With the laser, make a 360-degree incision through the skin edge around the claw (fig. 62-15).
5. Let the skin retract slightly, then make a second 360-degree incision through subcutaneous fascia around the claw to transect the fascia.
6. Distract the claw in a palmar direction to flex the joint and open it dorsally. Push the skin back (proximally) with a finger or instrument to expose the extensor tendon. Transect the tendon and elastic ligaments near their distal insertions and any underlying synovium (fig. 62-16).
7. Continue to distract the claw in a palmar direction to expose collateral ligaments. Transect the ligaments on each side, working dorsal to ventral with the beam perpendicular to the ligaments (fig. 62-17). Make sure the skin is pulled back and away from the ligaments as you cut.

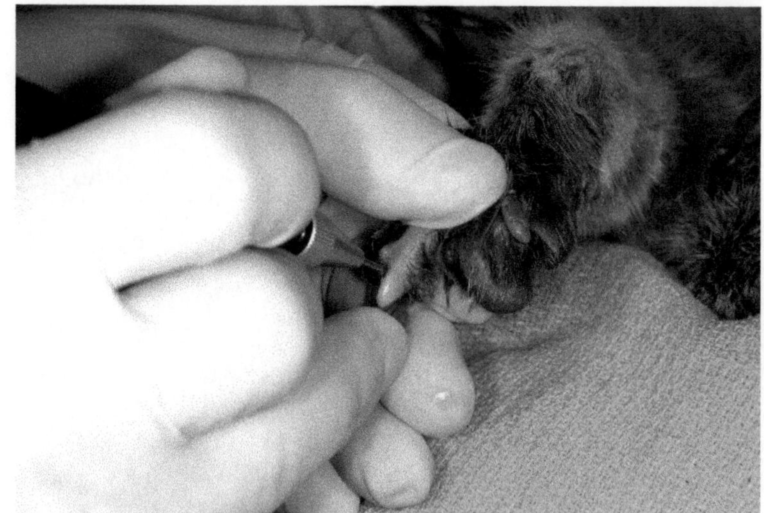

Figure 62-15 Incise the skin circumferentially around the claw.

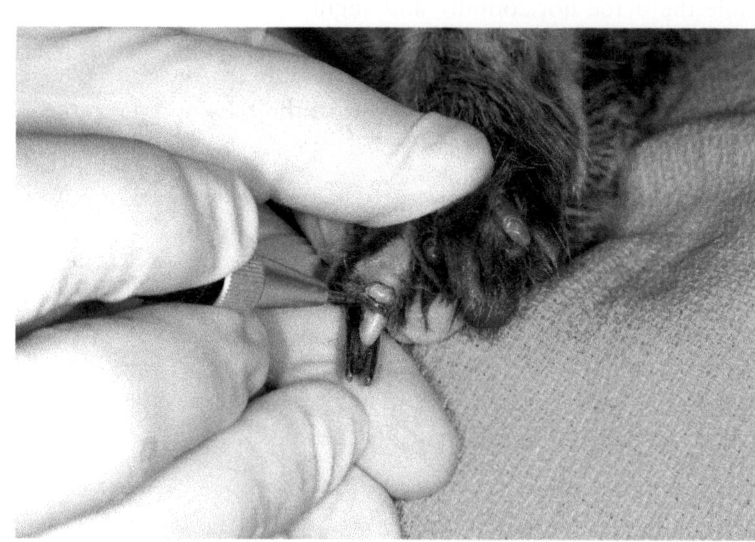

Figure 62-16 Flex the claw ventrally, and transect the extensor tendon and dorsal elastic ligaments.

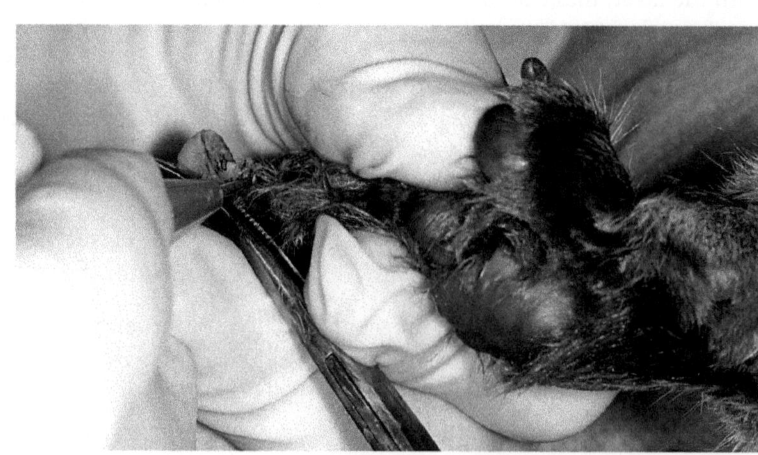

Figure 62-17 Flex the claw medially and laterally and then ventrally to open the joint while you cut the collateral ligaments and flexor tendon, respectively.

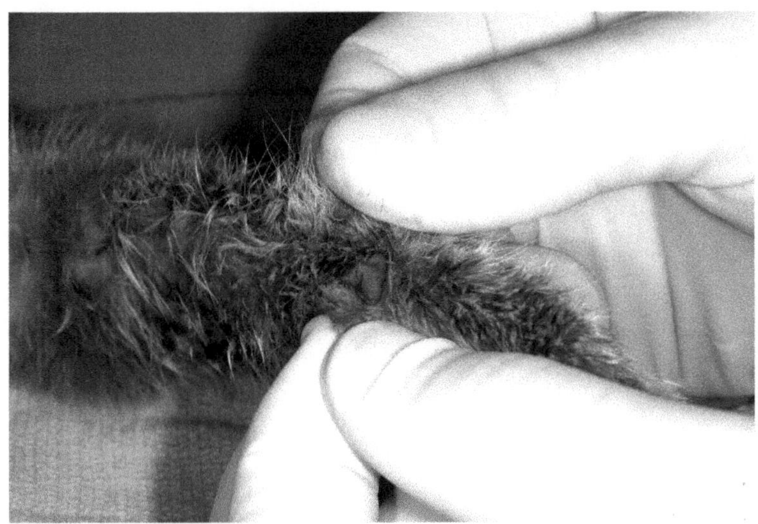

Figure 62-18 Final appearance before closure. Despite the lack of tourniquet, the site is free of hemorrhage.

8. With continued palmar traction, expose the flexor tendon. Transect the tendon, from dorsal to ventral, at its insertion to P3.
9. With extreme palmar rotation and distraction of the distal phalanx, expose remaining subcutaneous tissue attachments and transect them. Keep the laser beam close to P3 to prevent skin or pad trauma.
10. Remove any excess char and inspect the tissues for bleeding (fig. 62-18).

Surgical technique: tissue glue application

1. Evert the wound edges by grasping each side of the skin wound with thumb and index finger (fig. 62-19).
2. While continuing to hold the wound edges, press the pads of your index fingers together just above P2. This maneuver will cover the bone end with subcutis while leaving the edges of the skin everted (fig. 62-20).

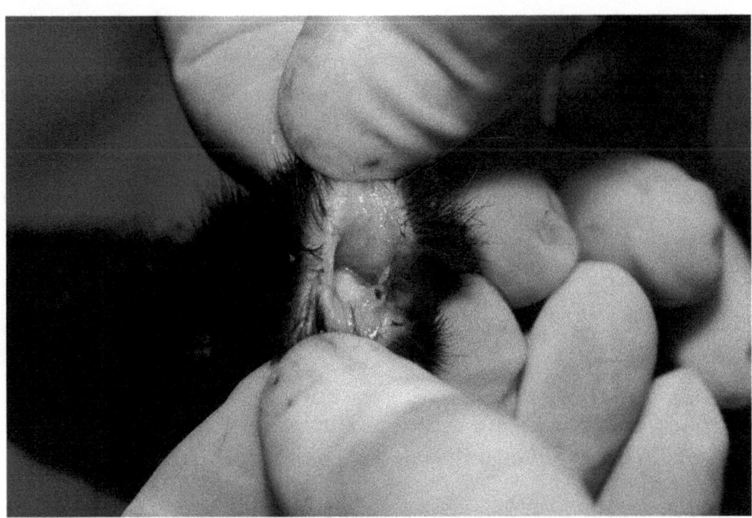

Figure 62-19 Grasp the skin edges with the thumb and index finger on each side. Remove any hair from the wound.

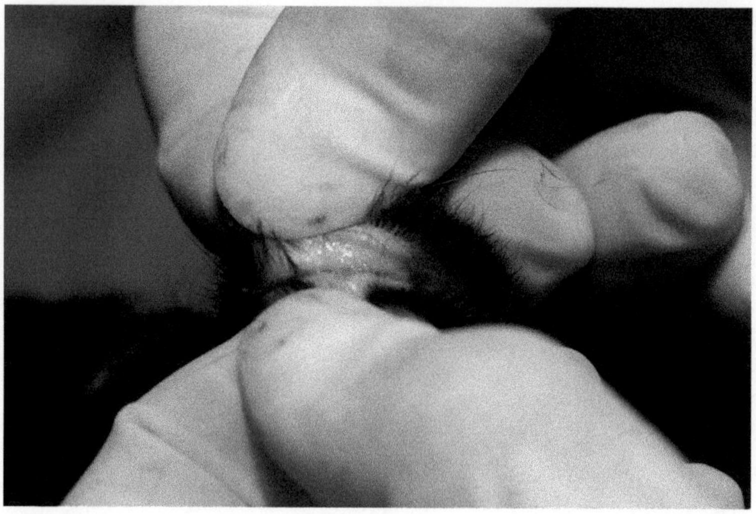

Figure 62-20 Press the tips of your index fingers together to appose the skin over the end of P2, leaving only the skin edges everted. A drop of glue will be placed on these edges.

3. Have an assistant place a small drop of tissue adhesive along the exposed wound. With your index fingers, immediately compress the remaining wound edges together from proximal to distal to force any glue out of the wound.
4. Hold the edges together for 10 seconds, then gently release. Repeat with the remaining toes.

Postoperative considerations

Analgesics are continued for at least 48 hours. Sedatives are recommended to reduce foot shaking and hemorrhage. Any bandages should be removed within 16 hours of placement; sedation is recommended during bandage removal since excitement may encourage hemorrhaging. Cats may require Elizabethan collars to prevent self-trauma. Shredded paper or compressed paper pellets should be used in the litter box until the wounds have healed. Cats should be kept indoors after onychectomy.

Postoperative complications are reported in up to 50% of cats and include pain, lameness, hemorrhage, swelling, dehiscence, infection, necrosis from incorrect laser usage or tight bandages, flexor tendon contracture, palmagrade stance, and behavior changes. Exposure of P2 through the healing surgical wound will cause persistent lameness, requiring amputation of the distal end of P2 and primary wound closure. Chronic lameness, infection, swelling, or fistula formation may occur from subcutaneous claw regrowth if the germinal tissue of P3 is not completely removed. If nail regrowth is suspected, the feet should be radiographed to determine whether more than one digit is affected. Remnants are removed by incision over the dorsal tip of each affected toe and transection of any ligamentous attachments with a blade.

Bibliography

Burns SM, Howerth EW, Rawlings CA, et al: Comparison of the carbon dioxide laser and the radiofrequency unit for feline onychectomies. J Am Anim Hosp Assoc 2010;46:375–384.

Clark K, Bailey T, Rist P, et al: Comparison of 3 methods of onychectomy. Can Vet J 2014;55:255–262.

Ellison GW: Feline onychectomy complications: prevention and management. NAVC Clinician's Brief 2003; April:29–31,47.

Enomoto M, Lascelles BDX, and Gerard MP: Defining the local nerve blocks for feline distal thoracic limb surgery: a cadaveric study. J Feline Med Surg 2016;1–8. DOI: 10.1177/1098612X15597967. Downloaded 8/19/2016.

Gaynor JS: Chronic pain syndrome of feline onychectomy. NAVC Clinician's Brief 2005;3:11–13,63.

Patronek GJ: Assessment of claims of short- and long-term complications associated with onychectomy in cats. J Am Vet Med Assoc 2001;219:932–937.

Robinson DA et al: Evaluation of short-term limb function following unilateral carbon dioxide laser or scalpel onychectomy in cats. J Am Vet Med Assoc 2007;230: 353–358.

Wilson DV, Pascoe PJ: Pain and analgesia following oncychectomy in cats: a systematic review. Vet Aneasthesia Analgesia 2016;43:5–17.

Clark K, Bailey T, Rist P, et al: Comparison of 3 methods of onychectomy. Can Vet J 2014;55:255–62.

Ellison GW: Feline onychectomy complications: prevention and management. NAVC Clinician's Brief 2003; April:29–31.4.

Enomoto M, Lascelles BDX, and Gerard MP: Defining the local nerve blocks for feline distal thoracic limb surgery: a cadaveric study. J Feline Med Surg 2016;1–8. DOI: 10.1177/1098612X15597967. Downloaded 8/15/2016.

Gaynor JS: Chronic pain syndrome of feline onychectomy. NAVC Clinician's Brief 2006;11–13,53.

Patronek GJ: Assessment of claims of short- and long-term complications associated with onychectomy in cats. J Am Vet Med Assoc 2001;219:932–937.

Robinson DA, et al: Evaluation of short-term limb function following unilateral carbon dioxide laser or scalpel onychectomy in cats. J Am Vet Med Assoc 2007;230:353–358.

Wilson DV, Pascoe PJ: Pain and analgesia following onychectomy in cats: a systematic review. Vet Anaesthesia Analgesia 2016;43:5–17.

Chapter 63
Dewclaw Removal

The first digit of the canine paw is called a dewclaw. In many dogs, this digit is absent from the hind limb. Dewclaws are often rudimentary structures consisting of an osseous, claw-bearing phalanx attached to the medial surface of the foot by skin alone. Some dogs have dewclaws containing a third (distal) phalanx with attached claw, a first (proximal) phalanx, and a metatarsal or metacarpal bone (fig. 63-1). In the hind limb, the metatarsal bone may be fused with the first tarsal bone. Occasionally, dogs have two dewclaws on each hind paw. Double dewclaws are considered desirable in some breeds, such as the Icelandic sheepdog and Great Pyrenees.

Surgical removal of dewclaws may be performed to conform to breed standards or to prevent injury. In these animals, dewclaws are amputated within several days after birth. Dewclaws are often removed in adult dogs to treat traumatic avulsion of the digit.

Preoperative management

A wide area around the digit is clipped and prepped. Clipping can be challenging because of the irregular surfaces, particularly between toes and around pads. Local nerve blocks can be performed before surgery or immediately after skin closure. Because contamination is likely, prophylactic antibiotics (e.g., first-generation cephalosporins) may be administered IV at induction.

Surgery

In adult dogs, rudimentary dewclaws are easily removed by transecting the skin attachment with scissors or a blade. The skin is closed with suture or tissue adhesive, and the site is covered with a bandage. Fully developed first digits require more extensive dissection; these surgical sites are prone to dehiscence from tension or self-trauma.

Surgical technique: dewclaw amputation

1. Make a teardrop-shaped or elliptical incision around the proximal phalanx and associated pad of the dewclaw (fig. 63-2). Leave excess skin to reduce tension on closure.

Manual of Small Animal Soft Tissue Surgery, Second Edition. Karen Tobias.
© 2017 John Wiley & Sons, Inc. Published 2017 by John Wiley & Sons, Inc.

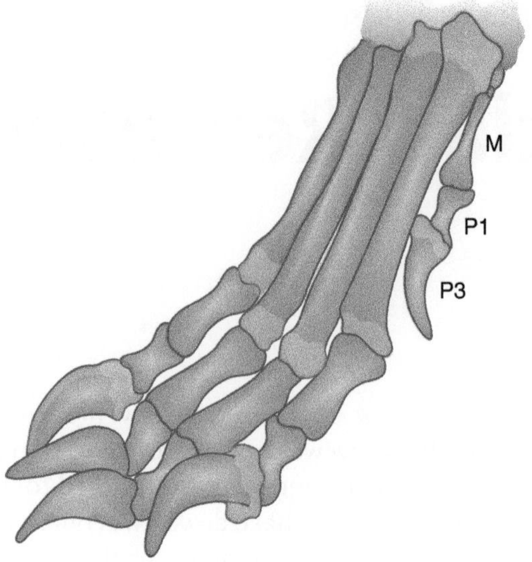

M

P1

P3

Figure 63-1 Right front paw of a dog. In this diagram, the dewclaw consists of a distal phalanx (P3), proximal phalanx (P1), and first metacarpal bone (M), which attaches to the first carpal bone.

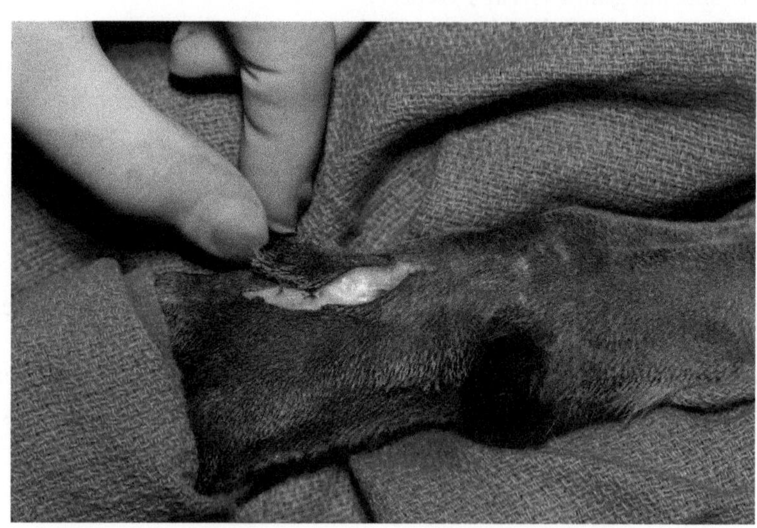

Figure 63-2 Make an elliptical incision around the proximal phalanx of the dewclaw. If the claw has boney attachments, extend the skin incision linearly up to the metatarsal- or metacarpal-phalangeal joint.

2. Extend the skin incision proximally, in a linear fashion, along the medial surface over the metatarsal or metacarpal bone if more bone exposure is required.
3. Dissect the subcutaneous tissues from the underlying bone (fig. 63-3) to expose the metatarsal- or metacarpal-phalangeal joint.
4. Ligate or cauterize the dorsal proper digital arteries medially and laterally as needed.
5. Transect tendons and ligamentous attachments between the proximal phalanx and the first metatarsal or metacarpal bone (fig. 63-4).
6. If the first metatarsal or metacarpal condyle is prominent and interferes with closure, remove it with rongeurs (fig. 63-5). Smooth the transected bone end with rongeurs or a file.

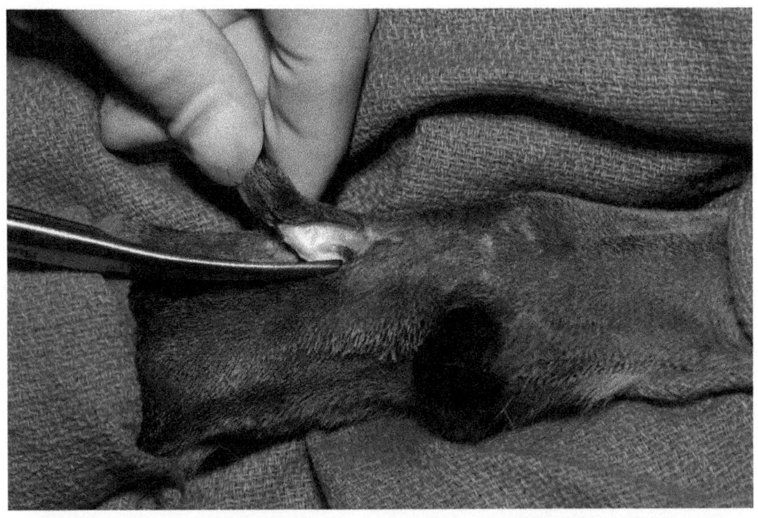

Figure 63-3 Dissect the subcutaneous tissues from underlying bone. If possible, ligate or cauterize the dorsal proper digital arteries before transecting them.

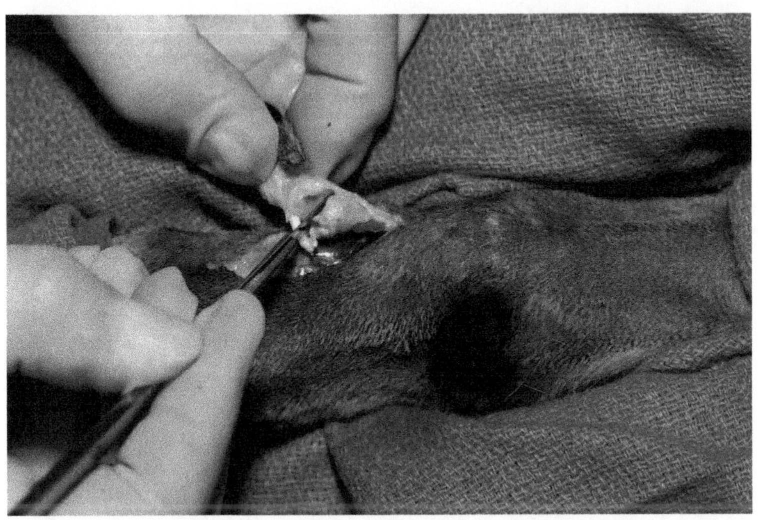

Figure 63-4 With a blade, transect the tendons and ligaments just proximal to the first phalanx.

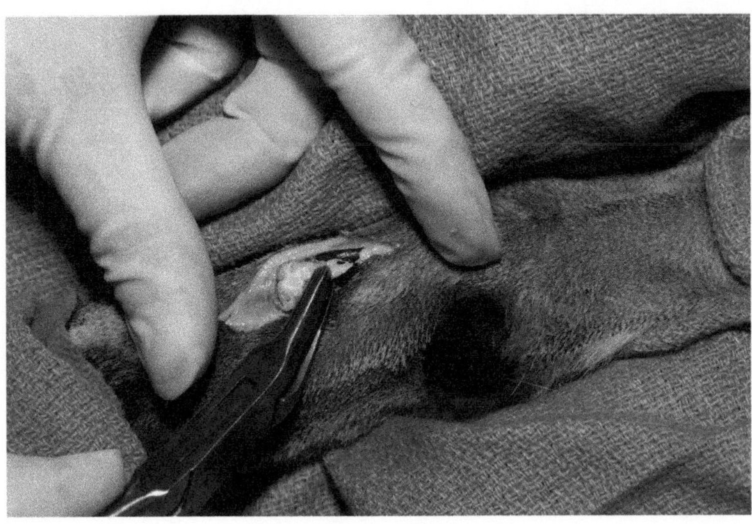

Figure 63-5 If the metatarsal or metacarpal condyle is prominent, remove it with rongeurs.

7. Appose subcutaneous tissues with buried interrupted sutures of 3-0 or 4-0 rapidly absorbable material (fig. 63-6). Tighten each throw by pulling the sutures longitudinally (along the length of the incision line) to bury the knots (fig. 63-7).
8. Close the skin with interrupted sutures (fig. 63-8). Cover the site with a padded bandage.

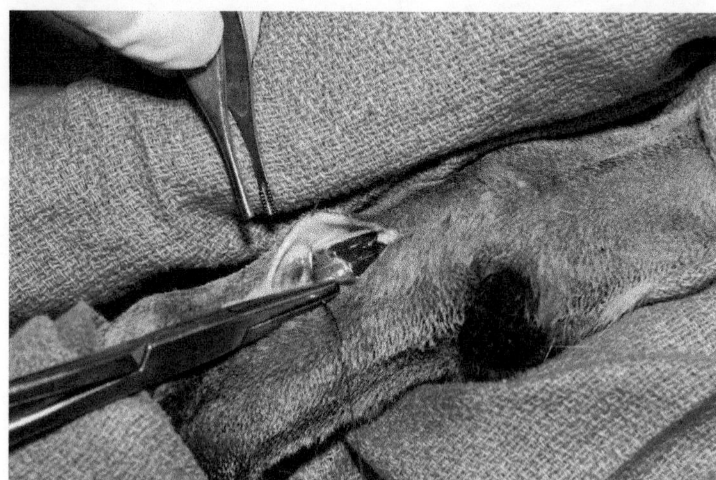

Figure 63-6 Close the initial layer with a buried intradermal pattern.

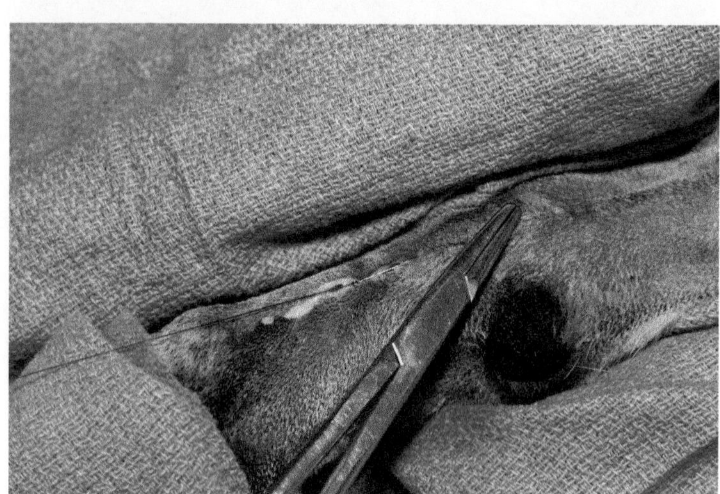

Figure 63-7 Pull lengthwise along the incision line to help bury the knots.

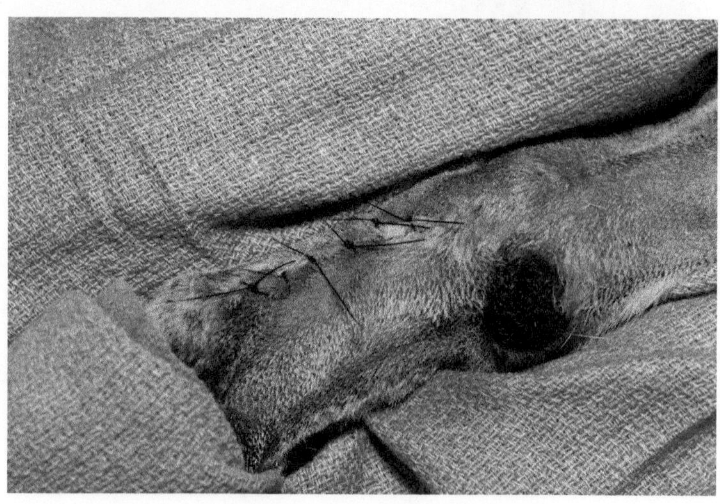

Figure 63-8 Final closure after placement of skin sutures.

Postoperative considerations

Bandages can be left in place for 1 to 7 days, and an Elizabethan collar should be kept on the dog until the surgery sites have healed. Analgesics should be administered for 1 to 3 days. Dehiscence is the most common surgical complication and is usually caused by self-trauma. Other complications include hemorrhage, infection, and scarring.

Bibliography

Mills KE, von Keyserlingk MAG, Niel L: A review of medically unnecessary surgeries in dogs and cats. J Am Vet Med Assoc 2016;248:162–171.

Chapter 64
Toe Amputation

In dogs and cats, weight bearing occurs primarily on digits 2 through 5, each of which consists of three phalangeal bones. Amputation of one or more of these toes is most commonly performed for treatment of injuries, malignant tumors, infection, or benign masses. In rare case, the bones of a toe are removed by "phalangeal fillet," producing a vascular compound flap that can be used to reconstruct the metacarpal or metatarsal pad or other parts of the foot.

In dogs, the most common neoplasms of the digits include squamous cell carcinoma, malignant melanoma, and mast cell tumors. Fortunately, metastases are uncommon with most types of canine digital tumors (except melanoma), and toe amputation provides a good chance for local control and long-term survival. In cats, the most common types of the digital tumors include squamous cell carcinoma and fibrosarcoma. Unfortunately, however, 20% of cats with digital neoplasia have "lung-digit" syndrome, in which a primary pulmonary tumor, particularly bronchogenic adenocarcinoma, metastasizes to one or more digits. Clinical signs of lung digit syndrome include lameness, digital swelling, and purulent nail-bed discharge, which can be confused with nail-bed infection. Amputation is usually not performed in these cats because of rapid and diffuse metastasis of their primary pulmonary neoplasia.

Preoperative management

For patients with suspected neoplastic disease, thoracic and distal limb radiographs should be taken. In cats, thorough examination of other feet, and even radiographs, should be performed, since more than one foot can be affected with lung-digit syndrome.

Usually, the entire foot must be clipped and prepped before surgery to reduce intraoperative contamination. Because it is difficult to thoroughly aseptically prepare the paw, prophylactic antibiotics (e.g., first-generation cephalosporins) are often administered IV at induction and again, if the surgery is still ongoing, 90 minutes to 2 hours later. Local nerve blocks can be performed before or during the surgery.

Surgery

Toe amputations are primarily performed at the metacarpophalangeal or metatarsophalangeal joint, although they can also be performed at the level

Manual of Small Animal Soft Tissue Surgery, Second Edition. Karen Tobias.
© 2017 John Wiley & Sons, Inc. Published 2017 by John Wiley & Sons, Inc.

of an interphalangeal joint. No matter the level, the procedures are essentially the same: an incision is made around the toe, leaving sufficient skin for closure, and the toe is dissected free from its softy tissue attachments. The toes have a rich vascular supply that primarily runs along the abaxial aspects of their dorsal and palmar/plantar surfaces. If the toe was a square on cross section, those vessels would be in each of the corners of that square. Most of the vessels are small enough to seal with bipolar cautery. Hemorrhage can be controlled during dissection by use of a tourniquet, which should be removed before closure so that any bleeding vessels can be cauterized or ligated.

Surgical technique: toe amputation

1. Make a circular incision around the base of the affected toe(s) and a linear incision over the distal half of the associated metacarpal or metatarsal bone (fig. 64-1).
2. Dissect the subcutaneous tissues down to the level of the metacarpo- or metatarso-phalnageal joint.
   a. Place a Penrose drain tourniquet above the carpus or tarsus to reduce bleeding during dissection (Fig. 64-2).
   b. Ligate or cauterize large vessels supplying the toe. Bipolar cautery is useful for precise hemostasis.
   c. Use a combination of blunt and sharp dissection with Metzenbaum scissors.
3. Transect the joint capsule and surrounding tendons and ligaments with a scalpel blade (Fig. 64-3) and remove the toe.
   a. Identify the joint by palpating for motion and thickness: the joints are wider than the bone shafts.
   b. If you can't identify the joint, hold the blade perpendicular to the dorsal surface of the toe and "walk" it down the distal portion of the metacarpal/metatarsal bone until the tip drops into the joint space.

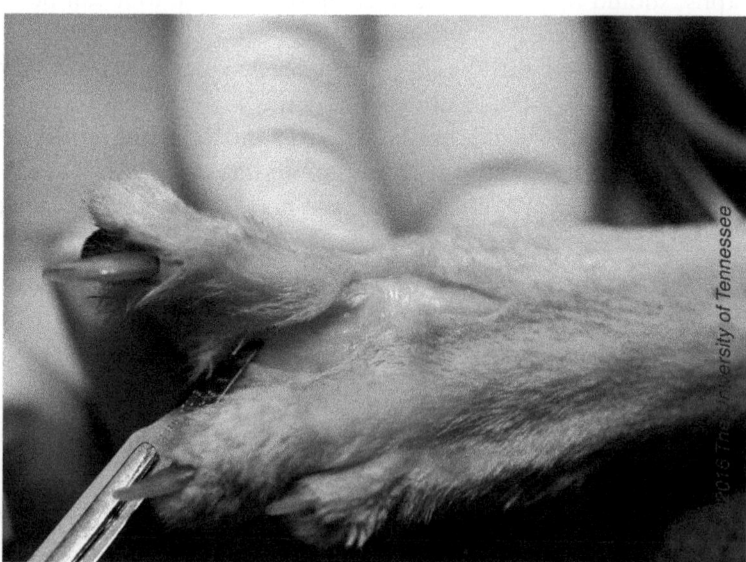

Figure 64-1 Incise the skin around the base of the toe and along the dorsal surface of the associated metacarpal or metatarsal bone. © 2016 The University of Tennessee.

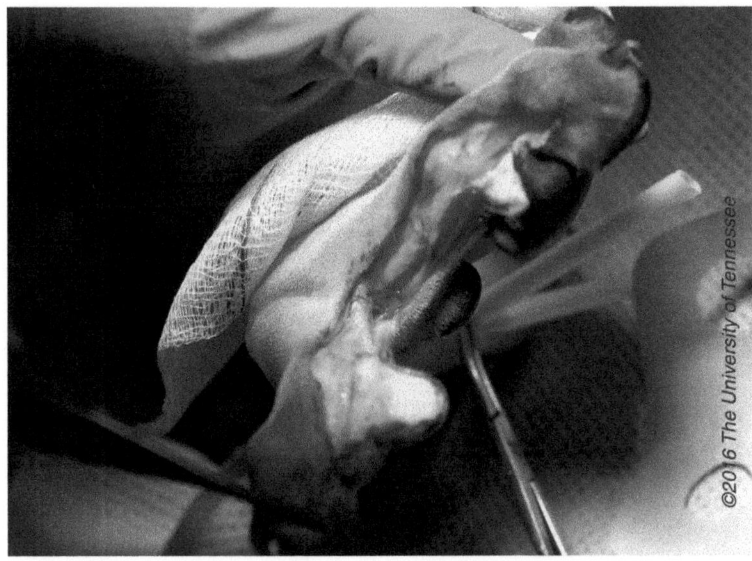

Figure 64-2 Branches of the common digital arteries are visible between the toes; a Penrose drain tourniquet controls the bleeding so that the blood vessels can be identified and cauterized or ligated. In this dog, skin resection included the medial surfaces of the adjacent toes. © 2016 The University of Tennessee.

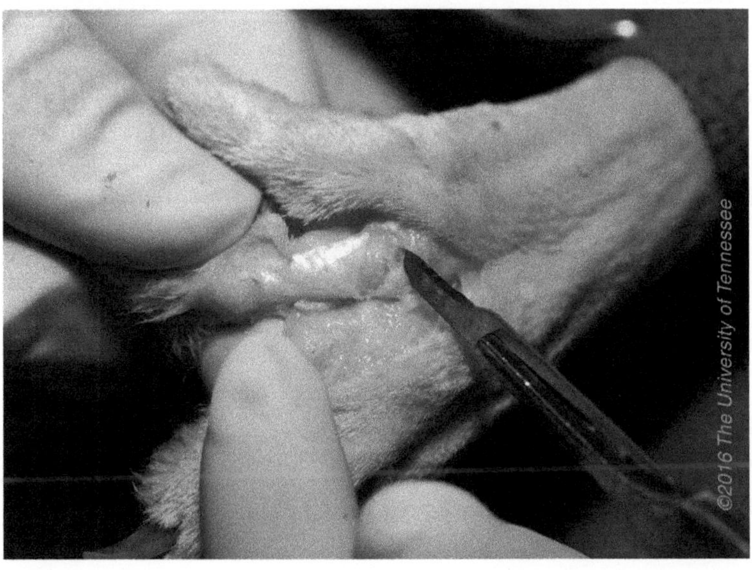

Figure 64-3 Amputate the toe at the joint. © 2016 The University of Tennessee.

   c. As you transect the tendons and ligaments on each side, pull the toe to the opposite side to open up the joint space.

4. Release the tourniquet and ligate or cauterize any bleeding vessels.
5. If possible, suture subcutaneous tissues together with simple interrupted sutures of 3-0 or 4-0 rapidly absorbable monofilament (fig. 64-4). In animals with thin skin or amputation of digit 2 or 5, there may be no subcutaneous tissues to appose.
6. Appose the skin with simple interrupted sutures.
   a. If sufficient skin is available, the dorsal edge of skin on each toe can be sutured to the palmar/plantar edge of skin on that same toe. This is most commonly used for closure of a digit 2 or 5 amputation.

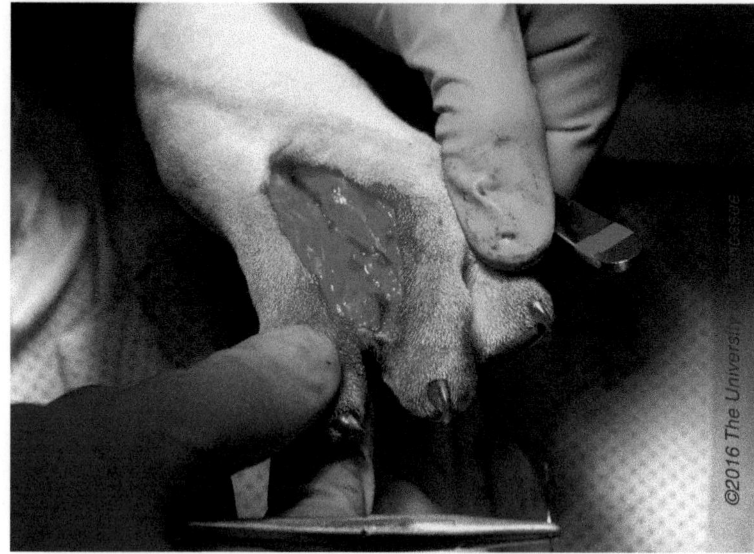

Figure 64-4 Appose subcutaneous tissues between the toes to reduce tension on the skin. © 2016 The University of Tennessee.

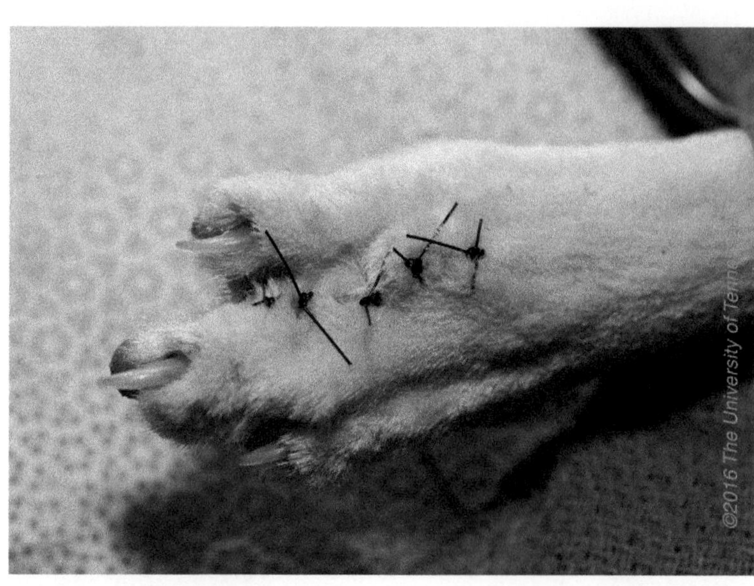

Figure 64-5 Appose the skin edges dorsally and ventrally to "fuse" the toes together. © 2016 The University of Tennessee.

b. If skin resection was more extensive, suture the toes together side to side in a "fusion podoplasty" by suturing the dorsal edges of skin together and the plantar/palmar edges of skin together (fig. 64-5). This is most commonly used when digit 3 or 4 is amputated.

Postoperative considerations

Bandages are commonly placed after surgery to provide mild compression for hemostasis and to protect the surgery site from trauma. Bandages should be changed or removed after 1 day or if they are wet or soiled. The animal should be kept in an Elizabethan collar or other restraint device, and exercise should be restricted until the surgery site has healed, since self-trauma is common. Dogs with tension along the suture line may benefit from splinting or use of a protective boot.

Complications are common after toe amputation and include lameness, infection, dehiscence, and swelling. Complications are more common after hind limb toe amputations. Postoperative lameness in dogs undergoing amputation of one or both central toes is expected but usually resolves within 8 weeks after surgery. Long term, most dogs and cats do well after toe amputation; however, larger dogs are more likely to have a permanent gait abnormality.

Bibliography

Goldfinch N, Argyle D: Feline lung-digit syndrome: Unusual metastatic patterns of primary lung tumors in cats. J Feline Med Surg 2012;14:202–208.

Henry CJ, Brewer WG, Whitley EM, et al: Canine digital tumors: a veterinary cooperative oncology group retrospective study of 64 dogs. J Vet Intern Med 2005;19:720–724.

Kaufman KL, Mann FA: Short- and long-term outcomes after digit amputation in dogs: 33 cases (1999–2011). J Am Vet Med Assoc 2013;242:1249–1254.

Liptak JM, Dernell WS, Rizzo SA, et al: Partial foot amputation in 11 dogs. J Am Anim Hosp Assoc 2005;41:47–55.

Shaw T, James F, Beierer L, et al: Bilateral phalangeal fillet technique for metacarpal pad reconstruction in a dog. Can Vet J 2014;55:955–960.

Complications are common after toe amputation and include lameness, infection, dehiscence, and swelling. Complications are more common after hind limb toe amputations. Postoperative lameness in dogs undergoing amputation of one or both central toes is expected but usually resolves within a few weeks after surgery. Long term, most dogs and cats do well after toe amputation; however, larger dogs are more likely to have a permanent gait abnormality.

Bibliography

[illegible] N, Argyle DJ. Feline lung-digit syndrome: Unusual metastatic patterns of primary lung tumours in cats. J Feline Med Surg 2012;14:202–208.

Henry CJ, Brewer WG, Whitley EM, et al. Canine digital tumors: a veterinary cooperative oncology group retrospective study of 64 dogs. J Vet Intern Med 2005;19:720–724.

Kaufman KL, Mann FA. Short- and long-term outcomes after digit amputation in dogs: 33 cases (1999–2011). J Am Vet Med Assoc 2013;242:1249–1254.

Liptak JM, Dernell WS, Rizzo SA, et al. Partial foot amputation in 11 dogs. J Am Anim Hosp Assoc 2005;41:47–55.

[illegible] J, [illegible] E, [illegible], et al. Bilateral phalangeal fillet technique for metacarpal pad reconstruction in a dog. Can Vet J 2015;[illegible].

Chapter 65
Rear Limb Amputation

Limb amputations are most frequently performed to provide wide resection of neoplastic lesions or as a treatment for severe trauma. Most dogs and cats do well on 3 legs, and most owners accept the cosmetic results of amputation once they see their pet adapt to the change in balance and weight bearing. However, musculoskeletal and neurologic issues in any of the remaining limbs and spine could interfere with mobility. Therefore, before an amputation is performed, the animal should be evaluated to determine whether ambulation with 3 limbs will be possible. Besides a thorough physical exam, suitability for amputation can also be tested by elevating the animal's affected leg with a sling or a bandage. Of course, many animals with osseous neoplasia or severe limb trauma are already successfully managing on three legs, so concern for postoperative mobility, at least in the short term, may not be an issue.

Preoperative management

Osseous neoplasia and nonrepairable limb fractures are usually diagnosed based on results of limb radiographs. For animals with limb neoplasia, three view-thoracic radiographs are performed to rule out metastatic disease. Animals that have suffered severe trauma should be examined for concurrent injuries such as pulmonary contusions, abdominal hemorrhage, spinal cord damage, and urinary tract rupture. Some of these patients will require an electrocardiogram, thoracic and abdominal radiographs and ultrasound, and even computed tomography. Blood work is usually performed in most patients. Anemic animals should be cross-matched, and coagulation should be evaluated in patients with thrombocytopenia, liver disease, or severe trauma.

If no infection is present, amputation is considered a clean procedure. However, surgeries lasting longer than 60 minutes will have increased infection rates, so prophylactic antibiotics are often administered intravenously at induction, with a second dose given 90 minutes after the first. Antibiotics do not need to be continued beyond the anesthesia period unless there was pre-existing infection or intraoperative contamination.

The limb and hemipelvis should be clipped and prepared widely and a purse string suture placed in the anus. Clipping should include the perineal, inguinal, and caudal abdominal regions and extend to the base of the tail, the level of umbilicus, and beyond midline dorsally and ventrally, especially if the animal

Manual of Small Animal Soft Tissue Surgery, Second Edition. Karen Tobias.
© 2017 John Wiley & Sons, Inc. Published 2017 by John Wiley & Sons, Inc.

has long hair. The foot is wrapped with a bandage that includes tape stirrups so that the leg can be suspended by a fluid stand or ceiling fixture during preparation and draping. Scrubbing of the limb is performed in stages with the goal of a five-minute contact time for all areas. Since the skin to be incised will be "downstream" of the suspended lower leg, any excess fluid left near the contaminated foot area will trickle down toward that site; this must be avoided during the final prep.

Options for perioperative analgesia include opioids delivered by injection or continuous rate infusion, preoperative epidural or regional block, direct injection of the nerves before transection, and placement of a fentanyl patch before or after the procedure. Some animals are already on nonsteroidal anti-inflammatory drugs before the procedure; these drugs provide good adjuncts to opioids during the postoperative period.

Fluid therapy is important during the procedure because of the risk for blood loss and is usually continued after surgery. After surgery, monitoring bladder size will be important, since many animals will not be able to immediately ambulate or posture appropriately during recovery.

Surgery

In patients with neoplasia, limb amputation is performed at least one joint above the involved bone. In animals with femoral neoplasia, the appropriate approach is therefore coxofemoral disarticulation (or even acetabulectomy or hemipelvectomy). When appropriate, midfemoral amputation may be considered for cosmetic reasons since it is more likely to conceal external genitalia. If the muscle over the femoral remnant atrophies, however, pressure necrosis of overlying subcutis and skin can occur if the animal frequently sits or lies on the amputation site.

For the procedure, the animal is positioned in lateral recumbency and, after a hanging limb prep, is draped in with surgical towels. For a coxofemoral disarticulation, the drapes should be wide enough to allow identification of the coxofemoral joint medially and laterally. The nonsterile portion of the limb (usually the foot) is covered during draping with a sterile self-adhesive wrap; sterility is easier to confirm and maintain if this wrap is a different color from any nonsterile wrap already on the foot. Once most of the nonsterile area is covered, the surgeon stabilizes the limb and a nonsterile assistant cuts the tape stirrups near the foot. The surgeon then covers the stirrup ends and any remaining nonsterile regions with the rest of the wrap. The top sheet is then placed over the leg, which is brought through a fenestration in that drape.

The major blood supply to the pelvic limb is the femoral artery, which lies superficially in the femoral triangle, cranial to the pectineus muscle and caudal to the caudal belly of the sartorius muscle. The femoral vein lies caudal and deep to the femoral artery. Each vessel is isolated and triple ligated so that two ligatures remain with the animal while one remains with the amputated leg. During ligature placement, at least 6 mm of space should be left between the distal 2 ligatures to leave an adequate stump of vessel beyond each ligature after transection. If vessels are large, the proximal and distal ligatures are placed in an encircling manner, and the middle ligature is placed as a transfixing encircling ligature. Some clinicians will use hemostats instead of the distal ligatures, but the hemostats interfere with subsequent muscle dissection and are easily knocked off during limb manipulation.

Muscles should be transected at least 3 cm away from any neoplastic or infected tissues. Muscle transection is facilitated by finger dissection: an index finger is worked between fascial planes and around a muscle belly until that muscle is isolated from other structures. The muscle is then severed with scissors, a blade, electrocautery, or a vessel-sealing device. Intramuscular vessels less than 1 mm can be cauterized, while larger vessels may require ligation. Mild bleeding often ceases once muscle ends are sutured together. Placement of a continuous suction drain may be necessary to close dead space and reduce seroma formation.

Surgical technique: amputation by femoral transection

1. Make two connected semicircular incisions in the skin, one lateral and one medial, starting cranially just distal to the level of the flank fold, extending down to the patella, and curving upward caudally to the same level as the cranial end of the incision (fig. 65-1)
    a. The resultant skin flaps can be made longer on one side of the leg (often the lateral side) so that the sutured incision is located away from the ventral surface of the stump once the amputation is complete.
2. With blunt and sharp dissection, transect subcutaneous tissues to elevate the skin flaps away from underlying muscle bellies (fig. 65-2).
3. With the leg abducted to expose its medial surface, transect the gracilis muscle and caudal belly of the sartorius muscle proximal to the patella.
    a. If the femoral artery and vein are visible once the caudal belly of the sartorius muscle has been transected, they can be ligated and divided before transecting the gracilis muscle.
4. With the leg still abducted, dissect the femoral artery and vein and saphenous nerve free of fascia. Isolate the saphenous nerve; block it with bupivacaine or lidocaine, and sever it distal to the local block.
5. With the leg still abducted, isolate, triple ligate, and transect the femoral artery and vein proximal to their saphenous branches and distal to their proximal caudal femoral branches (fig. 65-3).

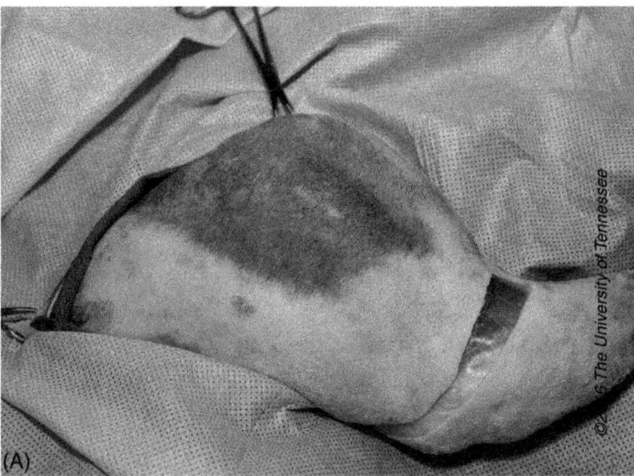

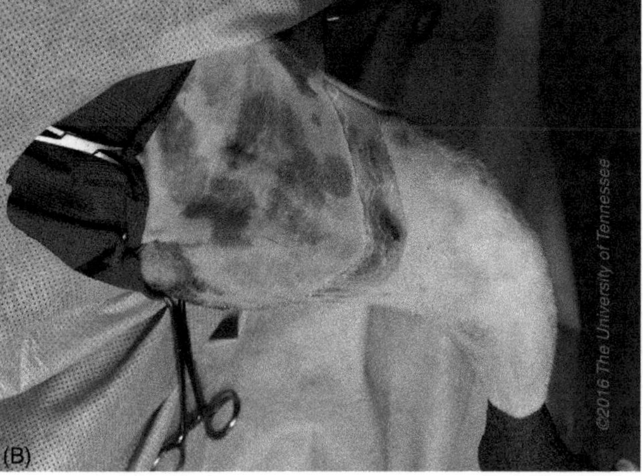

Figure 65-1 Lateral (A) and medial (B) skin incisions for a midfemoral amputation.

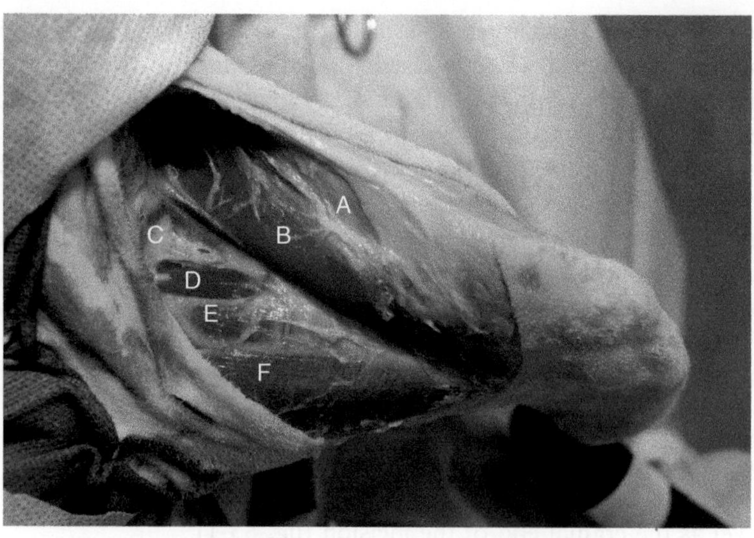

Figure 65-2 Muscles of the medial thigh. A, Cranial belly of the sartorius muscle; B, Caudal belly of the sartorius muscle; C, femoral head; D, pectineus muscle; E, adductor muscle; F, gracilis muscle

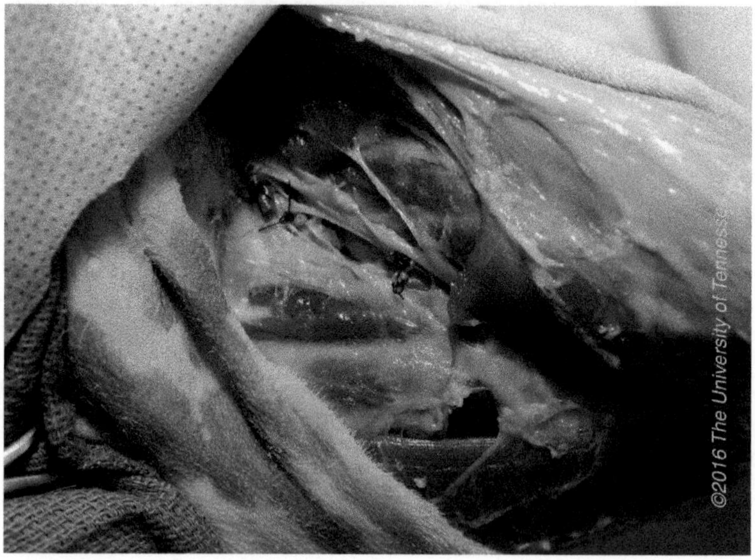

Figure 65-3 The caudal belly of the sartorius muscle has been transected and the femoral artery and vein individually ligated and transected.

6. Transect the pectineus muscle near its attachment to the femur, and transect the cranial belly of the sartorius muscle near the patella.
7. Transect the vastus medialis close to the patella.
   a. If the remaining quadriceps muscles can be reached from this exposure, they can be transected at this time.
   b. If the semimembranosus muscle is visible, it can be transected at this time.
8. Return the leg to its resting position so the lateral surface is exposed, and transect any remaining quadriceps muscles.
9. Proximal to the patella, incise the aponeurosis of the biceps femoris muscle and fascia lata, then isolate the biceps femoris muscle and transect it.

10. Retract the biceps femoris muscle dorsally, and isolate the sciatic nerve along the junction of the proximal and middle thirds of the femur. Block the nerve with local anesthetic, and transect it distal to the injection site (fig. 65-4).
11. Transect the abductor cruris caudalis, semitendinosus, and semimembranosus muscles proximal to the patella.
12. Using a periosteal elevator or blade, free the adductor muscle from the caudal aspect of the femur to the level of the proximal third of the femur (fig. 65-5), then transect the muscle belly. Transect any remaining muscle fibers to fully expose the femur.
13. Transect the femur with a bone saw or Gigli wire at the junction of its proximal and middle thirds (fig. 65-6).

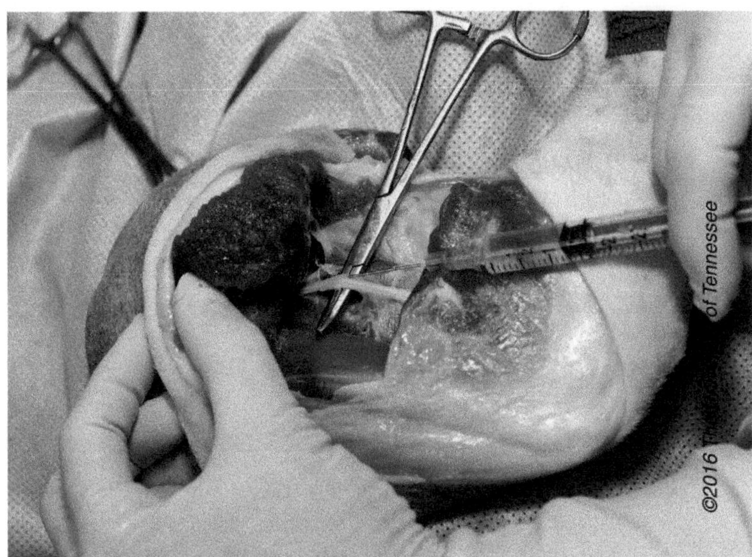

Figure 65-4 After the biceps femoris is transected, the sciatic nerve can be isolated and directly injected with 0.5% bupivacaine before transection.

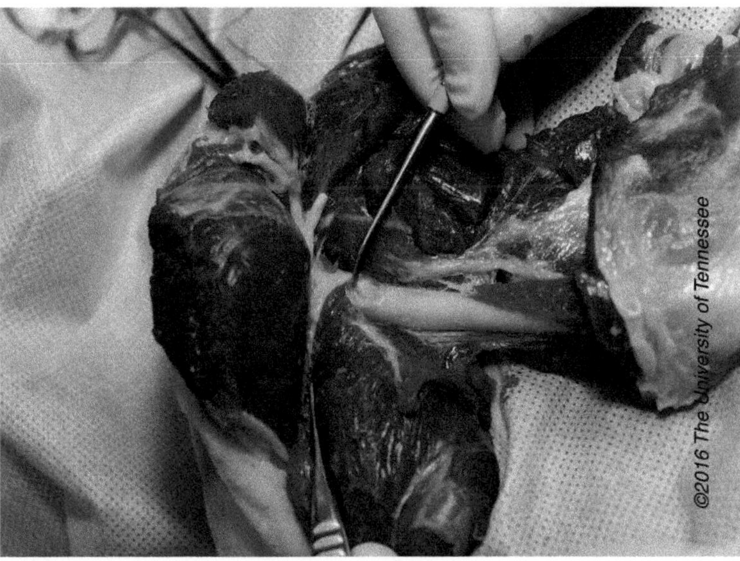

Figure 65-5 The adductor muscle is elevated from the femur and then transected.

a. The bone should be transected more proximally than the muscle so that it will be totally covered by muscle with closure.

b. If the osteotomy site is bleeding, pack the medullary cavity with bone wax.

c. If the edges of the bone are rough, smooth them with rongeurs or a metal file.

14. With 3-0 (or 2-0) absorbable monofilament suture, appose muscle ends to each other with simple interrupted or mattress sutures (fig. 65-7).

    a. Appose muscles from opposite sides of the femur (e.g., quadriceps to semitendinosus and adductor muscles, and biceps femoris to gracilis and semitendinosus muscles) so that the bone end is completely encased.

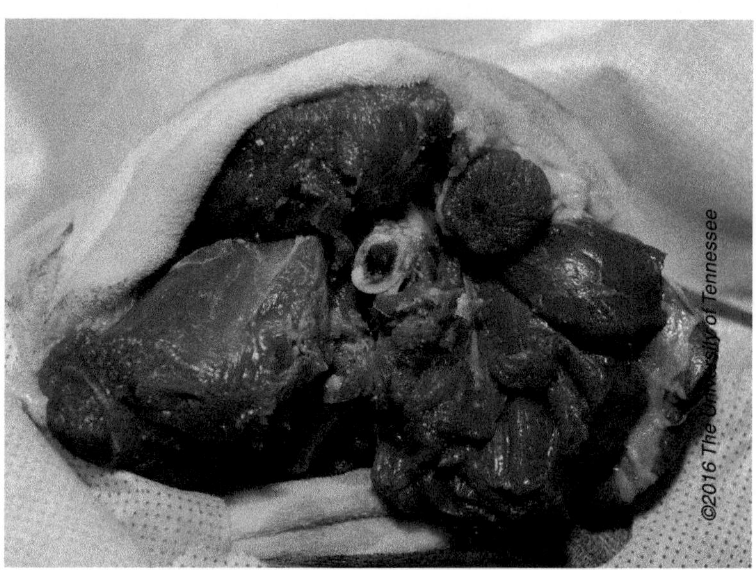

Figure 65-6 Transect the femur at its proximal third with a Gigli wire or bone saw. Note that sufficient muscle has been left to cover the bone remnant.

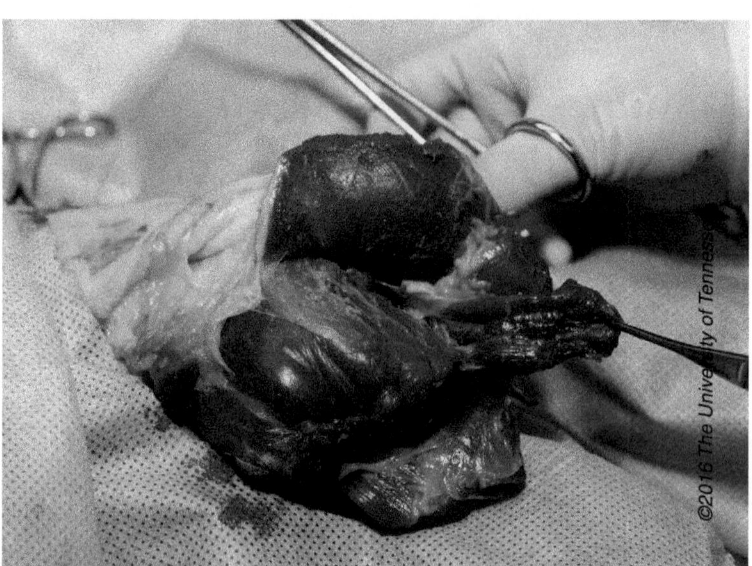

Figure 65-7 Appose transected muscle ends to one another so that the femoral remnant is completely covered.

b. To reduce postoperative hemorrhage, make sure all transected muscle bellies are sutured to other muscles or oversewn.

15. If dead space cannot be closed, place a continuous suction drain before completing the subcutaneous and skin closures.

Surgical technique: amputation by coxofemoral disarticulation

1. Make a semicircular incision on the lateral surface of the rear limb, starting and ending approximately level with the flank fold and with the midpoint reaching to the level of the midfemur or lower.
    a. If tension is a concern, make the skin incision more distal than necessary; excess skin can be removed at the time of closure.
    b. If skin on the lateral surface of the leg is unhealthy (e.g., traumatized or neoplastic), plan to make the medial incision longer so that the medial skin flap can be advanced to the lateral surface of the leg at closure.
2. Abduct the leg to expose its medial surface.
3. Make a semicircular skin incision along the medial surface of the leg (fig. 65-8).
4. Using a combination of blunt and sharp dissection, elevate the medial skin and reflect it proximally to the level of the proximal femur.
5. Dissect the femoral artery and vein free of surrounding fascia (fig. 65-9). Isolate each vessel and triple ligate it distal to its lateral circumflex branch, using encircling and transfixing-encircling ligatures. Transect the vessels.
    a. The lateral circumflex femoral artery originates from the caudal aspect of the femoral artery and will supply the residual muscle stumps.
6. Double ligate and transect the superficial circumflex iliac artery.

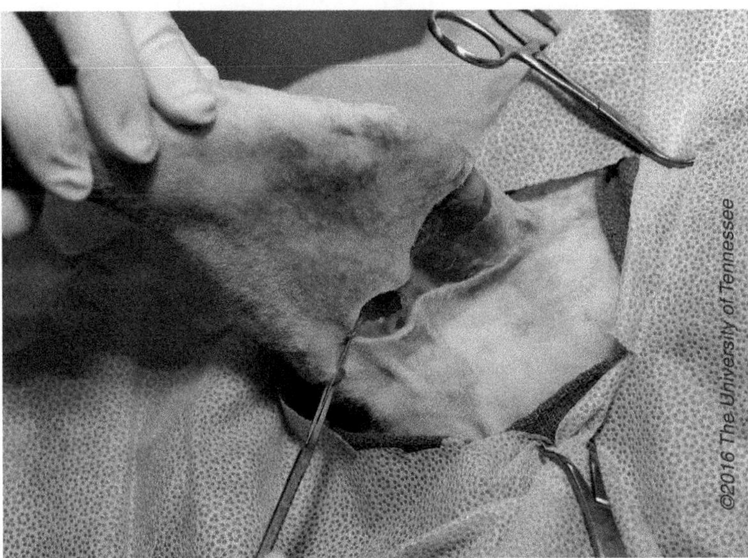

Figure 65-8 Medial incision for a coxofemoral disarticulation.

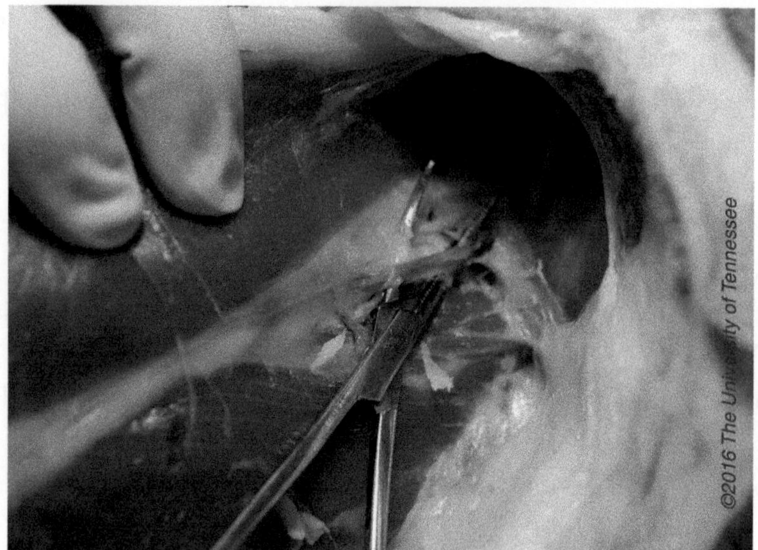

Figure 65-9 Isolate the femoral artery and vein distal to their lateral circumflex femoral branches. The surgeon's fingers are resting on the caudal belly of the sartorius muscle.

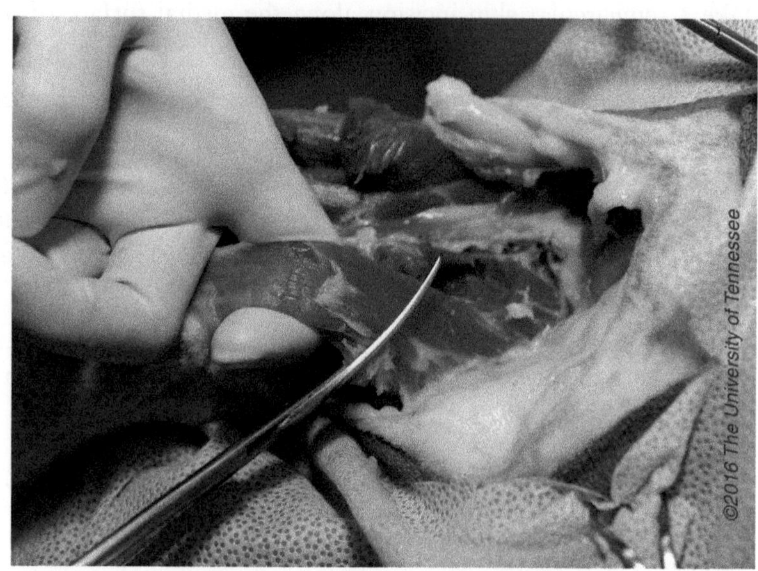

Figure 65-10 Transection of the gracilis muscle. During amputation, muscle bellies can be isolated by establishing a fascial place around them using digital dissection.

   a. The superficial circumflex iliac artery originates from the femoral artery just proximal to the origin of the lateral circumflex femoral artery, and runs cranial toward the caudal belly of the sartorius muscle and tensor fascia lata and rectus femoris muscles. Anastomosing branches may allow blood to flow retrograde in this vessel.

7. Transect both bellies of the sartorius muscle several cm distal to their origins on the ilium.
8. Transect the pectineus, gracilis, and adductor muscles at the same level as the sartorius muscles (fig. 65-10).
9. Double ligate and transect the medial circumflex femoral artery and vein.
   a. The medial circumflex femoral artery is a continuation of the deep femoral artery and is the principal blood supply to the femur. The

artery and accompanying vein cross the medial surface of the iliopsoas and vastus medialis muscles and lateral surface of the pectineus muscle proximal to the origins of the superficial circumflex iliac and lateral circumflex femoral vessels.

10. Transect the iliopsoas muscle (fig. 65-11) from its femoral attachment and retract it cranially to expose the saphenous and femoral nerves.
11. Inject the saphenous and femoral nerves with bupivacaine and transect them distal to the injection site.
12. Incise the medial joint capsule and the ligament of the head of the femur (fig. 65-12).
13. Adduct the limb and return it to a resting position to expose its lateral aspect. If necessary, transect the subcutaneous tissues to elevate the skin from underlying muscle.

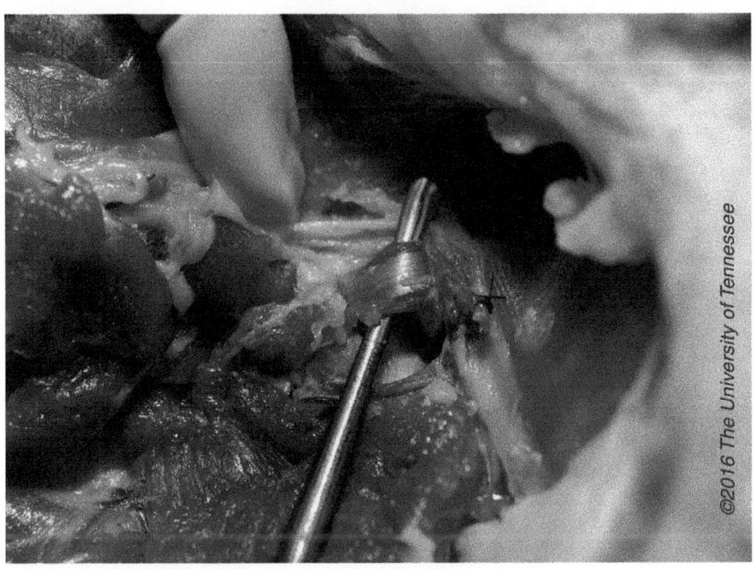

Figure 65-11 Transect the Iliopsoas muscle to expose the femoral head medially.

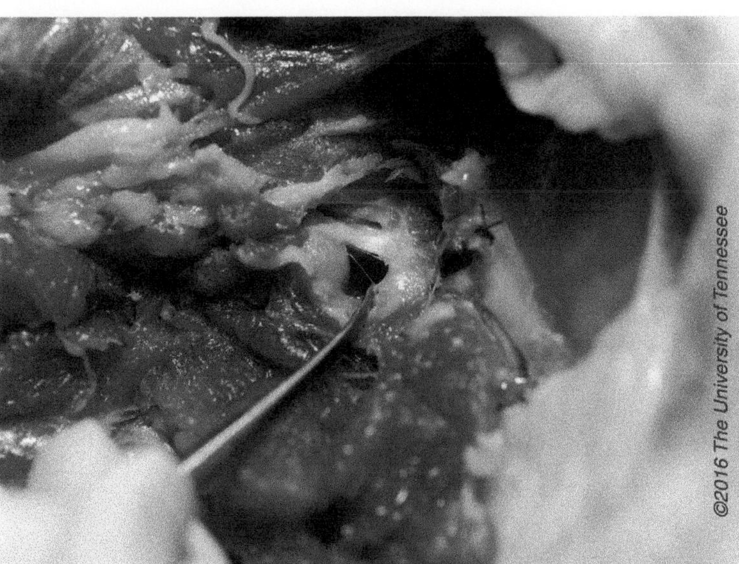

Figure 65-12 Transect the medial joint capsule and ligament of the head of the femur.

14. Transect the tensor fasciae latae muscle at the level of the junction between the proximal and middle thirds of the femur (fig. 65-13).
15. Continue the same incision to transect the biceps femoris and abductor cruris caudalis muscles.
    a. Note: The site for each muscle transection sites depends on the underlying condition. If neoplasia is present, deeper muscles may need to be transected more proximally to provide a clean margin of resection around the tumor.
16. Retract the tensor fasciae latae and biceps femoris muscles dorsally to expose the semimembranosus and semitendinosus muscles, and transect these muscles at the level of the junction between the proximal and middle thirds of the femur (fig. 65-14).

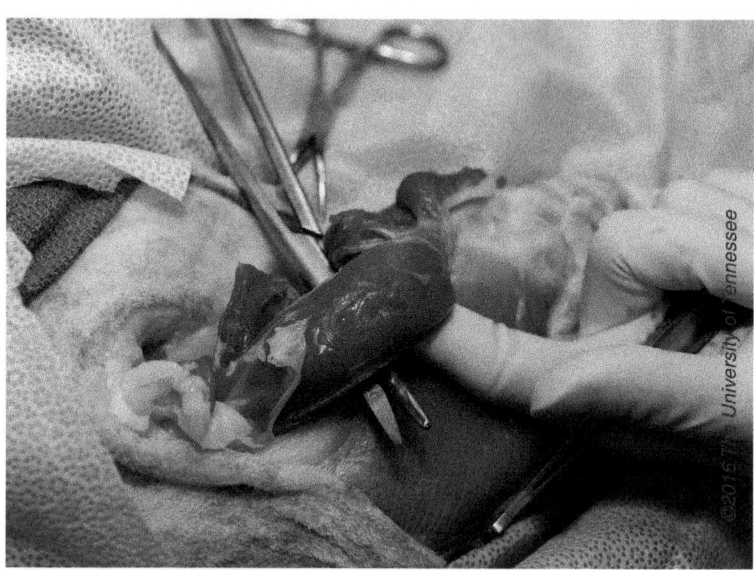

Figure 65-13 Transect the tensor fasciae latae muscles.

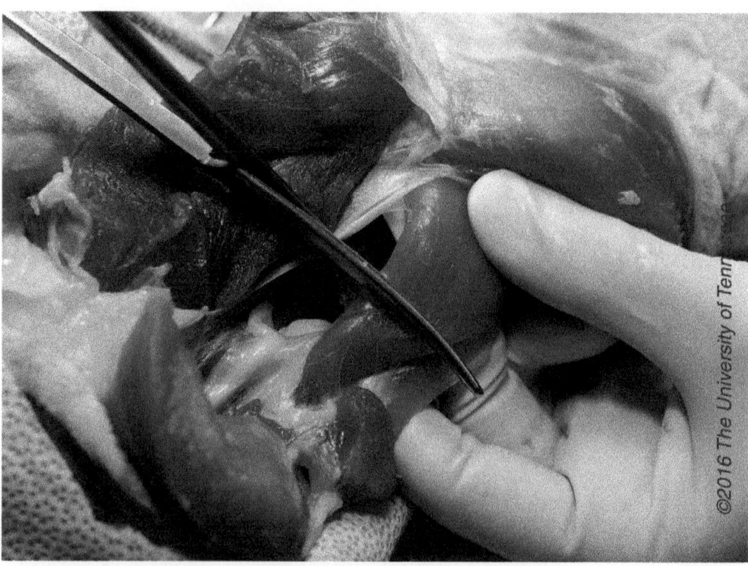

Figure 65-14 Transect the semimembranosus and semitendinosus muscles.

17. Expose and isolate the sciatic nerve distal to its branch supplying the semimembranosus, semitendinosus, and biceps femoris muscles. Inject the nerve with bupivacaine and transect it distal to the injection site.
    a. Some clinicians transect the sciatic nerve distal to its branch supplying the semimembranosus, semitendinosus, and biceps femoris muscle in an attempt to avoid neurogenic atrophy to the muscle stumps. Whether this actually prevents atrophy is unknown.
18. Flex and abduct the hip to expose the quadratus femoris muscle caudal to the joint, and transect it near its attachment to the third trocahanter.
19. With the limb in the same position, transect the internal obturator, external obturator, and gemelli muscles as they enter the trochanteric fossa.
20. Rotate the leg slightly inward to expose and transect the superficial gluteal, middle gluteal, and piriformis muscles.
21. Transect the deep gluteal muscle from the greater trochanter.
22. Transect the dorsal joint capsule and articularis coxae muscle to free the femur from the acetabulum.
23. Transect the rectus femoris muscle at its origin, and remove the limb (fig. 65-15).
24. With 3-0 (or 2-0) monofilament absorbable suture, appose muscle ends together to cover the acetabulum (fig. 65-16).
    a. The biceps femoris muscle can be sutured to the gracilis, semitendinosus, and semimembranosus muscles, and the tensor fasciae latae can be sutured to the iliopsoas muscle.
    b. In general, the goal is to cover any bone and to seal any raw, bleeding muscle ends by suturing them to each other or by oversewing them.
25. If dead space is likely to be an issue, place a continuous suction drain.
26. Align the skin, removing any excess as needed, and place a skin suture centrally to maintain position.

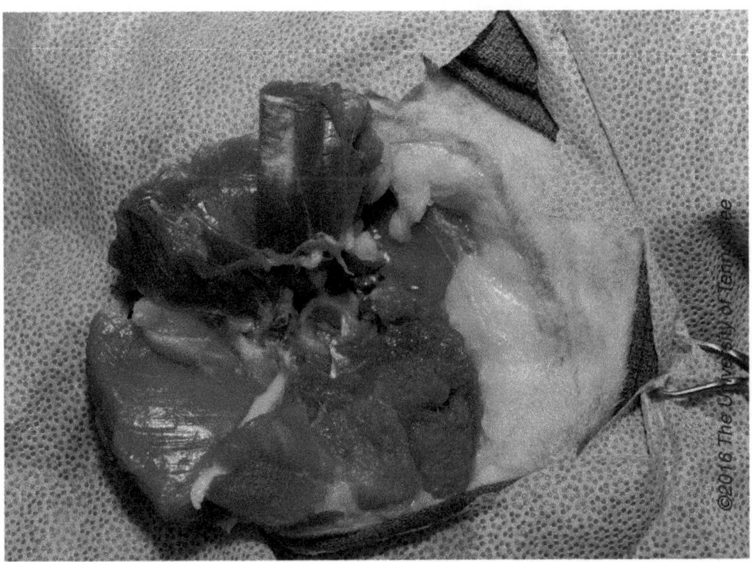

Figure 65-15 Appearance after removal of the hind leg.

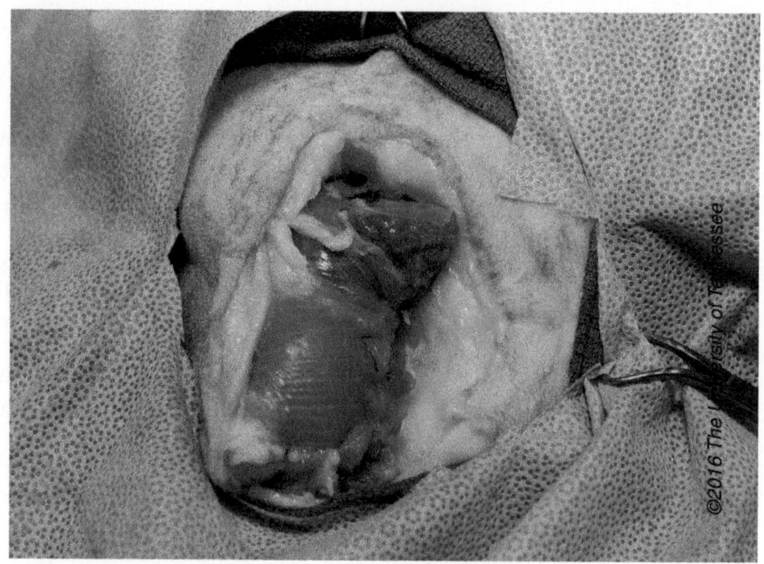

Figure 65-16 Suture muscle ends together to cover the acetabulum and seal and muscle ends

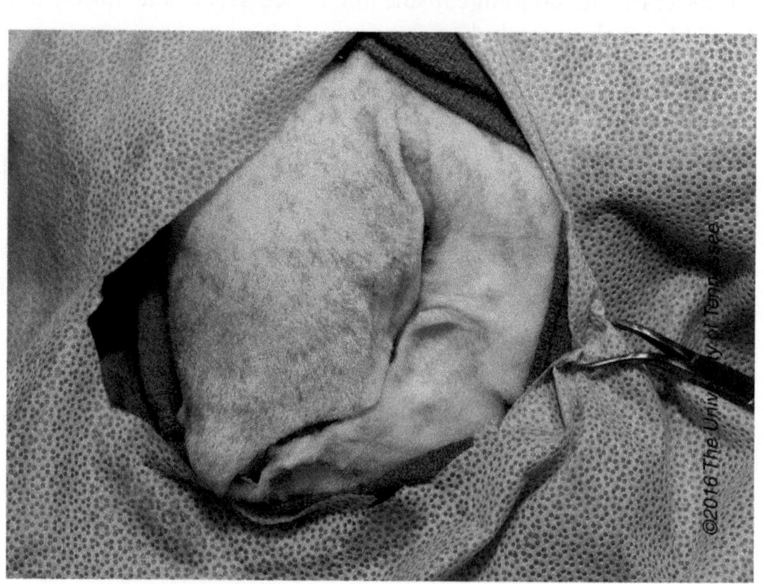

Figure 65-17 Skin flaps positioned for closure.

27. Once the skin is aligned (fig. 65-17), close the subcutaneous tissues with interrupted or continuous patterns, and close the skin with an interrupted pattern.
    a. In some animals, there is no subcutaneous fat along the center of the incision. Interrupted buried intradermal sutures can be placed to hold skin flaps in place before the skin is sutured.

Postoperative considerations

After surgery, a fentanyl CRI (1-8 mcg/kg/h, with lidocaine added at 25–50 mcg/kg/min for dogs) or an injectable opioid (e.g., buprenorphine, hydromorphone, or methadone) provides excellent analgesia during the initial recovery phase. Intravenous fluids are often continued to counteract intraoperative blood loss and provide hydration in animals too sleepy to drink. Urination must be monitored, since animals may be hesitant to stand and posture. Nonsteroidal anti-inflammatory drugs, if not already being administered, can be started postoperatively, with an initial dose given by injection immediately after the procedure. If a drain was placed, its exit site should be covered with a sterile dressing, and it is usually removed once fluid production has decreased to <4.8 mls/kg/day.

Use of a sling is helpful for supporting large dogs during standing and walking until they can adapt to the change in center of gravity. Flooring alternatives or toe grips may be necessary to provide traction at home. Balance can be improved by physical therapy with balance boards or uneven terrain. Weight management is important to reduce stress on the remaining limbs.

Short-term complications of amputation occur in 13–21% of animals and most commonly include surgical-site swelling, infection, and seroma formation. Less common complications include hemorrhage, dehiscence, breakthrough pain, incomplete tumor resection, and an inability to ambulate. Neuropathic (e.g., phantom limb) pain has been reported after hind-limb amputation and may be responsive to opioids and amitriptyline.

Delayed hemorrhage (36 to 72 hours after surgery) and subsequent severe bruising are reported in 28% of greyhounds after limb amputation. Affected dogs usually have normal platelet counts and coagulation panels; hemorrhage is thought to be a result of excess fibrinolysis. Intraoperative administration of blood products does not reduce the risk; instead, risk can be decreased by postoperative administration of epsilon-aminocaproic acid. An initial dose (15 to 40 mg/kg IV) can be given immediately after surgery, followed by 5 days of oral treatment (500–1000 mg total dose PO q8h).

Long-term complications of amputation may include decreased activity (dogs and cats) and stamina (dogs) and altered grooming habits (cats). Most owners are pleased with the outcome and feel their pets have regained a normal quality of life. Quality of life is better in dogs that are lighter, so weight management is an important part of lifelong care for amputees.

Bibliography

Dickerson VM, Coleman KD, Ogawa M, et al: Outcomes of dogs undergoing limb amputation, owner satisfaction with limb amputation procedures, and owner perceptions regarding postsurgical adaptation: 64 cases (2005–2012). J Am Vet Med Assoc 2015;247:786–792.

Forster LM, Wathes CM, Bessant D, et al: Owners' observations of domestic cats after limb amputation. Vet Rec 2010;167:734–739.

Goldner B, Fuchs A, Nolte I, et al: Kinematic adaptations to tripedal locomotion in dogs. Vet J 2015;204:192–200.

Marin LM, Iazbik MC, Zaldviar Lopez S, et al: Retrospective evaluation of the effectiveness of epsilon aminocaproic acid for the prevention of postamputation bleeding in retired racing Greyhounds with appendicular bone tumors: 46 cases (2003–2008) J Vet Emerg Crit Care 2012;22:332–340.

O'Hagan BJ: Neuropathic pain in a cat post-amputation. Aust Vet J 2006;84:83–86.

Raske M, McClaran JK, Mariano A: Short-term wound complications and predictive variables for complication after limb amputation in dogs and cats. J Small Anim Pract 2015;56:247–252.

Chapter 66
Forelimb Amputation

Each thoracic limb carries approximately 30% of a dog's body weight. Therefore, removal of one foreleg results in a greater shift of weight to the remaining legs and spine than a rear limb amputation. Despite this, quality of life is no different for thoracic limb amputees than those undergoing pelvic limb amputation. As with rear limb amputation, the animal should be evaluated for orthopaedic and neurologic issues that could interfere with postoperative ambulation. The affected limb can be secured to the animal's body with a bandage or sling to test ambulation before the procedure. Many animals are already carrying the affected leg, however, and thus do not require such a challenge.

Preoperative management

Preoperative diagnostics and use of prophylactic antibiotics are similar to those described for hind limb amputation (see Chapter 65). Intraoperative and postoperative analgesia can be supplemented by intraoperative nerve blocks or a preoperative regional block of the brachial plexus, which will provide analgesia from the elbow down. A needle is inserted medial to the shoulder joint and directed parallel to the vertebral column and toward the costochondral junction. The local anesthetic (maximum dose, 1.5 mg/kg of lidocaine or bupivacaine; usually 5 to 10 mls for medium to large dogs) is injected slowly as the needle is withdrawn. The block usually takes effect within 20 minutes and lasts for up to 2 hours.

Most complete forelimb amputations include scapulectomy. When the scapula is left in place, atrophy of overlying muscles results in visible and palpable bone, poor cosmetic results, and the potential for pressure sores. The area to be clipped should include the skin over the affected leg and scapula, distal cervical region, and cranial half of the thorax and should extend beyond midline dorsally and ventrally, especially in animals with long hair. As with rear limb amputations, a hanging limb prep is performed. The leg must be scrubbed and prepped with care to prevent contaminated fluids from trickling down toward the incisional area.

Surgery

The animal is positioned in lateral recumbency and, after a hanging leg prep, is draped in (see Chapter 65). Because the amputation includes the entire scapula, the animal is usually draped along the dorsal and ventral midlines.

Manual of Small Animal Soft Tissue Surgery, Second Edition. Karen Tobias.
© 2017 John Wiley & Sons, Inc. Published 2017 by John Wiley & Sons, Inc.

Electrocautery and vessel vessel-sealing devices are useful for controlling minor bleeding. If the scapula is unaffected, muscle insertions can be transected immediately adjacent to the bone to reduce haemorrhage from muscle bellies. Muscles should be transected several cm away from neoplastic, necrotic, or infected tissues, however. Drain placement (preferably a continuous suction drain) may be necessary to close dead space. Alternatively, a wrap can be placed around the chest and over the site to provide compression, as long as it does not compromise respiration.

Surgical technique: forelimb amputation

1. Incise the skin.
   a. Make an incision through the skin over the spine of the scapula from dorsal to ventral.
   b. At the level of the acromion process (the ventral end of the scapular spine), incise the skin caudoventrally toward the axillary fold.
   c. Continue the incision around the medial surface of the brachium.
   d. Start a connecting incision at the acromion process and incise cranioventrally toward the point of the shoulder, then around and medial to the brachium to meet the other incision. When completed, the lateral portion of the incision will be shaped like an inverted Y.
   e. If there is neoplasia near the proposed skin incisions, include overlying skin in the resection.
2. Incise the subcutaneous tissues with blunt and sharp dissection to expose underlying muscle.
   a. You may need to ligate the cephalic vein during subcutaneous tissue transection along the point of the shoulder.
3. Ligate (or cauterize) any visible superficial veins overlying muscles that will be transected (e.g., the omobrachial vein, which overlies the brachiocephalicus muscle).
4. Transect the brachiocephalicus muscle through the clavicular tendon.
   a. Before transecting muscle, dissect under it with scissors, Kelly hemostatic forceps, or a finger to isolate the muscle belly from the surrounding tissues.
5. With Mayo scissor or a blade, transect the trapezius and omotransversarius muscles.
   a. If the scapula is unaffected, insert scissors under the muscles and spread the blades to elevate and isolate the muscles, then transect the muscles along their insertion sites on the cranial border of the scapular spine (fig. 66-1).
   b. If the scapula is affected, elevate and transect the muscles at least 3 cm away from the diseased tissue.
6. Separate the latissimus dorsi muscle from the teres major muscle (fig. 66-2) and, if the proximal humerus is not affected, sever the muscle close to its insertion near the humerus.

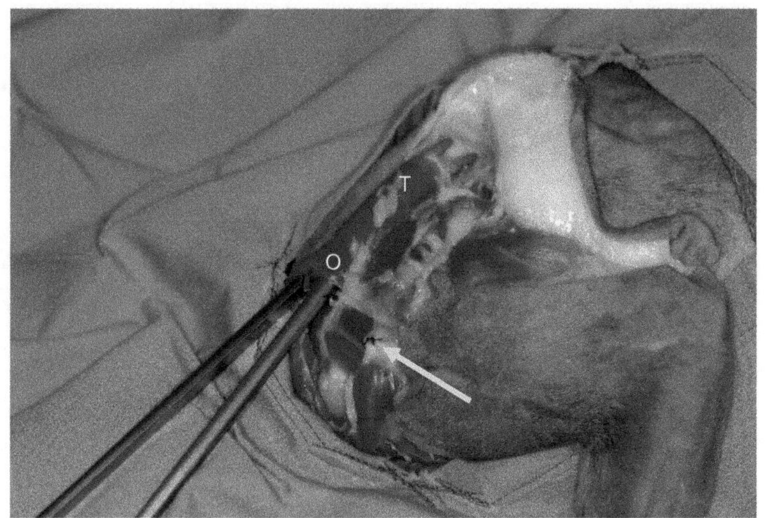

Figure 66-1 If the bone insertion side is unaffected (e.g., non-neoplastic), slide the closed scissors under the omotransversarius (O) and trapezius (T) muscles to elevate and isolate them, then transect them immediately adjacent to their bone insertion sites. The omobrachial vein has already been ligated (arrow).

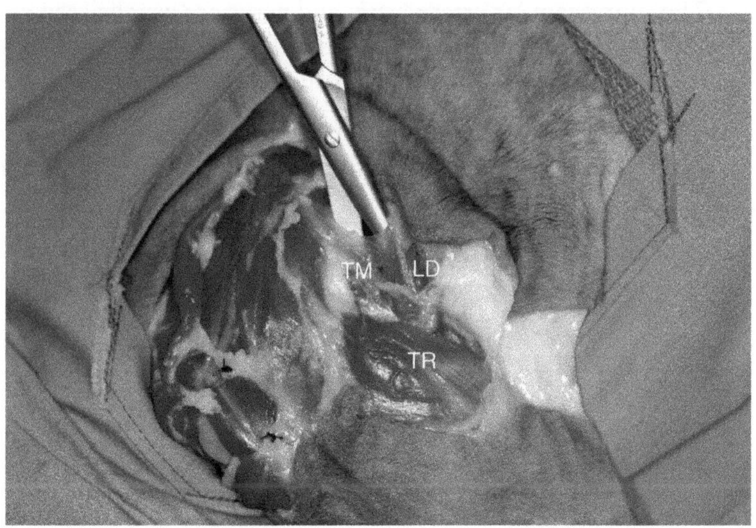

Figure 66-2 Separate the latissimus dorsi (LD) muscle from the teres major (TM) and transect the latissimus dorsi from its attachment to the humerus or its aponeurosis with the triceps (TR).

7. Grasp the cranial edge of the scapula and rotate it externally and caudally to expose its medial surface (fig. 66-3).
8. Transect the insertion of the rhomboideus and serratus ventralis muscles.
   a. The serratus ventralis muscles has a wide attachment along the dorsomedial margin of the scapula and sometimes can be elevated off the bone with a periosteal elevator instead of sharp transection.
   b. The rhomboideus muscle has a narrow attachment along the dorsal surface of the scapula and usually requires sharp transection with scissors or electrocautery. An instrument or finger can be slid under the muscle to isolate it before transection.
   c. As with all other muscles, if the scapula is neoplastic or infected, transect the muscles at least 3 cm away from the affected bone.

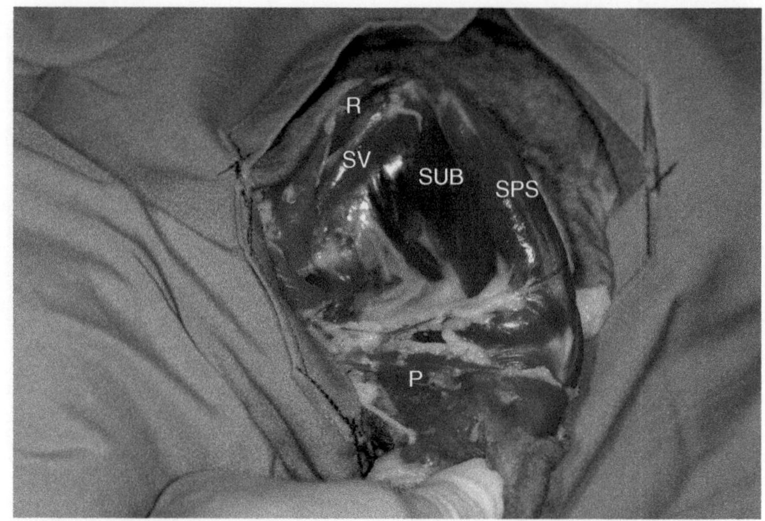

Figure 66-3 Rotate the scapula externally and caudally to expose the rhomboideus (R) and serratus ventralis (SV) muscle attachments along the dorsomedial surface of the scapula. SUB, subscapularis; SPS, supraspinatus; P, pectorals.

9. Ligate and transect the suprascapular artery and vein, and transect the adjacent suprascapular nerve.
   a. The suprascapular artery, vein, and nerve are usually seen cranial to the scapula near the point of the shoulder in a space bounded by the deep pectoral, subscapular, and supraspinatus muscles.
   b. If the nerve is large enough to accommodate a 25 gauge needle, it can be blocked with bupivacaine first and transected distal to the injection site.
10. Transect the humeral attachments of the superficial and deep pectoral muscles (fig. 66-4).
    a. Transect these muscles midbody if the humerus is neoplastic or infected.
11. Block and transect the subscapular nerve, which runs along the medial surface of the distal portion of the subscapularis muscle.

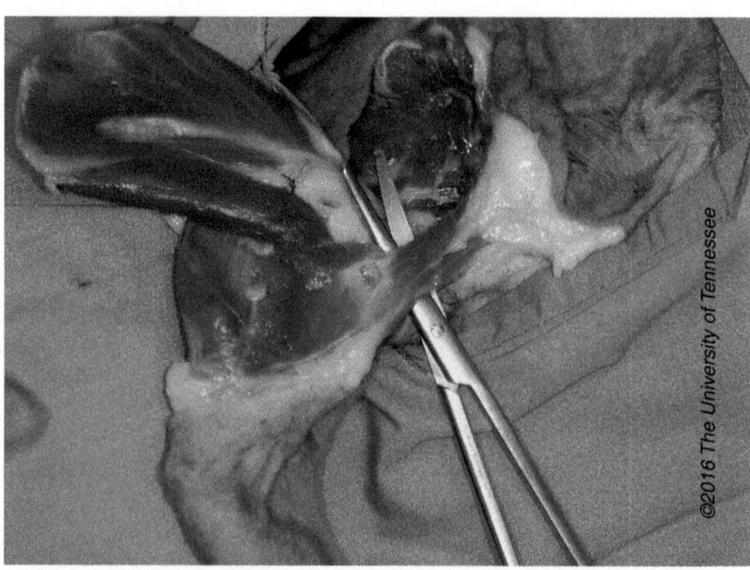

Figure 66-4 Transect the remaining muscle attachments, include the pectoral muscles.

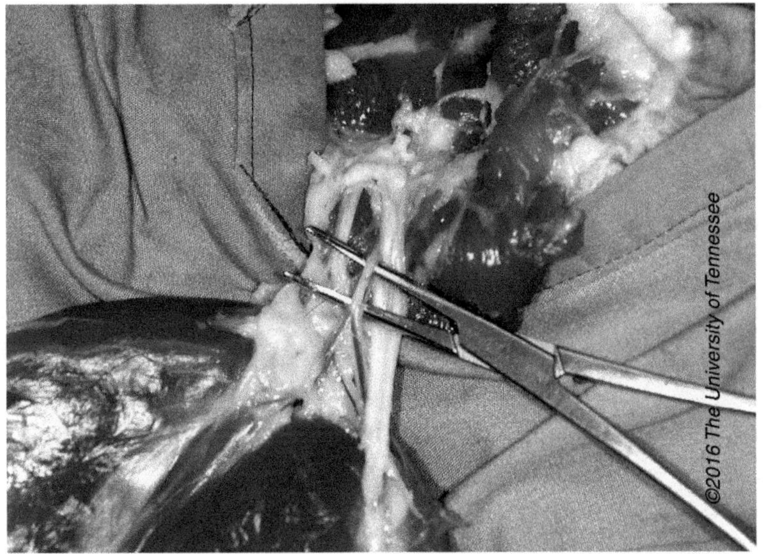

Figure 66-5 Isolate the vessels atraumatically by dissecting parallel to their length. Expose at least 1 cm of length to allow sufficient space for triple ligation and transection.

12. Identify the nerves of the brachial plexus and the axillary artery and vein.
    a. The axillary artery will usually be cranial to the axillary vein, and both vessels will be medial to the nerves.
13. Block and sever each nerve (see fig. 65-4).
    a. Isolate the nerve by dissecting around it with a hemostat.
    b. Insert a 25 gauge needle longitudinally into the nerve sheath.
    c. Inject a small bleb (up to 0.5 mls) of 0.5% bupivacaine into the nerve.
    d. Transect the nerve distal to the anesthetic bleb.
14. Triple ligate and transect the axillary artery.
    a. Dissect parallel to the artery with hemostatic forceps to isolate it atraumatically (fig. 66-5).
    b. Place 2 ligatures around the vessel and separate them so they are at least 1 cm apart before tying them.
    c. Place a third ligature in between the first two, spacing it closer to the proximal ligature (closest to the body wall).
        i. If the artery is large, place an encircling-transfixing ligature.
        ii. If the artery is small, place an encircling ligature.
    d. Transect the artery between the middle and distal ligatures, leaving a vessel stump of at least 3 mm beyond the middle ligature. This will reduce the risk of ligature slippage.
15. Triple ligate and transect the axillary vein as described for the artery.
16. Transect any remaining soft tissue attachments and hand the leg to a nonsterile assistant.

a. If the leg is being submitted for pathology, have the nonsterile assistant ink the cut margins.

17. Roll any cut edges of deep muscles (e.g., serratus ventralis) inward and suture the fascia from opposite sides of the muscle together to seal any raw edges and decrease bleeding.

    a. Use 3-0 absorbable monofilament in a continuous or interrupted pattern.

18. Suture the latissimus dorsi, trapezius, omotransversarius, and pectoral muscle together in a configuration that covers the rib cage and transected nerves (see fig. 65-16).

    a. Include muscle fascia in the suture bites.
    b. Use 3-0 absorbable monofilament in a continuous or interrupted pattern.

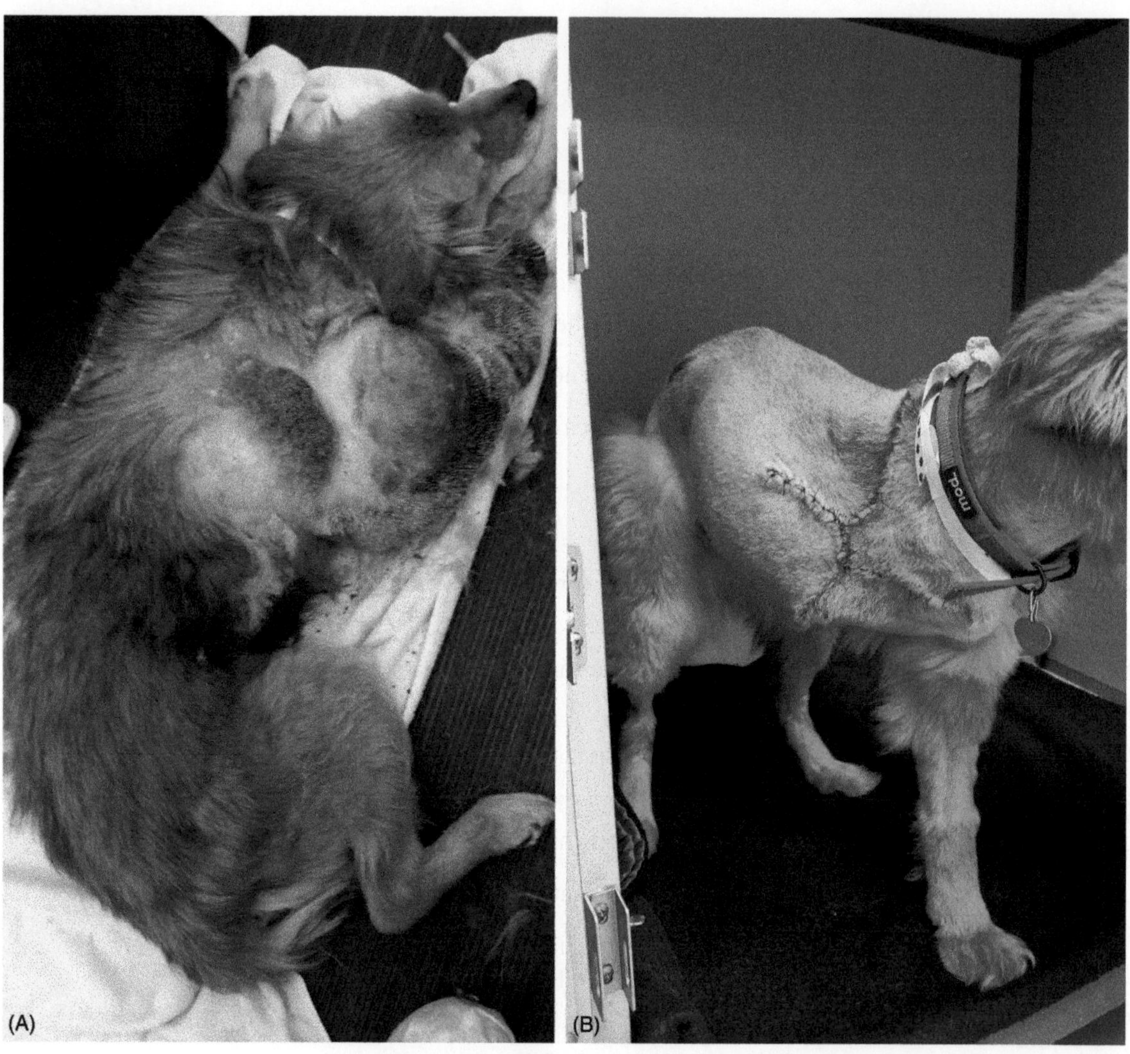

Figure 66-6 Infiltrating lipoma before (A) and after (B) amputation. Because of extensive skin removal, this closure required an X shape. Placement of a continuous suction drain, subcutaneous mattress or purse-string style sutures at all corners, and interrupted intradermal sutures in areas lacking subcutis reduced tension on the skin sutures and facilitated uncomplicated healing.

19. Place a continuous suction drain as needed to close dead space.
20. Adjust the skin edges to determine the best final position for skin closure (see Chapter 2).
    a. The final closure should have no tension.
    b. Dog ears (a fold caused by excess skin on one side of the incision) may need to be removed.
    c. Excess skin may need to be resected.
    d. The final closure often looks like an L, T, J, or inverse Y.
        i. Note: Y- and X-shaped incisions are more likely to have problems and should be avoided, if possible.
21. Once the final skin position is determined, place a few simple interrupted skin sutures at key points to maintain the skin position, then close the subcutaneous tissues.
    a. Appose the subcutaneous tissues in stages with interrupted sutures or with several continuous patterns.
    b. If a Y- or X-shaped closure must be used, the subcutaneous tissues at the junction of all the points should be held together with a mattress suture (see fig. 2-4) to reduce tension on the skin (fig. 66-6).
    c. In areas with no subcutaneous tissues, interrupted intradermal sutures can be added for skin support if tension is present.
22. Appose the skin edges with interrupted skin sutures.

Postoperative considerations

Postoperative care is similar to that described for rear limb amputations (see Chapter 65), including postoperative analgesics, fluids, sling walking, drain care, bladder monitoring, and long long-term weight management. Greyhounds can be started on epsilon epsilon-aminocaproic acid immediately after the surgery (15–40 mg/kg IV) and continued on the oral formulation (500–1000 mg [total dose] q8h) for 5 days to reduce the risk of severe postoperative bruising. Drains can often be pulled once fluid production decreases to less than 4.8 mls/kg/day.

Because it is more difficult to close dead space after a forelimb amputation, seroma formation is not unusual. Additionally, dogs are able to scratch their incisions with their ipsilateral hind legs, which can increase the risk of incision complications. In dogs, a thoracic bandage, t-shirt, or lycra body suit may help protect the area during healing. Cats, however, are not too keen on bandages and may be more likely to damage themselves if one is placed after recovery.

Bibliography

Dickerson VM, Coleman KD, Ogawa M, et al: Outcomes of dogs undergoing limb amputation, owner satisfaction with limb amputation procedures, and owner perceptions regarding postsurgical adaptation: 64 cases (2005–2012). J Am Vet Med Assoc 2015;247:786–792.

Forster LM, Wathes CM, Bessant D, Et al: Owners' observations of domestic cats after limb amputation. Vet Rec 2010;167:734–739.

Shaver SL, Hunt GB, Kidd SW: Evaluation of fluid production and seroma formation after placement of closed suction drains in clean subcutaneous surgical wounds of dogs: 77 cases (2005–2012). J Am Vet Med Assoc 2014;245:211–215.

Smeak DD, Lisano S: Forelimb amputation. Clinician's Brief 2012;10:69–74.

Section 10 Ophthalmic Techniques

Chapter 67
Enucleation

Removal of the eye is indicated in cases where the prognosis for vision is poor and the eye is a source of discomfort or difficulty for the animal or owner. Most domestic animals adapt well to monocular vision, and minimal overall visual deficits are to be expected with loss of one eye.

Preoperative management

Preparation of the area is accomplished by shaving a 2-inch (~5 cm) margin around the eye. The skin around the eye is alternately cleansed three times with cotton or gauze soaked in diluted (0.2%) povidone iodine solution and sterile saline. Following preparation of the skin, the conjunctival surfaces are gently swabbed with a moistened cotton-tipped applicator using the same alternating regimen of dilute povidone iodine and saline.

For recovery and analgesia, preoperative local blocks with lidocaine and bupivacaine injected into the retrobulbar space or as a splash block postoperatively, have been shown to have beneficial effects. Bupivacaine combined with epinephrine can also aid in hemostasis.

Surgery

Techniques for enucleation vary but can be broadly categorized as either transpalpebral or subconjunctival. These two categories refer to the initial approach of the enucleation: through the skin of the eyelid (transpalpebral) or through and under the conjunctiva (subconjunctival). The transpalpebral technique has no specific contraindications and can be used to remove an eye in most situations. It can be challenging, however, to find the appropriate plane of dissection and not disrupt the conjunctival sac formed by closure of the eyelids. If the plane of dissection is not immediately adjacent to the eye, more orbital tissue is typically removed with the transpalpebral technique than with the subconjunctival technique, leading to the potential for increased bleeding.

The subconjunctival technique enables the surgeon to immediately find the correct plane of dissection through the conjunctiva, close to the globe. Subconjunctival enucleation can be used for intraocular conditions such as glaucoma but is contraindicated if neoplasia or infection is present and not

Manual of Small Animal Soft Tissue Surgery, Second Edition. Karen Tobias.
© 2017 John Wiley & Sons, Inc. Published 2017 by John Wiley & Sons, Inc.

contained inside the globe. For a subconjunctival enucleation, a lateral canthotomy is performed, and the conjunctiva is incised along the limbus to expose the extraocular muscles and connective tissue attachments to the globe. Once the eye has been removed, all conjunctiva remaining in the orbit and along the eyelid margins must be resected to prevent formation of a mucocele from conjunctival goblet cells.

If nothing is placed into the orbit after the globe is removed, the skin will typically sink into the space left behind by removal of the eye. Ultimately, the animal is unaffected by this, but it can be cosmetically unappealing to the owner. One technique to ameliorate this effect is to place an orbital meshwork of nonabsorbable suture spanning the orbit to lessen the depression of the skin; the skin lies across this meshwork of suture, which acts like a hammock. The orbital meshwork alone still allows for some sinking of the skin, but it is potentially not as drastic. Another technique for cosmesis is to implant an intraorbital prosthesis (secured by a meshwork of suture) that will typically result in a more normal "closed-eye" appearance. The prosthesis achieves a more natural-looking outcome but also increases the risk for postsurgery complications: migration, extrusion, or seroma formation. Intraorbital prosthesis placement should be avoided in cases where the orbit is at risk for neoplasia or infection. Use in cats is also questionable due to potentially higher rates of failure or extrusion in this species.

Surgical Technique: Transpalpebral enucleation

1. Suture the eyelids closed with a simple continuous suture pattern (fig. 67-1), or clamp them closed with Allis tissue forceps, hemostats, or towel clamps.

    a. If suturing, the suture ends can be left long to allow for gripping in order to exert tension on the eyelids as needed later on in the procedure.

    b. The specific type of suture is immaterial because it will be removed with the eye. Typically, a 3-0 to 5-0 suture size is appropriate, depending on the thickness of the eyelids.

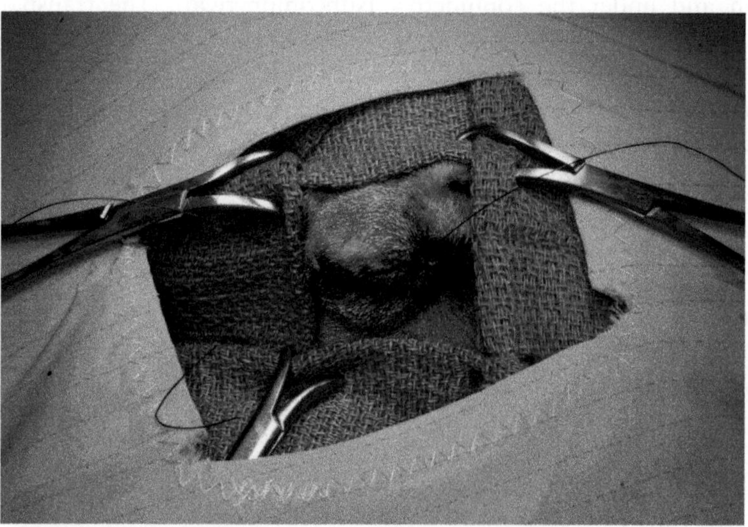

Figure 67-1 Suture the eyelids closed with a simple continuous pattern.

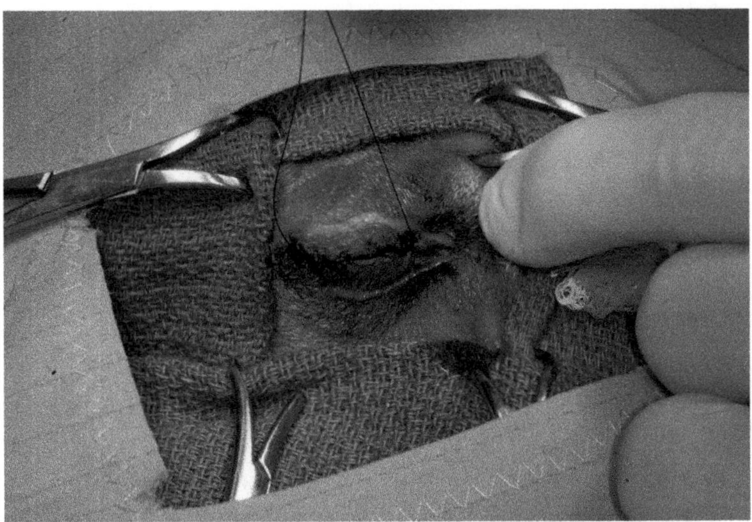

Figure 67-2 Make an elliptical incision around the eye 6 to 8 mm from the edges of the lids.

2. Using a 10 or 15 blade, create an oblong skin incision around the eyelids 6–8 mm away from the sutured or clamped edges, ensuring that there will be enough skin for closure over the orbit (fig. 67-2).
3. Using Metzenbaum scissors, sharply and bluntly dissect deep into the incision toward the eye (fig. 67-3), and create a plane of dissection separating the eyelids from the surrounding tissue so that the conjunctival sac is maintained 360° around the eye.
   a. The dissection goes through the subcutaneous tissue of the eyelid and the orbicularis oculi muscle, and then into the connective tissue surrounding the eye. Going any deeper can result in breaking into the conjunctival sac, which should be avoided if enucleation is being performed because of infection or neoplasia of the eyelids, conjunctiva, or cornea.
   b. If the conjunctiva is accidentally torn during dissection, note the proper plane of dissection (just above the tear in the tissue) and

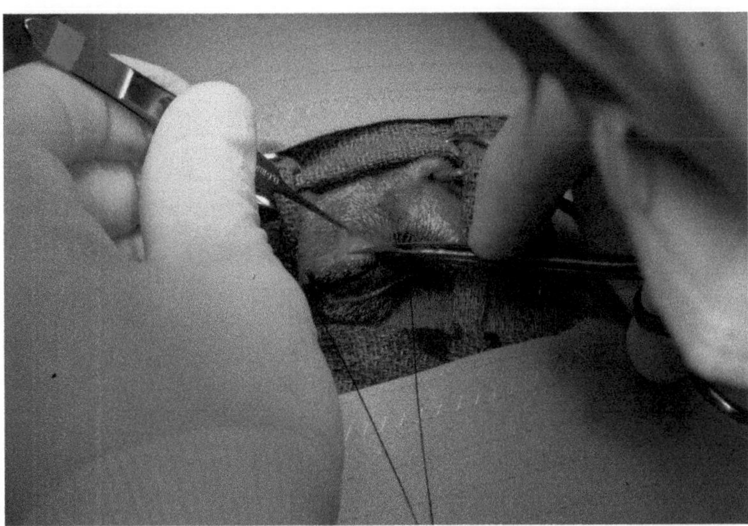

Figure 67-3 Dissect the subcutaneous tissues around the eye, leaving the conjunctiva intact.

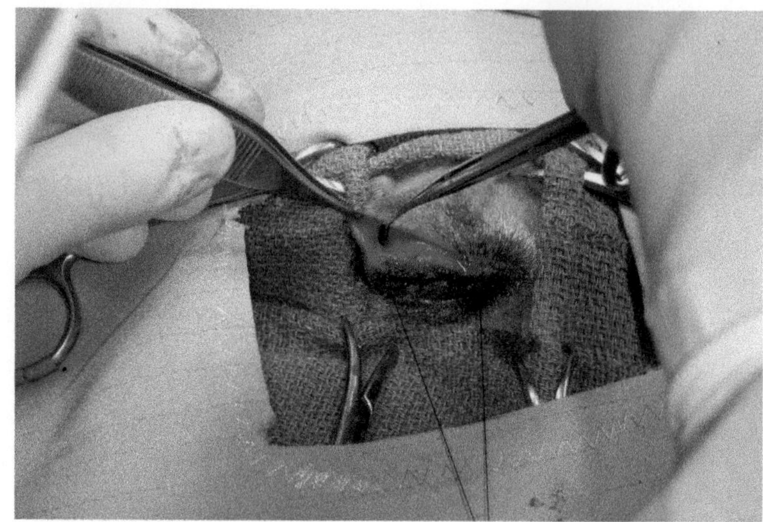

Figure 67-4 Subcutaneous dissection up to the level of the canthal ligaments.

maintain that level of dissection 360 degrees around the eye. The tear can be closed with a simple interrupted stitch to avoid contamination.

c. At the level of the conjunctiva, the globe can usually be seen slightly through the conjunctiva, and the cornea will appear as a dark area through the tissue.

4. Identify (fig. 67-4) and transect the ligaments at the lateral and medial canthi (palpebral commissures).

   a. These ligaments can typically be palpated by exerting some tension on the eyelids at the canthus with the suture or clamps and "strumming" across the band of tissue.

   b. Gently cut with a blade or scissors, taking care not to incise through the underlying conjunctiva (fig. 67-5).

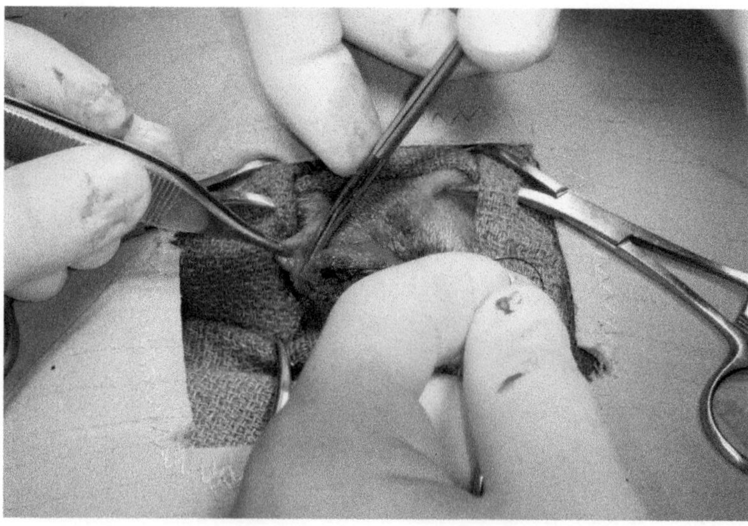

Figure 67-5 Transect the canthal ligaments with scissors.

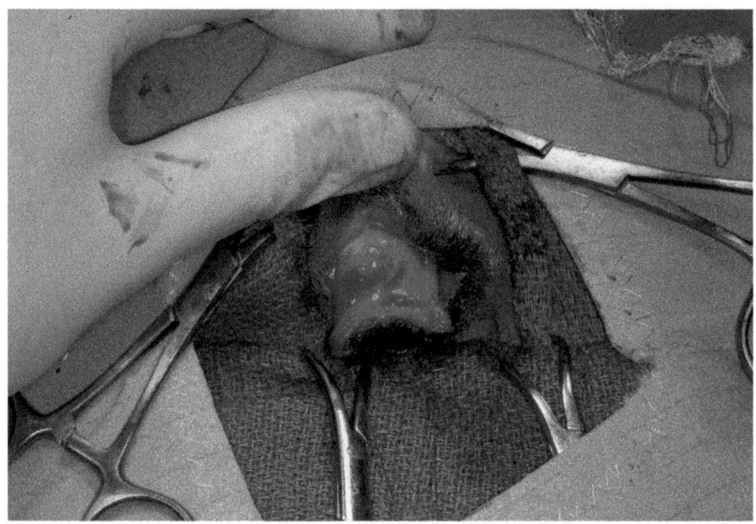

Figure 67-6 Retract the globe by pulling on the eyelid sutures to expose posterior soft tissue attachments.

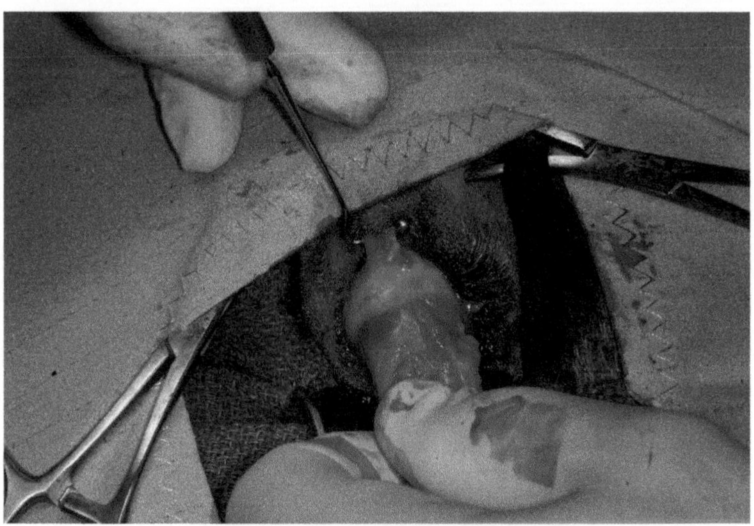

Figure 67-7 Identify and transect remaining extraocular muscle and connective tissue attachments.

5. Retract on the eyelid sutures (fig. 67-6) to expose connective tissue and extraocular muscle attachments (fig. 67-7), and sharply transect them with curved Metzenbaum scissors.
6. Sharply transect the optic nerve.
   a. The optic nerve can be felt posteriorly at the ventromedial aspect of the globe and can be sharply incised with scissors.
   b. Clamping of the nerve with hemostats (fig. 67-8) or suture ligation can be performed before transection but is not strictly necessary and may be difficult in deep orbits.
7. Remove the globe with the eyelids.
   a. The third eyelid and gland should be contained within the conjunctival sac.

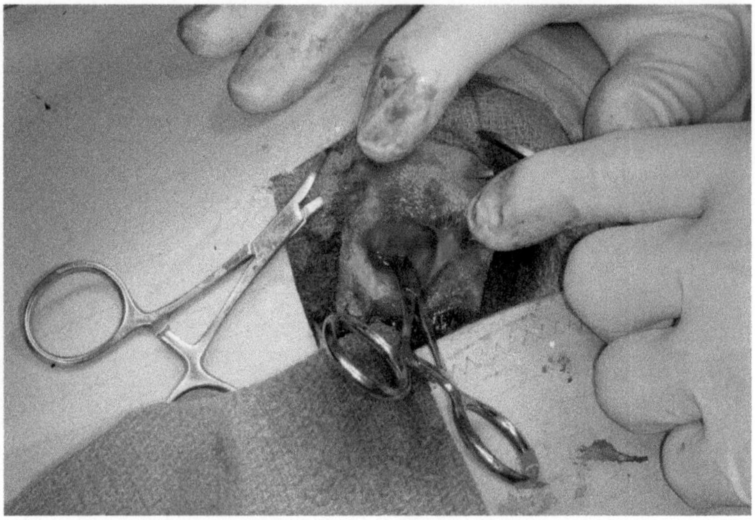

Figure 67-8 The optic nerve can be clamped with a hemostat and transected before or after ligation, or can be cut without clamping.

  b. If bleeding is noted at this point, the orbit can be packed with gauze and pressure applied for 5 minutes.

8. If desired, place an orbital meshwork or intraorbital prosthesis (see below).
9. Appose the deep edges of the subcutaneous layer of the eyelids with a simple continuous pattern of 3-0 to 5-0 absorbable suture (e.g., Vicryl), with the knots buried (fig. 67-9).
10. Appose the superficial layers of subcutis with a simple continuous or intradermal pattern, using 3-0 to 5-0 absorbable suture and burying the knots (fig. 67-10).
11. Appose the skin with an interrupted pattern of 3-0 to 5-0 monofilament, nonabsorbable suture on a cutting needle (fig. 67-11).

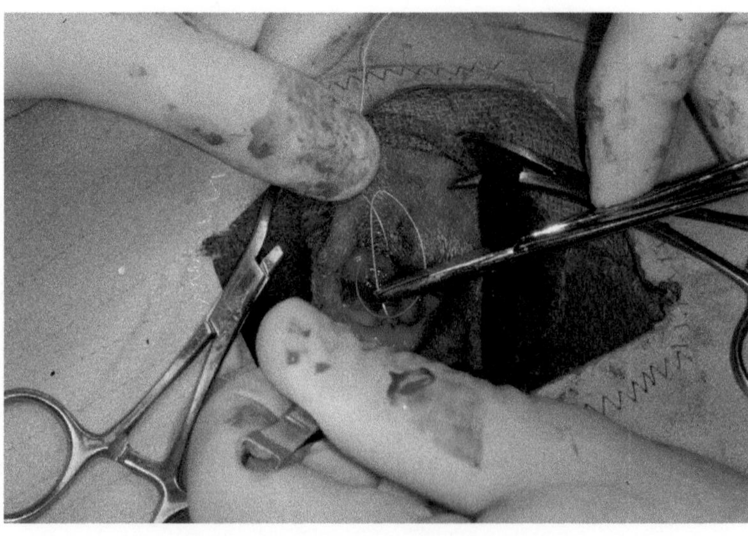

Figure 67-9 Appose the deep subcutaneous tissues of the eyelids with absorbable suture, burying the knots.

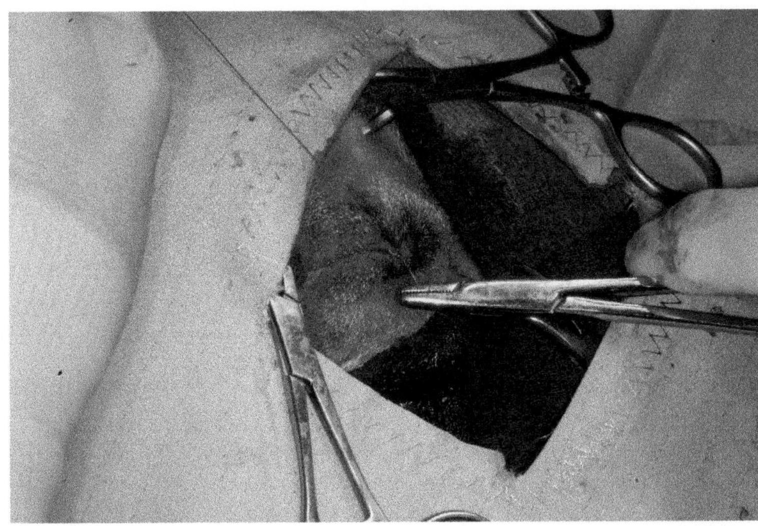

Figure 67-10 Appose the superficial subcutaneous layer with a simple continuous, horizontal mattress, or intradermal pattern, burying the knots.

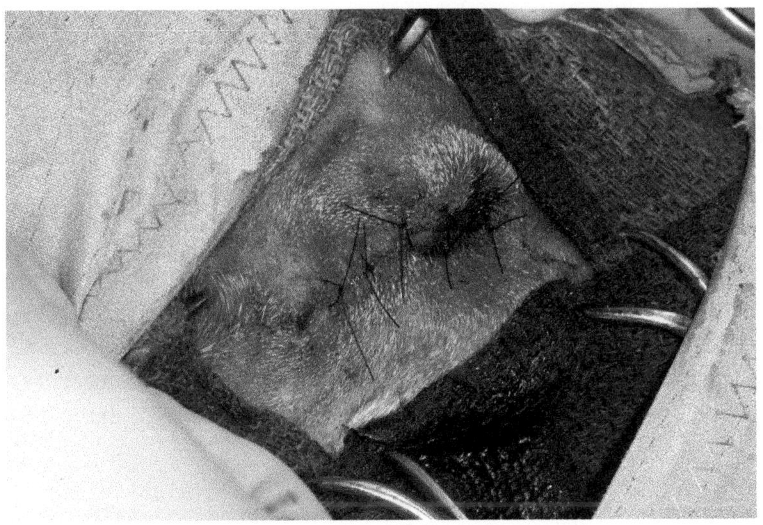

Figure 67-11 Final appearance after skin closure.

Surgical technique: intraorbital prosthesis

1. Estimate the size of the prosthesis, based on globe size.
   a. Prosthesis sizes vary between 14 mm and 22 mm.
   b. The prosthesis should not be so large as to exert undue tension against the skin nor so small that it prevents depression of the skin.
2. Insert the prosthesis into the orbit and hold it in place with simple interrupted or horizontal mattress sutures spanning the anterior periorbital fascial tissues.
   a. Use 3-0 or 4-0 nonabsorbable suture.
   b. The periorbital tissue included in each bite should be firmly adhered to the underlying bone; if the sutures are properly placed, the head can be shifted or moved with the suture bite.

c. The subcutaneous tissue underlying the eyelids should be avoided in these bites to prevent possible sinking of the skin into the orbit when the sutures are tightened.

3. Once the prosthesis is secured in place, suture the eyelids closed.

Surgical technique: orbital meshwork

1. Using 3-0 or 4-0 nonabsorbable suture, take a bite of the periorbital fascial tissue around the globe and secure an anchoring knot (4–6 throws). The bite should be firmly within the tissue closely adhered to the orbital bone.
2. Place a simple continuous pattern by taking bites of the periorbital tissue and spanning the orbit, dorsal to ventral. Continue the pattern so that a second layer of suture spans the orbit from one side of the orbit to the other (medial to lateral or vice-versa).
3. At the end of the suture pattern, tighten and secure the suture with another anchoring knot (4–6 throws). This can be performed by taking two bites of tissue immediately adjacent to one another for the loop and free-end.
4. Close the eyelids over this meshwork of suture.

Postoperative considerations

Oral nonsteroidal anti-inflammatory drugs and opioids (e.g., Tramadol) should be used for postoperative pain control if they can be given safely. Unless there is a concern for infection, most enucleations do not require systemic antibiotics postoperatively. An Elizabethan collar is necessary to prevent self-trauma and is typically left in place for at least 2 weeks. Complications from enucleation can include hemorrhage, infection, dehiscence, fistula or mucocele formation, and rarely, emphysema in brachycephalic breeds.

Bibliography

Chow DW, Wong MY, Westermeyer HD: Comparison of two bupivacaine delivery methods to control postoperative pain after enucleation in dogs. Vet Ophthalmol 2015;18 (5): 422–428.

Hamor RE, Roberts SM, Severin GA: Use of orbital implants after enucleation in dogs, horses, and cats: 161 cases (1980–1990). J Am Vet Med Assoc 1993;203 (5): 701–706.

Myrna, KE, Bentley E, Smith LJ: Effectiveness of injection of local anesthetic into the retrobulbar space for postoperative analgesia following eye enucleation in dogs. J Am Vet Med Assoc 2010;237 (2): 174–177.

Nasisse, MP et al., Use of methyl methacrylate orbital prostheses in dogs and cats: 78 cases (1980n1986). J Am Vet Med Assoc 1988;192 (4): 539–542.

Spiess BM, Pot SA: Diseases and surgery of the canine orbit. In Veterinary ophthalmology, K.N. Gelatt, (ed), Wiley-Blackwell, 2013, 816–820.

Chapter 68
Prolapsed Gland of the Third Eyelid

The membrana nictitans, or "third eyelid," consists of a T-shaped piece of cartilage covered entirely by conjunctiva. When the globe is in its normal position, the third eyelid rests within the orbit, with its free edge visible ventromedially. When the globe is retracted, the third eyelid sweeps across the globe, spreading tears across the surface of the cornea and protecting the eye from trauma. Surrounding the base of the cartilage is the gland of the third eyelid, which produces about a third of the tear volume in dogs.

Prolapse of the gland of the third eyelid is known colloquially as "cherry eye." The cause of the prolapse is unknown, although it is suspected to be a result of weakness of the ligamentous structures that normally anchor the gland to the periorbital tissues. Most affected dogs are less than 1 year old, and in about a third of dogs, both glands will be affected at some point. Predisposition for the condition has been reported in a variety of breeds, including cocker spaniels, English and French bulldogs, beagles, Lhasa apsos, and Shar Peis.

Removal of prolapsed glands should be avoided because of adverse changes in tear quality, stability of the tear film, and health of the conjunctival epithelium. In addition, many of the dog breeds predisposed to gland prolapse are also predisposed to developing keratoconjunctivitis sicca (KCS). Removal of the gland could accelerate the development or hinder the treatment of KCS. Instead, it is recommended that the gland be surgically returned to its normal position by tucking it back with a conjunctival fold to the base of the third eyelid ("pocket technique") or securing it to periorbital tissue or the third eyelid cartilage with suture ("anchor technique").

Preoperative management

As previously mentioned, breeds commonly affected with prolapse of the gland of the third eyelid are also predisposed to KCS or exposure keratitis from brachycephalic conformation. Tear production should therefore be measured in dogs presenting for prolapse; if low (< 15 mm/min), the dog should be

Manual of Small Animal Soft Tissue Surgery, Second Edition. Karen Tobias.
© 2017 John Wiley & Sons, Inc. Published 2017 by John Wiley & Sons, Inc.

started on a lacrostimulant (e.g., 0.2%–2% cyclosporine or 0.02%–0.03% tacrolimus). Likewise, fluorescein stain should be performed before and after surgical treatment to ensure that any corneal ulcerations are noted and properly treated.

Prior to surgery and in the absence of any corneal ulceration, treatment with a triple antibiotic-steroid combination (e.g., NeoPolyDex ointment) several times a day can be used to keep the gland lubricated and to reduce or prevent further swelling of the gland.

No surgical clip is required for the procedure; however, if lashes are very long, they can be shortened. Before cleansing the periorbital region, artificial tears or lubricant eye gel can be placed on the cornea to provide temporary protection. The skin around the eye is alternately cleansed three times with cotton or gauze soaked in diluted (0.2%) povidone iodine solution and sterile saline. Following preparation of the skin, the conjunctival surfaces, including the bulbar surface of the third eyelid, are gently swabbed with a moistened cotton-tipped applicator using the same alternating regimen of dilute povidone iodine and saline.

Surgery

The goal of surgery is to secure the prolapsed gland below the leading edge of the third eyelid without affecting the function of the gland and its ducts. For the pocket technique, two conjunctival flaps are elevated on either side of the gland and sutured together over the gland, leaving a gap at each end to allow tear secretions to exit the site, preventing cyst formation. For the anchor technique, the gland can be secured anteriorly to the ventral periorbital rim or posteriorly to the ventral oblique muscle, ventral equatorial sclera, ventral periorbital fascia, or to the base of the cartilage itself.

The benefit of the pocket technique is that it allows for natural movement of the third eyelid. This natural movement might be inhibited by the orbital anchoring technique, which will also result in some anterior movement of the third eyelid so that it protrudes forward. Some surgeons prefer to use anchoring techniques for chronically prolapsed and severely enlarged glands, however.

Surgical technique: pocket method

1. Retract and evert the third eyelid with two towel clamps, Allis tissue forceps, or mosquito hemostats placed at the medial and lateral aspects of the third eyelid to expose the bulbar conjunctival surface and the prolapsed gland (fig. 68-1).
2. With a 6400 Beaver blade or No. 15 Bard-Parker scalpel blade, make a curved conjunctival incision 120 degrees to 140 degrees around the gland, about 1–3 mm away from the edge of the gland, facing the free margin of the third eyelid (fig. 68-2).
   a. The incision should extend just through the conjunctiva so that the white connective tissue can be seen beneath.
   b. Conjunctival bleeding can be controlled with topical phenylephrine dropped directly on the site or applied with a cotton tip applicator.

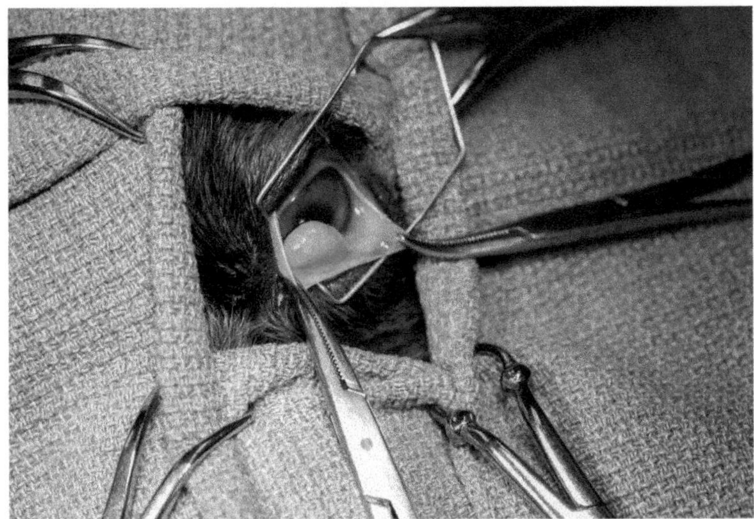

Figure 68-1 Retract and evert the third eyelid to expose the prolapsed gland.

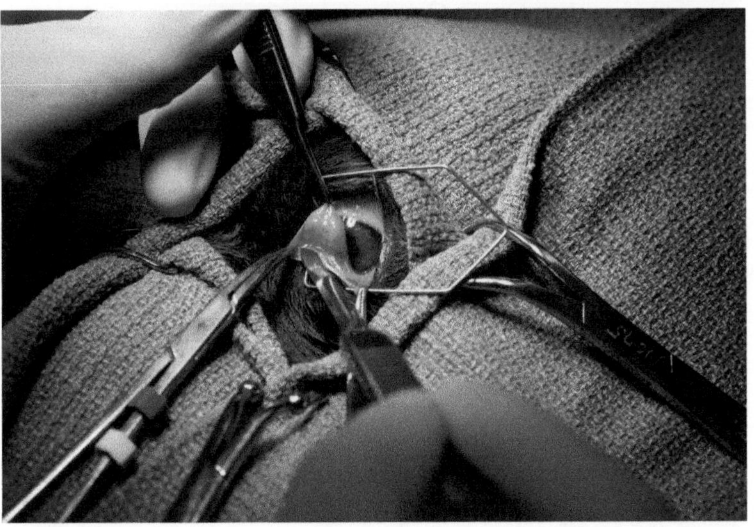

Figure 68-2 Make a semicircular incision through the conjunctiva along one side of the gland near the third eyelid margin.

3. Make a second, 120 degrees to 140 degrees, curved conjunctival incision (similar in depth to the first incision) along the edge of the gland closest to the bulbar conjunctival fornix (fig. 68-3).
   a. The final result will be two unconnected incisions facing each other across the gland.
4. With blunt-tipped tenotomy scissors, dissect the submucosa abaxial to each incision (fig. 68-4) to mobilize the conjunctiva along the incision edges away from the gland and to create the pocket at the fornix incision created in the previous step.
5. To facilitate suturing, push the gland into the fornix incision (the pocket) with a cotton-tipped applicator (fig. 68-5).
   a. If the gland is too large to enter the pocket easily or is prone to reprolapse out of the pocket, a continuous pattern can be started (as described below) and 3–4 stitches placed before attempting to reposition the gland into the pocket.

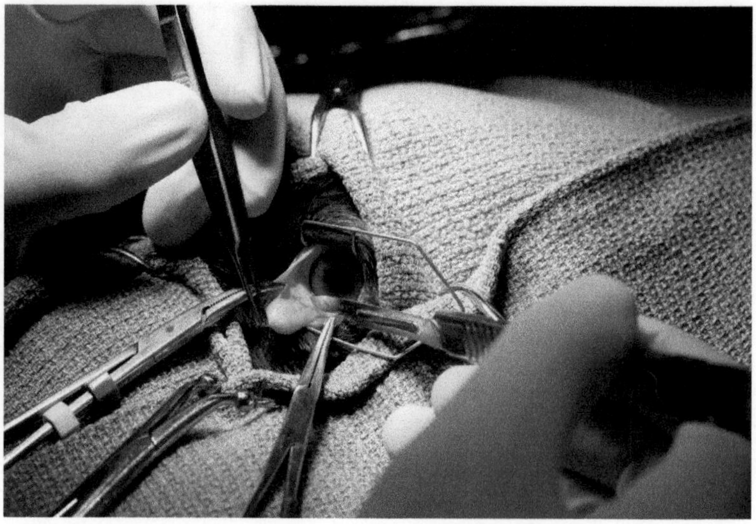

Figure 68-3 Make a semicircular incision through the conjunctiva along the opposite side of the gland near its base.

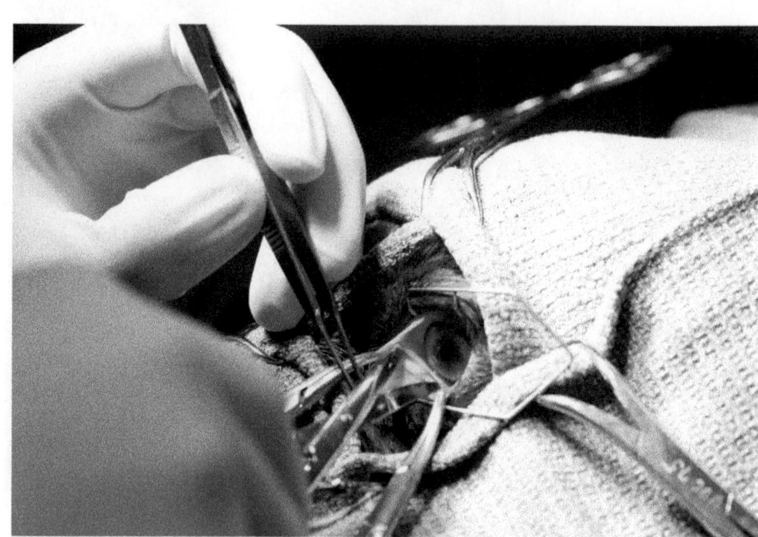

Figure 68-4 Elevate the conjunctiva away from the gland to create a pocket for the gland near the conjunctival fornix.

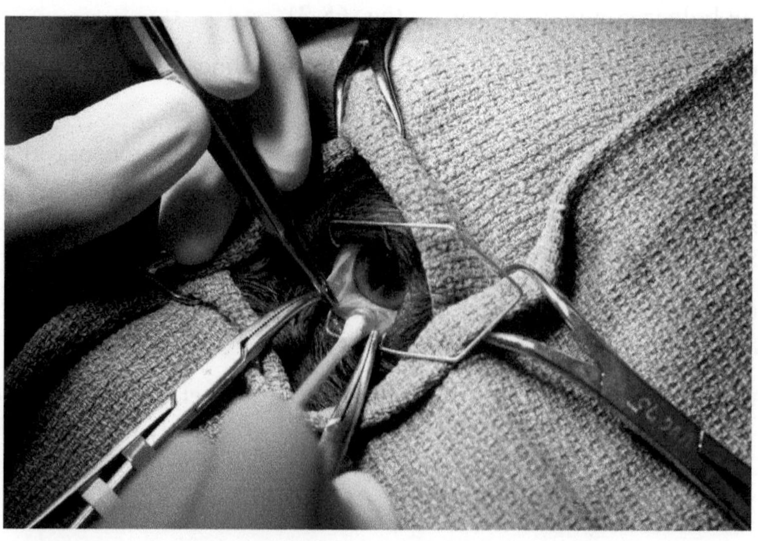

Figure 68-5 Reduce the gland into the conjunctival pocket near the fornix with a moistened cotton-tipped applicator swab.

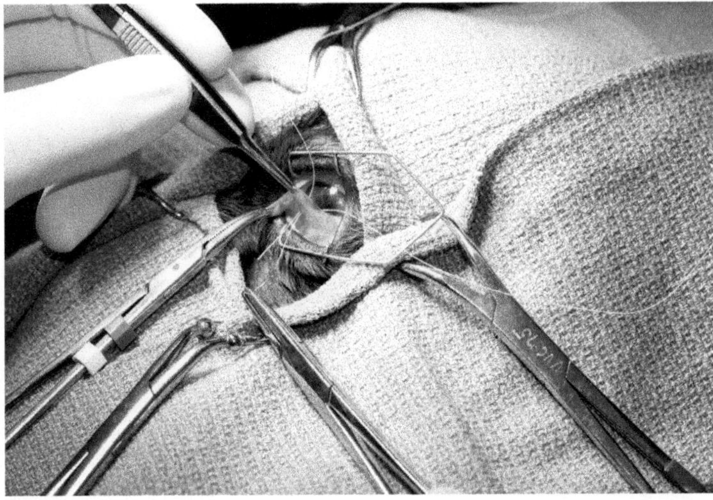

Figure 68-6 Start the continuous pattern by placing the knot on the external surface of the third eyelid so that it can't rub on the cornea.

6. Secure the gland in the pocket with 5-0 absorbable suture.
    a. To minimize the possibility of knot rubbing on the cornea, anchor the suture to the palpebral or exterior aspect of the third eyelid by first taking a full-thickness (outside to inside) bite through the third eyelid at the far end of the first incision (the one nearest the third eyelid margin) and then passing the suture back (inside to outside) and tying two square knots (fig. 68-6).
    b. Pass the suture again full thickness (outside to inside), then suture the abaxial edges of the conjunctival incisions together in a simple continuous pattern (figs. 68-7 and 68-8).
        i. This will leave a gap at the cranial and caudal ends of the gland to allow glandular excretions.
    c. Complete the closure by anchoring the suture again to the palpebral aspect of the third eyelid in a similar fashion as described in step 6a (fig. 68-9). Alternatively, double-back on the incision with a Cushing suture pattern and secure the suture with a knot adjacent to the original knot.

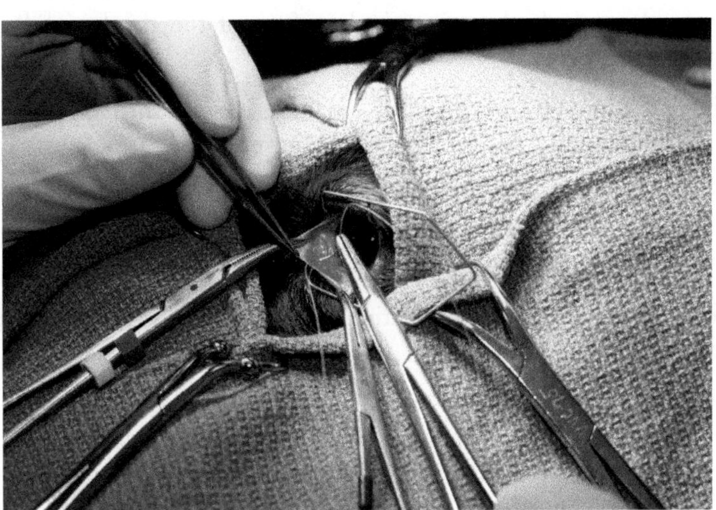

Figure 68-7 Appose the abaxial edges of the incisions together over the top of gland with a simple continuous pattern.

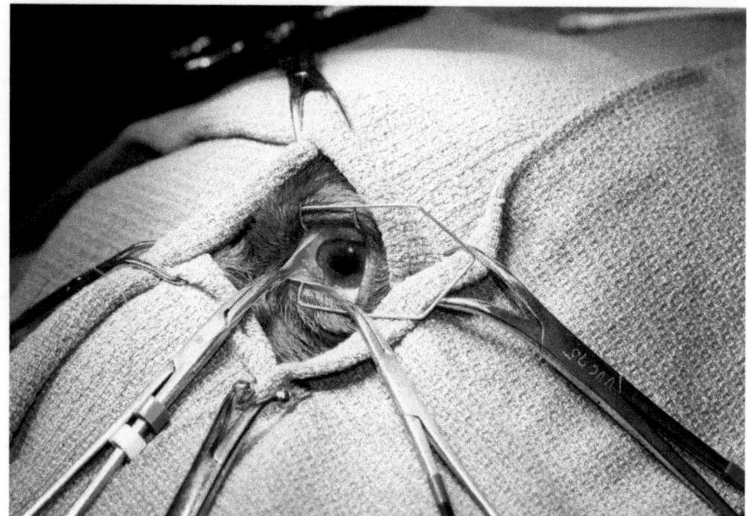

Figure 68-8 Simple continuous closure.

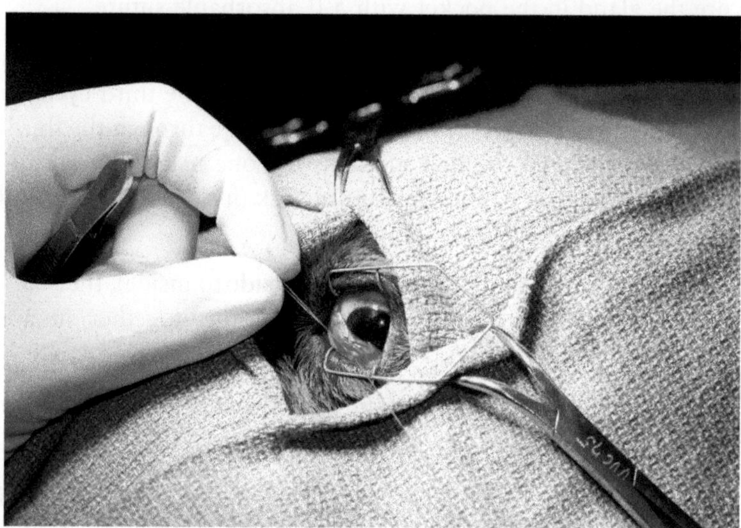

Figure 68-9 Exit the suture out the external surface of the third eyelid conjunctiva before tying it off.

Surgical technique: orbital rim suture anchor method

1. Retract the third eyelid out of the periorbital fossa with thumb forceps to expose the palpebral conjunctival surface of the third eyelid and the conjunctival fornix.
2. Using tenotomy scissors, make a 1-cm linear incision through the palpebral (anterior) conjunctiva over the orbital rim near the base of third eyelid.
    a. An alternative technique is to make a skin incision over the orbital rim, which may make passing the curved needle easier when it is further away from the eye.
3. Bluntly dissect the subconjunctival tissues to expose the ventromedial orbital rim.
4. With 3-0 or 4-0 nylon on a reverse cutting needle, take a bite of the periosteum of the ventromedial orbital rim and the gland, directing the needle dorsally to exit the top of the gland on one side (lateral or medial) of the gland (fig. 68-10A).

5. Reverse the needle and pass it back through the same suture exit hole in the gland and out the opposite side (medial or lateral) of the gland (fig. 68-10B).
   a. Passing the needle back through the same suture hole in the gland allows the suture to sink into the subconjunctival tissue.
6. Reinsert the needle through the second suture exit hole and direct the needle dow,n through, and out of the gland and into and through the periosteum (fig. 68-10C).
   a. This bite runs parallel to the first bite (taken in step 4).
7. Tighten the suture to return the prolapsed gland to its original position, and tie a knot to secure the gland.
8. Close the conjunctival mucosa with 5-0 or 6-0 absorbable suture in a simple, continuous pattern.
   a. If the original incision was in the skin, it can be closed with an interrupted pattern with nonabsorbable suture.

Postoperative considerations

A topical broad-spectrum antibiotic or antibiotic-steroid ointment is commonly used for 2 to 4 weeks after the procedure. The steroid component can be omitted in patients with ulceration or with KCS. In patients that have not received glucocorticoids, an oral nonsteroidal anti-inflammatory agent can be administered for 2 weeks to reduce pain and inflammation. An Elizabethan collar should be kept on the animal at all times to prevent self-trauma that could result in failure of the surgery. Treatment of KCS should be continued as needed.

Conjunctival hyperemia is to be expected after the procedure and should improve with topical and oral anti-inflammatories. If an anterior anchoring technique is used, the third eyelid will often be protruded forward until swelling subsides.

Complications of either technique include reprolapse and, less commonly, eversion of the nictitating cartilage, corneal ulcer formation from suture abrasion, and lacrimal cyst formation. If the surgery fails, repeating the same or any of the alternative techniques can be used to correct the prolapse.

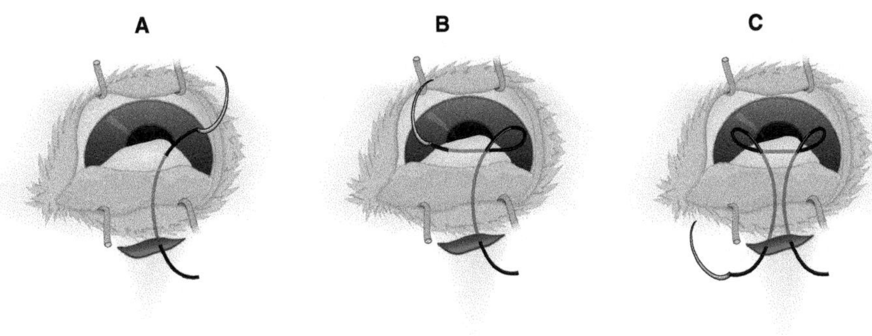

Figure 68-10 Orbital rim anchoring suture. **A.** Pass the needle through the skin incision and take the first suture bite through the periosteum of the ventromedial orbital rim and out of the medial or lateral edge of the top of the gland. **B.** Pass the needle back through the same suture hole and across the top of the gland to exit out the opposite side (lateral or medial edge, respectively). **C.** Pass the needle back through the second exit hole then down through the gland and orbital rim periosteum and out the skin incision. Courtesy of Samantha Elmurst.

Bibliography

Mazzucchelli S, Vaillant MD, Weverberg F, et al: Retrospective study of 155 cases of prolapse of the nictitating membrane gland in dogs. Vet Rec 2012;170:443.

Saito A, Izumisawa Y, Yamashita K, et al: The effect of third eyelid gland removal on the ocular surface of dogs. Vet Ophthalmol 2001;4:13–18.

Sapienza JS, Mayaordomo A, Beyer AM: Suture anchor placement technique around the insertion of the ventral rectus muscle for replacement of the prolapsed gland of the third eyelid in dogs: 100 dogs. Vet Ophthalmol 2014;17:81–86.

Chapter 69
Entropion Correction

Entropion is an inward rolling of the eyelid margin (fig. 69-1). Causes may include pain (termed spastic entropion), developmental abnormalities (conformational entropion), or scarring from trauma (cicatricial entropion). Developmental entropion is common in certain dog breeds, such as Shar Peis, Chow Chows, English bulldogs, and Rottweilers, and Persian cats. With inversion of the eyelid margin, eyelid hairs abrade the cornea, causing irritation, keratitis, pain, and corneal ulceration. Conformational and cicatricial entropion usually require some type of surgical intervention for permanent correction, while spastic entropion should be treated with a temporary "tacking" procedure or some other means to protect the cornea from the eyelashes (e.g., contact lens) until such time as the primary source of pain is healed or corrected.

Preoperative management

A diagnosis of entropion is typically made by observing the eyelid margin rolling inward toward the cornea. Wet hairs or eyelashes in the suspected area also are suggestive of entropion. Determining the etiology of the entropion is critical, as permanent surgical correction may not always be necessary. Since corneal pain can cause spastic entropion, the eyelid position should be evaluated before and after application of topical anesthetic. If the entropion partially or completely resolves with the anesthetic, permanent surgical correction to the eyelid may be unnecessary; instead, temporary tacking sutures should be placed.

If corneal ulceration is present, it may be the underlying source of the pain and subsequent entropion. Causes for ulceration or pain can include infection (e.g., bacterial/viral), ectopic cilia, distichiasis, or keratoconjunctivitis sicca. Ulcers can also be secondary to entropion, and temporary correction of the entropion may facilitate healing. A thorough ophthalmic exam, including Schirmer tear test, fluorescein staining, and examination of lid margins for cilia disorders, should be performed before entropion surgery is considered.

In cases where the underlying cause of entropion is conformational, clinical signs may occur when the animal is a puppy. Certain breeds, such as the Shar Pei and Chow Chow, may present with keratitis at a young age. In these instances, permanent correction is usually postponed until skull development is complete. These puppies can undergo temporary correction of entropion (tacking) as young as 2 to 4 weeks of age. Two or three vertical mattress sutures

Manual of Small Animal Soft Tissue Surgery, Second Edition. Karen Tobias.
© 2017 John Wiley & Sons, Inc. Published 2017 by John Wiley & Sons, Inc.

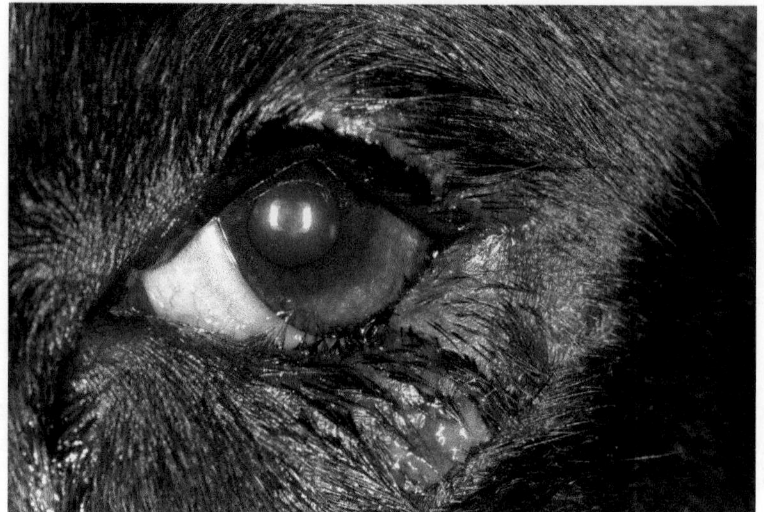

Figure 69-1 Entropion. The lower eyelid is rolled inward, and hair is contacting the cornea.

of nylon or absorbable multifilament are placed to roll the lid margin outward. The temporary sutures keep the eyelid margins in an overcorrected or normal position for 2 to 3 weeks while the puppy grows. In some cases, this may be the only procedure needed because of scar tissue formation from suture placement and improvement of conformation with skull growth.

For techniques requiring tissue resection, such as the modified Hotz-Celsus procedure, the amount and location of inward-rolling eyelid should be determined while the patient is awake and unsedated. Excess tissue can be visually estimated while the eyelid is manipulated. Alternatively, a dermal marker can be used to mark the highest point on the lower eyelid or the lowest point on the upper eyelid. The amount of correction needed is equivalent to the distance between the mark and the eyelid margin. Some surgeons prefer to undercorrect the defect by 0.5 to 1 mm to account for postoperative contraction associated with fibrosis.

Before surgery, ophthalmic lubricant gel or an artificial tear ointment is placed on the eye to protect the cornea and collect loose hairs and debris during clipping and prepping. For dogs undergoing permanent correction, the surgical area is clipped with a fine clipper blade. The area is prepped in an alternating fashion with a 0.2% povidone iodine solution and sterile saline, with a final saline rinse to flush away the povidone iodine, and the area is draped.

Surgery

For eyelid surgery, specialized instruments are preferred. Incisions are usually made with a Beaver blade (e.g., No. 6400) or a no. 15 blade. Dissection and suture cutting are performed with tenotomy scissors or small, straight or curved strabismus scissors. A locking ophthalmic (e.g., Castroviejo) or small conventional (e.g., Derf) needle holder, Bishop-Harmon thumb forceps, and magnification are recommended. Use of a lid plate will stabilize lid skin to make incising the tissue easier and more accurate.

Although eyelids are extremely vascular, use of cautery should be minimized and limited to bipolar or point application because excess scarring could result in conformational changes to the eyelid. Multifilament absorbable suture (e.g., polyglactin 910 or polyglycolic acid) is often used because of its excellent handling characteristics and knot security, and because it softens when wet, reducing the risk of corneal irritation. Additionally, these sutures may not need to be removed. A cutting needle is preferred when working on eyelids.

In some animals, entropion must be repaired with a combination of techniques, including skin resection, lateral canthal closure, and full-thickness lateral eyelid wedge resection. Complicated entropion is best managed by an experienced ophthalmic surgeon.

Temporary tacking can be performed with sedation and local anesthetic. If any lidocaine is administered in the area, the surgeon should be aware that this alone can cause the lid to swell and may make it difficult to gauge the degree of eversion. Fortunately, excessive eversion (ectropion) is not undesired as long as the owner is prepared for the postprocedure appearance.

In both the modified Hotz-Celsus and temporary tacking procedure, special attention should be paid to the location of the suture and incision. Everting the lid is most effective when the traction that is asserted by the suture is as close to the lid margin as possible but not close enough to damage the margin or for any knots or suture material to touch the cornea. A rule of thumb for everting the lid is to place the suture approximately at the haired/nonhaired junction along the eyelid, which is typically 1–2 mm from the margin.

Surgical technique: temporary tacking

1. Pull the eyelid away from the eye so the majority of the lid is in a normal position but with the margin everted.
2. Using 4-0 or 5-0 nylon or multifilament absorbable suture on a cutting needle, take a bite through the eyelid skin, close to the eyelid margin (at the haired/nonhaired junction or 1–2 mm from the eyelid margin), and pass the suture through.
3. Take another bite of skin tissue to create a vertical mattress pattern a short distance away (~1 cm) from the first bite (fig. 69-2).
4. Tie the suture, and note the degree of eversion that results. If there is not sufficient eversion, the suture can be withdrawn and replaced or more stitches placed adjacent to the originally placed suture.

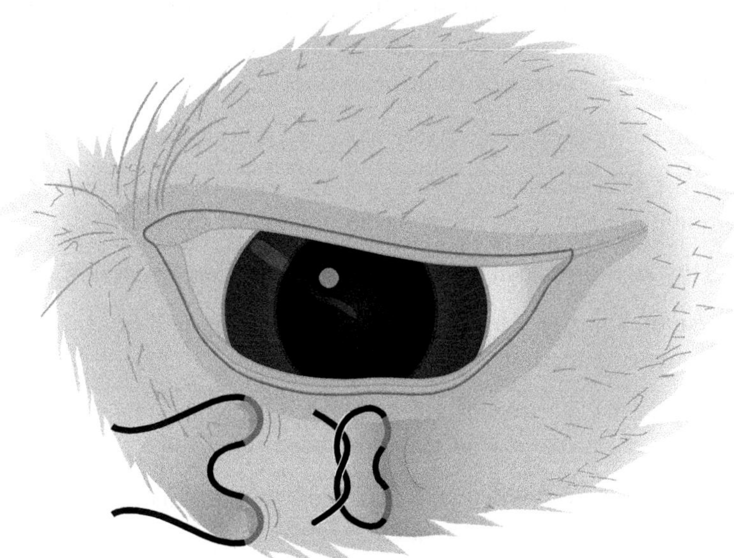

Figure 69-2 Temporary tacking sutures. Take a bite through the eyelid perpendicular to the eyelid margin and then a second bite in line with the first but starting about 1 cm away. Tie the suture to evert the lid margin.

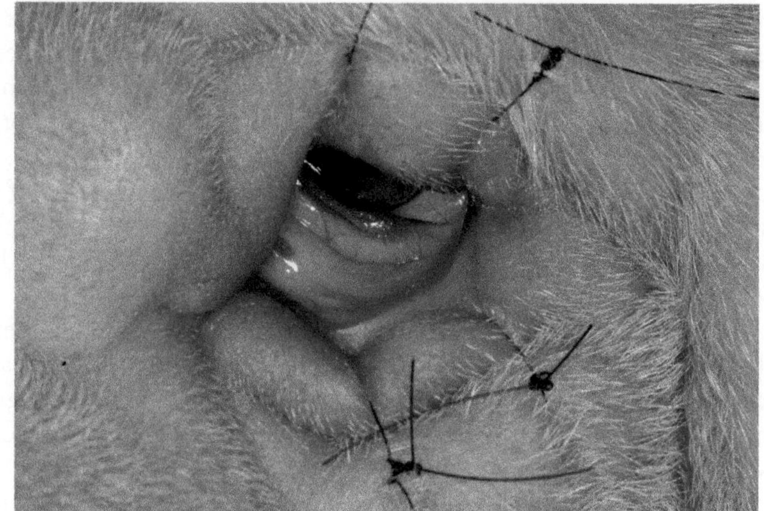

Figure 69-3 Temporary tacking sutures in a Shar Pei. This puppy's entropion may be permanently resolved with the temporary tacking sutures or with skull growth.

5. Cut the suture end that is closest to the eye short so that it is not at risk for rubbing on the cornea. The suture end farthest away can be kept long to allow for visualization and for grasping for removal at a later date, if necessary.
6. Place additional sutures to evert the eyelid along the segment of entropion. Typically, 2–3 sutures can be placed to evert most entropions, but more could be necessary if the area of entropion occupies more of the length of the lid (fig. 69-3).

Surgical technique: modified Hotz-Celsus procedure

1. Identify the region of entropion and the amount of tissue to be removed.
   a. With the lid inverted in its entropic position, make a mark on the eyelid skin where it is closest to the globe. For the lower lid, this is the highest point of rolled skin, and for the upper lid, this is the lowest point of rolled skin.
   b. Manually place or roll the lid out to a normal position, and measure the distance between the lid margin and the mark. That will be the maximum amount of skin removed.
   c. Alternatively, remove a crescent that is 5 mm wide at its maximum width.
2. Incise the skin about 1–2 mm from, and parallel to, the lid margin and extending the length of the inverted portion of the eyelid.
   a. This incision is usually at the haired/nonhaired junction.
   b. Use of a Jaeger lid plate or entropion clamp will hold the skin taut, facilitating incision.
3. Make a second, crescent-shaped skin incision abaxial to the first incision to outline the piece of skin to be removed (fig. 69-4).
   a. The incisions should meet at each end, with the maximum width of the crescent at the site of greatest lid inversion.

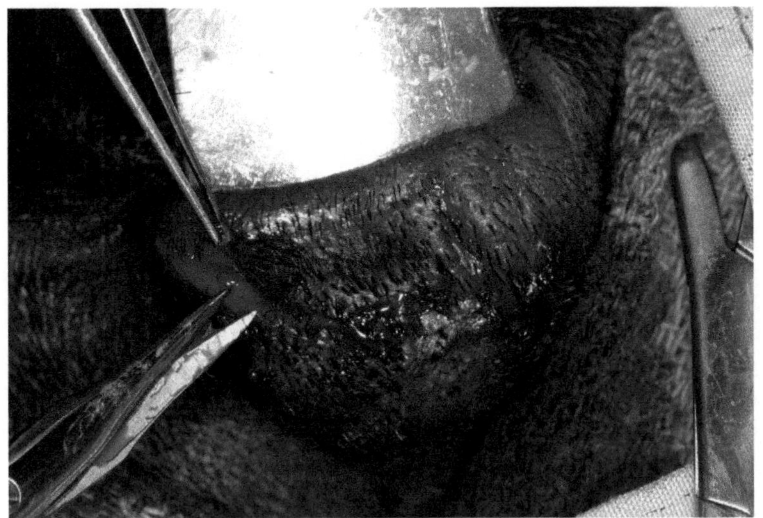

Figure 69-4 After the skin has been incised, tenotomy scissors are used to elevate and resect the skin and superficial portion of the orbicularis oculi muscle. A Jaeger lid plate protects the cornea during incision and dissection as well as provides the necessary tension to the eyelid when making the initial incisions with a blade.

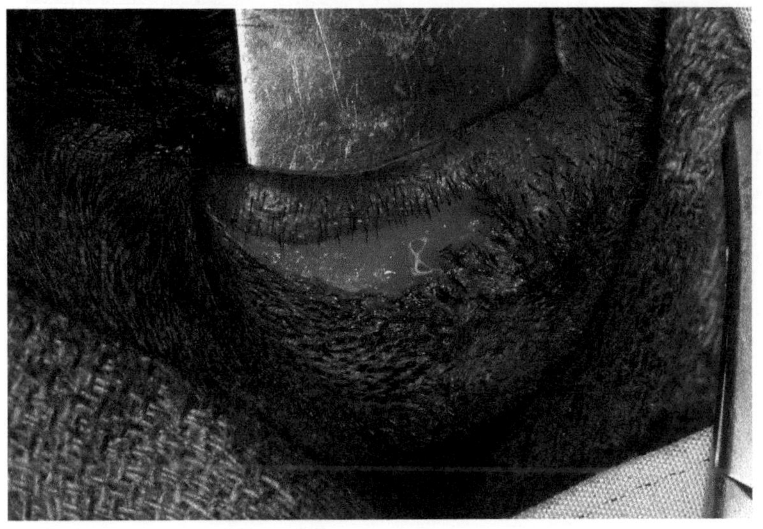

Figure 69-5 Skin flap and superficial muscle removed. For a routine entropion, the skin edges will be sutured together at this point.

4. With tenotomy scissors, excise the skin and superficial portion of the orbicularis oculi muscle (figs. 69-4, 69-5, and 69-6).
5. Appose the skin edges with simple interrupted sutures of 4-0 or 5-0 absorbable multifilament (figs. 69-7 and 69-8).
    a. Sutures should be split thickness to appose the tissue edges.
    b. Place each skin suture so it is perpendicular to the wound margin. This may require taking a bite at one side of the incision, pulling the needle and suture through, and then taking the second bite.
    c. Place the central suture first, then bisect the remaining gaps with additional sutures until the skin is apposed. Skin sutures will be about 2–3 mm apart.
    d. Cut suture ends short.

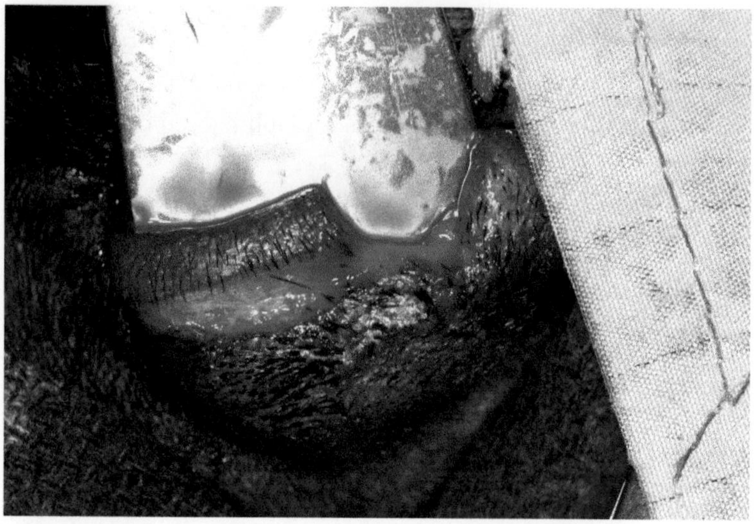

Figure 69-6 In this dog, the lower lid was deemed overly long, and a portion was resected full thickness to allow shortening and to facilitate entropion correction.

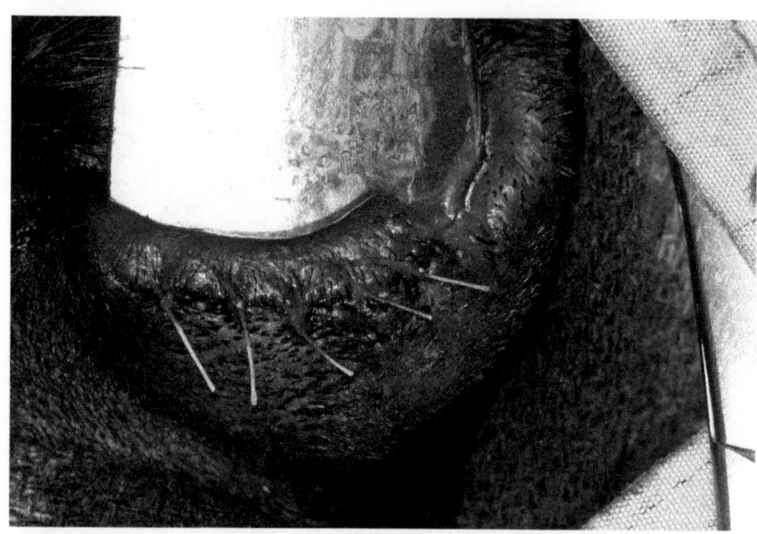

Figure 69-7 The margins of the skin defect are apposed with fine absorbable monofilament sutures.

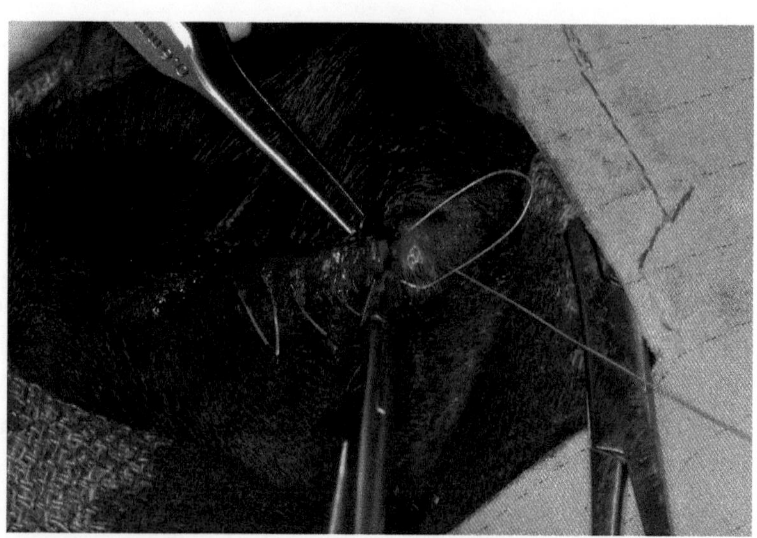

Figure 69-8 The full thickness resection site is closed with a figure-8 suture at the margin (see Chapter 71).

Postoperative considerations

Elizabethan collars are recommended to prevent self-trauma after eyelid surgery. A topical broad-spectrum antibiotic ophthalmic ointment is applied for 2 weeks to help lubricate the eye and prevent infection.

In Shar Pei puppies, temporary sutures may cut through and pull out within a few days because of abnormal subdermal tissue. If this occurs, the sutures should be replaced. For spastic entropions, the sutures can be removed once the eye is pain-free or left to fall out on their own. Some spastic entropions may resolve, only to recur if there is some cicatricial or conformational component that is not readily apparent, or if the dog is especially prone to entropion or is sensitized to squint. The owners should be warned of this possibility and be prepared to pursue permanent correction if the dog starts to squint or produce excess tear fluid after the temporary sutures are removed.

In about 6% of animals undergoing permanent surgical correction of entropion, a second surgery may be required because of recurrence of entropion at the same site or a new occurrence along the same eyelid. Overcorrection to the point where the eyelid becomes ectropic is cosmetically displeasing but usually does not cause as much damage to the cornea or vision as entropion. Exposure conjunctivitis from ectropion can occur, and surgical correction for the ectropion could be performed in these cases.

Bibliography

Johnson BW, Gerding PA, McLaughlin SA, et al: Nonsurgical correction of entropion in Shar Pei puppies. Vet Med 1988;83:482–483.

Read RA, Broun HC: Entropion correction in dogs and cats using a combination Hotz-Celsus and lateral eyelid wedge resection: results in 311 eyes. Vet Ophthalmol 2007;10:6–11.

White JS, Grundon RA, Hardman C, et al: Surgical management and outcome of lower eyelid entropion in 124 cats. Vet Ophthalmol 2012;15:231–235.

Chapter 70
Temporary Tarsorrhaphy

A temporary tarsorrhaphy is a procedure wherein the eyelids are sewn together. It is a useful technique to maintain globe (eyeball) position after proptosis, protect the cornea after conjunctival graft placement, or facilitate healing of corneal ulcers or exposure keratopathy from lagophthalmos (inability to close the eyelids) or facial nerve paralysis.

Suture apposition of the eyelids can be either complete or partial. Partial closure allows for medications to be applied to the surface of the eye and also for continued observation of the eye. Complete closure of the eyelids can be turned into partial closure with removal of one or more sutures, if indicated.

Another option for covering the cornea is a third eyelid flap. Third eyelid flaps provide adequate protection but can interfere with monitoring of the cornea and hamper dispersion of topical medications to the corneal surface. In addition, third eyelid flaps are more difficult to place properly than a temporary tarsorrhaphy.

Preoperative management

Temporary tarsorrhaphy is usually performed under anesthesia. The procedure itself does not require clipping and aseptic preparation, so the need for aseptic preparation should be based on any concurrent procedures.

Surgery

Temporary tarsorrhaphy is performed with fine, 4-0 to 6-0 nylon or multifilament nonabsorbable suture on a ½ or ¾ cutting micropoint needle. Sutures enter and exit the lid at, or just anterior to, the Meibomian gland openings and should not penetrate the conjunctiva; magnification is extremely helpful for accurate suture placement. Sutures can be placed over stents made of tubing or rubber bands to spread out pressure and decrease the chance of suture cut-through. The sutures should be knotted firmly to prevent inadvertent separation of the eyelids and subsequent corneal exposure and damage. Knots tied over the upper lids may be less likely to become coated with ocular secretions.

Manual of Small Animal Soft Tissue Surgery, Second Edition. Karen Tobias.
© 2017 John Wiley & Sons, Inc. Published 2017 by John Wiley & Sons, Inc.

Surgical technique: temporary tarsorrhaphy

1. Take a partial-thickness bite of the skin of the upper eyelid.
    a. Use 4-0 to 6-0 monofilament or multifilament nonabsorbable suture.
    b. If stent sutures are desired, pass the needle first through a stent (e.g., short piece of rubber band or tubing).
    c. Start the eyelid bite a few millimeters away from the eyelid margin.
    d. Take a vertically oriented bite, exiting the tip of the needle at or anterior to the opening of the Meibomian glands along the lid margin.
2. Directly across from the exit site of the first bite, take a vertically oriented bite in the lower eyelid, entering through the eyelid margin at or anterior to the Meibomian gland openings, and exiting several mm away through the skin.
3. If stent sutures are desired, pass the needle and suture through one side of a second stent and back through it, so the suture will rest horizontally along the external surface of the stent.

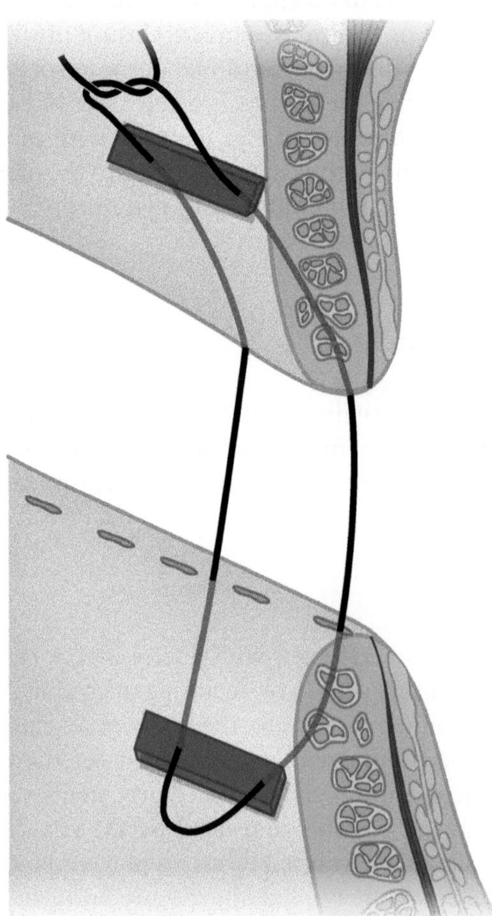

Figure 70-1 Temporary tarsorrhaphy suture over stents. The sutures are placed in a horizontal mattress pattern, entering and exiting the lid margins at or just anterior to the Meibomian gland openings.

4. With the needle directed dorsally, take bites of the lower and upper eyelids, as described in steps 1 and 2, to create a horizontal mattress suture (fig. 70-1).
5. Pass the needle and suture through the opposite end of the first stent.
6. Tie the suture over the stent.
   a. The knot should be tight enough for apposition of the eyelid but not so tight that it can result in damage to the eyelid.
7. Add additional sutures to completely close the eyelid, or leave the medial or lateral canthal areas open.
   a. An average dog will usually have 2 to 4 horizontal mattress sutures placed over the length of the eyelid.

Postoperative considerations

Elizabethan collar use is recommended to prevent self-trauma and subsequent suture disruption. Other potential complications include suture reaction, eyelid swelling, suture loosening with subsequent corneal irritation from rubbing of sutures, and eyelid necrosis if the sutures are placed too tightly.

Temporary tarsorrhaphies can be left in place for a few days to a few weeks, as long as regular monitoring is provided. If the ends of the suture are left long, adjustments can be made later (e.g., sutures retightened after loosening). Individual sutures can be removed one at a time as dictated by clinical progress of the underlying disease.

Bibliography

Chow DW, Westermeyer HD: Retrospective evaluation of corneal reconstruction using ACell Vet alone in dogs and cats: 82 cases. Vet Ophthalmol 2016;19:357–366.

Gilger BC, Hamilton HL, Wilkie A, et al: Traumatic ocular proptoses in dogs and cats: 84 cases (1980–1993). J Am Vet Med Assoc 1995;206(8):1186–1190.

Pederson, SL, Pizzirani S, Andrew SE, et al: Use of a nictitating membrane flap for treatment of feline acute corneal hydrops: 21 eyes. Vet Ophthalmol 2016;19:61–68.

Chapter 71
Eyelid Wedge Resection

Eyelid wedge resection is used to excise eyelid margin tumors (fig. 71-1), which are common in older dogs, and to treat ectropion or entropion that occurs from excessive lid length (see fig. 69-6). In dogs, most tumors of the eyelid margin are benign, with the most common being Meibomian adenoma, squamous papilloma, and benign melanoma. These masses can be removed with minimal margins (e.g., 1 mm). In cats with poorly pigmented eyelids, squamous cell carcinoma is of greatest concern.

For function to be maintained, the portion of eyelid removed should not exceed one-third of the total length of the lid. If resection of a diseased area requires a length greater than this, alternative methods for eyelid reconstruction (e.g., advancement, transpositional, and lid-to-lip flaps) or even enucleation, in cases of malignancy, may be required. Referral is recommended for advanced procedures.

Preoperative management

If malignancy is a concern, biopsy is recommended, since marginal excision may be insufficient for cure. Before eyelid wedge resection, ophthalmic lubricant gel or an artificial tear ointment is placed on the eye to protect the cornea and collect loose hairs and debris during clipping and prepping. The surgical area is clipped with a fine clipper blade. The area is prepped in an alternating fashion with a 0.2% povidone iodine solution and sterile saline, with a final saline rinse to flush away the povidone iodine. The area is then draped.

Surgery

For eyelid surgery, specialized instruments are preferred. Incisions are usually made with a Beaver blade (e.g., No. 6400) or a no. 15 blade. Dissection and suture cutting are performed with tenotomy scissors or small, straight or curved strabismus scissors. A locking ophthalmic (e.g., Castroviejo) or small conventional (e.g., Derf) needle holder, Bishop-Harmon thumb forceps, and magnification are recommended. Use of a lid plate will stabilize lid skin to

Manual of Small Animal Soft Tissue Surgery, Second Edition. Karen Tobias.
© 2017 John Wiley & Sons, Inc. Published 2017 by John Wiley & Sons, Inc.

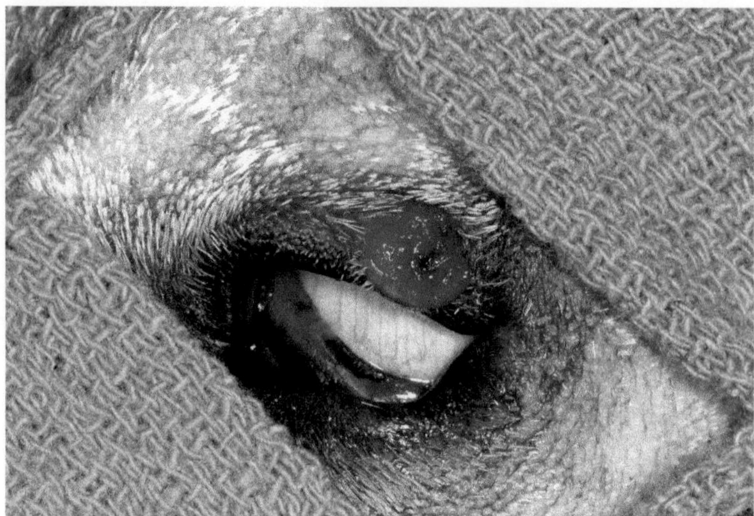

Figure 71-1 Eyelid mass in a dog.

make incising the tissue easier and more accurate. Although eyelids are extremely vascular, use of cautery should be minimized and limited to bipolar or point application because excess scarring could result in conformational changes to the eyelid.

The goal of eyelid wedge resection is to remove the affected tissue and reappose the eyelid margin so that the margin edges are continuous with each other and the chance of rubbing of the suture on the cornea is minimized. If the resection site is large and thus likely to experience tension, a two-layer closure can be used. The deeper layer can be a single mattress suture or a continuous pattern; this suture should not penetrate the conjunctiva or skin. A figure-8 suture is used to align and appose skin at the lid margin. Its suture ends can be left long and tucked under each subsequent skin suture, working away from the lid margin, so the suture ends are trapped and directed away from the cornea.

Multifilament absorbable suture (e.g., polyglactin 910 or polyglycolic acid) is often used in deeper tissues and skin because of its excellent handling characteristics and knot security, and because it softens when wet, reducing the risk of corneal irritation. Additionally, these sutures may not need to be removed since they may fall out on their own. A cutting needle is preferred when working on eyelids. When more than one skin suture is needed, sutures are usually spaced approximately 2 mm apart.

Surgical technique: wedge resection with single-layer closure

1. To exert some tension on the skin, insert a Jaeger lid plate behind the eyelid associated with the mass or area of eyelid to be excised.
2. Using a no. 15 or Beaver blade, create two partial-thickness or full-thickness incisions at angles that encompass the mass (fig. 71-2), removing a small margin of normal tissue.
   a. The area to be resected can be shaped like a triangle or pentagon.
   b. If the first incisions are partial-thickness, complete the incision full-thickness with small scissors and forceps or with a blade.

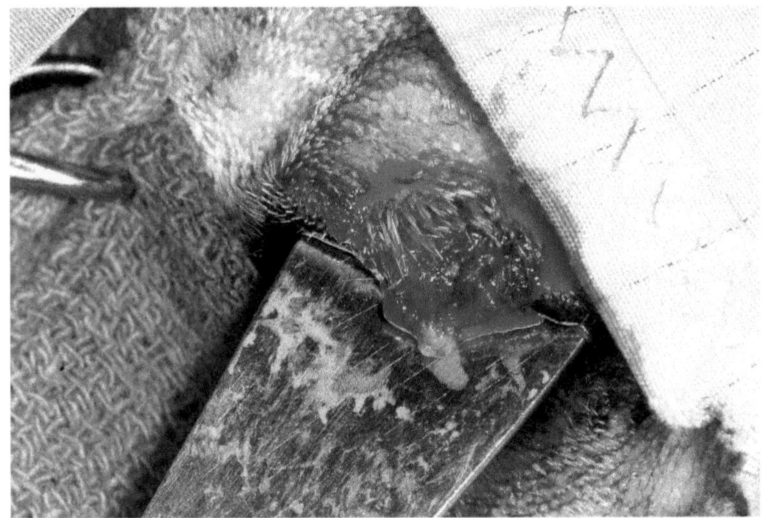

Figure 71-2 Partial-thickness skin incision around the mass. A Jaeger lid plate is used to tense the eyelid, provide a platform for incision, and protect the cornea.

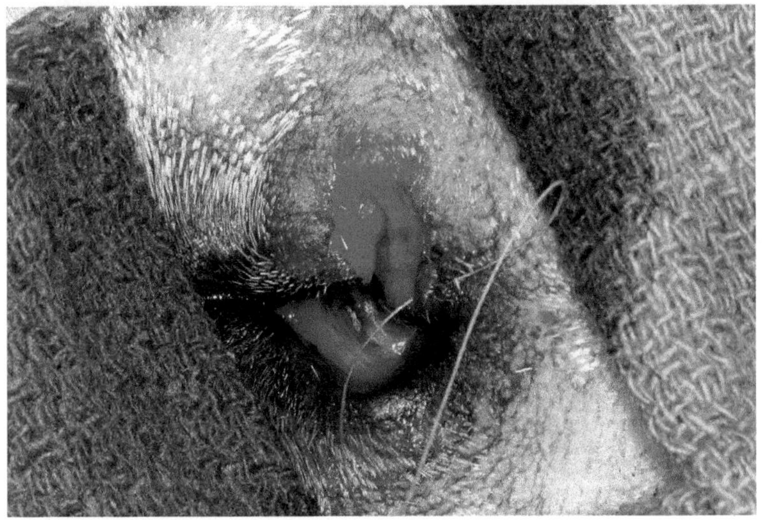

Figure 71-3 Start the figure-8 suture by taking a bite through the skin along one margin of the resection and exiting the subcutis in the cut margin.

3. Using 4-0 to 6-0 suture, appose the eyelid margins using a figure-8 suture.
   a. On one side of the incision, take a partial-thickness skin bite a few millimeters from the eyelid margin and exit out the cut edge within the subcutaneous tissues (fig. 71-3).
   b. Cross over to the opposite skin edge, and take a bite that enters the subcutaneous tissue at the cut edge and exits out the eyelid margin at or anterior to the Meibomian gland openings (fig. 71-4).
   c. Return to the original skin edge, and take a bite mirroring the bite in step 3b.
      i. Enter the eyelid margin at or anterior to the Meibomian gland openings and exit the subcutaneous tissue at the cut edge.
   d. Cross over to the opposite side and take the last bite, mirroring the bite in step a.

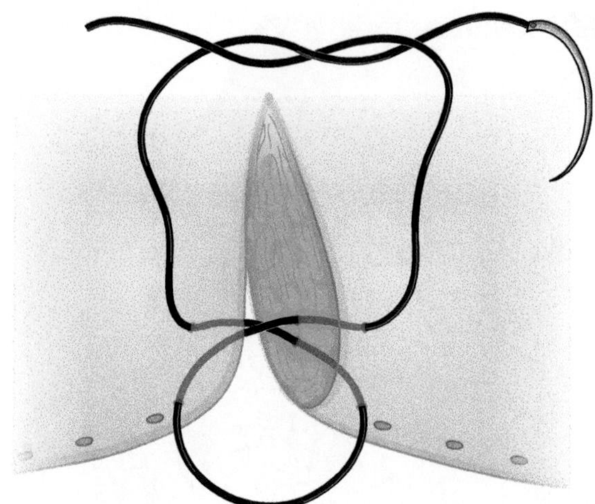

Figure 71-4 The completed figure-8 suture requires a total of 4 tissue bites.

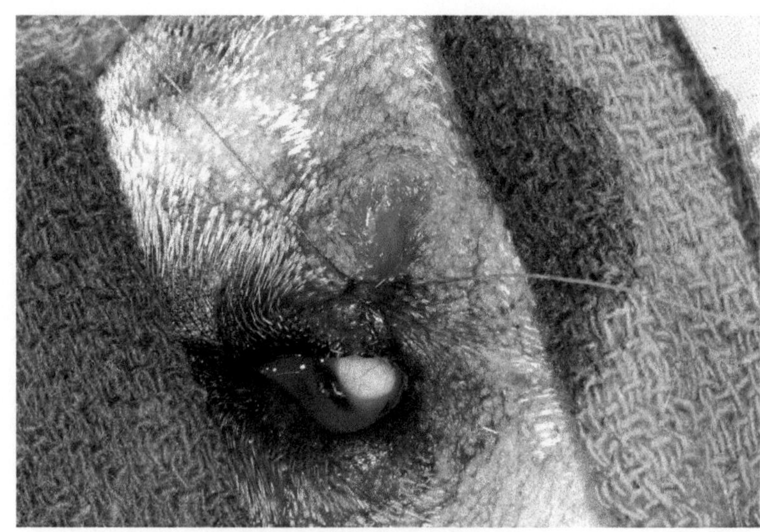

Figure 71-5 Tighten the figure-8 suture and examine the lid margin for any defects. Leave the suture ends long after tying.

   i. Enter the subcutaneous tissue at the cut edge, and exit through the skin.

e. Pull on the suture ends to appose the skin, then evaluate the eyelid margin.

   i. The margins should form a continuous line from one side to another (fig. 71-5).

   ii. If there is any overriding tissue or a step defect, remove the suture and try again.

f. If the edges are apposed appropriately, secure the suture with 2 knots (4 throws).

4. Place additional simple interrupted sutures to appose the defect.

   a. Place sutures closest to the lid first and work distally.

   b. Tuck the long ends of each suture under each subsequent suture to keep them directed away from the cornea. (fig. 71-6).

Postoperative considerations

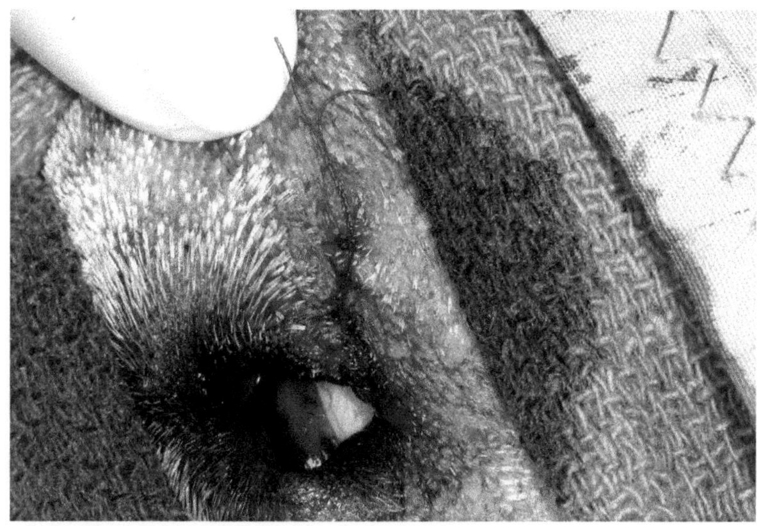

Figure 71-6 Tuck the suture ends of the figure-8 suture under subsequent skin sutures.

If resection of adequate tissue margins is a concern, the cut edges of the resected tissue should be inked and allowed to dry before placement in formalin. The pathologist can then determine the proximity of the tissue margins to the tumor. The animal should wear an Elizabethan collar for at least 2 weeks to ensure proper healing. Triple antibiotic ointment can be applied topically to the eye 2 to 3 times daily, if tolerated. Skin sutures can be removed in 2 weeks after healing is complete. Complications of wedge resection may include suture dehiscence, regrowth of the mass, and iatrogenic ulcer formation from suture rubbing or poor technique.

Bibliography

Brightman AH, Helper LC: Full thickness resection of the eyelid. J Am Anim Hosp Assoc. 1978;14:483–485.

Gelatt, KN, Blogg JR. Blepharoplastic procedures in small animals. J Am Anim Hosp Assoc 1969;5:67–78.

Gwin RM, Gelatt KN, Williams LW Ophthalmic neoplasms in the dog. J Am Anim Hosp Assoc 1982;18:853–866.

Read, RA, Broun HC: Entropion correction in dogs and cats using a combination Hotz-Celsus and lateral eyelid wedge resection: results in 311 eyes. Vet Ophthalmol 2007;10(1):6–11.

Appendix

Absorbable Suture Materials

Suture	Brand Name	Monofilament Braided	% of Original Strength Remaining	Effective Wound Support	Absorption Time
Polyglycolic acid	Dexon II	Braided, Coated	65% at 2 weeks 35% at 3 weeks	21 days	60–90 days
Polyglactin 910	Vicryl, Vicryl Plus	Braided, Coated	75% at 2 weeks 50% at 3 weeks 25% at 4 weeks	30 days	56–70 days
	Vicryl Rapide	Braided, Coated	50% at 5 days 0% at 14 days	10 days	42 days
Glycomer 631	Biosyn	Monofilament	75% at 2 weeks 40% at 3 weeks	21 days	90–110 days
Poliglecaprone 25	Monocryl	Monofilament	Dyed: 60% at 1 week 30% at 2 weeks 0% at 4 weeks Undyed: 50% at 1 week 20% at 2 weeks 0% at 3 weeks	20 days	90–120 days
Polygytone 6211	Caprosyn	Monofilament	50–60% at 5 days 20–30% at 10 days	10 days	56 days
Polyglyconate	Maxon	Monofilament	75% at 2 weeks 65% at 3 weeks 50% at 4 weeks 25% at 6 weeks	42 days	180 days
Polydioxanone	PDS II	Monofilament	3-0 or larger: 80% at 2 weeks 70% at 4 weeks 60% at 6 weeks 4-0 or smaller: 60% at 2 weeks 40% at 4 weeks 35% at 6 weeks	60 days	180–210 days

Manual of Small Animal Soft Tissue Surgery, Second Edition. Karen Tobias.
© 2017 John Wiley & Sons, Inc. Published 2017 by John Wiley & Sons, Inc.

Index

Manual of Small Animal Soft Tissue Surgery, Second Edition. Karen Tobias.
© 2017 John Wiley & Sons, Inc. Published 2017 by John Wiley & Sons, Inc.